Robert L. Allen M.D.
4/6/94

PEDIATRIC AND ADOLESCENT SPORTS MEDICINE

PEDIATRIC AND ADOLESCENT SPORTS MEDICINE

Volume 3

Carl L. Stanitski, M.D.
Professor of Orthopaedic Surgery
Wayne State University
Chief, Department of Orthopaedic Surgery
Children's Hospital of Michigan
Detroit, Michigan

Jesse C. DeLee, M.D.
Associate Clinical Professor of Orthopaedics and
Director, University of Texas Health Science Center
at San Antonio Sports Medicine Fellowship Program
San Antonio, Texas

David Drez, Jr., M.D.
Clinical Professor of Orthopaedics and
Head, Louisiana State University Knee and
Sports Medicine Fellowship Program
Louisiana State University
Lake Charles, Louisiana

W.B. SAUNDERS COMPANY
A Division of Harcourt Brace & Company
Philadelphia   London   Toronto   Montreal   Sydney   Tokyo

W.B. SAUNDERS COMPANY
A Division of
Harcourt Brace & Company

The Curtis Center
Independence Square West
Philadelphia, Pennsylvania 19106

Library of Congress Cataloging-in-Publication Data
(Revised for vol. 3)

Orthopaedic sports medicine.

Vol. 3 edited by: Carl L. Stanitski, Jesse C. DeLee, David Drez, Jr.

Includes bibliographical references and indexes.

Contents: v. 1–2 [without special title]—v. 3 Pediatric and
adolescent sports medicine.

1. Sports injuries.   2. Musculoskeletal system—wounds and
   injuries.   3. Sports medicine.   I. DeLee, Jesse.   II. Drez,
   David.   III. Stanitski, Carl L.   [DNLM: 1. Sports
   Medicine.   2. Athletic Injuries.   3. Orthopedics.
   4. Athletic Injuries—in infancy & childhood.   5. Athletic
   Injuries—in adolescence.   QT 260 077 1994]

RD97.078 1994   617.3′008′8796   93–28370

ISBN 0–7216–2834–6 (v. 1)
ISBN 0–7216–2835–4 (v. 2)
ISBN 0–7216–3216–5 (v. 3)

Pediatric and Adolescent Sports Medicine

Volume 3 ISBN 0–7216–3216–5
3 Volume set ISBN 0–7216–5602–1

Last digit is the print number: 9   8   7   6   5   4   3   2   1

This book is dedicated to my children,
Michael, Ann, John, and Kate, who, through
their vigorous participation in crew, field
hockey, lacrosse, skiing, soccer, and
swimming, taught me the benefits and joys of
''other'' sports

C.L.S.

CONTRIBUTORS

A. Leland Albright, M.D.
Professor of Neurosurgery, University of Pittsburgh School of Medicine; Chief of Pediatric Neurosurgery, Children's Hospital of Pittsburgh, Pittsburgh, Pennsylvania

Brandon G. Bentz, M.D.
Resident in Otolaryngology, Head and Neck Surgery, Northwestern University Medical Center, Chicago, Illinois

James P. Bradley, M.D.
Clinical Assistant Professor, University of Pittsburgh School of Medicine; Team Physician, Pittsburgh Steelers Football Club, Pittsburgh, Pennsylvania

Frank M. Chang, M.D.
Associate Clinical Professor, University of Colorado School of Medicine; Director, Orthopaedic Surgery, The Children's Hospital, Denver, Colorado

Ralph J. Curtis, Jr., M.D.
Clinical Assistant Professor of Orthopaedic Surgery, University of Texas Health Science Center at San Antonio, San Antonio, Texas

Jesse C. DeLee, M.D.
Associate Clinical Professor of Orthopaedics and Director, University of Texas Health Science Center at San Antonio Sports Medicine Fellowship Program, San Antonio, Texas

Paul G. Dyment, M.D.
Director, Tulane University Student Health Center, and Vice-Chancellor for Academic Affairs, Tulane University Medical Center, New Orleans, Louisiana

Gerald A.M. Finerman, M.D.
Professor and Acting Chief, Division of Orthopedic Surgery, University of California at Los Angeles, Los Angeles, California

Frances L. Geigle-Bentz, Ph.D.
Associate Professor, University of Pittsburgh School of Health and Rehabilitation Sciences, Pittsburgh, Pennsylvania

William A. Grana, M.D.
Clinical Professor, Department of Orthopaedic Surgery and Rehabilitation, University of Oklahoma Health Sciences Center, Oklahoma City, Oklahoma

Letha Y. Griffin, M.D., Ph.D.
Team Physician, Georgia State University; Team Physician, Agnes Scott College, Atlanta, Georgia

George W. Gross, M.D.
Associate Professor of Radiology and Pediatrics, Jefferson Medical College of Thomas Jefferson University, Philadelphia, Pennsylvania

Richard H. Gross, M.D.
Professor of Orthopaedic Surgery and Pediatrics, Medical University of South Carolina, Charleston, South Carolina

James J. Irrgang, M.S., P.T., A.T.C.
Assistant Professor, Department of Physical Therapy, University of Pittsburgh School of Health and Rehabilitation Sciences; Clinical Instructor, Department of Orthopaedic Surgery, University of Pittsburgh School of Medicine; Director, Outpatient Physical Therapy and Sports Medicine, University of Pittsburgh Medical Center, Pittsburgh, Pennsylvania

Frank A. Kulling, Ed.D.
Associate Professor and Director of Human Performance Laboratories, Department of Health, Physical Education, and Leisure, Oklahoma State University, Stillwater, Oklahoma

Jeffrey L. Lovallo, M.D.
Assistant Professor, Department of Orthopedics, University of Connecticut School of Medicine, Farmington, Connecticut

Lyle J. Micheli, M.D.
Associate Clinical Professor of Orthopaedic Surgery, Harvard Medical School; Attending Physician, the Boston Ballet, Boston, Massachusetts

Michael B. Millis, M.D.
Assistant Clinical Professor in Orthopaedic Surgery, Harvard Medical School; Associate in Orthopaedics, The Children's Hospital, Boston, Massachusetts

Michael A. Nelson, M.D.
Associate Clinical Professor of Pediatrics, University of New Mexico Medical School, Albuquerque, New Mexico

Peter D. Pizzutillo, M.D.
Professor of Orthopaedic Surgery, Jefferson Medical College of Thomas Jefferson University, Philadelphia, Pennsylvania

Rajiv Sawhney, M.S., P.T., O.C.S.
Oakland Rehabilitation Associates, Pittsburgh, Pennsylvania

Barry P. Simmons, M.D.
Associate Professor, Department of Orthopedics, Harvard Medical School; Chief of Hand and Upper Extremity Service, Brigham and Women's Hospital, Boston, Massachusetts

Carl L. Stanitski, M.D.
Professor of Orthopaedic Surgery, Wayne State University; Chief, Department of Orthopaedic Surgery, Children's Hospital of Michigan, Detroit, Michigan

Keith L. Stanley, M.D.
Associate Clinical Professor and Co-Coordinator, Primary Care Sports Medicine Fellowship, Oklahoma University College of Medicine, Tulsa, Oklahoma

J. Andy Sullivan, M.D.
Professor and Chair, Department of Orthopaedic Surgery and Rehabilitation, University of Oklahoma, College of Medicine, Oklahoma City, Oklahoma

Daniel C. Wascher, M.D.
Assistant Professor and Chief, Sports Medicine Division, Department of Orthopaedics and Rehabilitation, University of New Mexico School of Medicine, Albuquerque, New Mexico

Peter M. Waters, M.D.
Instructor, Orthopaedic Surgery Department, Harvard Medical School; Assistant, Department of Orthopaedic Surgery, Children's Hospital Medical Center, Boston, Massachusetts

Kaye E. Wilkins, M.D.
Clinical Professor of Orthopaedics and Pediatrics, University of Texas Health Science Center at San Antonio; Chief, Pediatric Orthopaedics, Children's Hospital, Santa Rosa Medical Center, San Antonio, Texas

Robert A. Yancey, M.D.
Pediatric Orthopedic Surgeon, Mary Bridge Children's Hospital, Tacoma, and Children's Hospital and Medical Center, Seattle, Washington

PREFACE

The school-age athlete has always been a major segment of the athletic population. Although the injuries and care of professional and collegiate athletes have become well known because of their increasing visibility in the print and electronic media, it is on the school-age athlete that this book's efforts are concentrated. These athletes encompass a wide and changing spectrum of ages, sizes, athletic potential, interest, and abilities.

As bodies mature at varying rates, sports demands on the musculoskeletal system of the school-age athlete produce different effects. Adolescence is a physiologic "never-never land" and an especially vulnerable time for musculoskeletal injury to occur because sport, like other aspects of life, has a risk–benefit ratio, with some sports producing greater risks than others. With the large variety of sports currently offered to children (scholastic competitive sports, intramurals, physical education, community programs, free play), injuries are a common occurrence. Most of these, fortunately, are minor contusions, sprains, abrasions, and lacerations, which cause little time to be lost from activity and have no significant long-term sequelae. Unfortunately, the media have emphasized catastrophic acute injuries associated with sports, but these uncommon events do not reflect the broad picture of the athletes we care for.

The initial description of the genre of injury now known as "overuse" was of "Little League elbow," a pediatric injury resulting from excessive pitching, often with little form and/or supervision. The long-term effects of most overuse problems are currently unknown. Certainly the potential for overuse problems has risen with the prolongation of the sports season, intense sports camps, and almost year-round training demanded for certain sports excellence, allowing little time for resolution of musculoskeletal stresses in a growing system.

Several significant areas of sports participation have emerged over the past decade. These include women's embracement of and involvement in sports—women's participation in scholastic athletics has seen an almost 800% increase over the past two decades. Another equally fast-growing field is that of sports for the disabled, where the injuries must be recognized as sports related and not disability related.

This text is designed to provide orthopaedic surgeons with a compendium of current musculoskeletal concepts, including historical background, pathophysiology, and up-to-date diagnostic and therapeutic techniques for sports injuries in a skeletally immature patient. These principles of treatment take into account the effects of growth, both current and future. The basic concepts of preventing disuse and misuse are the same in the nonathlete, but in athletes, the time course is compressed. Often the school-age athlete's goals and aspirations are to attain immediate accomplishments equivalent to those of the professionals, and this prompts family, coach, community, and peer pressures for the athlete to return to play prematurely.

I hope this book will provide the needed guidelines for proper diagnosis, treatment, rehabilitation, and preventive measures that will reduce not only the immediate sequelae of musculoskeletal injury, but also prevent development of long-term disabling conditions.

I would like to offer a heartfelt thank you to Lewis Reines, President of the W.B. Saunders Company, for his encouragement; to my chapter authors, who so graciously gave of their time and talents; to Ron Filer, our illustrator; and to Wilda Ward, Linda Simon, and Patricia Stevens, my secretaries, whose work capacity and ability enabled them to meet the many deadlines placed before them. Special thanks also are given to Clifford Roberts and Janet McMahon, Educational Services, Audiovisual Section, Department of Orthopaedic Surgery, Children's Hospital of Michigan, for their superb photographic work..

CARL L. STANITSKI, M.D.

CONTENTS

EXERCISE PHYSIOLOGY

Frank A. Kulling, Ed.D.

Increasing attention is being devoted to the topic of children and physical activity. The reasons are numerous, diverse, and at times based on subjective reasoning. An evolving technology continually increases personal time and then produces sedentary prone "gadgetry" to occupy leisure pursuits. Persistent economic woes have affected public education curricula, necessitating a "bare bones" approach that has increasingly forced the removal of activity or activity-related classes. Reports of children's fitness seem to imply incessantly that our young people are not as fit as they once were or should be. Finally, scientific studies continue to establish an ever stronger connection between hypokinesis and a number of degenerative diseases that continue to ravish our population—diseases whose pathophysiologic inception may occur in childhood.

These concerns and others prompted publication of a recent federal document establishing national health, fitness and exercise objectives [68]. Much attention was devoted to the subjects of determining, assessing, and improving children's fitness through physical activity. If, as the document recommends, more than 90% of children and adolescents are to be regularly engaged in appropriate physical activities, it is prudent to review research directed toward assessing their capacity for, and response to, physical activity. This initial chapter purports to examine those physiologic systems, organs, and tissues and their related measures that could be considered as contributing to health-related fitness [6].

TANNER CLASSIFICATION

The author wishes to acknowledge the material in this section as derived from the classic work of J. M. Tanner [67]. Interpretation of physiologic phenomena is heavily age- and sex-dependent. For this reason, it often is necessary to identify developmental bench marks to impart meaning to physical findings and measures. Often, this is accomplished by using chronologic age; however, be-

cause children vary so widely in attaining adolescent and adult maturation stages, other systems involving the skeleton, dentition, morphology, and secondary sex characteristics have evolved. Because of its close correlation with skeletal maturation and clear delineation of adolescent development, the secondary sex classification system devised by Tanner [67] has received wide acceptance in the medical field. Boys and girls grow and mature at different intervals along a chronologic continuum as depicted in Figure 1–1. Tanner, therefore, devised a system for both sexes that adjudged maturation based on development of the male genitalia, female breasts, and pubic hair. Development of each variable occurs in five stages based on size, shape, appearance, and relative changes therein (Table 1–1). Tanner stage 1 represents preadolescence, stages 2 through 4 various levels within adolescence, and stage 5 adulthood. The recommended method of assigning a Tanner stage is to

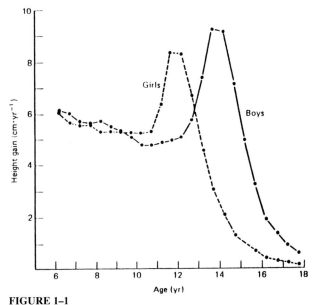

FIGURE 1–1
Growth curves for boys and girls. (From Tanner, J. M. *Growth at Adolescence.* Oxford, Blackwell Scientific Publications, 1962.)

TABLE 1–1
Tanner Stage Ratings for Boys and Girls

Pubertal Stage	Pubic Hair	Genital Development	Breast Development
1	None	Testes, scrotum about same size and proportions as in early childhood	Elevation of papilla only
2	Sparse growth of long, slightly pigmented downy hair, straight or only slightly curled, appearing chiefly at base of penis or along labia	Enlargement of scrotum and testes; skin of scrotum reddens and changes in texture; little or no enlargement of penis at this stage	Breast bud stage; elevation of breast and papilla as small mound; enlargement of areolar diameter
3	Considerably darker, coarser, and more curled; hair spreads sparsely over junction of pubes	Enlargement of penis, which occurs at first mainly in length; further growth of testes and scrotum	Further enlargement and elevation of breast and areola, with no separation of their contours
4	Hair now resembles adult in type, but area covered is still considerably smaller than in adult; no spread to medial surface of thighs	Increased size of penis with growth in breadth and development of glans; further enlargement of testes and scrotum; increased darkening of scrotal skin	Projection of areola and papilla to form a secondary mound above the level of the breast
5	Adult in quantity and type with distribution of horizontal (or classically "feminine") pattern; spread to medial surface of thighs but not up the linea alba or elsewhere above the base of the inverse triangle. In about 80% of Caucasian men and 10% of women, pubic hair spreads further, but this takes some time to occur after stage 5 is reached. This may not be completed until the mid-twenties or later	Genitalia adult in size and shape; no further enlargement after stage 5 is reached	The mature stage; projection of papilla only, due to recession of areola to general contour of breast

Adapted from Larson, L. *Fitness, Health and Work Capacity.* New York, Macmillan, 1974, pp. 516–517.

average the levels for genitalia or breasts and pubic hair; however, assignment based solely on pubic hair evaluation is often practiced, especially when limited observation precludes relative change comparisons.

Using pubic hair as a maturation variable, the chronologic age ranges that encompass 95% of the population in beginning adolescence (Tanner stage 2) are 10 to 15 years for boys and 8 to 14 years for girls. The progression from Tanner stage 2 to Tanner stage 5 (adulthood) encompasses 4 years on average but may vary by plus or minus 2 years. From this summary it can be seen that in some cases children with the same chronologic age may vary from Tanner stage 1 to Tanner stage 5. Subsequent chapters in this book often mention the Tanner developmental stages, and it is hoped that this cursory introduction will prove beneficial to the reader's understanding. The study of exercise physiology has not relied heavily on the Tanner system, and this author cannot arbitrarily assign such stages to original contributions

devoid of such references. For the purposes of this chapter, therefore, ages and maturation levels are reported as they occur in the literature reviewed.

DIFFERENCES AMONG CHILD, ADOLESCENT, AND ADULT

Cardiorespiratory Factors

Information in this section encompasses the cardiovascular and pulmonary organs, tissues, and related measures associated with activity.

Cardiorespiratory Potential

A requirement for activity sustained beyond a few moments is the delivery and utilization of oxygen (O_2);

moreover, the salient associated physiologic variable is maximal O_2 uptake (VO_2 max) [26]. Although it is commonly included in the cardiorespiratory or cardiovascular category, VO_2 max requires the integrated and effective functioning of several body systems. The heart must provide adequate cardiac output (Q); alveolar tissue must be adequately perfused with air and capillary blood; the circulatory system must deliver O_2 and remove the metabolic byproducts of oxidation; and active tissue must be capable of oxidizing food substrates to produce energy. When expressed in absolute terms (L/min), VO_2 max increases concomitantly with growth in children until age 18 in boys and age 14 in girls [9]. Until age 12, absolute VO_2 max values increase at the same rate in both sexes, although boys have higher values as early as age 5 [74].

Since activity requires the movement of body and body segments through space, VO_2 max values are often examined relative to body size (ml/kg/min) for comparative purposes. With these relative measures as a criterion, Pate and Blair [54], Krahenbuhl and colleagues [42], and Bar-Or [9] all reviewed laboratory studies of children and adolescents and found that VO_2 max (ml/kg/min) values were significantly in excess of those recorded for an average American adult population. Additionally, Pate and Blair [54] found that children's values were historically consistent for two decades, and Bar-Or [9] found that values in boys remained stable for ages 6 to 17 and values in girls were less than those in boys and remained stable until the age of 11 or 12 and then declined each year thereafter. Adult values for a sedentary male tend to remain stable until sometime during the third decade, when progressive decline, averaging somewhat less than 1% per year, begins and continues throughout life [26].

In Bar-Or's review [9], boys' values encompass a 45- to 57-ml/kg/min range throughout childhood and adolescence, whereas girls' values are approximately 5 ml/kg/min lower until the age of 11 or 12, when a decline begins. An acceptable scientific explanation elucidating the VO_2 max differences between boys and girls has not been found; however, differences in body composition, particularly during and after adolescence (Tanner stages 2 to 4) constitute a plausible hypothesis. Average relative VO_2 max values for adults are age- and sex-dependent; however, using Cooper's data [20], an average 30- to 39-year-old American male would be expected to possess a VO_2 max of between 30.2 and 39.1 ml/kg/min. Using weight-adjusted VO_2 max as a criterion, one would likely conclude that children and adolescents are at least the aerobic equals of their adult counterparts.

In addition to VO_2 max, the anaerobic threshold (AT) is often mentioned as a measure of activity potential because it represents the upper limits of activity intensity that can be maintained without subsequent accumulation of endurance-limiting lactate [71]. The reasons for activity cessation in response to lactate accumulation are not completely understood; however, impairment of cellular enzyme activity in response to lowered tissue pH is a possible explanatory factor. When Cooper and colleagues tested 109 boys and girls between the ages of 6 and 17, they found that mean AT was 58% of VO_2 max [19]. This compares with the results of Davis and colleagues, who found that the mean AT of college-age males was 58.6% of VO_2 max [25]. A number of studies have shown that AT in adult males ranges from 49% to 63% of VO_2 max, and values for adult women range between 50% and 60% of VO_2 max [71].

Acute Cardiorespiratory Response

In a closer examination of the acute hemodynamic and ventilatory changes that provide O_2 uptake (VO_2) in support of activity, children respond in a manner that is qualitatively similar to that of adults; however, some quantitative differences may affect activity of high intensity. Specifically, children and adolescents have somewhat higher heart rates (HR) and arteriovenous oxygen differences (AV-O_2 diff) and somewhat lower systolic and diastolic blood pressures (SBP, DBP), stroke volumes (Sv), and Q at any given level of VO_2 [9, 10, 28]. Although research has yet to elucidate the exercise limitations, if any, these differences portend, one could speculate that decreases in Q might be offset by the increased AV-O_2 diff at submaximal activity levels. The same line of reasoning would predict exercise limitations at maximal or near-maximal activity levels at which AV-O_2 extraction rates cannot increase and also during hot, humid conditions, which require increased peripheral blood flow in support of heat dissipation.

Children's ventilatory response to exercise is relatively tachypneic with lower relative tidal volumes (Tv) and higher breathing rates (f), ventilation rates (Ve), and ventilatory equivalents (Ve/VO_2) than those occurring in adults [9]. Interpretation of these findings leads to the conclusion that children have a higher relative energy cost associated with breathing and, in this regard, are somewhat inefficient in breathing compared with adults. Changes in these ventilatory variables toward adult equivalents occur both continuously and progressively with growth during childhood and adolescence [9]. This is not surprising because the variable most closely associated with ventilatory volumes is body size.

Although children possess more than adequate VO_2 max and AT levels relative to body size and qualitatively similar hemodynamic and ventilatory responses to acute exercise, they are nonetheless metabolically inefficient at comparable workloads [9]. Daniels and colleagues found that 10-year-old boys expend 26% more energy (VO$_2$ ml/kg/min) than 18-year-olds while running 12 km/hr [23]. Based on the treadmill tests of Astrand [5, 9], it appears this metabolic inefficiency applies to both boys and girls over a wide range of walking and running speeds until they reach adulthood (Fig. 1–2). Although research has yet to explain satisfactorily these energy differences occasioned by walking and running, possible contributing factors include inefficiencies in gait [23] and the previously discussed ventilatory inefficiencies.

Musculoskeletal Factors

Information in this section includes factors relating to muscle, bone, joint, and connective and adipose tissue and the related measures commonly associated with activity. The musculoskeletal system provides for movement by converting foodstuffs into chemically usable energy in the form of adenosine triphosphate (ATP). ATP is then used to provide energy for muscle cell contraction. If the movement lasts longer than a few moments, this process must be aided by O$_2$ delivered by the cardiorespiratory system; however, short-term intense activity is possible in the relative absence of O$_2$.

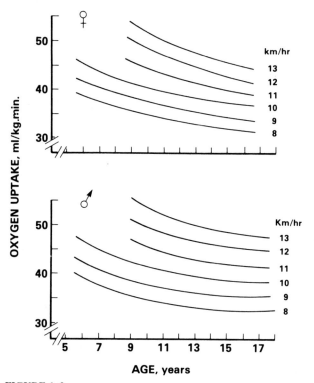

FIGURE 1–2
VO$_2$ and age for young males and females walking at various treadmill speeds. (From Astrand, P. O. *Experimental Studies of Working Capacity in Relation to Sex and Age.* © 1952 Munksgaard International Publishers Ltd., Copenhagen, Denmark.)

Morphology

It has been known for some time that very young children possess muscle fiber numbers, types, and distribution ratios similar to those of adults [12]. Likewise, resting energy substrates and sources, such as creatine phosphate (CP), ATP, and glycogen, are also similar [27]. Because growth is characterized by a protein anabolic state to support tissue synthesis, children are not likely to be as musculoskeletally stable as adults [41]. The developing tissues most potentially susceptible to instability are bone, articular cartilage, and tendon-bone junctions [16]. At particular risk is the open epiphysis because it is three to five times weaker than the capsular and ligamentous tissues that surround it [47]. Additionally, epiphyseal damage is likely to be of greater consequence in children because it can result in various stages of growth reduction in the affected long bone [41]. The probability of such injury is likely to be the result of a number of inter-related factors in addition to activity itself [46]. The subject of injury will be more completely addressed in subsequent chapters.

Strength, Endurance, and Power

Muscular strength, endurance, and power are highly desired attributes in many activities. Maximal muscle strength is usually considered to be the maximum one-effort force that can be exerted against a resistance [26]. Muscle endurance, on the other hand, is the ability to apply repeatedly or sustain a submaximal force over a period of time [26]. Power refers to the amount of work that can be accomplished over time [26]. Although these related concepts are obviously different, many field tests that measure endurance (e.g., sit-ups, chin-ups, pull-ups) are incorrectly labeled as strength measures. Investigators consistently find increases in muscular strength accompanying growth, with maximum values attained during early adulthood in both sexes [26].

Increased strength is almost entirely due to concomitant increase in muscle tissue growth [59]. The rate of decline in muscle strength in an adult population depends in part on the specific muscle groups tested and on continuing activity levels; however, the decline is generally considered to be somewhat less than 1% per year from the middle of the third through the sixth decades of life [26]. Males tend to be stronger than females at any age, particularly with regard to the muscle groups of the upper extremity; however, differences in muscle strength reported by sex and age can be virtually eliminated if strength is expressed per unit of cross-sectional muscle area (kg/cm^2) [26]. Measured as the ability to sustain isometrically a percentage of a maximum voluntary contraction (MVC) before fatigue occurs, studies

FIGURE 1–3
Adiposity in young males and females during growth and maturation. Boys' values (%): 10.1, 10.1, 11.1, 12.1, 12.1, 14.1, 13.2, 13.2, 12.1, 12.1, 12.1, 13.2, 13.2. Girls' values (%): 14.1, 15.2, 16.1, 17.1, 18.0, 19.0, 19.0, 19.8, 23.1, 23.8, 23.8, 25.3, 25.3. (Skinfold sums (50th percentile) from AAHPERD. *Test Manual: Health Related Physical Fitness.* 1900 Association Dr., Reston, VA, American Alliance for Health, Physical Education, Recreation, and Dance (AAHPERD), 1980; Percent fat from AAHPERD. *Technical Manual: Health Related Fitness.* 1900 Association Dr., Reston, VA, AAHPERD, 1984.)

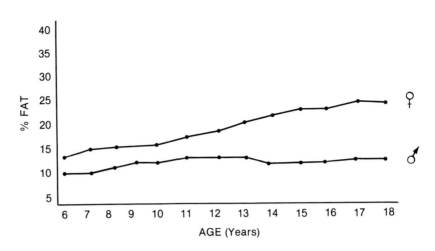

of muscle endurance in relation to age are inconclusive [30, 55]. Tests of muscle endurance in both sexes generally show males as superior [1]; however, most field tests involve only the upper body musculature.

One area in which children are markedly inferior to adults is that of anaerobic power production, even when weight-adjusted measures are considered. Using kcal/kg/hr as an objective measure, research has shown that boys are capable of producing more anaerobic power than girls and both steadily progress to adult levels by the end of adolescence [9]. The primary reason for this anaerobic deficiency appears to be the limited phosphofructokinase (PFK) activity that occurs in children and early adolescents [26]. Because PFK is a key enzyme in glycolysis, this factor alone may cause the reduced anaerobic capacity of children.

Although children cannot emulate the activity of adults under anaerobic conditions, the potential detriment may be less than anticipated for a number of reasons. First, most ''aerobic'' activities are not significantly above the AT. Second, during activity transitions from a lower to a higher submaximal intensity, children do not require as much time to reach an O_2 steady state [44].

Body Composition

Body composition is a difficult area in which to make comparisons because the variables are highly age- and sex-specific in an adult population and because acceptable and comparable field methods of collecting and assessing data are lacking. As an example, adult skinfold measures commonly employ three to seven sites, whereas children's skinfold measures seldom use more than two. With these shortcomings in mind, if two-site skinfold measures are compared from ages 6 to 18, boys at the 50th percentile show virtually no change, whereas

girls show a gradual increase to age 15 [1]. Using Lohman and colleagues' equations [2] to estimate body fat from the skinfold sums, it can be shown that body fat in boys at the 50th percentile increases from 10% to 13%, whereas body fat in girls increases from 14% to 25% during the 6- to 18-year time frame. These results are depicted in Figure 1–3. These figures remain relatively constant during the college years [51], but by middle age (40 to 49 years), American males average 20% to 25% body fat, whereas similarly aged American women average 30% to 35% body fat [63]. Using the midpoints of these figures, we can calculate an approximate 8% to 10% increase in body fat between the ages of 25 and 45 for both sexes; therefore, the average increase is approximately 4% to 5% per decade. These figures may be somewhat misleading, however, since body composition comprises lean tissue constituents, primarily muscle and bone, in addition to adipose tissue. Brozek depicted adult changes in body composition as a combination of increasing adiposity and decreasing lean tissue mass [14]. This changed combination could easily be the result of a slowly declining basal metabolic rate [26] and hypokinesis.

Flexibility

Flexibility encompasses two basic measures: static or range of motion flexibility and dynamic or motion resistance flexibility [26]. A number of studies [40, 56, 58] indicate that children become less statically flexible as they age, reaching minimal levels between 10 and 12 years of age and then improving again toward early adulthood but not sufficiently to emulate childhood results [26]. Since limitations on static flexibility are imposed by muscle, bone, and soft tissue, the early adolescent growth spurt may occasion a short-term ''tightness'' about the joints, perhaps as a result of increased tension in connective tissue. Girls appear to be more flexible than boys [40, 56, 58], an advantage that is likely sustained in adulthood [26]. Static flexibility tends to decrease progressively after early adulthood, and dynamic flexibility decreases with age from childhood [26].

Heat and Cold Adaptability

Heat is a metabolic byproduct of energy production; therefore, the ability to dissipate heat quickly and effectively is crucial to continuance of activity. Because children possess a larger surface area relative to body mass [9] and less subcutaneous fat [1, 51, 63], one might suspect that they have a disadvantage in dissipating heat and adapting to cold. Additionally, although children possess a higher sweat gland density than adults, they produce far less sweat for evaporative heat dissipation [8]. The result is that children respond with significantly higher skin and rectal temperatures when confronted with heat stress [9]. Additionally, children do not acclimatize to heat as quickly [70] or perceive exercise as intensely as adults [7]. With respect to cold adaptation, a study involving trained male and female swimmers in cold water (20.3°C) showed a linear inverse relationship between core temperature reduction and age [65].

PHYSIOLOGIC RESPONSE TO TRAINING

This section examines documented changes at the systemic, organic, and tissue levels and their associated measures in response to training. Unless otherwise specified, ''training'' is assumed to mean those activities that produce the greatest beneficial response in the affected area—i.e., endurance activities and cardiorespiratory endurance, resistance activity and musculoskeletal strength, and so on.

Cardiorespiratory Function

In response to training, children's absolute performance measures are likely to improve, but VO_2 max may not [22, 66]. When Rowland examined this subject, he found that increases in VO_2 max ($\bar{x} = +14\%$) occurred if exercise intensity and duration were commensurate with adult aerobic prescriptive criteria [60]. VO_2 max changes experienced in a healthy adult population depend on age, sex, starting fitness and habitual activity levels, intensity, duration, and frequency of activity, and, most important, heredity. Expected VO_2 max increases in an average American adult population range from 5% to 25% [3]. Declines in VO_2 max normally experienced

in a sedentary adult population can be effectively forestalled for decades through continued activity [39]. Although more work needs to be done in understanding the pediatric response to endurance exercise, one might speculate that possible improvements in VO_2 max would tend to be proportionately less because of the relatively high starting values [9, 42, 54].

In both children and adults training results in lowered heart rates, at rest and at submaximal workloads, while stroke volume tends to increase [13, 26, 37, 66]. The resulting combination allows a given Q at a reduced heart rate and an increased Q at maximal and near-maximal workloads [26, 29, 33]. The bottom line, simply put, is attainment of increased physical work capacity (PWC), that is, the ability to be active at previously unattainable intensities or to be active for longer periods at similar intensities. Biochemical and cellular explanations supporting increased PWC response in adults include oxidative cellular shift, increased number and volume of oxidative mitochondria, increased potency of oxidative enzymes, increased glycogen storage, increased efficiency and endurance of accessory ventilatory muscles, increased blood volume, increased total circulating hemoglobin, increased erythrocytic production of 2,3-diphosphoglycerate, increased capillarization of active tissue, increased cellular myoglobin content, increased production of endorphins and enkephalins, and myocardial hypertrophy [26, 51]. Although much needs to be done in determining which activity-induced changes are responsible for increased PWC in children, the available evidence indicates that increased glycogen stores and oxidative enzyme activity [32] as well as increased left ventricular mass [18, 34] are contributing factors.

Training has been shown to be capable of increasing both absolute and proportionate (%VO_2 max) AT values in adult males [24]. Although more research needs to be done in this area in children and adolescents, at least one study indicated that no such improvement occurred in trained children [11].

Because pulmonary ventilation is so highly correlated with body size, it is difficult to distinguish growth from training-induced changes; moreover, studies involving adequate control group inclusion are few. With these limitations in mind, it appears that children respond in much the same way as adults, showing increases in Tv, f, Ve, and possibly Ve/VO_2 [9]. Since these improvements are manifest primarily during the activity bout, one suspects that the increased endurance and efficiency of the accessory ventilatory muscles enhance changes in thoracic volume.

Musculoskeletal Function
Morphology

Skeletal muscle hypertrophy has been reported among adolescents participating in endurance training but not sprint training [32]. Although endurance training facilitates a muscle fiber shift toward more oxidative fibers in adults [26], no such shift has been noted in children [38]. Studies indicate that activity elicits a hypertrophic response in the most heavily loaded areas of immature bone [4, 45].

Strength, Endurance, and Power

A number of investigators have found that most subjects, regardless of age and sex, experience proportionately similar increases in strength in response to a resistive training program [50, 61, 62, 72, 73]. However, corresponding increases in muscle hypertrophy are significantly less in females and immature males [31, 72, 73]. A likely explanation for this different hypertrophic response is low circulating androgen levels. Increased strength in the absence of hypertrophy can be hypothesized to result from neural adaptations [36] or changes in the rate and sequence of motor unit innervation [21].

It has long been known that endurance activities increase the endurance of the muscle groups involved. Cardiorespiratory endurance has been discussed previously; however, we are concerned here with musculoskeletal endurance. The ability of any given activity to induce muscle endurance depends on how closely it incorporates the principles of "overload" and "specificity" with respect to the muscles in question [26]. Perhaps the best illustration of these concepts is the fact that a healthy untrained person can increase the number of push-ups, pull-ups, or sit-ups he or she can perform simply by regularly completing such exercises to or near the point of exhaustion. Clarke and Vaccaro [17] found that 9- to 11-year-old boys and girls completing a 7-month swimming program improved arm endurance as measured through push-ups and pull-ups; however, hand grip endurance was not changed. Despite the research that has been accomplished, there is ample room for additional work in this area, particularly in understanding the inter-relationship between strength and endurance activities and the extent to which one can influence the other.

Body Composition

In adults, activity tends to have both anabolic and metabolic effects and results in increases in lean body tissue and decreases in adipose tissue. The effect of activity on this variable in children is unclear because studies have failed to control for the possibly confounding variables of growth and the amount and composition of food intake. It does appear, however, that obese youths respond to exercise with greater beneficial changes in body composition [49] than their nonobese counterparts [35].

Flexibility

Static stretching can be demonstrated to increase static flexibility in both children and adults [26]. Attempts to elucidate the effects of common activities and exercises on flexibility are likely to be confounded by the fact that they incorporate static stretching as part of their regimen. Connective tissues tend to shorten when placed in a shortened position; therefore, to the extent that hypokinesis reduces motion opportunities among opposing muscle groups, flexibility will tend to decrease. More needs to be done in determining the effects of various activities on flexibility in children, particularly during the growth spurt when flexibility decreases [26].

Heat and Cold Adaptability

Children and adults become more efficient at dissipating heat when they are exposed to periods of increased activity in a hot environment; however, young adults showed better thermoregulatory responses than either children or older men [70]. More needs to be done in this area, particularly studies that include inactive controls subjected to the same environmental conditions as the subjects of the study.

Health and Disease

Epidemiologic studies conducted in adults show a strong inverse relationship between physical activity and coronary heart disease (CHD) risk [52, 57, 64]. One study has established an inverse relationship between occupational activity and colon cancer [69]. Finally, it is conceded that 90% of adult-onset diabetes is preventable through proper dietary and exercise regimes [15]. Despite the fact that manifestation of heart disease does not usually occur until later adulthood, CHD is increasingly considered pediatric in origin [43]. Additionally, there is evidence of an inverse relationship between physical activity and CHD risk factors among children [48]. With respect to myocardial infarction, Paffenberger and colleagues found that sedentary Harvard alumni, even those who were physically active as students, were at greater risk than previously sedentary students who became active later [53]. The message here seems to be that children can reduce the risk of at least some degenerative diseases by being active; however, the carryover of this effect into adulthood is likely to depend on maintenance of activity. In this respect, increased attention should be devoted to activities with carryover potential in the hope of increasing adult compliance.

BASELINE DATA FOR TREATMENT CONSIDERATIONS

The vast majority of diseases, illnesses, and conditions that limit activity for children and adolescents are obvious and are diagnosed. Subsequent chapters deal with adapted activities for these special populations; however, it might be beneficial to establish "baseline" data for some of the measures discussed in this initial chapter. *Baseline* is interpreted to mean values that encompass the lowest 5% of an age-specific population. Although these values are not in themselves indicative of limiting conditions, they are indicative of limited capacity or undesirable morphology. As such, they should elicit review and investigation by competent personnel with regard to developing an appropriate course of subsequent action. These data include only values for children and adolescents and only values that are applicable by age; therefore, variables correlated with body size are not included. Baseline data are presented in Table 1–2.

SUMMARY AND RECOMMENDATIONS

The purpose of this introductory chapter is to examine the physiologic systems, organs, and tissues and their related measures that contribute to health-related fitness

[6] in our children and adolescents. The examination is directed toward better understanding the capacity for and response to the increased physical activity thought to be important for children [68].

The Tanner classification system [67] permits distinction of various maturational levels based on secondary sex characteristics. Using VO_2 max and AT measures as indicators of cardiorespiratory potential, children and adolescents appear to be at least the equal of their adult counterparts [9, 19, 20, 25, 42, 51, 71]. In response to a single exercise bout, children exhibit cardiorespiratory responses that are qualitatively similar to those of adults [9, 10, 28]. Notable quantitative exceptions include reduced Q [10] and increased Ve, f, and possibly Ve/VO_2 [9]. Partially as a result of these differences, children demonstrate an inverse relationship between relative energy expenditure (VO_2, ml/kg/min) and age while walking and running [5, 9, 23]. This portends difficulty for young children who attempt to emulate absolute adult activity levels.

Anaerobically speaking, children are inferior to adults, even when weight-adjusted measures are considered; moreover, progression to adult levels is continuous with growth and maturation [9]. This anaerobic inefficiency is largely due to the limited activity of PFK [26], a key enzyme in the anaerobic glycolytic process. This limitation is not significant at aerobic intensities or during activity transitions within aerobic intensities.

Children's muscle tissue is similar to that of adults with respect to the numbers, types, and distribution ratios of muscle fibers [12]; however, children may be at increased risk of musculoskeletal injury, particularly at

TABLE 1–2
Baseline Data (Lowest 5 Percentile) for Health-Related Physiologic Data

Measure	Sex	Age (Years)											
		6	7	8	9	10	11	12	13	14	15	16	17
VO_2 max (ml/kg/min)	M	32								37			
	F	26						27					
AT (ml/kg/min)	M	18								17			
	F	16						14					
AT (%VO_2 max)	ALL	40%											
Skinfold Triceps (mm)	M	13	14	17	20	20	22	23	23	21	21	20	20
	F	16	17	20	22	23	23	25	26	27	29	30	29
Skinfold Triceps and	M	20	24	28	34	33	38	44	46	37	40	37	38
Subscapularis (mm)	F	26	28	36	40	41	42	48	51	52	56	57	58
% Body Fat	M	18	21	24	28	27	30	32	29	30	29	30	30
	F	25	26	31	32	33	33	35	35	36	36	36	36
Sit-Ups (in 1 min)	M	6	10	15	15	15	17	19	25	27	28	28	25
	F	6	10	12	14	15	19	19	18	20	20	20	19
Sit and Reach (cm) 23 cm	M	16				12	12	13	12	15	13	11	15
equals level of feet	F	18	16	17	17	16	16	15	17	18	19	14	22

the epiphysis [47]. The probability of such injury involves a number of factors in addition to activity itself [46]. Strength continues to increase with growth to early adulthood, and males tend to be stronger than females at any age, particularly with respect to the upper body musculature [1, 26]. However, when strength is expressed per unit of cross-sectional muscle area (kg/cm²), age and sex differences are virtually eliminated [26].

The percentage of body fat tends to increase with age from at least childhood through middle age, with females possessing greater adipose tissue than males throughout life [1, 2, 51, 63]. Flexibility tends to decrease with age, and females are more flexible than males [1, 26, 40, 56, 58]. Because of their relatively large surface area [9], diminished sweat production [8], and less subcutaneous fat [1, 51, 63], children do not adapt to heat [8, 9, 70] or cold [65] as well as adults. Additionally, children do not perceive the intensity of exercise as do adults [7].

In response to appropriate training, children and adolescents also receive most of the beneficial physiologic and performance changes documented for adults [9, 17, 26, 29, 33, 34, 50, 51, 61, 62, 72, 73], although there are some questions about the improvements or lack thereof associated with VO_2 max [22, 60, 66], AT [11], and body composition [35, 49].

Investigators continue to establish inverse relationships between physical activity and degenerative disease risk factors in adult populations [15, 52, 57, 64, 69]. Available evidence indicates that at least CHD may originate in childhood [43]; moreover, physically active children possess fewer risk factors [48]. The health protective effects of activity are optimized when activity is continued during the adult years [15, 53]. Finally, PWC and strength, previously thought to decline inevitably with aging, can be maintained at or near maximal levels into the sixth decade of life [39, 55].

Recommendations

Based on the preceding information, it is this author's opinion that children and adolescents have much to gain from beginning and then maintaining an exercise or activity regimen. To optimize the potential benefits and minimize risk, the following recommendations are offered to those involved in the planning and administration of activity programs:

1. An initial physical examination should be required for participants. Ideally, contraindicating or limiting conditions will have been previously diagnosed and known; however, this examination can uncover those conditions that are not known. The examination should include orthopaedic evaluation of the musculoskeletal system and components at greatest risk for injury.

2. "Conservative" adult citeria should be employed as guides to activity. Activity should be undertaken at the conservative end of relative adult ranges for intensity, duration, frequency, and progression [3, 51, 75]. This author recommends using conservative component ranges owing to proven pediatric metabolic [5, 9] and anaerobic inefficiencies [9, 26] and the increased risk of musculoskeletal injury in children [16, 41, 47].

3. Activity bouts should include "warm-up" and "cool-down" periods. Activity should be preceded and followed by activity of a lesser intensity. Since children do not perceive exercise as intensely [7] and experience shorter O_2 uptake transitions [44], they are more likely to forego warm-ups and cool-downs, thus increasing the risk of musculoskeletal injury.

4. Avoid activity during climatic extremes. Because of their limited response to heat stress [9, 70], children should restrict their activity during hot, humid conditions. If this is not possible, the intensity and duration of exercise should be reduced, frequent rest periods should be given, and approximately 150 ml of water should be consumed every 15 to 30 minutes [9, 75]. Drinks containing more than 2.5% solutes should be avoided because gastric emptying will be delayed [51]. Additionally, because children experience greater core body temperature reductions in cold water [65], exposure to cold water under these conditions should be avoided.

5. Collision or high-risk sports activity should be supervised. To an extent, this is somewhat age-dependent. Supervision should be adequate to minimize extraneous hazards and provide required medical attention.

6. The activity environment should emphasize adult "carryover" potential. Activities should be planned to maximize the participant's potential involvement. Achievement should be rewarded and recognized for as many participants as possible. Injuries and limiting conditions should receive immediate and appropriate attention, and, if necessary, activity should be suspended to permit proper resolution of problems. Educational components should be included concerning the physiologic and health benefits of the activity. Perhaps the most important attribute of an activity program is its potential for producing active adults.

References

1. American Alliance for Health, Physical Education, Recreation, and Dance. *Test Manual: Health Related Physical Fitness.* 1900 Association Dr, Reston, VA, AAHPERD, 1980.
2. American Alliance for Health, Physical Education, Recreation, and Dance. *Technical Manual: Health Related Fitness.* 1900 Association Dr, Reston, VA, AAHPERD, 1984.
3. American College of Sports Medicine. Position statement on the

recommended quantity and quality of exercise for developing and maintaining fitness in healthy adults. *Med Sci Sports Exerc* 10:VII-X, 1978.

4. Alekseev, B. A. The influence of skiing races on the hand and foot skeleton of young sportsmen. *Arch Anat Hist Embryol* 72:35–39, 1977.
5. Astrand, P.O. *Experimental Studies of Working Capacity in Relation to Sex and Age.* Copenhagen, Munksgaard, 1952.
6. Bar-Or, O. A commentary to children and fitness: A public health perspective. *Res Q* 58:304–307, 1987.
7. Bar-Or, O. Age related changes in exercise prescription. *In* Borg, G. (Ed.), *Physical Work and Effort.* New York, Pergammon Press, 1977, pp. 255–266.
8. Bar-Or, O. Climate and the exercising child—A review. *Int J Sports Med* 1:53–65, 1980.
9. Bar-Or, O. *Pediatric Sports Medicine for the Practitioner: From Physiologic Principles to Clinical Applications.* New York, Springer-Verlag, 1983.
10. Bar-Or, O., Shephard, R. J., and Allen, C. L. Cardiac output of 10–13 year old boys and girls during submaximal exercise. *J Appl Physiol* 30:219–223, 1971.
11. Becker, D., and Vaccaro, P. Anaerobic threshold alterations caused by endurance training in young children. *J Sports Med* 23:445–449, 1983.
12. Bell, R. D., MacDougall, J. D., Billeter, R., et al. Muscle fiber type and morphometric analysis of skeletal muscle in six-year-old children. *Med Sci Sports Exerc* 12:28–31, 1980.
13. Brown, C. H., Harrower, J. R., and Deeter, M. F. The effect of cross country running on pre-adolescent girls. *Med Sci Sports* 4:1–5, 1972.
14. Brozek, J. Changes in body composition in man during maturity and their nutritional implications. *Fed Proc* 11:784–793, 1952.
15. Cantu, R. C. *Diabetes and Exercise.* Ithaca, Monument Publications, 1982.
16. Clain, M. R., and Hershman, E. B. Overuse injuries in children and adolescents. *Physician Sportsmed* 17:111–123, 1989.
17. Clarke, D., and Vaccaro, P. The effect of swim training on muscular performance and body composition in children. *Res Q* 50:9–17, 1979.
18. Cohen, J. L., and Segal, K. R. Left ventricular hypertrophy in athletes: An exercise–echocardiographic study. *Med Sci Sports Exerc* 17:695–700, 1985.
19. Cooper, D. M., Weiler-Ravell, D., Whipp, B.J., et al. Aerobic parameters of exercise as a function of body size during growth in children. *J Appl Physiol* 56:628–635, 1984.
20. Cooper K. H. *The New Aerobics.* New York, M. Evans, 1970.
21. Coyle, E. F., Feiring, D. C., Rotkins, T. C., et al. Specificity of power improvements through slow and fast isokinetic training. *J Appl Physiol* 51:1437–1442, 1981.
22. Daniels, J., and Oldridge, N. Changes in oxygen consumption of young boys during growth and running training. *Med Sci Sports* 3:161–165, 1971.
23. Daniels, J., Oldridge, N., Nagle, F., et al. Differences and changes in VO$_2$ among young runners 10 to 18 years of age. *Med Sci Sports* 10:200–203, 1978.
24. Davis, J. A., Frank, M. H., Whipp, B. J., et al. Anaerobic threshold alterations caused by endurance running in middle aged men. *J Appl Physiol* 46:1039–1046, 1979.
25. Davis, J. A., Vodak, P., Wilmore, J. H., et al. Anaerobic threshold and maximal aerobic power for three modes of exercise. *J Appl Physiol* 41:544–550, 1976.
26. DeVries, H. *Physiology of Exercise for Physical Education and Athletics* (4th ed.). Dubuque, Wm. C. Brown, 1986.
27. Erikkson, B. Muscle metabolism in children—a review. *Acta Paediatr Scand* (Suppl.) 283:20, 1980.
28. Erikkson, B. O., Grimby, G., and Saltin, B. Cardiac output and arterial gases during exercise in pubertal boys. *J Appl Physiol* 31:348–352, 1971.
29. Erikkson, B. O., and Koch, G. Effect of physical training on hemodynamic response during sub-maximal and maximal exercise in 11–13 year old boys. *Acta Physiol Scand* 87:27–39, 1973.
30. Evans, S. J. An electromyographic analysis of skeletal neuromus-

cular fatigue with special reference to age (Thesis). Los Angeles, University of Southern California, 1971.
31. Fahey, T., Del Valle-Zuris, A., Oehlsen, G., et al. Pubertal stage differences in hormonal and hematological responses to maximal exercise in males. *J Appl Physiol* 46:825–833, 1979.
32. Fournier, M., Ricci, J., and Taylor, A. Skeletal muscle adaptation in adolescent boys: Sprint and endurance training and detraining. *Med Sci Sports Exerc* 14:453–456, 1982.
33. Gatch, W., and Byrd, R. Endurance training and cardiovascular function in 9 and 10 year old boys. *Arch Phys Med Rehabil* 60:574–577, 1979.
34. Geenan, D. L., Gilliam, T. B., Crowley, D., et al. Echocardiographic measures in 6 to 7 year old children after an 8-month exercise program. *Am J Cardiol* 49:1990–1995, 1980.
35. Glick, Z., and Kaufmann, N. Weight and skinfold thickness changes during a physical training course. *Med Sci Sports* 8:109–112, 1976.
36. Hakkinen, K., and Komi, P. Electromyographical changes during strength training and detraining. *Med Sci Sport Exerc* 15:455–460, 1983.
37. Hamilton, P., and Andrew, G. M. Influence of growth and athletic training on heart and lung functions. *Eur J Appl Physiol* 36:27–38, 1976.
38. Jacobs, I., Sjodin, B., and Svane, B. Muscle fiber type, cross sectional area and strength in boys after 4 years endurance training (abstract). *Med Sci Sports Exerc* 14:123, 1982.
39. Kasch, F. W., Wallace, J. P., VanCamp, S. P., et al. A longitudinal study of cardiovascular stability in active men aged 45 to 65 years. *Physician Sportsmed* 16:117–123, 1988.
40. Kirchner, G., and Glines, D. Comparative analysis of Eugene, Oregon, elementary school children using the Kraus-Weber test of minimum muscular fitness. *Res Q* 28:16–25, 1957.
41. Kozar, B., and Lord, R. M. Overuse injury in the young athlete: Reasons for concern. *Physician Sportsmed* 11:117–122, 1983.
42. Krahenbuhl, G. S., Skinner, J. S., and Kohrt, W. M. Developmental aspects of maximal aerobic power in children. *In* Terjung, R. L. (Ed.), *Exercise Science and Sports Research.* New York, Macmillan, 1985, pp. 503–538.
43. Laver, R. M., Conner, W. E., Leaverton, P. E., et al. Coronary heart disease risk factors in school children: The Muscatine Study. *J Pediatr* 86:697–706, 1975.
44. Macek, M., and Vavra, J. The adjustment of oxygen uptake at the onset of exercise: A comparison between pre-pubertal boys and young adults. *Int J Sports Med* 1:75–77, 1980.
45. Malina, R. M. Exercise as an influence upon growth. *Clin Pediatr* 8:16–26, 1969.
46. Micheli, L. J. Lower extremity injuries: Overuse injuries in the recreational adult. *In* Cantu, R. C. (Ed.), *The Exercising Adult.* Lexington, MA, Collamore Press, 1982, pp. 115–120.
47. Micheli, L. J., Santore, R., and Stanitski, C. L. Epiphyseal fractures of the elbow in children. *Am Fam Physician* 22:107–116, 1980.
48. Montoye, H. I. Risk factors for CVD in relation to physical activity in youth. *In* Burkhaust, R. A., Keruber, H. C. G., and Soris, W. H. (Eds.), *Children and Exercise XI.* Champaign, IL, Human Kinetics, 1985, pp. 3–25.
49. Moody, D. L., Wilmore, J. H., Girandola, R. N., et al. The effect of a jogging program on the body composition of normal and obese high school girls. *Med Sci Sports* 41:210–213, 1972.
50. Moratani, T., and De Vries, H. Neural factors versus hypertrophy in the course of muscle strength gain in young and old men. *J Gerontol* 36:294–297, 1981.
51. Neiman, D. C. *The Sports Medicine Fitness Course.* Palo Alto, CA, Bull Publishing, 1986.
52. Paffenberger, R. A., and Hyde, R. T. Exercise in the prevention of coronary heart disease. *Prev Med* 13:3–22, 1984.
53. Paffenberger, R. A., Hyde, R. T., Wing, A. L., et al. A natural history of athleticism and cardiovascular health. *JAMA* 252:491–495, 1984.
54. Pate, R. R., and Blair, S. N. Exercise and the prevention of atherosclerosis: Pediatric implications. *In* Strong, W. (Ed.), *Pediatric Aspects of Atherosclerosis.* New York, Grune & Stratton, 1978, pp. 255–286.

55. Petrofsky, J. S., and Lind, A. R. Aging, isometric strength and endurance, and cardiovascular response to static effort. *J Appl Physiol* 38:91–95, 1975.

56. Phillips, M. Analysis of results from the Kraus-Weber test of minimum fitness in children. *Res Q* 26:314–323, 1955.

57. Poole, G. W. Exercise, coronary heart disease and risk factors: A brief report. *Sports Med* 1:341–349, 1984.

58. Public Health Service: Summary of findings from National Children and Youth Fitness Study. *Journal of Health, Physical Education, and Recreation,* 56:44–90, 1985.

59. Rodahl, K. Physical work capacity. *Arch Environ Health* 2:499–510, 1961.

60. Rowland, T. Aerobic responses to endurance training in prepubescent children: A critical analysis. *Med Sci Sports Exerc* 17:493–497, 1985.

61. Sailors, M. S., and Berg, K. Comparison of responses to weight training in prepubescent boys and men. *J Sports Med* 27:30–37, 1987.

62. Sewall, B. S., and Micheli, L. J. Strength training for children. *J Pediatr Orthop* 6:143–146, 1986.

63. Shephard, R. J. Physiologic changes over the years. *In* Blair, S. N., Painter P., Pate, R. R., et al. (Eds.), *Resource Manual for Guidelines for Exercise Testing and Prescription.* Philadelphia, Lea & Febiger, 1988, pp. 297–304.

64. Siscovik, D. S., Laporte, R. E. and Newman, J. M. The disease specific benefits and risks of physical activity and exercise. *Public Health Rep* 100:180–188, 1985.

65. Sloan, R. E. G., and Keating, W. R. Cooling rate of young people swimming in cold water. *J Appl Physiol* 35:371–375, 1973.

66. Stewart, K., and Gutin, B. Effects of physical training on cardiorespiratory fitness in children. *Res Q* 47:110–120, 1985.

67. Tanner, J. M. *Growth at Adolescence.* Oxford, Blackwell Scientific Publications, 1962.

68. U.S. Department of Health and Human Services. *Promoting Health/Preventing Disease: Objectives for the Nation.* Washington, D.C., U.S. Government Printing Office, 1980.

69. Vena, J. E., Graham, S., Zielezny, M., et al. Lifetime occupational exercise and colon cancer. *Am J Epidemiol* 122:357–365, 1985.

70. Wagner, J. A., Robinson, S., Tzankoff, S. P., et al. Heat tolerance and acclimatization to work in the heat in relation to age. *J Appl Physiol* 33:616–622, 1972.

71. Wasserman, K., Whipp, B. J., Koyal, S., et al. Anaerobic threshold and respiratory gas exchange during exercise. *J Appl Physiol* 35:236–243, 1973.

72. Weltman, A., Janney, C., Rian, C. B., et al. The effects of hydraulic resistance strength training in pre-pubertal males. *Med Sci Sports Exerc* 18:629–638, 1986.

73. Wilmore, J. H. Alterations in strength, body composition and anthropometric measurement consequent to a 10 week weight training program. *Med Sci Sports Exerc* 6:133–138, 1974.

74. Yoshizawa, S., Ishizaki, T., and Honda, H. Physical fitness in children aged 5 and 6 years. *J Hum Ergol* 6:41–51, 1977.

75. Zwiren, L. D. Exercise prescription for children. *In* Blair, S. N., Painter, P., Pate, R. R., et al. (Eds.), *Resource Manual for Guidelines for Exercise Testing and Prescription.* Philadelphia, Lea & Febiger, 1988, pp. 309–314.

SPORTS AND THE NEURODEVELOPMENT OF THE CHILD

Paul G. Dyment, M.D.

Children undergo neurologic and physical development in a fairly consistent pattern, and when groups of children are observed, a steady progression of stages can be described. The early research literature on this phenomenon concentrated on motor skills using *quantitative* data—e.g., at what age can a child sit up, stand, run, and catch a ball? Studies have shown that most children have developed an adult style of walking by age 4 years, running by age 5 to 6 years, climbing by age 6 years, and galloping by age 6½ years. But knowing these average ages is of little help to the clinician who is attempting to decide whether a particular child should be encouraged to participate in a certain athletic activity that requires a degree of motor development the child may or may not have achieved.

By the 1920s *qualitative* differences in motor skills began to be studied, although most of these studies were cross-sectional in design. During the past two decades Seefeldt and Haubenstricker's group in Michigan evaluated two cohorts of children over a period of time and demonstrated both the relative stability of selected motor skills and the "norms" for the ages at which those skills were developed [6]. By stability we mean that from year to year the degree of performance compared to that of the peer group remains consistent, i.e., there is an acceptable correlation coefficient.

Seefeldt and Haubenstricker's motor performance study looked at eight fundamental skills (Fig. 2–1) and subdivided them descriptively into four or five stages of development [6]. An example of this is their subdivision of the skill of throwing a ball (Fig. 2–2). During stage 1 the throwing motion is essentially posterior-anterior in direction, and there is no trunk rotation. The distinctive feature of stage 2 is the rotation of the body about an imaginary vertical axis. Stage 3 is characterized by the forward motion of the leg ipsilateral to the throwing arm; if the contralateral leg moves forward, this is stage 4. When the weight shifts entirely to the rear leg, which pivots in response to the rotating joints above it, stage 5 begins. The ages by which 60% of boys and girls could perform these specific stages are shown in Figure 2–1. Although it had been widely believed that prior to age 7 or 8 years children could not perform tasks requiring much coordination and therefore that early instruction and repetitive practice would have little or no effect on improving athletic skills, their study indicated that the preschool and early elementary school years are appropriate times for children to learn to refine these motor skills through repetitive action. Almost all of the children in their study followed the same sequence in progressing through the stages of motor skill acquisition. The same sequence was observed even in blind children who could not observe other children performing these tasks, so there must be an ingrained progression of motor skill acquisition.

Ball-handling skills (dribbling, catching, and aiming) of boys of different ages have been studied, and incremental improvements have been found until puberty, when skills reached a plateau [2]. Branta and colleagues reviewed the data concerning the ages at which athletic motor skills are achieved and concluded that a gender difference begins to appear at puberty, with boys continuing to improve in skills requiring strength, endurance, and power, and girls reaching a plateau or actually declining in certain skills such as the flexed-arm hang, timed sit-ups, and leg lifts [3]. This gender difference may be due to different environmental stimulants during childhood (i.e., "nurture"), to biologic predeterminism

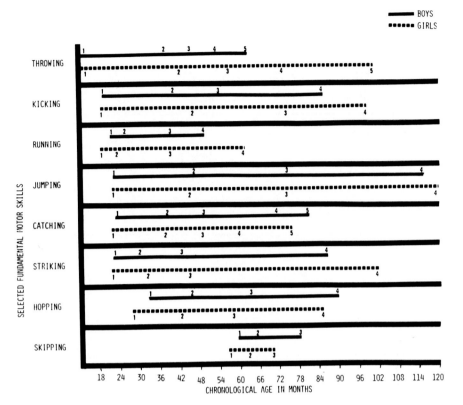

FIGURE 2–1
Age at which 60% of the boys and girls were able to perform a specific developmental level for selected fundamental motor skills. Numbers refer to developmental stage of that motor skill. (From Seefeldt, V., and Haubenstricker, J. Patterns, phases, or stages: An analytical model for the study of developmental movement. *In* Kelso, J.A.S., and Clark, J.E. (Eds.), *The Development of Movement Control and Coordination.* Copyright 1982 by John Wiley & Sons. Reprinted by permission of John Wiley & Sons, Ltd.)

"SPORTS READINESS"

There have been many scientific studies of age changes in motor skills during childhood and adolescence, but they offer little help to the physician who is asked by a parent, "Is my 8-year-old ready to play football?" [3]. Far easier to answer is whether it is *safe* for that 8-year-old to play football. (The prepubertal years are actually the safest age for boys to play that particular sport.) One cannot predict the readiness of school-age children to learn specific motor skills based on age, body size, or assessment of physical maturation. However, success in certain sports such as ice hockey can be predicted by sport-specific tests of certain motor skills [4]. These tests predict *proficiency* in that sport rather than sports readiness, and they were devised by subjecting players to a wide battery of tests of athletic motor skills, comparing these results with eventual sport proficiency, and then selecting the discriminating motor tests.

Sports readiness implies that the child's growth, maturity, and development are *all* at the stage where the child can acquire the necessary athletic skills and emo-

tional drive to compete successfully [5]. In this definition *growth* refers to body size, muscle strength, and endurance; *maturity* refers to the child's age (both chronologic and physiologic) and previous acquisition of basic motor skills; and *development* includes social, emotional, and cognitive competence. The first two factors, growth and maturity, are basically biologic phenomena and hence genetic in origin, whereas development is either biologic (i.e., cognitive competence), social (i.e., social competence), or both (i.e., emotional competence). All of these factors affect a child's ability to compete in a sport, so predicting sports readiness requires a biosocial perspective and not just a simple assessment of motor development.

A child may be neurodevelopmentally ready for a certain sport, but if he or she is having emotional difficulties that prevent him from accepting the team discipline insisted on by the coach, then the experience may well be a negative one for the coach and the team and a disaster for the child. A common condition in boys, the attention deficit hyperactivity disorder (ADHD), affects at least 10% of all elementary school boys and can affect their ability to compete athletically, especially in team sports. This is a neurologic condition characterized by a short attention span, hyperactivity, restlessness, impulsive behavior, learning disability, and a behavior problem secondary to school failure. A child with this con-

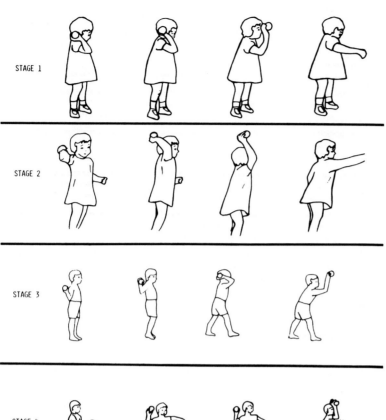

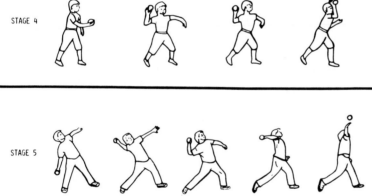

FIGURE 2–2
Developmental sequence of throwing behavior. (From Seefeldt, V., and Haubenstricker, J. Patterns, phases, or stages: An analytical model for the study of developmental movement. *In* Kelso, J.A.S., and Clark J.E. (Eds.), *The Development of Movement Control and Coordination.* Copyright 1982 by John Wiley & Sons. Reprinted by permission of John Wiley & Sons, Ltd.)

dition may be developmentally ready to play baseball, but his attention span is so short that he gets bored playing out in the field and may well become a sports dropout. A wise coach should try to have him play as catcher, a position in which something is happening most of the time. Fortunately, many of the symptoms of ADHD improve with treatment with methylphenidate, and this drug may be as important for athletic success for these boys as an albuterol inhaler is for a player with exercise-induced bronchospasm [1].

So what should a physician do when asked to predict "sports readiness" in a child? This review has indicated that there are no objective tests that can guide the clinician, so we are left with relying on our *clinical judgment* or, even better, our *common sense.* Even applying a biosocial perspective as described above is fraught with

the probability of error, so it is probably better to err in the liberal direction with "If your child wants to play, let him try" than to arbitrarily prevent participation because of a vague feeling that the child is "too young" or "too immature."

References

1. Alexander, J.L. Hyperactive children: Which sports have the right stuff. *Physician Sportsmed,* 1990.
2. Bodie, D.A. Changes in lung function, ball-handling skills, and performance measures during adolescence in normal schoolboys. *In* Binkhorst, R.A., et al. (Eds.), *Children and Exercise XI.* Champaign, IL, Human Kinetics Pub, 1985, pp. 260–268.
3. Branta, C., Haubensticker, J., and Seefeldt, V. Age changes in motor skills during childhood and adolescence. *Exerc Sport Sci Rev* 12:467–520, 1984.

4. Hermiston, R.T., Gratton, and Teno, T. Three hockey skills tests as predictors of hockey playing ability. *Can J Appl Sport Sci* 4:95–97, 1979.

5. Malina, R.M. Readiness for competitive sports. Unpublished manuscript.

6. Seefeldt, V., and Haubenstricker, J. Patterns, phases, or stages: An analytical model for the study of developmental movement. *In* Kelso, J.A.S., and Clark, J.E. (Eds.), *The Development of Movement Control and Coordination.* New York, John Wiley & Sons, 1982, pp. 309–318.

THE YOUNG FEMALE ATHLETE

Letha Y. Griffin, M.D., Ph.D.

THE CHANGING ABILITIES OF THE FEMALE ATHLETE DURING DEVELOPMENT FROM CHILDHOOD THROUGH ADOLESCENCE

In discussing anatomic and physiologic variations in young male and female athletes, it is important to consider the athlete during the three stages of development because athletic abilities differ in each stage. These stages are the child, the adolescent, and the young adult. For the purposes of this discussion, the adolescent period is termed the pubertal period; the child is then the prepubertal athlete, and the young adult is the postpubertal athlete.

Little boys and little girls are most equal in their athletic abilities during childhood [63]. Therefore, in grade school or up until about the sixth grade it is reasonable to have coeducational physical education classes. Similar recreational soccer, basketball, softball, and baseball teams may be organized, with boys and girls participating together on a team rather than having separate male and female leagues. It is at about the sixth grade level (approximately age 12) that pubertal development is seen. Since puberty is a continuum with a variable age of onset, not all children are at the same stage of development at the same age. Onset of puberty in males occurs from ages 13 to 15, whereas puberty in girls begins usually between the ages of 11 and 13 years.

During the pubertal years, schools and leagues should consider basing their sports programs on weight rather than on age. If two girls or boys are both 13 years old, but one has gone through puberty and the other is just starting this developmental process, their sizes (both height and weight) are very different and their sport interaction should be adjusted accordingly.

Postpubertal differences occur in males and females that were not present in childhood. Males undergo large increases in height, weight, and muscle mass, whereas in females lesser increases in height and weight occur without a comparable increase in muscle mass [39]. The result is that postpubertal males are taller and heavier than females of equal age.

Differences in body percentage of muscle mass and fat in males and females begin to occur during puberty. These differences are not present in children. In equally conditioned postpubertal males and females, the females have only 23% of body weight in muscle, whereas the males have 40% [35]. Females have 15% body fat compared to 5% in males. Thus, the female is at a slight physiologic disadvantage in sports because she has less muscle mass to propel greater body weight [31, 32, 43, 68, 71, 72].

Also, in terms of physiologic parameters, postpubertal females have a smaller heart size, smaller rib cage, smaller vital capacity, and a greater respiratory rate than equally well conditioned postpubertal males. So although childhood abilities are similar, following puberty differences in athletic potential become evident between the sexes. At this developmental stage, the aim should be equal opportunity for sport participation for boys and girls but not necessarily coeducational sport participation.

As a consequence of pubertal development, not only are women no longer competitive with men in certain sports due to differences in height, weight, muscle mass, and cardiac and pulmonary capacities, but also women may find it more difficult to excel in the same sports they participated in prior to puberty. One must consider the dilemma of being too big for some sports and not big enough for others.

For example, if a young elite gymnast, dancer, or skater who has practiced her sport 3 to 4 hours a day 5 days a week since early childhood goes through puberty and experiences a marked change in physique, growing markedly taller, developing thick rather than slender muscles, and experiencing significant breast development, she may find that because of body type alone she is less proficient in her sport. Often girls who "grow out of their sport" during puberty find it difficult to communicate to their parents their frustration in continuing to try to participate in that sport. These girls know how much time and effort the parents have devoted to their sport development and how the parents look forward to their child's continued participation. These athletes may use physical complaints as an excuse to avoid participating. The treating physician must be sensitive to these clues of frustration and depression expressed by the athlete. It is the physician who may need to suggest to the parents that these girls may no longer wish to participate in the sport for which they have been groomed.

During puberty, youngsters may grow out of a sport psychologically as well as physically. Although ideas in our culture are changing, traditionally boys "prove" their masculinity through sports participation, whereas many female athletes, especially those involved in contact sports, have to justify their femininity [24, 65]. These additional psychological demands placed on teens involved in sports occur during that crucial pubertal time when these young women are trying to find themselves and their place in the world. It should be emphasized to these girls that athletics and femininity are not separate entities but in fact overlap. Girls who play a hard game of basketball on Friday night can look just as feminine as any other girl on a Saturday night date.

Not only is there a perception factor for young women engaged in sport, but time limitations exist as well. It is during the teenage years that girls typically begin paying more attention to their appearance and experimenting with hair styles, make-up, and trends in clothing styles. They may no longer want or feel that they have the time to spend every night in the gymnasium practicing their sport.

ADVANTAGES OF SPORT PARTICIPATION BY FEMALES THROUGHOUT DEVELOPMENT AND INTO ADULTHOOD

Many positive effects have resulted from the increased female participation in sports. It is acceptable these days for women to be tall, tough, and competitive [40]. Fathers teach sport skills to their daughters as well as to their sons, leading to a closer father-daughter relationship [5]. In previous years, "pretty" had a certain connotation and was frequently the major criterion on which popularity for girls during the teenage years was based. Now recognition through athletic ability is as possible

for women as is popularity based on scholastic and leadership abilities. Moreover, many believe that women in the future will be more effective in the workplace because of team skills learned through sports participation in their youth.

SPECIAL AREAS OF CONCERN IN THE PREPARTICIPATION PHYSICAL EXAMINATION FOR WOMEN

History

Family History. An athlete's medical history should include a family history. In screening women athletes, one should ask if anyone in the family has had scoliosis because there is a familial tendency to this spinal deformity. Not only is scoliosis slightly more common in females, but also females have a greater tendency for progression of a curve once it develops. If a teenager has a family history that is positive for scoliosis, she should be followed very carefully during her rapid growth years (ages 11 to 13).

A history of familial cardiovascular disease is also important, especially in the college and elite athlete. Although coronary artery disease is more common in males, premenopausal women may also be affected. Elite athletes who are maximizing performance may need to have stress electrocardiograms as early as the late teens if there is a strong family history of arteriosclerotic heart disease.

Mitral valve prolapse is more common among females and has a familial tendency. Diagnosis is suspected when a midsystolic click associated with a late systolic murmur is heard and is confirmed by echocardiogram. The presence of mitral valve prolapse alone does not preclude sports participation, but if it is associated with syncope, disabling chest pain, complex ventricular arrhythmias, significant mitral regurgitation, a prolonged Q–T interval, Marfan's syndrome, or a family history of sudden death, further investigation is warranted.

Past Medical History. When reviewing the past medical history of a female athlete, it is important to include questions on the urogenital system. If a woman gives a history of prior urinary tract infections, the need for frequent fluids, especially water, should be discussed. Some athletes tend to diminish their fluid intake when traveling. They should be cautioned not to do so.

One should document the date of the first menses, the date of the last period, the average length of the period, the presence of dysmenorrhea, and the pregnancy history. Athletes may experience a delay in menarche [21]. The average age of menarche in nonathletes is reported to be 12.5 years, whereas in athletes it is 13.5 to 15.5

years [18, 42]. The athlete who has not had a period by age 16 is considered to have primary amenorrhea and should be referred to her physician for further evaluation to confirm that sports participation and not other diseases has delayed menstrual periods (Table 3–1) [68].

The normal menstrual cycle is 28 days, with a range of 25 to 35 days. Many athletes (as many as 46% of runners) have oligomenorrhea or infrequent periods (cycles greater than 35 days but less than 90 days) [13, 41]. Five to fifteen percent of athletes are reported to have secondary amenorrhea, or cessation of menses for more than 3 months. Secondary amenorrhea is more common in sports such as running and ballet and less common in sports such as swimming and cycling [57, 62].

Physical stress, emotional stress, and weight loss appear to be the most common contributing factors to the development of secondary amenorrhea [4, 7, 12, 14, 20, 22, 45, 58, 60, 61, 69]. Athletes who have not had a menstrual period in a year should not assume that a prolonged period of amenorrhea is secondary to athletic participation but should be evaluated to exclude other abnormalities.

Some gynecologists advocate estrogen replacement in women with low-estrogenic secondary amenorrhea because they believe that prolonged low-estrogen states may result in early osteoporosis [8, 9, 15, 25]. A decrease in cancellous bone of the vertebral bodies of women athletes who have been amenorrheic for a year or longer has been reported. The amount of cortical bone in these athletes did not change [44, 48]. The significance of the cancellous bone loss is not clear. Estrogen replacement is certainly not without consequences and side effects [51]. Moreover, many women athletes have a psychological aversion to replacement therapy even if it is recommended [56]. Therefore, more documentation of the need for estrogen replacement in low-estrogenic secondary amenorrheic athletes is needed.

Girls should be reminded that secondary amenorrhea is no guarantee against pregnancy [54]. The amenorrheic athlete may start ovulating normally at any time. Contraceptive methods can be discussed with the athlete when obtaining her history.

Dysmenorrhea, or painful periods, are less common in athletes than in nonathletes [17]. If dysmenorrhea does occur during competition it can be disabling to the ath-

lete. Menstrual cramps are caused by endometrial release of prostaglandins, which then act on the myometrium to cause contractions. Prostaglandin inhibitors such as naproxen sodium (Anaprox), ibuprofen (Motrin), and naproxen (Naprosyn) may be used to treat dysmenorrhea. Persistent disabling dysmenorrhea deserves further gynecologic evaluation to rule out endometriosis, pelvic infection, and other diseases.

Frequent vaginal infections should be noted as a part of the history. If antibiotics need to be used in athletes who are prone to candidal vaginitis, preventive douches or medicated suppositories may be recommended to avoid development of the candidal infection.

Physical Examination

Cardiovascular System. Particular emphasis should be given to listening to the midsystolic click and late systolic murmur in patients with mitral valve prolapse [28]. As already discussed under family history, mitral valve prolapse occurs with greater frequency in women, although it is by no means limited to them. Prophylactic antibiotics should be given to athletes with mitral valve prolapse who experience severe abrasions, dental work, or gastrointestinal instrumentation.

Breast Examination. Should a breast examination be done as part of a preparticipation physical assessment? This depends on the age of the athlete. In the athlete of college age or older, a breast examination should be done if this is the only physical the athlete will have. If the preparticipation physical examination is a sport-specific examination done to augment a routine physical examination performed by the athlete's personal physician, then the breast examination can be deleted. Also, if an athlete is very large-breasted, counseling about the use of sports bras can be given during this part of the examination.

Pelvic Examination. Most physicians do not perform pelvic examinations as part of preparticipation physicals unless they are family physicians and are doing the preparticipation examination as part of a complete physical examination. If one discovers something unusual or abnormal about the athlete's menstrual history while taking her medical history, one can refer her to her own physician for additional gynecologic evaluation.

Musculoskeletal Examination. Women have been reported to have greater joint laxity than men [55]. In preseason physical examinations it is important to document the degree of laxity of the major joints, including the shoulders, knees (anterior-posterior, medial-lateral, patellar laxity), and ankles so that if an injury occurs the preinjury laxity is available for comparison. Furthermore, if excessive joint laxity compared with age-related norms is discovered, preseason conditioning exercises

TABLE 3–1
Gynecologic Facts

Average age of menarche:
　Nonathletes　　　　　12.5 years
　Athletes　　　　　　　13.5–15.5 years
Normal menstrual cycle: 28 days (range 25–35 days)
Primary amenorrhea: no menses by age 16
Secondary amenorrhea: lack of normal menses for 3 months

can be developed to emphasize strengthening of the muscles about these joints.

The Spine. The configuration of the cervical spine is always assessed. Women frequently have long, slender necks. In football players we emphasize strengthening of the cervical paravertebral muscles. We should do the same thing for athletes engaged in other sports, particularly contact sports.

Note should be taken of excessive lumbar lordosis. Certain sports, such as women's gymnastics, women's diving, roller skating, ice skating, and ballet, emphasize lumbar hyperextension. Girls participating in these sports should strengthen their abdominal and paravertebral muscles to minimize the occurrence of lumbar pain and the potential for stress fractures of the pars interarticularis.

The Knee. During the knee examination the physician should note patellar laxity as well as patellar tracking patterns during active and passive extension of the knee. With the athlete standing, the examiner should look at the configuration of the lower extremities as a whole. If femoral anteversion, foot pronation, and a laterally tracking patella are observed, the physician should recommend that the athlete's conditioning program include quadriceps muscle–strengthening exercises, especially exercises that strengthen the vastus medialis [33].

A biking program to supplement the routine sports program may be excellent for the girl with patellar pain or abnormal patellar tracking. Biking can increase quadriceps strength at low patellofemoral forces. The seat of the bicycle should be maximally elevated and the wheel tension should be minimal during the exercise. Stair-climbing drills should be avoided in women found to have subluxable or laterally tracking patellas as well as in those who have parapatellar or retropatellar tenderness or evidence of patellar crepitance on physical examination.

Girls found to have excessive pronation may benefit from an arch support, but the physician should be careful about prescribing arches or orthotics in the asymptomatic athlete who has performed without symptoms for a number of years. These women probably have adjusted successfully to the biomechanics of the lower extremity and may become symptomatic if these mechanics are altered.

If the patella subluxes easily with gentle pressure on the medial side, a patellar stabilizing brace made with a lateral restraining pad may be helpful. It is unusual to find junior college, college, or elite women athletes with patellar instability because this condition typically disables an athlete early in her career.

The Foot. In examining the foot of the athlete, one should note the presence of soft or hard corns or thickening of the bursa over the first metatarsal head medi-

ally, the fifth metatarsal head laterally, or the superior prominence of the calcaneus posteriorly. Such findings usually indicate that the athlete is wearing an improperly fitting shoe. Many girls have slender heels but a proportionately wider forefoot. Shoes fitted to the hindfoot may be too narrow for the forefoot. Alternatively, shoes wide enough for the forefoot may be too wide for the heel, causing the foot to slide forward in the shoe and impinging on the forefoot. Foot pain secondary to improper shoewear can be disabling to an athlete. Symptoms ranging from bursitis to corns and blisters are slow to resolve once they occur, so prevention must be emphasized.

Hallux primus varus is more frequent in girls than in boys. In most athletes this deformity is asymptomatic. However, if it is symptomatic, shoe modification rather than surgery should be tried initially to relieve symptoms. Surgical correction of bunions can alter foot mechanics disadvantageously. Bunionectomies often result in shortening of the first metatarsal and can shift the axis of weight bearing to the center of the foot, resulting in stress fractures or metatarsalgia of the middle metatarsals.

Laboratory Tests. The preparticipation physical examination of the high school or junior high school athlete rarely includes laboratory testing of blood or urine because such tests have not proved cost effective. If the preparticipation physical is done by the athlete's own physician as part of a yearly physical examination, a blood count and urinalysis may be obtained.

Some clinicians believe that in women athletes, especially athletes at the college and elite levels, tissue iron as well as hematocrit should be measured because tissue iron may be depleted before an athlete's hematocrit falls. Iron is important not only in oxygen transport [26] but also in oxidative enzyme function. Depleted iron stores may adversely affect performance by decreasing strength and endurance, resulting in easy fatigability [11, 30, 49, 52, 66]. Altered visual perception has also been blamed on depleted tissue iron. Measuring serum ferritin levels is a reasonable way of assessing tissue iron [47].

Menstruating women need an extra 10 mg of iron per day. Fifty percent of women have been reported to have iron deficiencies in their basic diet. Women should be counseled about the need to include in their diet iron-rich foods, such as meats (liver, oysters, turkey, pork, beef), dried fruits (apricots, dates, prunes, raisins), and beans (baked, lima, kidney, refried) [53]. A multivitamin pill that includes iron can provide about 12 mg of iron.

Fitness Evaluation. Assessment of physical fitness for both male and female athletes includes evaluation of muscle strength, muscle power, speed, agility, flexibility, and cardiovascular endurance. In evaluating the results of such an examination in postpubertal athletes, one cannot use the same parameters to assess men's and women's performances because the anatomic and physiologic differences between the sexes influence the results (Figs. 3–1 and 3–2) [23].

CONDITIONING TECHNIQUES AND THEIR EFFECT ON INJURY RATES IN THE YOUNG FEMALE ATHLETE

With the growth of women's athletics, many observers predicted an increase in the number and types of injuries in women as they became more aggressive and competitive in sports. In fact, early injury studies of female athletes reported increases in the number of injuries sustained compared with male athletes [16, 36]. As women have become more serious in their participation in sports, however, training and conditioning techniques have improved, and injury rates have decreased [10, 29, 70]. Injuries are now felt to be more sport-specific than sex-specific; that is, injury types and rates are similar for men and women in the same sport but differ for athletes participating in different sports.

Conditioning programs result in improvements in strength, endurance, and flexibility and hence decrease the chance of injury [1, 54]. Although at one time it was feared that girls would become "muscle bound" if they participated in weight-training programs as part of their conditioning programs, it is now realized that weight training is beneficial to girls because it increases their strength and does not result in large increases in muscle bulk unless the athlete is genetically predisposed to such increases [3]. Most girls can increase their strength up to 40% through weight-training programs without demonstrating a marked increase in muscle bulk.

NUTRITIONAL CONCERNS

With regard to nutritional concerns, one must remember that after puberty the basal metabolic rate is lower in women than in men. Hence, women need fewer calories to sustain the same level of activity as their male counterparts, yet all the required dietary components must be included within these total calories [2]. Women athletes have a higher incidence of eating disorders (principally anorexia nervosa and bulimia) than men. Perhaps this occurs because with the image changes brought by puberty the athlete may find that her "new" body is undesirable for sports such as track, ice skating, and ballet, in which the lean look is appreciated.

ATHLETIC FITNESS SCORE CARD—Boys and Men

Test	0 = Below Athlete Level	1 = Above Average	2 = Good	3 = Very Good	4 = Excellent
1. *Strength—* Pull-ups (no.)	fewer than 7	7 to 9	10 to 12	13 to 14	15 or more
2. *Power—*Stand. long jump (ins.)	fewer than 85	85 to 88	89 to 91	92 to 94	95 or more
3. *Speed—* 50-yd. dash (secs.)	slower than 6.7	6.7 to 6.4	6.3 to 6.0	5.9 to 5.6	5.5 or less
4. *Agility—* 6-ct. agility (cts.)	fewer than 5-5	5-5 to 6-3	6-4 to 7-2	7-3 to 8-1	8-2 or more
5. *Flexibility—*Forward flexion (ins.)	not reach ruler	1 to 2	3 to 5	6 to 8	9 or more
6. *Muscular Endurance—* Sit-ups (no.)	fewer than 38	38 to 45	46 to 52	53 to 59	60 or more
7. *Cardiorespiratory Endurance—*12-min. run (miles)	fewer than 1½	1½	1¾	2	2¼ or more

YOUR SCORE

	Strength	Power	Speed	Agility	Flexibility	Muscular Endurance	Cardiorespiratory Endurance
Your Score							
Rating (0–4)							

FIGURE 3–1
Athletic fitness score card for boys and men. (From Gaillard, B., Haskell, W., Smith, N., and Ogilvie, B. (Eds.), *Handbook for the Young Athlete.* Palo Alto, CA, Bull Publishing, 1978.)

ATHLETIC FITNESS SCORE CARD—Girls and Women

Test	0 = Below Athlete Level	1 = Above Average	2 = Good	3 = Very Good	4 = Excellent
1. *Strength*—Pull-ups (no.)	fewer than 2	2 to 3	4 to 5	6 to 7	8 or more
2. *Power*—Stand. long jump (ins.)	fewer than 63	63 to 65	66 to 68	69 to 71	72 or more
3. *Speed*—50-yd. dash (secs.)	slower than 8.2	8.2 to 7.9	7.8 to 7.1	6.9 to 6.0	5.9 or less
4. *Agility*—6-ct. agility (cts.)	fewer than 3-5	3-5 to 4-3	4-4 to 5-2	5-3 to 6-2	6-3 or more
5. *Flexibility*—Forward flexion (ins.)	fewer than 3	3 to 5	6 to 8	9 to 11	12 or more
6. *Muscular Endurance*—Sit-ups (no.)	fewer than 26	26 to 31	32 to 38	39 to 45	46 or more
7. *Cardiorespiratory Endurance*—12-min. run (miles)	fewer than 1¼	1¼	1½	1¾	2 or more

YOUR SCORE

	Strength	Power	Speed	Agility	Flexibility	Muscular Endurance	Cardiorespiratory Endurance
Your Score Rating (0–4)							

FIGURE 3–2

Athletic fitness score card for girls and women. (From Gaillard, B., Haskell, W., Smith, N., and Ogilvie, B. (Eds.), *Handbook for the Young Athlete*. Palo Alto, CA, Bull Publishing, 1978.)

Anorexia is defined as a ''severe and prolonged inability or refusal to eat, sometimes accompanied by spontaneous or induced vomiting.'' Bulimia is ''the marked fear of becoming obese, with uncontrolled binges followed by purging, vomiting, laxatives, or excessive exercise.'' Anorexia is more than the practice of simply starving oneself to ''make weight.'' It is a psychological disorder in which one perceives oneself as much, much heavier than is actually the case.

The incidence of eating disorders has been estimated at 13% to 17%. Eating disorders occur primarily in the middle and upper classes and are nine times more common in females than in males. The typical age range is 15 to 26 years of age. Girls with eating disorders may be more prone to injury and thus they seek treatment from their sports physician. It is important for the physician to recognize the scope of the illness and encourage the athlete and her parents to seek help. The parents may not even realize that their child has an eating disorder, or if they do, they may not know how to deal with it.

At the other extreme, anabolic steroids combined with high-protein diets and rigorous weight-training regimens have been used by some girls to increase muscle bulk [34, 38, 73]. These athletes should realize that the use of anabolic steroids is not without side effects. Some side effects are reversible and others are not. Side effects include acne, excessive facial hair, menstrual irregularities, male-pattern baldness, deepening of the voice, enlarged clitoris, fluid retention, increased blood pressure, and increased risks of heart attack, stroke, and liver abnormalities (Table 3–2) [37]. The use of anabolic steroids should be condemned.

TABLE 3–2
Side Effects of Anabolic Steroids in Women

Acne
Excessive facial hair
Menstrual irregularities
Male-pattern baldness
Enlarged clitoris
Deepening of voice
Fluid retention
Increased blood pressure
Increased risk of heart attack, stroke, liver abnormalities

References

1. American Academy of Orthopaedic Surgeons. Basic principles of conditioning programs. *In Athletic Training and Sports Medicine*

(2nd ed.). Park Ridge, American Academy of Orthopaedic Surgeons, 1991, pp. 721–750.

2. Anderson, J. Women's sports and fitness programs of the U.S. Military Academy. *Physician Sportsmed* 7(4):72–78, 1979.

3. Benas, D. Special considerations in women's rehabilitation programs. *In* Hunter, L., and Funk, F. (Eds.), *Rehabilitation of the Injured Knee.* St. Louis, C.V. Mosby, 1984, pp. 393–405.

4. Bonen, A., and Keizer, H. Athletic menstrual cycle irregularity: Endocrine response to exercise and training. *Physician Sportsmed* 12(8):78–94, 1984.

5. Boutilier, M., and SanGiovanni, L. *The Sporting Woman.* Champaign, IL, Human Kinetics, 1983.

6. Butts, N. Physiological profile of high school female cross country runners. *Physician Sportsmed* 10(11):103–111, 1982.

7. Calabrese, L., Kirkendall, D., Floyd, M., et al. Menstrual abnormalities, nutritional patterns, and body composition in female classical ballet dancers. *Physician Sportsmed* 11(2):86–98, 1983.

8. Caldwell, F. Light boned and lean athletes: Does the penalty outweigh the reward? *Physician Sportsmed* 12(9):139–149, 1984.

9. Carr, C., Gevant, H., Ettinger, B., et al. Spinal mineral loss in oophorectomized women. *JAMA* 244(18):2050–2059, 1980.

10. Clarke, K., and Buckley, W. Women's injuries in collegiate sports. *Am J Sports Med* 8(3):187–191, 1980.

11. Cooter, G., and Moribray, K. Effect of iron supplementation and activity on serum iron depletion and hemoglobin levels in female athletes. *Research* 49:114–117, 1978.

12. Dale, E. Exercise and the menstrual cycle. *Emory University Department of Obstetrics and Gynecology Bulletin,* 6(1):48–53, 1984.

13. Dale, E., Gerlach, D., and Wilhote, A. Menstrual dysfunction in distance runners. *Obstet Gynecol* 54:47, 1979.

14. Diddle, A. Athletic activity and menstruation. *Sports-medicine* 76(5):619–624, 1983.

15. Drinkwater, B., Nilson, K., Chesnut, C., et al. Bone mineral contents of amenorrheic and eumenorrheic athletes. *N Engl J Med* 311(5):277–280, 1984.

16. Eisenberg, T., and Allen, W. Injuries in a women's varsity athletic program. *Physician Sportsmed* 6(3):112–116, 1978.

17. Erdelyi, G. Gynecological survey of female athletes. Presented at the Second National Conference on Medical Aspects of Sports Sponsored by the American Medical Association, Washington, D.C., November 27, 1960, pp. 174–178.

18. Erdelyi, G. Effects of exercise on the menstrual cycle. *Physician Sportsmed* 4(3):79–81, 1976.

19. Ferstle, J. Christine Wells: Asking the right questions. *Physician Sportsmed* 10(7):157–160, 1982.

20. Frisch, R. Food intake, fatness, and reproductive ability. *In* Virgersky, R. (Ed.), *Anorexia Nervosa.* New York, Raven Press, 1977, pp. 149–160.

21. Frisch, R. Delayed menarche and amenorrhea of college athletes in relation to age of onset of training. *JAMA* 246:1559, 1982.

22. Frishe, R., and McArthur, J. Menstrual cycle: Fitness as a determinant of minimal weight for height necessary for maintenance or onset. *Science* 185(9):949–961, 1976.

23. Gaillard, B., Haskell, W., Smith, N., et al. *Handbook for the Young Athlete.* Palo Alto, Bull Publishing, 1978.

24. Gerber, E., Felshin, J., Berlin, P., et al. *The American Woman in Sport.* Reading, MA, Addison Wesley, 1974.

25. Gonzalez, E. Premature bone loss found in some nonmenstruating sportswomen. *JAMA* 24(5):513–514, 1983.

26. Hale, R. Factors important to women engaged in vigorous physical activity. *In* Strauss, R. *Sports Medicine.* Philadelphia, W.B. Saunders, 1984, pp. 250–269.

27. Haymes, E. Physiological response of female athletes to heat stress: A review. *Physician Sportsmed* 12(3):45–59, 1984.

28. Haycock, C. *Sports Medicine for the Athletic Female.* Oradell, NJ, Medical Economics, 1980.

29. Haycock, C., and Gillette, G. Susceptibility of women athletes to injury: Myths versus reality. *JAMA* 236:163–165, 1976.

30. Haymes, E. Iron deficiency and the active woman. *American Alliance for Health, Physical Education and Recreation Research Report* 2:91–97, 1973.

31. Higdon, R., and Higdon, H. What sports for girls? *Today's Health* 10:21, 1967.

32. Hoffman, T., Stauffer, R., and Jackson, A. Sex differences in strength. *Am J Sports Med* 7(4):265–267, 1979.

33. Hunter, L., Andrews, J., Clancy, W., et al. Common orthopaedic problems of the female athlete. *Instr Course Lect* 31:126–152, 1982.

34. Johnson, L., and O'Shea, J. Anabolic steroids: Effects on strength development. *Science* 164:957–959, 1969.

35. Klafs, C., and Lyon, J. *The Female Athlete* (2nd ed.). St. Louis, C.V. Mosby, 1978.

36. Kosek, S. Nature and incidence of traumatic injury to women in sports. *In Proceedings of the National Sports Safety Congress,* Cincinnati, Ohio, 1973, pp. 50–52.

37. Lamb, D. Anabolic steroids in athletes: How well do they work and how dangerous are they? *Am J Sports Med* 12(1):31–38, 1984.

38. Lamb, D. Anabolic steroids and athletic performance. *Sportsmed Dig* 6(7):1, 1984.

39. Lesmes, G., Fox, E., Stevens, C., et al. Metabolic responses of females to high intensity interval training of different frequencies. *Med Sci Sports Exerc* 10(4):229–232, 1978.

40. Lindgren, A. Is it feminine to be fit? *Melpomene J* 8(3):2–4, 1989.

41. Lutter, J., and Cushman, S. Menstrual patterns in female runners. *Physician Sportsmed* 10(9):60–72, 1982.

42. Malena, R. Age at menarche in athletes and nonathletes. *Med Sci Sports* 5(1):11, 1973.

43. Malena, R., Harper, H., and Avent, H. Physique of female track and field athletes. *J Am Coll Sports Med* 3:32, 1982.

44. Marcus, R., Cann, C., Madvig, P., et al. Menstrual function and bone mass in elite women distance runners: Endocrine and metabolic features. *Ann Intern Med* 102:158–163, 1985.

45. McArthur, J., Bullen, B., and Beitens, I. Hypothalamus amenorrhea in runners of normal body composition. *Endocrine Res Commun* 7:13–27, 1980.

46. McWhirter, N. *Guiness Book of Women's Sports Records.* New York, Sterling Publishing, 1979.

47. Mirkin, G. Nutrition for sports. *In* Shangold, M., and Mirkin, G. *Women and Exercise: Physiology and Sports Medicine.* Philadelphia, F.A. Davis, 1988.

48. Nelson, M., Fisher, E., Castos, P., et al. Diet and bone status in amenorrheic runners. *Am J Clin Nutr* 43:910–916, 1986.

49. Nilson, K., and Schoene, R. Iron repletion decreases maximal exercise lactate concentration in female athletes with minimal iron deficiency anemia. *J Lab Clin Med* 102:306–312, 1983.

50. Nunnaley, S. Physiological response of women to thermal stress: A review. *Med Sci Sports* 10(4):250–255, 1978.

51. Parrish, M. Exercising to the bone. *Women's Sports* 5(4):25–32, 1983.

52. Pate, R. Sports anemia: A review of the current research literature. *Physician Sportsmed* 11(2):115–126, 1983.

53. Pate, R., Maguire, M., and Wyk, J. Dietary iron supplementation in women athletes. *Physician Sportsmed* 7(9):81–86, 1979.

54. Pipes, T. Strength training modes: What's the difference? *Scholastic Coach* 46(10):96, 1977.

55. Powers, J. Title IX Knee. Hilton Head Symposium, American Academy of Orthopaedic Surgeons, April, 1977.

56. Puhl, J., and Brown, C. (Eds.). *The Menstrual Cycle and Physical Activity.* Champaign, IL, Human Kinetics, 1986.

57. Sanborn, C., Martin, B., and Wagner, W. Is athletic amenorrhea specific to runners? *Am J Obstet Gynecol* 143:859–861, 1982.

58. Shangold, M. Sports and menstrual function. *Physician Sportsmed* 8(8):66–70, 1980.

59. Shangold, M. Evaluating menstrual irregularity in athletes. *Physician Sportsmed* 10(2):21–24, 1982.

60. Shangold, M. Exercise and the adult female: Hormonal and endocrine effects. *Exerc Sport Sci Rev* 12:53, 1984.

61. Shangold, M., and Levine, H. The effect of marathon training upon menstrual function. *Am J Obstet Gynecol* 143:862, 1982.

62. Speroff, L., and Redwine, D. Exercise and menstrual function. *Physician Sportsmed* 8(5):42–52, 1980.

63. Thomas, C. Special problems of the female athlete. *In* Ryan, A., and Allman, F. (eds.), *Sports Medicine.* New York, Academic Press, 1974, pp. 347–373.

64. Thomas, C. Factors important to women participants in vigorous athletics. *In* Strauss, R. (Ed.), *Sports Medicine and Physiology*. Philadelphia, W.B. Saunders, 1979, pp. 304–319.
65. Twin, S. *Out of the Bleachers*. Old Westbury, Feminist Press, 1979.
66. Ullyot, J. *Women's Running*. Mountain View, CA, World Publications, 1976.
67. Walker, C. The crone and the lady. *Melpomene J* 8(3):7–8, 1989.
68. Wells, C. *Women, Sport and Performance*. Champaign, IL, Human Kinetics, 1985.
69. Wentz, A. Psychogenic amenorrhea and anorexia nervosa. *In* Givens, R. (Ed.), *Endocrine Causes of Menstrual Disorders*. Chicago, Year Book, 1977.
70. Whiteside, P. Men's and women's injuries in comparable sports. *Physician Sportsmed* 8(3):130–140, 1980.
71. Wilmore, J., and Brown, C. Physiological profile of women distance runners. *Med Sci Sports Exerc* 6(3):178–181, 1974.
72. Wilmore, J., Brown, C., and Davis, J. Body physique and composition of the female distance runner. *In* Milvy, P. (Ed.), *The Marathon: Physiological, Medical, Epidemiological, and Psychological Studies*. New York, New York Academy of Sciences, 1977, pp. 764–776.
73. Wright, J. Anabolic steroids and athletes. *Exerc Sports Sci Rev* 8:149–202, 1980.
74. Zaharieva, E. Survey of sportswomen at the Tokyo Olympics. *J Sports Med Physical Fitness* 5:215–219, 1965.

PREPARTICIPATION EVALUATION OF THE YOUNG ATHLETE

Keith L. Stanley, M.D.

Health care of the healthy adolescent population in the United States is largely crisis oriented. The only youths who have regular encounters with a physician generally are those with congenital or chronic medical illnesses such as congenital heart disease, type I diabetes mellitus, and asthma. One exception is the preparticipation physical examination performed on the more than 20 million young people involved in organized athletics. As a result, interest in this examination is increasing among team physicians and other health care professionals involved in the care of young athletes in this country.

The importance of the preparticipation physical examination was recognized by the American Medical Association's Committee on Medical Aspects of Sports, as evidenced by their statement that every athlete has the right to a thorough preseason evaluation [1]. Although most physicians agree on the necessity for an examination, there are many controversies and conflicts about the content of the preparticipation evaluation and the best way to conduct it. As a result, this examination has undergone quite an evolution during the last several years. Many sports medicine physicians, including this author, remember the locker room line-up examination. Fortunately, this has evolved into a better organized and even sports-specific examination. In many areas of the country, the examination now includes the expertise not only of primary care physicians but also of those in all specialties, both in and out of the sports medicine arena. Some athletic programs even include exercise physiolo-

gists, physical therapists, and athletic trainers to evaluate performance and maturity components.

PURPOSE OF THE PREPARTICIPATION EXAMINATION

Several authors have offered statements concerning the purpose or goal of this examination [6, 14, 15, 18, 19, 28, 29, 31, 34, 40]. Most agree that, in general terms, the focus of the examination is to ensure the health and safety of the athlete. In his review, Jones [15] noted that examining and profiling young athletes involves gathering medical and physiologic information that helps to determine each child's suitability for participation in sports activities. Linder and associates [18] stated that the major purpose of the preparticipation examination is to screen for conditions that could predispose the athlete to injury or death. Evaluating health risks and relieving the school systems of the legal implications of sports participation by their students were applications of the examination noted by Rowland [28]. Runyan [29] noted that some authors want the examination to serve as a comprehensive interval evaluation; however, this does not appear to be the prevailing attitude among most sports medicine physicians. Strong and Linder [34] mention the identification of conditions that need rehabilitation before sports participation and matching young athletes with an appropriate sport or position as important purposes of the examination. Lombardo [19] summarizes the purposes of the preparticipation examination very nicely in the following six points: (1) to detect additional risks; (2) to detect medical contraindications; (3) to indicate which sports are safe for the individual;

This chapter has been abstracted from the following source: Stanley, K.L. Preparticipation evaluation of the young athlete. *Adv Sports Med Fitness* 3:69–87, 1990. Reprinted with permission of Year Book Publishing Company, Chicago.

(4) to serve as a limited general health screening; (5) to meet legal and insurance requirements; and (6) to evaluate physical maturation.

As can be seen from these statements, the purpose of the preparticipation sports examination has undergone significant transition. With the increasing interest in identifying conditions that require rehabilitation before performance and in obtaining performance measurements, it appears that the evolution of the preparticipation examination will continue for some time.

All states require that physical examinations be performed before young athletes participate in interscholastic sports in order to identify conditions that may increase the risk of injury [9]. Feinstein and colleagues [11] conducted a survey of all 50 states and the District of Columbia. Out of the 45 replies that they received, they found that 35 states require a yearly examination, three states require an examination every 3 years, one state requires examination only once, and six did not specify their requirements.

Several authors now have spoken out in support of requiring only two comprehensive examinations, one to be performed in junior high school and one in senior high school, and annual medical history reviews. If the history indicates something of significance or if there is an injury, a medically specific examination is then recommended. Risser and associates [27] found that, because of the low frequency of significant findings and unfavorable cost-benefit ratio of annual examinations, the University Interscholastic League recommended that the annual examination be required only once or twice in the secondary school years. In the American Academy of Pediatrics publication, Smith [31] proposed that examinations be performed every 2 years. Other authors support similar requirements [19, 40]. Wood [40] described a pilot program in which examinations are done once in junior high and once in senior high, with the school nurse conducting annual reviews of the medical histories. The school nurse then refers athletes with significant interval histories to a physician. Therefore, although most states still require an annual examination, a growing body of data and an increasing number of sports medicine physicians advocate a reduction in the frequency of the preparticipation examination to two times during the secondary school years. Exceptions are made for athletes who experience an illness or injury that requires an updated examination.

Other data that support less frequent preparticipation examinations are those of Thompson and associates [37], who found that only 1.2% of 2670 athletes had medical problems that excluded them from sports participation. During 2 consecutive years, Linder and associates [18] found that none of 562 athletes were diagnosed with an exclusionary illness or injury the first year, and only 2 (0.3%) of 706 athletes were excluded from sports partic-

ipation the following year. Of 701 athletes in a study done by Goldberg and colleagues [12], only 1.3% were excluded from sports participation. Thus, because of the low frequency of significant findings, the trend is to move away from the traditional annual preparticipation examination.

METHOD OF EXAMINATION

The preparticipation examination also has undergone a significant evolution in the manner in which it is conducted. The three most commonly identified means of conducting the examination are having it performed by the personal family physician, as a locker room examination, and using a station-type method. However, most sports medicine physicians feel that the locker room examination has no place in the evaluation of athletes. Although many authors point out that an examination performed by the family physician offers the advantages of continuity of care, a readily available complete medical history, and better doctor-athlete rapport [5, 6, 19, 28, 34], there can be drawbacks to this type of examination. Lombardo [19] notes that the accuracy of this type of examination may be limited by the level of interest and knowledge of the private physician. Strong and Linder [34] indicate that an examination done by the private physician may not be sports-oriented or sports-specific and all too often may be performed in a cursory manner [34].

The group or station method appears to be the type favored by most sports medicine physicians. It is possible to include specialty physicians as well as flexibility and performance testing in this type of examination, and it also appears to be more sports oriented [36]. In addition, at least one study indicates that this type of examination is more sensitive in uncovering significant illness or injury [5]. DuRant and associates [5] found that fewer diagnoses were recognized with single physician examinations than with multiple physician examinations done in a station-type method. Multiple examiners found a higher percentage of abnormalities in 20 of 21 examination categories. The differences were statistically significant in six categories. These included diagnoses of the mouth, teeth, hips, thighs, knees, and ankles. They also noted that only 2.4% of athletes seen by a single physician were referred for further evaluation compared to 6.4% of those seen by multiple physicians. This study lends support to the station method of examination.

There is general agreement among sports physicians about the timing of the preparticipation examination. Most agree that it is best to do the examination or medical history review (if an institution is not conducting annual examinations) 6 to 8 weeks prior to the beginning of the sports season [17, 19, 31, 33, 34, 37]. In most cases, this leaves adequate time for any additional evaluations that may be needed. It also gives the athlete time to rehabilitate an injury or illness before the start of the season. Special cases may arise in which an athlete may need to be evaluated much earlier than 6 to 8 weeks before the start of the season. This is especially true when significant surgery involving the musculoskeletal system has been performed. Thus, it is important for the sports physician to have a close working relationship with the coaching staff and the athletic trainer.

Organization and Set-Up

Before going into detail about each area of the medical history and physical examination, some suggestions on how to organize and set up the examination may be timely. First, the number of athletes that will be examined is established. The athletes and their parents are notified of the date, time, and place in advance. This may actually be done by the school administration, athletic directors, or coaches. Second, the number of people that will be participating as staff for the examinations is determined. Their capabilities are analyzed, and their appropriate responsibilities are assigned on that basis. If one has fewer personnel, one may have to combine some stations. Also, it is important to ask the athletes to dress in gym shorts and loose-fitting T-shirts to ease and expedite the examination.

If possible, one may ask the athlete to complete the medical history form in advance. If this is not possible, then the first station is a check-in to pay the examination fee (if charged) and to get the examination form. This may be staffed by a parent, teacher, or coach. Next in line is the station to review the medical history. As discussed below, this process is very important in the preparticipation evaluation and should be conducted by a nurse, nurse clinician, or physician.

Vision testing may follow if it has not been done previously by the school nurse. This can be done at the time of the preparticipation examination by a nurse or other trained personnel.

Next, height and weight are obtained. If one is also evaluating the percentage of body fat, it could be done at this station. This station may be manned by a parent. If percentage of body fat is being measured, the staff would have to include an exercise physiologist, nurse, trainer, or some qualified person. Blood pressure and pulse are obtained next. Appropriate personnel include a nurse, trainer, or emergency medical technician.

At the next station the athlete enters the physical examination itself. It is recommended that the ear, nose, and throat examination be conducted first, followed by a dental examination if a dentist is available at this station. The cardiovascular and pulmonary systems are evaluated next. It is imperative to have a quiet room for this part of the examination.

The athlete then goes on to the abdominal examination. Tables are needed to allow comfortable recumbency during this examination. For male athletes, hernia and genitourinary evaluations are done at this station.

If flexibility testing is part of the program, it can be done just prior to the orthopedic examination. This testing could be conducted by an exercise physiologist, physical therapist, or athletic trainer.

The final part of the examination is the orthopedic assessment. Shoes and socks should be removed. One may also have male athletes remove their T-shirts. Female athletes should wear halter tops or swim suits. Part of the orthopaedic examination should include evaluation for spinal deformity. The final examiner may also be responsible for reviewing the status of the athlete's sports participation.

Again, it should be emphasized that one may have to be flexible depending on the number of personnel available. If stations have to be combined, consolidate those that lead to a smooth-flowing operation (e.g., combine the cardiovascular and pulmonary examination with examination of the abdomen).

MEDICAL HISTORY

A complete medical history is important in every area of medical care, and the sports preparticipation examination is no exception. Runyan [29] indicates that the sports medical history should have a limited scope and should attempt to identify those conditions that are significant to sports participation. Taken in this manner, a medical history can be brief yet effective in identifying potential problems.

Ascertaining the accuracy of information given in an athlete's medical history can prove difficult. The athlete himself may neglect to indicate on the history form an illness or injury that he fears might exclude him from participation. He also may not deem significant something that may in fact be essential to his protection or rehabilitation. Another problem may lie in discrepancies between the medical history provided by the athlete and that provided by the parent. In the study by Risser and colleagues [27], only 39% of the athletes' histories agreed with those of their parents. Another problem that may sabotage the acquisition of a good medical history is the possible inability of the athlete or his parents to read or understand the history form. With illiteracy as high as 25% to 30% in some areas, this can be a significant problem. One solution may be to have one station in the examination include a physician who takes the history [18, 27]. Smith [31] suggests that history taking be assisted by a physician, nurse, or trainer; Wood [40] used the school nurses to obtain the medical history in his program.

Other side issues may be important in the medical history. As Lombardo [19] indicates, it is very important to ascertain a history of chemical or substance abuse in a young athlete. He also notes that obtaining a menstrual history in female athletes may be critical in view of the growing concern about exercise amenorrhea and its relationship to bone density and the prevention of osteoporosis in women. The medical history should also include questions about the potential existence of eating disorders.

Overall, most sports physicians agree that the medical history should be sports-specific and include certain targeted areas. Areas most often noted include musculoskeletal injuries, neurologic injuries, infectious diseases, cardiac disease, pulmonary disease, hospitalizations, medicine allergies, and surgical procedures [5, 9, 29, 31, 34]. In their study, Strong and Linder [34] indicated that the most frequently reported problems in the medical history were previous injury, hospitalization, and joint problems.

Many authors have formulated medical history forms to include those items that they feel are important [5, 15, 17, 31, 33, 34]. Feinstein and colleagues [11] found that 25 states have a standardized medical history questionnaire. Although medical history forms do vary, they all have several areas that consistently are viewed as significant by sports physicians. A question relating to sudden death or myocardial infarction in family members under the age of 50 years is found on most forms. This means of discovering an athlete with hypertrophic-obstructive cardiomyopathy [3, 8, 20, 22, 23, 24, 35] may be even more sensitive than the physical examination. The responses obtained to an inquiry about syncope or even near-syncope during exercise are deemed important. The ability to complete a quarter- or half-mile run without stopping is also questioned on most forms. The inclusion of questions about arrhythmias, murmurs, hypertension, and previous cardiac surgery on these forms is vital. All of these are necessary for proper screening of an athlete's cardiovascular medical history.

A neurologic history is also critical, especially as it pertains to head and neck injuries. Since a neurologic deficit can result from the cumulative effect of cerebral contusions, specific questions should be asked about loss of consciousness associated with head injury or any history of diagnosed concussions. A history of a seizure disorder should prompt inquiries about medication because the maintenance of good seizure control must be established.

Most forms contain inquiries about infectious diseases, but no specific diseases are usually mentioned. This places the burden on the examiner to be specific and inquisitive about infectious diseases.

The most significant question with regard to pulmonary disease in the athletic population is the one relating to asthma or exercise-induced bronchospasm. If the medical history is positive for either of these conditions, the examiner should inquire about any medications being used and their availability during practices and events should they be needed.

Inquiries should be made about medications being taken, medication allergies, and environmental allergies. One question that is rarely found on medical history forms for athletes is the presence of allergies to insect stings. In view of the life-threatening potential of these allergies, this question should be included, especially for athletes involved in outdoor sports.

Surgeries should be recorded; if any are recent, a proper release should be obtained from the surgeon of record to be included in the athlete's health record.

Any history of chronic illness should be elucidated. If chronic illness exists and requires constant monitoring (as is the case with diabetes mellitus), the medication history is necessary.

The musculoskeletal history is of utmost importance when evaluating the athlete. A history of sprains, strains, dislocations, or fractures is often uncovered in the preparticipation examination. DuRant and colleagues [5] found that the most frequent musculoskeletal problems discovered in the health history were previous fractures (22.1%). Other injuries of the musculoskeletal system comprised 20.9% of the responses. The examiner taking the medical history should indicate clearly the presence of any previous musculoskeletal injuries. This allows the physician doing the orthopedic examination to give special attention to these areas of previous injury.

Many other questions may be included in the medical history. However, it should be kept in mind that the questionnaire should be sports-specific, easily understood, and constructed for efficient use by both the athlete and the examiner. Table 4–1 is a compilation of sports medical history questions that this author views as significant. Although this list is not comprehensive, the questions listed should be found consistently on all medical history formats.

The importance of the medical history for sports participation is underscored by the results of two studies. Risser and colleagues [27] found that 67% of all medical problems and 63% of all orthopedic problems were referred to specialists for further care after being noted in the history. Goldberg and colleagues [12] similarly found that 74% of significant medical and orthopedic problems were reported. Further, in Goldberg and colleagues' study, seven of nine athletes excluded from participation would have been so excluded on the basis of the history alone.

Many have recommended that the sports preparticipation physical examination be sports-specific [15, 17,

TABLE 4–1
Medical History Questions

1. Are you taking medications?
2. Any medication allergies?
3. Any environmental allergies?
4. Any allergies to insect stings?
5. Any hospitalizations?
6. Any surgeries?
7. Has any family member had sudden death or heart attack before age 50?
8. Have you had any heart disease, murmur, extra beats, or high blood pressure?
9. Have you ever been dizzy or passed out from exercise?
10. Have you ever been knocked out or had a concussion?
11. Any joint injuries (fractures, sprains, strains, or dislocations)?

_____ Neck	_____ Arm	_____ Thigh
_____ Back	_____ Hand	_____ Knee
_____ Shoulder	_____ Fingers	_____ Ankle
_____ Elbow	_____ Hip	

12. Any organs missing?
13. Any chronic illness?
14. Any chemical or substance use?
15. Any menstrual irregularities?
16. Have you ever induced vomiting, engaged in binge eating or purging?
17. Have you ever been disqualified from participation?
18. Date of last tetanus shot?
19. Do you wear eye glasses, contact lenses, or dental appliances?
20. Any history of seizure disorder?

34]. Because most significant findings on the sports preparticipation physical examination involve the musculoskeletal system, emphasis should be placed on this area during the examination [5, 27, 28, 37]. This topic will be addressed in more detail later in this chapter. Another area of emphasis should be the cardiovascular examination because most causes of sudden death are cardiac in origin [3, 8, 10, 23, 24]. This subject will also be addressed in more detail later.

SPECIFIC AREAS

General Data

Most examinations begin with measurements of height, weight, blood pressure, and pulse. Some also include body fat determination. Goldberg and co-workers [12] found that 32% of the athletes in their study had excessive body fat. Blood pressure parameters, suggested by Smith [31], are less than 130/75 mm Hg for children aged 6 to 11 years and less than 140/85 mm Hg for children 12 years and older. As pointed out by Strong and Linder [34], an athlete should not be labeled hypertensive until three abnormal readings are obtained at different times. If hypertension in a child is documented, Strong and Lindner further recommend testing the blood pressure response to exercise. They state that no data have been published indicating that hypertension causes any direct morbidity or mortality during athletic participation. A rapid or irregular pulse should be correlated with the cardiovascular examination to determine its clinical significance.

Head and Neck

Vision screening should be performed, and an uncorrected vision of less than 20/40 should be referred for further evaluation [31]. This is the time to note whether corrective lenses have been prescribed already.

Certain findings in the head, eyes, ears, nose, and throat examination should be noted. Unequal or unreactive pupils should be documented because this finding may be very important later should the athlete incur a head or neck injury. For athletes participating in water sports, the condition of the external auditory canal and tympanic membranes is important. Proper treatment should be given and proper hygiene practiced by those who have chronic external otitis due to their constant water exposure. A new area of interest among young athletes is the sport of scuba diving. These young people require a more intense examination of the ear, nose, and throat [2, 4], because, as noted by Dembert and Keith [4], most injuries sustained in scuba diving are related to barotrauma or decompression sickness. On inspection the physician looks for polyps, a deviated septum, or evidence of a necrotic or perforated septum that might indicate substance abuse. Inspection of the mouth should include the teeth. Dentition abnormalities are some of the findings reported most frequently on the physical examination [34]. Note should be made of any dental appliance being worn by the athlete.

Skin and Lymphatics

A dermatologic assessment is vital, especially in those participating in contact or collision sports. As Lombardo [19] noted, clearance should not be given to those athletes who have such dermatologic pathologies as herpes, scabies, louse infestations, or impetigo. Other dermatologic conditions such as acne and fungal dermatophytic infections require referral for proper care. Assessment of the lymphatics and abdomen is recommended also. The cervical, supraclavicular, axillary, and inguinal lymph nodes should be checked for any enlargement or tenderness. The abdomen should be palpated for hepatomegaly or splenomegaly. Should any lymphadenopathy or organomegaly be discovered, referral should be initiated for further evaluation.

Genitourinary System

The genitourinary examination has to a great extent been conducted in males and neglected in females. Females with a significant menstrual history, such as primary or secondary amenorrhea, should be referred to their private physicians for further evaluation. A female nurse or female physician may also need to check pubic hair and breast development to assess maturation (this will be discussed later). Examination of male athletes should establish the presence or absence of a hernia and whether or not both testes are present and descended. Thompson and associates [37] found three previously undiagnosed cases of cryptorchidism in more than 1700 males examined. Three cases of inguinal hernia were also diagnosed. Strong and Linder [34] reported that 6.5% of all abnormalities found were discovered in the genital and hernia examination. If a hernia is present and an additional risk would be incurred by continued sports participation, surgical correction should be performed before clearance is given [19]. The issue of participation by athletes who are missing a paired organ will be discussed later.

Cardiovascular System

Because most catastrophic situations involving young athletes are related to sudden death and cardiovascular pathology, an in-depth discussion of this topic is appropriate. The highly conditioned athlete is viewed as the epitome of health, and sudden death is such an alarming and unexpected event that it may cause overreaction in an entire community. Because of this, sports physicians and cardiologists have tried to search for the best screening methods to minimize the risk of this tragic occurrence.

However, cost containment is one major problem with an extensive cardiovascular screening examination. Another difficulty lies in targeting certain areas in the medical history and physical examination to create the most sensitive protocol. Maron and associates [22] conducted a cardiovascular screening of 501 intercollegiate competitive athletes. The screening protocol included personal and family history, a physical examination, and a 12-lead electrocardiogram. One hundred and two athletes had positive findings on one or more of the three parameters. Of the 90 who submitted to further evaluation, 75 (84%) had no definitive evidence of cardiovascular disease. Of the other 15, one had mild systemic hypertension and 14 had mild mitral valve prolapse. The

TABLE 4–2
Clinical Complaints in Cases of Sudden Death

Reported Symptoms	Number
Syncope	3
Presyncope	1
Chest pain	2
Periodic mild fatigue	1
Mild fatigue, presyncope, palpitations	1

Reprinted with permission from the American College of Cardiology (Journal of the American College of Cardiology, 1980, Vol. 8, pp. 382–385).

authors concluded that performance of an electrocardiogram did not appreciably enhance the sensitivity of the informed history and physical examination and further, that it was responsible for a high number of false-positive observations.

In a study of sudden death that included necropsy in highly conditioned, competitive athletes, cardiovascular abnormalities were found in 28 of 29 athletes (97%) and almost certainly were the cause of death in 22 of the athletes (76%) [23]. In only 7 of the 29 patients was cardiac disease suspected, and in only two of the seven had the correct diagnosis been made. Table 4–2 lists the clinical complaints noted by family members of eight of the athletes when questioned retrospectively, and Table 4–3 lists the cardiac abnormalities that were found. Hypertrophic-obstructive cardiomyopathy was found in 14 athletes and was the most common cause of death by far. Other diagnoses that were made in more than one athlete included anomalous origin of the left coronary artery from the right sinus of Valsalva, idiopathic concentric left ventricular hypertrophy, coronary heart disease, and ruptured aorta. Other authors have mentioned other, less common causes of sudden death such as prolonged Q–T syndrome, mitral valve prolapse, valvular heart disease, myocardial and pericardial diseases, sarcoidoses, and abnormalities in the cardiac conduction

TABLE 4–3
Probable Cause of Death in Cases of Sudden Death

Probable Cause of Death	Number
Hypertrophic cardiomyopathy	14
Idiopathic concentric LVH	5
Anomalous origin of the left coronary artery	3
Atherosclerotic coronary disease	3
Ruptured aorta	2
Hypoplastic coronaries	1
No cardiovascular disease	1

Reprinted with permission from the American College of Cardiology (Journal of the American College of Cardiology, 1980, Vol. 8, pp. 382–385).

system [3, 8, 20, 24, 34, 38]. Thus far, no author on the subject of sudden death has recommended including an electrocardiogram or echocardiogram in the screening of athletes. The most cost-effective screening method apparently is an informed medical history and physical examination.

The cardiovascular examination should include inspection, palpation (especially of the femoral pulses and precordium), and auscultation of heart sounds [35]. Strong and Steed [35] note that unusual facies and body habitus that are characteristic of syndromes associated with cardiac defects should be recognized. Palpation of the brachial and femoral pulses should be done to rule out the presence of coarctation. A bifid pulse should be recognized as a possible abnormal finding consistent with hypertrophic cardiomyopathy. The carotids and precordium should be palpated for trills. Auscultation should be done to identify S_1 and S_2 heart sounds. An S_3 may be a normal finding in young athletes, but an S_4 is always considered pathologic [35]. Murmurs should be identified as systolic or diastolic in origin. The intensity of a murmur itself may not be indicative of either a pathologic or nonpathologic state; the murmur associated with hypertrophic cardiomyopathy may be very soft [23]. Therefore, the intensity of the murmur should not be the only parameter by which one determines the necessity of referral for further evaluation. Most innocent murmurs should diminish with the Valsalva maneuver; however, the murmur of hypertrophic cardiomyopathy increases in the sitting and standing positions as well as with exercise. These parameters may help the examiner determine which athletes should be referred for further evaluation.

Auscultation of premature beats or frequent dysrhythmias also is an indication that further cardiac evaluation is needed. If the arrhythmia is suppressed with mild exercise, most likely it is benign. But if there is any question, referral for probable exercise testing and 24-hour Holter monitoring may be necessary. The cardiovascular examination should be emphasized during the sports preparticipation physical examination to attempt to identify those athletes who may be at risk for sudden death from cardiovascular disease.

Musculoskeletal System

The musculoskeletal system is another area that should undergo close inspection during the preparticipation examination. Strong and Linder [34] found that 38.3% of abnormal findings on the physical examination were musculoskeletal in origin. Thompson and colleagues [37] reported a much higher incidence of musculoskeletal problems in their series (67%). Although the incidence of musculoskeletal abnormalities identified on a sports preparticipation physical examination may vary, they are still the findings that are most frequently identified and referred for further evaluation in every series. One exception is a study by Goldberg and colleagues [12] in which 60 athletes were reported to have medical problems needing further consultation, 35 of whom had musculoskeletal problems. However, it should be noted that 40 of the athletes in the medical category were referred for proteinuria. The knees and ankles appear to be the most frequently injured joints in athletes. Linder and colleagues [18] reported findings related to the knee in 6.9% and 8.8% of athletes and to the ankle in 2.1% and 2.5% in two consecutive years, respectively. DuRant and co-workers [5] observed that in the multiple-examiner station examination method, more musculoskeletal problems were identified in more athletes (67%) than in the single-physician examination (5.4%). This fact illustrates the necessity of having an examining physician who is trained in musculoskeletal evaluation and understands a sports-specific examination.

Table 4–4 describes a functional orthopedic screening examination that is similar to that used by Thompson and colleagues [37] in their series. This type of examination is very efficient in terms of both time and sensitivity in identifying problems. Any problem identified by the screening examination or the medical history may require a more specific, in-depth evaluation. At the time of the examination it is important to identify problems that require rehabilitation so that a program can be initiated that will allow the athlete to be prepared in time for the sport season. Special emphasis should be placed on those who have had previous surgery. If the surgery has been recent, it is necessary to coordinate the athlete's return to his sport with the surgeon of record.

In general, laboratory tests have been found to cause added expense with little return in the preparticipation examination. Urinalysis has not proved effective in identifying significant problems; in fact, it creates much anxiety because of the number of referrals it prompts for further evaluation [31]. Hematocrit and hemoglobin determinations also have been found unnecessary; they may be normal even in athletes who are iron-deficient. Tissue iron depletion is best determined biochemically with serum ferritin levels. However, this test should be reserved for athletes who have indications for such evaluation (endurance athletes or female athletes with fatigue or diminished performance).

Maturation Indexing

Currently, areas that are generating interest for inclusion in the sports preparticipation examination include maturation indexing and physiologic testing such as tests

TABLE 4–4
Orthopedic Screening Examination*

The orthopedic screening examination requires about 90 seconds. Time studies indicate that it is most efficiently done one athlete at a time rather than in small groups. It is designed to reveal previous inadequately rehabilitated injuries or those few previously unrecognized orthopedic conditions that might be adversely affected by participation in a sports activity. Positive findings require a more extensive examination and/or history. A more detailed examination *should not* be attempted at the screening examination.

Athletic Activity (Instructions)	Observation
Stand facing examiner	Acromioclavicular joints; general habitus
Look at ceiling, floor, over both shoulders; touch ears to shoulders	Cervical spine motion
Shrug shoulders (examiner resists)	Trapezius strength
Abduct shoulders 90% (examiner resists at 90%)	Deltoid strength
Full external rotation of arms	Shoulder motion
Flex and extend elbows	Elbow motion
Arms at sides, elbows 90% flexed; pronate and supinate wrists	Elbow and wrist motion
Spread fingers; make fist	Hand or finger motion and deformities
Tighten (contract) quadriceps; relax quadriceps	Symmetry and knee effusion; ankle effusion
"Duck walk" four steps (away from examiner with buttocks on heels)	Hip, knee, and ankle motion
Back to examiner	Shoulder symmetry; scoliosis
Knees straight, touch toes	Scoliosis, hip motion, hamstring tightness
Raise up on toes, raise heels	Calf symmetry, leg strength

*May require reflex hammer, tape measure, pin, and examination table.
From Smith, N. J. (Ed.), *Sports Medicine: Health Care for Young Athletes.* Evanston, IL, American Academy of Pediatrics, 1983.

of endurance, agility, strength, flexibility, and body composition [12, 15, 19, 30, 34].

Maturation indexing, following guidelines by Tanner [36], has been recommended to profile athletes to allow them to compete with others who are at similar maturity levels. Proponents believe that this will minimize the higher potential for injury in those with a lower maturity level [13, 26]. However, they also acknowledge that no data have been reported to indicate that such an increased risk exists. For the clinician, knowing that peak height velocities occur at Tanner stage 2 breast development in girls and at Tanner stage 4 genital development in boys may aid in predicting or even preventing certain injuries that occur with rapid growth [15]. This is especially true of injuries related to inflexibility or diminished agility.

In an effort to develop some type of screening method to aid in indexing maturity, Kreipe and Gewanter [16] used a handgrip strength measurement and self-assessed Tanner staging levels. They reported that only 67 of 364 males (18%) had grip strength and self-assessed Tanner staging levels that were discordant. Tanner stage 3 was considered immature. The data indicated a break between Tanner stages 3 and 4 at about 55 pounds of grip strength as measured by a Jamar hand dynamometer. By their data, when self-assessed Tanner staging levels and grip strength were performed together to test for imma-

turity, the false-negative ratio was 5%. When testing for maturity, the false-positive rate was 1%.

Maturity indexing may become a more important part of the preparticipation examination, especially if profiling becomes accepted more widely. This concept is probably very important for many young athletes. In his discussion about the uniqueness of young athletes, Martens [25] lists six major reasons why young athletes drop out of sports. Two of these six are not getting to play and being mismatched. Maturation assessment may prove to be very helpful in screening young athletes and placing them in a healthier sports environment.

Physiologic Assessment

Flexibility assessment is being used more often in the preparticipation evaluation also. Goldberg and colleagues [12] have described a flexibility screening technique. Some protocols have included goniometer measurements for selected joints and sit-and-reach measurements. The method described by Goldberg and colleagues is more comprehensive but may not fit into each program's framework of evaluations. As a result, the sports physician may want to have the coaching staff and athletic trainer conduct this protocol at another time and then assess the results with them.

Body composition has already been mentioned in the discussion on the physical examination. Body composition can be measured quickly by skin calipers. This measurement is important from the perspective of athletic performance and also may provide an opportunity for counseling an athlete about health issues that have a lifelong impact. It also may provide important information to wrestlers about the amount of weight loss that is feasible and medically safe.

Strength and endurance measurements as well as assessments of agility also are potentially valuable aspects of a preparticipation examination. However, each physician or school system may have to develop its own program in these areas because many of these tests do not have well-defined standards. Except for the 12-minute or 1.5-mile run, standards for comparison may not be readily available.

CLASSIFICATION OF SPORTS READINESS

The final step in the preparticipation examination is the classification of the young athletes according to the safety of their participation. Most authors recommend three clearance options [19, 34, 37]. Clearance A permits unrestricted participation, clearance B permits participation after further evaluation or rehabilitation is completed, and clearance C defers clearance because a high-risk medical contraindication to participation has been detected. The final results should be discussed with the athlete, his parents, and coaches if clearance B or C is selected for that particular examination. Much has been written and considerable debate has arisen about which sports are safe for young athletes with certain medical conditions. The American Academy of Pediatrics [7] recently published a statement classifying sports and listing recommendations for the participation of athletes with specific medical conditions in competitive sports (see Tables 5–2 and 5–3). Sports are classified as contact or collision, limited contact or impact, and noncontact (which has three levels: strenuous, moderately strenuous, and nonstrenuous).

Sports participation by athletes who are missing one part of a paired organ is a controversial topic. Although many physicians and school districts have refused to approve participation in these cases, the courts sometimes have intervened to allow the athlete to perform [38]. Thus, the ultimate decision may not rest with the physician in many cases. In athletes with loss of vision in one eye, an approved eye protection device must be worn for participation in any sport that poses a risk to the eyes. In athletes with an absent testicle, the risks should be discussed with the athlete and his parents, and proper protection should be included in the athletic gear

[21]. Athletes with a solitary kidney that demonstrates an abnormal anatomic variant (i.e., ectopic location or a ureteropelvic junction abnormality) or any degree of obstruction or impairment of function, according to Mandell and colleagues [21], are not allowed to participate in contact or collision sports. It is evident, therefore, that any decision about inclusion or exclusion from participation in sports activities must be made on an individual basis. In tenuous cases extensive discussion with the athlete, parents, coaches, school administrators, and physician should take place before a decision is made.

It must be recognized that the preparticipation examination does not replace regular continuous care by the athlete's private physician, even though this is the view currently held by most athletes and parents and even by some physicians.

The goal of the preparticipation examination should be to ensure as much as possible the health and safety of young athletes. The sensitivity design should be such that potential health risks and medical contraindications to sports participation by the athlete are identified. The examination should be regarded not as an examination designed to exclude young people from participation but as a means of including all young people who can participate safely in athletic endeavors. In addition, the examination should be sport-specific, not only designed for the athletic population as a whole but also emphasizing the sport or sports of choice. The examination should convey a positive image of the physician and his role in the care of athletes. The athlete should be made to feel comfortable in the relationship that may be built from this encounter. It is also a means by which to bring the physician, athletic trainer, and coaching staff together in a cooperative effort to provide a healthy, safe environment in which young athletes can compete. It should provide an opportunity for each professional involved to gain a better understanding of his or her role in the care of the total person, not just the athlete. Alienation of any of these components is not in the best interest of the young athlete.

The preparticipation evaluation is a small but significant investment in our young people. Directly or indirectly, these evaluations affect the physical, psychological, and emotional development of young athletes and provide an opportunity to exert a positive and rewarding influence on their lives.

References

1. American Medical Association. *Medical Evaluation of the Athlete: A Guide* (Revised ed.). Chicago, American Medical Association, 1976.
2. Becker, D., and Parell, G.J. Medical examination of the sport scuba diver. *Otolaryngol Head Neck Surg* 91:246–250, 1983.
3. Braden, D.S., and Strong, W.B. Preparticipation screening for the

sudden cardiac death in high school and college athletes. *Physician Sportsmed* 16:128–140, 1988.

4. Dembert, M.L., and Keith, J.F. Evaluating the potential pediatric scuba diver. *Am J Dis Child* 140:1135–1141, 1986.

5. DuRant, R., Seymore, C., Linder, C.W., et al. The preparticipation examination of athletes: Comparison of single and multiple examiners. *Am J Dis Child* 139:657–661, 1985.

6. Dyment, P.G. Another look at the sports preparticipation examination of the adolescent athlete. *J Adolesc Health Care* 7:130S–132S, 1986.

7. Dyment, P.G., Goldberg, B., Haefele, S.B., et al. Recommendations for participation in competitive sports. *Pediatrics* 81:737–739, 1988.

8. Epstein, S.E., and Maron, B.J. Sudden death and the competitive athlete: Perspectives on preparticipation screening studies. *J Am Coll Cardiol* 7:220–230, 1986.

9. Esquivel, M.T., and McCormick, D.P. Preparticipation sports evaluation, part 1: The station-method examination. *Fam Pract Recert* 9:41–60, 1987.

10. Esquivel, M.T., and McCormick, D.P. Preparticipation sports evaluation, part 2: Recommendations for student participation. *Fam Pract Recert* 9:107–118, 1987.

11. Feinstein, R.A., Soilean, E.J., Daniel, W.A. A national survey of preparticipation physical examination requirements. *Physician Sportsmed* 16:51–59, 1988.

12. Goldberg, B., Saranit, A., Witman, P., et al. Preparticipation sports assessment—an objective evaluation. *Pediatrics* 66:736–745, 1980.

13. Goldberg, B., and Boiardo, R. Profiling children for sports participation. *Clin Sports Med* 3:153–169, 1984.

14. Hunter, S.C. Screening high school athletes. *J Med Assoc G* 74:482–484, 1985.

15. Jones, R. The preparticipation, sport-specific athletic profile examination. *Semin Adolesc Med* 3:169–175, 1987.

16. Kreipe, R.E., and Gewanter, H.L. Physical maturity screening for participation in sports. *Pediatrics* 75:1076–1080, 1985.

17. Kulund, D.N. *The Injured Athlete*. Philadelphia, J. B. Lippincott, 1982.

18. Linder, C.W., DuRant, R.H., Seklecki, R.M., et al. Preparticipation health screening of young athletes. *Am J Sports Med* 9:187–193, 1981.

19. Lombardo, J.A. Preparticipation physical evaluation. *Prim Care* 11:3–21, 1984.

20. Luckstead, E.F. Sudden death in sports. *Pediatr Clin North Am* 29:1355–1362, 1982.

21. Mandell, J., Cromie, W.J., Caldemore, et al. Sports-related genitourinary injuries in children. *Clin Sports Med* 1:483–493, 1982.

22. Maron, B.J., Bodison, S.A., Wesley, Y.E., et al. Results of screening a large group of intercollegiate competitive athletes for cardiovascular disease. *J Am Coll Cardiol* 10:1214–1221, 1987.

23. Maron, B.J., Roberts, W.C., McAllister, H.A., et al. Sudden death in young athletes. *Circulation* 62:218–229, 1980.

24. Maron, B.J., Epstein, S.E., Roberts, W.C. Causes of sudden death in competitive athletes. *J Am Coll Cardiol* 7:204–214, 1986.

25. Martens, R. The uniqueness of the young athlete: Psychologic considerations. *Am J Sports Med* 8:382–385, 1980.

26. Nicholas, J.A. The value of sports profiling. *Clin Sports Med* 3:3–10, 1984.

27. Risser, W.L., Hoffman, H.M., and Bellah, G. Frequency of preparticipation sports examinations in secondary school athletes: Are the university interscholastic league guidelines appropriate? *Tex Med* 81:35–39, 1985.

28. Rowland, T.W. Preparticipation sports examination of the child and adolescent athlete: Changing views of an old ritual. *Pediatrician* 13:3–9, 1986.

29. Runyan, D.K. The pre-participation examination of the young athlete. *Clin Pediatr* 22:674–679, 1983.

30. Smith, N.J., and Garrick, J.G. Pre-participation sports assessment. *Pediatrics* 66:803–806, 1980.

31. Smith, N.J. (Ed.). *Sports Medicine: Health Care for Young Athletes*. Evanston, IL, American Academy of Pediatrics, 1983.

32. Stanley, K.L. Pre-participation evaluation of the young athlete. *Adv Sports Med Fitness* 3:69–87, 1990.

33. Strauss, R.J. (Ed.). *Sports Medicine*. Philadelphia, W. B. Saunders, 1984.

34. Strong, W.B., and Linder, C.W. Preparticipation health evaluation for competitive sports. *Pediatr Rev* 4:113–121, 1982.

35. Strong, W.B., and Steed, D. Cardiovascular evaluation of the young athlete. *Pediatr Clin North Am* 29:1325–1338, 1982.

36. Tanner, J.M. *Growth at Adolescence* (2nd ed.). Springfield, IL, Charles C Thomas, 1962.

37. Thompson, T.R., Andrish, J.T., and Bergfeld, J.A. A prospective study of preparticipation sports examinations of 2670 young athletes: Method and results. *Cleve Clin Q* 49:226–233, 1982.

38. Tucker, J.B., and Marron, J.T. The qualification-disqualification process in athletics. *Am Fam Physician* 29:149–154, 1984.

39. VanCamp, S.P. Exercise-related sudden death: Cardiovascular evaluation of exercises: Part 2. *Physician Sportsmed* 16:47–54, 1988.

40. Wood, I.R. A new approach to athletic physicals. J Sch Health 57:346–348, 1987.

THE CHILD ATHLETE WITH CHRONIC DISEASE

Michael A. Nelson, M.D.

There are an estimated 10 million children and adolescents in the United States with chronic disease of varying severity. A variety of studies have revealed an overall prevalence of all chronic disorders ranging from 10% to 20% [3]. Data from the 1981 National Health Interview Survey indicate that there are 2 million children (3.8% of those less than 17 years old) who have limited physical activity secondary to chronic disease [57]. Between 1960 and 1981 the percentage of children with activity-limiting chronic illness doubled [56].

Disability refers to the limitation of activity that may be experienced by an individual. Disability that occurs in association with chronic disease has several determinants including severity of the disease, associated handicaps, and limitations imposed by society, physicians, family, or the chronically ill child. Restrictions on sports and regular exercise are among the many disabilities experienced by children with chronic disease. Recent advances in medical care and in the understanding of the impact of sports and exercise on the natural history of certain diseases may serve to lessen or eliminate the disability associated with many childhood chronic diseases. Disability can be modified by knowledgeable physicians who provide accurate information to children and their families.

In 1976 the American Medical Association (AMA) published guidelines for conditions disqualifying an individual from sports participation [7]. Since that time advances in medical management have occurred, and our understanding of disease pathophysiology, natural history, mechanisms of injury, and the role of exercise in therapy has improved. Changes in rules, safety equipment, and sports pedagogy have lessened the risk for all children participating in competitive sports. In 1988 the American Academy of Pediatrics (AAP) published new guidelines for participation in competitive sports [5] (Tables 5–1 and 5–2). These new guidelines include

previously unknown diseases and reflect the current understanding of some chronic diseases as well as the practitioner's need for more latitude in making decisions regarding the participation of individual athletes. The number of indications for disqualification from sports activities is significantly lessened in the current guidelines. The practitioner should become familiar with these new AAP guidelines and disregard the previous AMA guidelines. What follows is a more detailed discussion of the management of children with chronic diseases for participation in sports.

DIABETES MELLITUS TYPE I

Glucose Homeostasis Associated with Exercise: Normal Children

At rest approximately 15% to 20% of circulating glucose is used by muscle tissue. In the resting state most energy for muscle function is derived from fatty acids and amino acids [1]. Carbohydrate utilization increases dramatically in response to exercise through hepatic glycogenolysis and gluconeogenesis as well as increased glucose uptake from the circulation. Exercise also stimulates lipolysis, resulting in release of free fatty acids (FFA). At low to moderate levels of exercise, glucose and FFA supply the fuel for exercising muscle. After 2 to 3 hours of low to moderate exercise fatty acid oxidation becomes the major source of fuel. However, as exercise intensity increases, the proportion of energy arising from carbohydrate oxidation increases. Muscle use during intense exercise ($>80\%$ VO_2 max) relies predominantly on carbohydrate utilization.

Exercise increases sensitivity to insulin, which leads to decreased insulin requirements and lowered plasma insulin levels. A lower insulin level facilitates hepatic

TABLE 5–1
Classification of Sports

| | | Noncontact | | |
Contact/Collision	Limited Contact/Impact	*Strenuous*	*Moderately Strenuous*	*Nonstrenuous*
Boxing	Baseball	Aerobic dancing	Badminton	Archery
Field hockey	Basketball	Crew	Curling	Golf
Football	Bicycling	Fencing	Table tennis	Riflery
Ice hockey	Diving	Field		
Lacrosse	Field	Discus		
Martial arts	High jump	Javelin		
Rodeo	Pole vault	Shot put		
Soccer	Gymnastics	Running		
Wrestling	Horseback riding	Swimming		
	Skating	Tennis		
	Ice	Track		
	Roller	Weight lifting		
	Skiing			
	Cross-country			
	Downhill			
	Water			
	Softball			
	Squash, handball			
	Volleyball			

Reproduced by permission of *Pediatrics*, Vol. 81, page 737. Copyright 1988.

glucose production and provides more circulating glucose to fuel muscles. Other neuroendocrine responses to exercise have been extensively reviewed [29, 73] elsewhere and will not be discussed here.

Short-term moderate exercise is associated with decreasing levels of plasma glucose. However, high-intensity exercise ($>80\%$ VO$_2$ max) may lead to increased blood glucose levels. These elevations gradually return to normal within 1 hour [55]. If an athlete consumes an adequate diet, muscle glycogen stores are replaced preferentially to exercised muscle within 12 to 24 hours [51].

Effect of Exercise in the Insulin-Dependent Diabetic

Plasma insulin levels do not decrease in response to exercise in the diabetic athlete. In fact, insulin levels may paradoxically increase. Exercise that uses muscles at the insulin injection site, if performed within 1 hour of the injection, may release insulin to the circulation more rapidly than normal [13]. The major effect of sustained levels of insulin during exercise is inhibition of hepatic glucose production. Both during and after prolonged exercise, decreased hepatic glucose production and relative hyperinsulinemia may result in hypoglycemia.

The blood glucose level preceding exercise has a major effect on the regulatory responses to falling glucose [8]. Many diabetics have hypoglycemic reactions secon-

dary to increased insulin sensitivity several hours after exercise. MacDonald demonstrated that 16% of 300 participants developed postexercise late-onset hypoglycemia (within 24 hours), often at night during sleep [50].

In type I diabetics blood glucose may rise in response to intense exercise ($>80\%$ VO$_2$ max), especially if the preexercise glucose level is high. This effect may last several hours. If exercise is undertaken in the presence of severe insulin deficiency (i.e., missed insulin dose), hyperglycemia and ketosis may result [12]. Many sport programs require short-duration, high-intensity activity, which may induce hyperglycemia, particularly if the preexercise blood glucose was greater than 250 mg/100 ml.

Knowledge of these possible metabolic changes with exercise is important for proper management. However, individual responses to exercise have been shown to be quite variable [18]. Assessment of the individual's response to exercise is necessary to develop an optimum plan for each athlete.

Intervention Strategies

Prior to participation in sports or exercise programs the diabetic athlete should undergo a thorough physical examination with particular attention paid to assessment of diabetic risk factors. To lessen the occurrence of vitreous hemorrhage, individuals with diabetic retinopathy should avoid maximum weight lifting or sports associ-

TABLE 5–2
Recommendations for Participation in Competitive Sports

	Contact/ Collision	Limited Contact/Impact	Noncontact		
			Strenuous	*Moderately Strenuous*	*Nonstrenuous*
Atlantoaxial instability	No	No	Yes*	Yes	Yes
*Swimming; no butterfly, breast stroke, or diving starts					
Acute illnesses	*	*	*	*	*
*Needs individual assessment, eg, contagiousness to others, risk of worsening illness					
Cardiovascular					
Carditis	No	No	No	No	No
Hypertension					
Mild	Yes	Yes	Yes	Yes	Yes
Moderate	*	*	*	*	*
Severe	*	*	*	*	*
Congenital heart disease	†	†	†	†	†
*Needs individual assessment.					
†Patients with mild forms can be allowed a full range of physical activities; patients with moderate or severe forms, or who are postoperative, should be evaluated by a cardiologist before athletic participation.					
Eyes					
Absence or loss of function of one eye	*	*	*	*	*
Detached retina	†	†	†	†	†
*Availability of American Society for Testing and Materials (ASTM)-approved eye guards may allow competitor to participate in most sports, but this must be judged on an individual basis.					
†Consult ophthalmologist					
Inguinal hernia	Yes	Yes	Yes	Yes	Yes
Kidney: Absence of one	No	Yes	Yes	Yes	Yes
Liver: Enlarged	No	No	Yes	Yes	Yes
Musculoskeletal disorders	*	*	*	*	*
*Needs individual assessment					
Neurologic					
History of serious head or spine trauma, repeated concussions, or craniotomy	*	*	Yes	Yes	Yes
Convulsive disorder					
Well controlled	Yes	Yes	Yes	Yes	Yes
Poorly controlled	No	No	Yes†	Yes	Yes‡
*Needs individual assessment					
†No swimming or weight lifting					
‡No archery or riflery					
Ovary: Absence of one	Yes	Yes	Yes	Yes	Yes
Respiratory					
Pulmonary insufficiency	*	*	*	*	Yes
Asthma	Yes	Yes	Yes	Yes	Yes
*May be allowed to compete if oxygenation remains satisfactory during a graded stress test					
Sickle cell trait	Yes	Yes	Yes	Yes	Yes
Skin: Boils, herpes, impetigo, scabies	*	*	Yes	Yes	Yes
*No gymnastics with mats, martial arts, wrestling, or contact sports until not contagious					
Spleen: Enlarged	No	No	No	Yes	Yes
Testicle: Absence or undescended	Yes*	Yes*	Yes	Yes	Yes
*Certain sports may require protective cup.					

Reproduced by permission of *Pediatrics*, Vol. 81, page 738. Copyright 1988.

ated with head jarring (i.e., football, hockey). The athlete with peripheral neuropathy must take extra care in selecting shoes for running to avoid blisters, abrasions, and overuse syndromes. Autonomic neuropathy requires the athlete to devote special attention to fluid and electrolyte replacement.

Several factors should be considered prior to participation in sports (Table 5–3). Consideration of the impact of sports participation on the lifestyle of the athlete and his or her family facilitates management during the sport season. Carbohydrate and insulin requirements during exercise depend on the frequency, intensity, and duration of exercise, prior training, and insulin levels and glucose levels preceding the activity.

Insulin should be given at least 1 hour before exercise. If this is not possible, injection into areas that will be least involved during the activity will minimize excess absorption. Meals should be consumed 1 to 3 hours prior to competition. Routine monitoring of blood glucose levels immediately before participation decreases the likelihood of hypo- or hyperglycemia. Maintenance of precompetition blood glucose levels between 100 and 250 mg/100 ml is ideal. In those with elevated precompetition blood glucose levels a urine check for ketosis should be performed. The athlete should always have supplemental simple carbohydrates such as sugar cubes, candy bars, or fruit juice available.

Because of individual variation in response to exercise, monitoring of blood glucose levels is most helpful. Using home monitoring equipment, the athlete should measure blood glucose immediately before and at frequent intervals during sports participation as well as immediately after exercise. Monitoring during the 24 hours following exercise reveals potential problems with postexercise hypo- or hyperglycemia. Nocturnal measurements should be included. After a few cycles of test-ing it should not be necessary to continue this intense level of monitoring, assuming that there is some day-to-day consistency in dietary intake and sport participation. However, many athletes practice during the day and compete at night. In this situation, monitoring should be done in both settings. Potential adjustments in the management program to allow sports participation may include splitting the insulin dose, decreasing or increasing the amount of short-acting insulin given during the competitive season, and consuming increased carbohydrates before, during, or after exercise. More detailed descriptions of these potential adjustments are available elsewhere [62].

Scuba diving is considered by some authorities to have too great a risk to allow participation by the insulin-dependent diabetic. Recognition of hypoglycemic symptoms and access to exogenous glucose may be impaired in this sport [38].

Therapeutic Value of Exercise in Insulin-Dependent Diabetes

Diabetics can enjoy the same positive benefits of exercise as normal individuals. Decreases in cholesterol, low-density lipoprotein (LDL), and blood pressure as well as increases in high-density lipoprotein (HDL) and aerobic capacity have all been demonstrated in diabetics [38]. Whether or not a properly planned exercise program enhances diabetic control is controversial. Some studies have shown no improvement in control as reflected in unchanged levels of glycosylated hemoglobin [76, 78]. Others, using glycosylated albumin or hemoglobin levels as measures, indicate that improved control is possible [71]. Among the studies performed to date on the long-term effect of exercise on diabetes there has been great variability in protocol. The therapeutic value of exercise for diabetic control remains to be clarified by future research.

ASTHMA

Prevalence

Asthma is probably the most common chronic disease among athletes. Asthma occurs in 6% to 9% of children [49]. Exercise-induced asthma (EIA) occurs in approximately 10% of all children regardless of whether or not they suffer from other forms of asthma. EIA has been demonstrated in the laboratory in 60% to 80% of children with asthma [53] and should be considered a universal feature of asthma. Youth with a history of croup, cystic fibrosis, bronchopulmonary dysplasia, and allergic

TABLE 5–3
Preparticipation Considerations in Type I Diabetes

Sport
Consistency:
    Practices and competitions at same time of day?
Timing relative to:
    Regular meals and snacks
    Routine insulin doses
Will participation result in a large change in daily energy
    expenditure?
Diabetes Management
Current degree of control (glycosylated hemoglobin?)
Current monitoring:
    Methodology; blood glucose?
    Compliance?
Willingness to increase monitoring during sport participation?
Family involvement and support in management?

rhinitis are at risk for developing EIA [53]. The success of Olympic athletes with this disorder attests to the capacity to modify the disabilities that often accompany asthma to allow successful participation in sports.

In normal individuals some degree of bronchodilation accompanies exercise [70]. Among asthmatics there may be a lack of bronchodilation in mild cases or frank bronchoconstriction and associated changes in mucous composition and production during exercise. Bronchoconstriction can be precipitated by low temperature and humidity of inspired air, pollen, airborne pollutants, medications, and infectious agents [53] (Fig. 5–1). Cold dry air is more likely to precipitate airway obstruction than warm humidified air. Exercise performed during periods of high pollen count or environmental pollution is more likely to be associated with EIA in selected individuals. Therefore, it is not surprising that symptoms may appear inconsistently while performing the same type and amount of exercise under different environmental conditions. The purported mechanisms for the pathophysiology of EIA have been reviewed extensively elsewhere [53].

In acute-onset EIA airway obstruction generally starts after 10 to 12 minutes of intense exercise. If the individual stops exercising, symptoms usually disappear within 30 minutes. In a minority of athletes the symptoms may become worse for up to 60 minutes before gradually improving [53]. In late-onset EIA, following resolution of the symptoms from the acute phase, a second episode of airway obstruction may occur 2 to 8 hours later with no further exposure to exercise [16]. This phenomenon may occur in approximately 30% of adults [16] and seems to be more common in children [48]. After an episode of acute EIA as many as 50% of athletes dem-

onstrate a refractory period of approximately 2 hours during which they are partially resistant to developing EIA while performing an identical exercise task [68].

Recognition

Children and adolescents may not recognize the symptoms of EIA as being abnormal. Some simply believe they are "out of shape." The symptom complex of EIA may include cough, sharp chest pain, shortness of breath, wheezing, dyspnea, and even headache or abdominal pain [25]. Some patients may not report the onset of symptoms in acute EIA until after they stop the exercise activity. Awareness of symptoms after exercise probably coincides with the peak period of airway obstruction and lack of recognition of earlier symptoms.

Pulmonary function tests and "challenge" tests using bronchoconstrictors are probably not necessary in patients with a good history for EIA. Exercising these patients in the physician's office in an attempt to recreate symptoms is likely to be futile. For the majority of these patients a trial of effective pharmaceuticals for EIA is the most cost-effective form of diagnosis and management. However, children with more severe forms of airway insufficiency, including severe asthma, cystic fibrosis, and other forms of chronic pulmonary disease, may have significant alterations in ventilation–perfusion ratios leading to oxygen desaturation during exercise. These patients should probably undergo exercise stress testing for desaturation prior to participating in moderate to intense exercise (>60 VO$_2$ max).

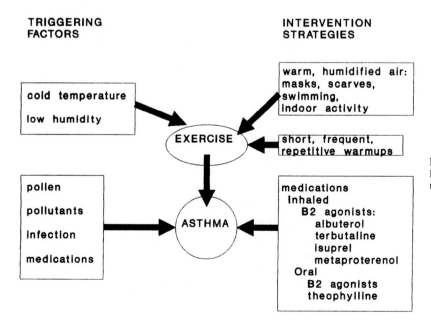

TRIGGERING FACTORS

INTERVENTION STRATEGIES

FIGURE 5–1
Factors precipitating bronchoconstriction and treatment of exercise-induced asthma.

Management

Treatment of EIA is primarily preventive and may include modification of the environment, use of warm-up periods, changing the exercise type or intensity, and initiating the use of medication (see Fig. 5–1). The particular mix of treatment modalities that prove most effective in an individual athlete is variable.

Warm moist air is least likely to cause EIA. Exercising outdoors during warm seasons and indoors during the winter months may be helpful. The use of surgical masks and, particularly in young children, scarves worn loosely around the nose and mouth will warm and humidify inspired air.

Athletes with refractory EIA may be encouraged to select specific sports to minimize their symptoms. Swimmers breathe maximally humidified air just above the water surface. Studies have demonstrated less airway obstruction during swimming compared to equivalent exercise on land [17]. Sports that require short moderate to intense periods of effort are less likely to induce EIA. Wrestling, gymnastics, football, baseball, softball, and track and field events (e.g., shot put, discus, pole vault) are typical of such sports.

Adequate warm-up before exercise will help to diminish airway obstruction during participation. Because the refractory period of EIA may last up to 2 hours, short, frequent, repetitive warm-up drills may induce a refractory state that allows symptom-free exercise. Individuals with mild forms of EIA may be able to "run through" their period of peak airway obstruction and reach a point where no further symptoms occur with continued exercise.

Pharmacologic Management

The use of medication to prevent EIA is the most common form of treatment. Categories of medications found to be useful in treatment are listed in Figure 5–1.

Cromolyn sodium inhaled in either capsular Spinhaler form or nebulized solution before exercise has been shown to be at least partially effective in preventing EIA in up to 73% of patients [30]. Chronic use of cromolyn sodium may enhance the acute effect of preventing EIA [22]. The duration of action has been shown to be quite variable between patients. In general, a protective effect beginning 15 to 30 minutes after inhalation and lasting up to 2 hours has been demonstrated [11].

Beta-adrenergic agonists are excellent bronchodilators and probably are most effective for preventing EIA. Although oral beta-adrenergic agonists have been shown to be helpful in preventing EIA, the inhalation form has been shown to be superior. Isoproterenol and metaproterenol have been available in the United States for several years. Both have been shown to inhibit EIA within 5 minutes after inhalation and have a duration of action of up to 2 hours [49].

Newer agents such as albuterol, terbutaline, and fenoterol are thought to be more selective of beta-2 receptors and therefore potentially less cardiotoxic. Terbutaline and fenoterol have been shown to be effective within 10 to 15 minutes of inhalation and inhibit EIA for up to 1 to 2 hours [43, 65]. Albuterol has a duration of protection ranging from 4 to 6 hours [69]. For this reason, it may be the drug of choice for the prevention of EIA. All of these newer beta-2 agonists are reported to be significantly more effective for prophylaxis of EIA than cromolyn sodium [49].

Athletes should be taught to medicate themselves with inhaled beta-2 agonists or cromolyn sodium 10 to 15 minutes before exercise begins. Children as young as toddler age can take inhaled medications through the use of spacing devices. The majority of young children maintain fitness through involvement in unstructured play activity. Toddlers and early school-age children with asthma should be encouraged to use these medications before play activities that typically induce symptoms.

Oral theophylline, a methylxanthine, is effective in partially preventing EIA in approximately 80% of individuals [24]. It has positive inotropic effects on the heart, pulmonary vascular bed, and skeletal muscle that could potentially enhance athletic performance. However, many individuals cannot tolerate the negative effects commonly associated with theophylline such as headache, nausea, irritability, and insomnia. Methylxanthines are acceptable for use by the International Olympic Committee as long as urinary caffeine levels do not exceed 15 μg/ml [19].

Antihistamines have a minimal effect on the airway response to exercise and inspired cold air [61]. Inhaled corticosteroids have shown variable effects on EIA [49]. The role of these medications in the treatment of EIA at this time is minimal.

Other drugs have shown some benefit in preventing EIA. Cholinergic antagonists such as ipratropium bromide may have some limited usefulness [28]. Calcium channel blockers such as nifedipine and verapamil have demonstrated some protective benefit in individuals with EIA [9]. Experience with these medications is limited, and their routine use is not recommended at this time.

Therapeutic Benefit

Children with asthma who participate in long-term exercise programs including swimming and running have fewer days of nonexercise-induced asthma, decreased medication use, decreased school absenteeism,

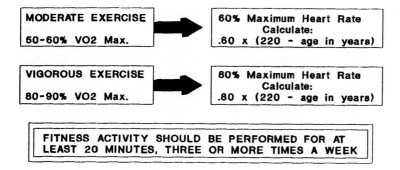

FIGURE 5–2
Exercise intensity levels in children and adolescents.

and decreased hospitalization [74]. Psychological benefits and increased self-esteem result from participation in sport and exercise programs [49]. Pulmonary function studies have not been shown to change in response to physical training.

Research on the impact of training on EIA has produced conflicting results. Some studies have shown decreased airway obstruction using the same pre- and post-exercise tests following a training program [49]. No harm has resulted from asthmatics participating in physical training. Because of their potential benefits and lack of harmful effects, all children and adolescents with asthma should be encouraged to participate in exercise programs and competitive sports.

Although the exact amount of exercise needed is unknown, participation in moderate or vigorous physical activity (Fig. 5–2) at least three times a week for 20 minutes or more per session should be adequate.

HYPERTENSION

Hypertension affects 15% to 20% of the adult population. Estimates of its prevalence in children vary depending on the methodology and criteria used for defining elevated blood pressure. Various studies have demonstrated that 0.6% to 11% of children are hypertensive [63]. The American College of Cardiology has developed guidelines defining mild, moderate, and severe hypertension [27] (Table 5–4). Criteria for defining the severity of hypertension in children must be inferential because the long-term consequences of elevated blood pressure levels in children are unknown. The National Heart, Lung and Blood Institute Task Force on Blood Pressure Control in Children has established a classification of hypertension in children based "not upon risk data but upon clinical experience and consensus" [56] (see Table 5–4). Significant hypertension is defined as values that are persistently between the 95th and 99th percentiles for age. Severe hypertension refers to persistent values at or above the 99th percentile for age.

Hypertension in adults is associated with increased risk of stroke, coronary artery disease, and renal disease. It is reasonable to assume that childhood hypertension that persists into adult life would be associated with the same risks as adult hypertension. Evidence that adult hypertension has its origin in childhood includes the

TABLE 5–4
Classifications of Hypertension

Adult Hypertension* (mm Hg)	Children and Adolescents Hypertension†		
	Age (years)	Significant 95th–99th Percentiles	Severe 99th Percentile and Above
Mild >90 diastolic	6–9	S >122	S >130
Moderate >105 diastolic		D >78	S >86
Severe >115 diastolic			
	10–12	S >126	S >134
Isolated		D >82	D >90
Systolic >160			
	13–15	S >136	S >144
		D >86	D >92
	16–18	S >142	S >150
		D >92	D >98

*Adapted from Frolich, E. D., et al. Task Force IV: Systemic arterial hypertension. *J Am Coll Cardiol* 6:1218–1221, 1985.

†Adapted from National Heart, Lung and Blood Institute. Report of the Second Task Force on Blood Pressure Control in Children—1987. *Pediatrics* 79:1–25, 1987.

maintenance of rank order of blood pressure percentiles throughout childhood and adolescence [35] and familial aggregation of blood pressure [42].

The predictive power of blood pressure levels for future hypertension in the individual child has some limitations. Prediction of future height and weight based on measurements at an early age is more precise than prediction of future blood pressure based on measurements at an early age [20]. Among children whose blood pressure exceeds the 95th percentile, 30% to 50% return to a normotensive state within 2 years without therapy [27].

Critical aspects of the methodology of obtaining blood pressure are reviewed elsewhere [56]. In no case should the diagnosis of hypertension be made without serial measurements on at least three occasions using proper methodology. Tall, large children as well as children who progress through puberty more rapidly than age-matched peers may have blood pressure measurements higher than the 90th percentile but still be considered normal. The clinician should be very cautious in labeling a child hypertensive.

Sports Participation

Recommendations for sports participation should not be based solely on blood pressure levels. If a child has hypertension based on accurate measurements taken on at least three separate occasions, evaluation should be undertaken in regard to its etiology and target organ involvement [63]. Hypertensive individuals with polycystic kidneys, renal parenchymal disease, or solitary kidneys should not participate in contact or collision sports [27]. The risk of renal trauma in limited contact or impact sports and noncontact strenuous sports is unknown. Common sense indicates that the risks would be similar to or less than those associated with unsupervised recreational play activities. Participation in these sports should be individualized based on patient and family desires and an understanding of the theoretical risks.

Blood pressure in children during isometric (static) and dynamic exercise is significantly higher than resting blood pressure. Children with resting blood pressures in the higher percentiles have correspondingly higher blood pressure elevations during exercise than children with resting blood pressures in the lower percentiles [67]. Adolescents with sustained hypertension have been shown to have significantly higher blood pressure levels during maximal exercise than normotensive controls [58]. Isometric exercise appears to produce greater degrees of diastolic blood pressure elevation and peripheral resistance than does dynamic exercise [72]. Systolic blood pressure can rise above 250 mm Hg in adolescents participating in maximal exercise [58]. When performing double leg presses, mean systolic blood pressures in

adults may rise to 350 mm Hg and sometimes to above 400 mm Hg [47].

The significance of the dramatically elevated pressures that occur during exercise is unknown. Stroke and cerebral hemorrhage without regard to blood pressure have occurred during maximum weight lifting [47]. However, there is no direct evidence linking hypertension and sudden death during sports participation. Exercise stress testing may eventually prove to be helpful in making recommendations for participation in sports. However, studies indicating how such test results can be utilized in making judgments about participation are not available [77]. At this time, exercise stress testing is not recommended as part of an evaluation to determine readiness for competitive sports participation.

When properly performed, strength training has a long-term effect, similar to that of aerobic training, of lowering blood pressure [34]. Adherence to the AAP position statement, *Strength Training, Weight and Power Lifting and Body Building by Children and Adolescents* [6], will provide a safe program of strength training for normal children as well as those with mild or significant hypertension. Because of an increased risk of injury, all prepubertal children should avoid maximum lifts and lifts involved in Olympic or power-lifting sports such as the clean and jerk, snatch, dead lift, overhead lift, bench press, and squat.

The American College of Cardiology has recommended that all adolescents with mild or moderate essential hypertension (adult standard 90 to 115 mm Hg diastolic) without target organ involvement be allowed to participate in all competitive sports [27]. Comparative categories of adult mild, moderate, and severe hypertension have not been established for prepubertal children. However, it is reasonable to allow children with significant hypertension [56] to participate in all competitive sports.

Children and adolescents with severe hypertension should not participate in exercise or sports with high static demands. Prudence should be used in recommending participation in moderately strenuous exercise because of the possible dramatic elevations in blood pressure that occur during these activities. However, there is no demonstrated evidence to indicate any immediate risk related to participation in these sports by children and adolescents.

Therapy

There is ample evidence in children and adolescents showing an inverse relationship between blood pressure and physical activity. Children who have achieved improved physical fitness reveal concomitant lowered blood pressure [37, 59]. Hypertensive adolescents exposed to vigorous aerobic training programs (running, swimming, cycling) for 6 weeks demonstrated significant decreases in both systolic and diastolic blood pressures [34]. Six of these same adolescents demonstrated maintenance of reduced blood pressure during strength training performed 3 days a week for 5 months. Cessation of strength training resulted in a return to preexercise blood pressure values. Studies in obese adolescents demonstrated similar results [64]. Children whose blood pressure is in the upper percentiles for age should be encouraged to participate in an aerobic exercise training program.

Participation in moderate physical exercise (see Fig. 5–2) three times a week for at least 20 minutes seems reasonable. Continuous maintenance of this type of program is necessary to ensure a long-term beneficial effect on blood pressure. Decisions about exercise at more intense levels should be based on the previously mentioned recommendations for participation in sports.

CONGENITAL HEART DISEASE

Heart disease in children includes structural abnormalities, conduction disturbances, inflammatory changes, and myopathic disturbances. Studies detailing the participation of children with heart disease in recreational play or competitive sports in the United States are lacking, but data from Norway are encouraging. The percentage of children with heart disease participating in sports and physical education is similar to or higher than the percentage of normal children in these activities [40]. However, these children have a tendency to select sports with a lower aerobic demand. Every attempt should be made to encourage these children to participate in sports and exercise programs to the degree that their individual disease allows.

Sports Participation

A complete review of participation in sports and the therapeutic value of exercise for children with congenital heart disease is beyond the scope of this chapter. Extensive guidelines are available elsewhere [26, 33, 54].

Sudden death in sports is often not preventable because many individuals are asymptomatic or do not have abnormal physical findings on examination. However, reviews of cases of sudden death reveal that many individuals showed previous symptoms. Children and adolescents with a history of exertional syncope, chest pain, or palpitations should be considered for an expanded work-up including chest radiograph, electrocardiography, echocardiography, and electrocardiographic stress testing prior to being allowed to participate in sports.

Cardiac lesions associated with sudden death in sports include hypertrophic cardiomyopathy, anomalies of the coronary vessels, myocarditis, certain arrhythmias, and severe aortic stenosis (>40 mm Hg gradient at rest) [75]. Children with these abnormalities should be proscribed from participation in all but nonstrenuous sports.

Children with premature atrial or ventricular beats in the resting state are common. If the premature contractions are not associated with structural heart disease, are unifocal, and disappear with exercise (adequate to raise the heart rate to between 120 and 140 beats/minute), further evaluation is not required. These children may participate in all competitive sports [26].

Children with congenital heart disease generally have decreased exercise tolerance compared to normal children when evaluated on treadmill exercise tests [21]. After surgical correction of the disease, decreased exercise tolerance often persists to a lesser degree [52]. Even children with postoperative ostium secundum atrial septal defects and ventricular septal defects may have some residual deficits in exercise tolerance. Several authors and organizations have made recommendations for sports participation and exercise for youngsters with congenital heart disease [26, 52, 54]. The defects that, with certain qualifications, allow participation in all competitive sports are summarized in Tables 5–5 and 5–6. Treadmill exercise testing is necessary for most of these individuals who desire to compete in strenuous sport programs. In both the pre- and postoperative states there is a wide range of severity for each heart defect, which makes generalized recommendations for the individual patient impossible. Decisions about the sport participation of youth with more severe forms of congenital heart disease should probably be made under the direction of a cardiac specialist.

Therapeutic Recommendations

Participation in sports and exercise may have psychosocial benefits through increased peer interaction and enhanced self-esteem. Exercise training in normal children may produce decreases in heart rate and increases in cardiac muscle and chamber size, maximum oxygen consumption, stroke volume, and blood volume [15].

Studies of the value of exercise training in children with cardiac disease are limited. Children who qualify for participation in all competitive sports should be able to complete moderate and vigorous fitness activities (see Fig. 5–2) without difficulty. Therapeutic exercise programs for others should be done under the direction of a cardiologist.

OBESITY

Between 1965 and 1980 there was a 54% increase in the prevalence of obesity in 6- to 11-year-old children

TABLE 5–5
Congenital Heart Disease Participation in all Competitive Sports

Defect	Qualifiers		
	American College of Cardiology	*Freed*	*American Heart Assoc.*
ASD	No pulmonary hypertension	Normal pulmonary artery pressure	No pulmonary obstructive disease
VSD	Small Normal EKG, CXR	Normal pulmonary artery pressure	No pulmonary obstructive disease
PDA	Normal EKG, CXR	Normal pulmonary artery pressure	No pulmonary obstructive disease
Pulmonary stenosis	<50 mm Hg gradient	<40 mm Hg gradient	Mild
Aortic stenosis	<20 mm Hg gradient, no arrhythmia Normal 24-hr EKG Normal exercise stress test Normal echocardiogram, CXR	<20 mm Hg gradient	Mild

ASD = Atrial septal defect
VSD = Ventricular septal defect
PDA = Patent ductus arteriosus
CXR = Chest x-ray

and a 39% increase in obesity in 12- to 17-year-olds [31] (Fig. 5–3). These estimates are based on triceps skinfold measurements, which clearly demonstrate the trend toward increasing body adiposity in American children.

There has, however, been some debate about the significance of these findings.

Obesity in children and adults may be associated with significant psychosocial consequences. Other children

TABLE 5–6
Postoperative Congenital Heart Disease Participation in All Competitive Sports

Defect	Qualifiers		
	Matthys 1989	*American College of Cardiology 1985*	*Freed 1984*
ASD		Pulm. artery pressure <20 mm Hg No sinus node dysfunction Normal x-ray No complete AV block	Normal pulmonary artery pressure
	1. Normal blood pressure parameters		
VSD		Pulm. artery pressure <20 mm Hg Mild or no EKG hypertrophy Normal exercise stress test Normal 24-hr EKG	Normal pulmonary artery pressure
	2. Normal exercise stress test		
PDA		Normal cardiac examination Normal CXR	Normal pulmonary artery pressure
Coarctation of aorta		No gradient Normal: Echo, EKG, CXR Normal peak BP with exercise stress test	Normal pressure gradient at rest (<10 mm Hg)
	3. No associated lesions	>1 yr postoperative	
Pulmonary stenosis		Gradient <50 mm Hg Normal RV function	Gradient: <40 mm Hg

ASD = Atrial septal defect   VSD = Ventricular septal defect
AV = Atrioventricular   PDA = Patent ductus arteriosus
BP = Blood pressure   CXR = Chest x-ray
Echo = Echocardiogram   RV = Right ventricular

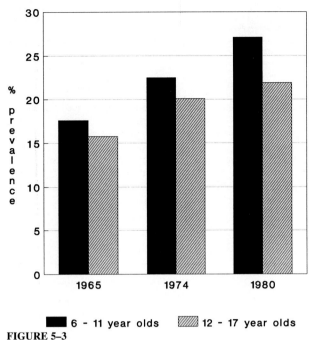

■ 6 - 11 year olds ▨ 12 - 17 year olds

FIGURE 5–3

Prevalence of obesity in children and adolescents. (Adapted from Gortmaker, S.L. Increasing pediatric obesity in the United States. *Am J Dis Child* 141:535–540, 1987. Copyright 1987, American Medical Association.)

often view obese individuals as overindulgent and lazy [45]. The concept that obese children have poor dietary habits and are less physically active than other children is open to serious question. In children, many studies have failed to show a significant relationship between overeating and obesity [59]. Other factors including heredity, metabolic rates, various enzyme levels, and physical activity may be more important determinants of obesity.

The question of whether or not obese children are less physically active than nonobese children is controversial. Differences of opinion may be related to the difficulties of methodology encountered in measuring children's activity and movement. Hypoactivity has been shown to precede the onset of obesity in newborns and infants [14]. Obese children aged 5 to 16 years in Finland participated less in sports clubs, and their sports grades at school were lower than those of nonobese children [39]. However, the same children showed no differences in routine daily physical activities compared to nonobese children.

Sports Participation

The risks of sports participation for obese children are limited. Obesity predisposes to a greater risk of heat-related disorders. See Chapter 1. Obese children may have fewer opportunities to learn sports skills [39]. Their level of proficiency in sports skills may therefore be lower than that of their nonobese peers, which could theoretically place them at greater risk for physical injury. The obese child may also be ridiculed by peers and coaches for poor sports performance. However, because the cardiovascular and respiratory systems respond to exercise in the same fashion regardless of whether the athlete is obese or nonobese [36, 39, 64], and because the risk factors are minimal, obese children and adolescents should be encouraged to participate in any sport program.

Therapy

Most successful weight control studies have included exercise in their protocols. In studies in which caloric intake has been controlled during periods of increased activity, weight reduction was greater than in programs in which no such restrictions were used [59]. Caloric intake tends to rise with increasing intensity of exercise unless provisions are made for controlling dietary intake.

When obese children do participate in team sports, they tend to select sports in which strength and power are valued (i.e., football, wrestling) over endurance skills. Most community team sports available for children do not provide significant endurance training [10]. Individual sports such as running, cycling, and swimming provide greater endurance enhancement than team sports and may prove to be more useful for obese children.

The intensity of exercise recommended for a weight control program should be at least as high as the level needed to promote fitness. Moderate physical activity (see Fig. 5–2) performed three times a week for at least 20 minutes is the minimum level of intensity that should be prescribed for weight control. Encouragement of activity that raises the heart rate to 80% of VO_2 max performed more frequently is likely to be more successful in weight control. The obese child or adolescent who participates in such a program can reasonably expect not only weight reduction but decreases in blood pressure and circulating insulin levels and increases in VO_2 max [64].

SICKLE CELL DISEASE OR TRAIT

Sickle cell disease (homozygosity for sickle cell genes) is associated with production of concentrations of sickle hemoglobin that are usually greater than 90%. These high levels predispose the athlete to severe hemolytic anemia and vaso-occlusive phenomena that may have fatal consequences [66]. Cardiovascular responses to exercise testing in children with sickle cell disease include altered heart rate and blood pressure and ischemic electrocardiographic (ECG) changes [3]. The ECG changes occurred in 15% of patients studied but reverted to normal with cessation of exercise. The occurrence of these altered responses correlated best with the severity of anemia. There does not, however, appear to be any progressive deterioration in cardiac function in children over a period of several years [2]. None of the children tested experienced arrhythmias or vaso-occlusive phenomena. If proper attention is directed to heat stress and hydration there is no reason to limit arbitrarily the participation of children with sickle cell anemia in sports. However, consideration should be given to exercise stress testing before participation in very strenuous activity for all children with sickle cell anemia and is strongly recommended for those with severe disease (<8 g/dl Hgb).

Children and adolescents with sickle cell trait generally have only 30% to 40% sickle hemoglobin. In the past, health risks for individuals with sickle cell trait were thought to be minimal [66]. The most commonly reported hazard is splenic infarction, which can occur at high altitudes [46], but the magnitude of infarction and its clinical importance are not thought to be significant [23].

In 1987 a study was published that described a 28% increase in sudden death in black military recruits with sickle cell trait compared with black recruits without sickle cell trait [41]. Nearly all the deaths occurred during the strenuous exercise involved in basic training. Questions were then raised about the potential risk for athletes with sicle cell trait. However, there have been no reports of disproportionate numbers of sudden death among black athletes. The studies performed on military recruits may not be applicable to athletes; it is likely that the preconditioning of athletes is significantly different from that of military recruits.

Common sense indicates that all athletes should gradually become conditioned and acclimatized to altitude changes, maintain adequate fluid intake for hydration, and decrease exercise in hot humid environments. The athlete with sickle cell trait should pay particular attention to these recommendations for sport participation. However, at this time, athletes with sickle cell trait should be allowed to participate in all competitive sports.

EPILEPSY

In the past, children with epilepsy have too often been excluded from sports participation. Reasons for disqualifying them fall into two general categories. Head trauma is known to be associated with the onset of seizures in any children. Assuming that the brain of an epileptic child is more vulnerable than that of a normal child, further trauma from contact or collision sports might worsen the disease. Injury or death could result from hazards inherent in some sports if a seizure were to occur during participation. Although there may be some credence to these arguments, they have been too widely applied in the past.

Recent recommendations are more appropriate. The AAP recommended restricting epileptic children from underwater swimming, rope climbing, parallel bars, or high diving or any activity in which there is a high risk of a fall [4]. Theoretically, the risk of significant injury or death if a seizure occurs during these activities is high. Any swimming activity should be carried out using a ''buddy system'' with adequate supervision.

For the child with epilepsy, medical management, seizure control, and available supervision during the sport activity should be considered part of the decision-making process in regard to participation. Responsibility for the decision about athletic participation should be shared by the physician, parents, and child.

There is a paucity of reports about seizures and participation in other sports or exercise activity [44]. There should be no absolute disqualification for sports other than those mentioned earlier. For children with incompletely controlled seizures, strict exclusion from other sports, including those classified as contact or collision sports, may be more harmful than a rare seizure that could occur during participation in such activities. Most states allow driving privileges if a patient has been seizure-free for 1 to 2 years regardless of treatment status. If adolescents are allowed to drive a motor vehicle under that guideline, participation in all competitive sports (except those mentioned above) is reasonable. If a child has been seizure-free without treatment for at least 2 years, participation in all sports should be considered.

CONCLUSION

Advances in medical science and competitive sports allow greater participation of children with chronic illness in sport and exercise programs than in the past. In 1988 the American Academy of Pediatrics published new guidelines for participation of children in sports [5]. Recognition of the therapeutic value of exercise for many chronic illnesses has increased. In spite of these changes, data from the early part of the 1980s indicate that increasing numbers of children with chronic disease are limited in their activities [51]. Physician recognition of increased safeguards in competitive sports and the benefits of exercise in chronic disease should allow many of these children to live a healthier, fuller lifestyle. Physicians are encouraged to promote both sports participation and fitness activity for their patients who have chronic disease.

References

1. Ahlborg, G.P., Felig, L., Hagenfeldt, R., et al. Substrate turnover during prolonged exercise. *J Clin Invest* 53:1080–1090, 1974.
2. Alpert, B.S., Dover, V., Strong, W.B., et al. Longitudinal exercise hemodynamics in children with sickle cell anemia. *Am J Dis Child* 138:1021–1024, 1984.
3. Alpert, B.S., Gilman, P.R., Strong, W.B., et al. Hemodynamic and ECG responses to exercise in children with sickle cell anemia. *Am J Dis Child* 135:362–366, 1981.
4. American Academy of Pediatrics Committee on Children with Handicaps and Committee on Sports Medicine. Sports and the child with epilepsy. *Pediatrics* 72:884–885, 1983.
5. American Academy of Pediatrics Committee on Sports Medicine. Participation in competitive sports. *Pediatrics* 81:737–739, 1988.
6. American Academy of Pediatrics Committee on Sports Medicine. Strength training, weight and power lifting and body building by children and adolescents. *Pediatrics* 86:801–803, 1990.
7. American Medical Association. *Medical Evaluation of the Athlete: A Guide* (Rev. ed.). Chicago, IL, American Medical Association, 1976.
8. Amiel, S.A., Tamborlane, W.V., Sacca, L., et al. Hypoglycemia and glucose counterregulation in normal and insulin-dependent diabetic subjects. *Diabetes Metab Rev* 4:71–89, 1988.
9. Barnes, P.J. Clinical studies with calcium antagonists in asthma. *Br J Clin Pharmacol* 20:289S–298S, 1985.
10. Bar-Or, O. *Pediatric Sports Medicine for the Practitioner, from Physiologic Principles to Clinical Application.* New York, Springer Verlag, 1983, pp 38–53.
11. Bar-Yshay, E., Gur, I., Levy, M., et al. Duration of action of sodium cromoglycate on exercise-induced asthma: Comparison of two formulations. *Arch Dis Child* 58:624–627, 1983.
12. Berger, M., Berchtold, H.J., Cuppers, H., et al. Metabolic and hormonal effects of muscular exercise in juvenille type diabetics. *Diabetologia* 13:355–365, 1977.
13. Berger, M., Cuppers, H.J., Hegner, H., et al. Absorption kinetics and biological effects of subcutaneously injected insulin preparations. *Diabetes Care* 5:77–91, 1982.
14. Berkowitz, R.I., Agras, W.S., Korner, A.F., et al. Physical activity and adiposity: A longitudinal study from birth to childhood. *J Pediatr* 106:734–738, 1985.
15. Braden, D.S., and Strong, W.B. Cardiovascular responses and adaptations to exercise in childhood. *In* Gisolfi, C. V., and Lamb, D.R. (Ed.). *Perspectives in Exercise Science and Sports Medicine. Vol. 2. Youth, Exercise and Sport.* Carmel, IN, Benchmark Press, 1989, pp. 293–333.
16. Boulet, L., Legris, C., Turcotte, H., et al. Prevalence and characteristics of late asthmatic responses to exercise. *J Allergy Clin Immunol* 80:655–662, 1987.
17. Carlsen, K., Oseid, S., Odden, H., et al. The response of children with and without bronchial asthma to heavy swimming exercise. *In International Series on Sports Sciences. Vol. 19. Children and Exercise XIII.* Champaign, IL, Human Kinetics, 1989.
18. Caron, D., Poussier, P., Marliss, E.B., et al. The effect of postprandial exercise on meal-related glucose intolerance in insulin-dependent diabetic individuals. *Diabetes Care* 5:364–369, 1982.
19. Clarke, K.S. Sports medicine and drug control programs of the U.S. Olympic Committee. *J Allergy Clin Immunol* 73:740–744, 1984.
20. Clarke, W.R., Schrott, H.G., Leaverton, P.E., et al. Tracking of blood lipids and blood pressure in childhood: The Muscatine Study. *Circulation* 58:626–634, 1978.
21. Cummings, G. Maximal exercise capacity of children with heart defects. *Am J Cardiol* 42:613–619, 1978.
22. Eggleston, P.A., Bierman, W.C., Pierson, W.E., et al. A double blind trial of the effect of cromolyn sodium on exercise-induced bronchospasm. *J Allergy Clin Immunol* 50:57–62, 1972.
23. Eichner, E.R. Sickle cell trait, exercise and altitude. *Physician Sports Med* 11:144–157, 1986.
24. Ellis, E. Inhibition of exercise-induced asthma by theophylline. *J Allerg Clin Immunol* 73:690–692, 1984.
25. Exercise and asthma, a round table. *Physician Sports Med* 12:59–77, 1984.
26. Freed, M.D. Recreational and sports recommendations for the child with heart disease. *Pediatr Clin North Am* 31:1307–1320, 1984.
27. Frohlich, E.D., et al. Task Force IV: Systemic arterial hypertension. *J Am Coll Cardiol* 6:1218–1221, 1985.
28. Furukawa, C.T. Other pharmacologic agents that may affect bronchial hyperreactivity. *J Allergy Clin Immunol* 73:693–698, 1984.
29. Galob, H. *Hormonal and Metabolic Adaptation to Exercise.* New York, Thieme-Stratton, 1983.
30. Godfrey, S., and Konig, P. Inhibition of exercise-induced asthma by different pharmacological pathways. *Thorax* 31:137–140, 1976.
31. Gortmaker, S.L., Dietz, W.H., Sobol, A.M., et al. Increasing pediatric obesity in the United States. *Am J Dis Child* 141:535–540, 1987.
32. Gortmaker, S.L., and Sappenfield, W. Chronic childhood disorders: Prevalence and impact. *Pediatr Clin North Am* 31:3–18, 1984.
33. Gutgesell, H.P., Gessner, I.H., Vetter, V.L., et al. American Heart Association. Recreational and occupational recommendations for young patients with heart disease. *Circulation* 74:1195A–1198A, 1986.
34. Hagberg, J.M., Ehsani, A.A., Goldring, D., et al. Effect of weight training on blood pressure and hemodynamics in hypertensive adolescents. *J Pediatr* 104:147–151, 1984.
35. Hait, H.I., Lemeshow, S., and Rosenman, K.D. A longitudinal study of blood pressure in a national survey of children. *Am J Pub Health* 72:1285–1287, 1982.
36. Hayashi, T., Fujino, M., Shindo, M., et al. Echocardiographic and electrocardiographic measures in obese children after an exercise program. *Int J Obesity* 11:465–472, 1987.
37. Hofman, A., Walter, H.J., Connelly, P.A., et al. Blood pressure and physical fitness in children. *Hypertension* 9:188–191, 1987.
38. Horton, E.S. Exercise and diabetes in youth. *In* Gisolfi, C.V., and Lamb, D.R. (Ed.), *Perspectives in Exercise Science and Sports Medicine. Vol. 2. Youth, Exercise and Sport.* Carmel, IN, Benchmark Press, 1989, pp. 539–574.
39. Huttunen, N.P., Knip, M., and Paavilainen, T. Physical activity and fitness in obese children. *Int J Obesity* 10:519–525, 1986.
40. Kahrs, N. A survey of the physical activity of 926 Norwegian schoolchildren with congenital heart disease. *In* Oseid, S., and Carlsen, K. (Ed.), *International Series on Sport Sciences. Vol. 19. Children and Exercise XIII.* Champaign, IL, Human Kinetics, 1989.
41. Kark, J.A., Posey, D.M., Schumacher, H.R., et al. Sickle-cell trait as a risk factor for sudden death in physical training. *N Engl J Med* 317:781–787, 1987.
42. Klein, B.E., Hennekens, C.H., Jesse, M.J., et al. Longitudinal studies of blood pressure in offspring of hypertensive mothers. *In* Paul, O. (Ed.), *Epidemiology and Control of Hypertension.* New York, Grune & Stratton, 1977.
43. Konig, P., Hordvik, N.L., and Serby, C.W. Fenoterol in exercise-induced asthma. Effect of dose on efficacy and duration of action. *Chest* 85:462–464, 1984.
44. Korczyn, A.D. Participation of epileptic patients in sports. *J Sports Med* 19:195–198, 1979.
45. Korsch, B. Childhood obesity. *J Pediatr* 109:299–300, 1986.
46. Lane, P.A., and Githens, J.H. Splenic syndrome at mountain altitudes in sickle cell trait. Its occurrence in nonblack persons. *JAMA* 253:2251–2254, 1985.
47. Lauer, R.M., Burns, T.L., Mahoney, L.T., et al. Blood pressure in children. *In* Gisolfi, C.V., and Lamb, D.R. (Eds.), *Perspectives in Exercise Science and Sports Medicine. Vol. 2. Youth, Exercise and Sport.* Carmel, IN, Benchmark Press, 1989, pp. 431–463.
48. Lee, T.H., Nagakura, T., Papageorgiou, N., et al. Exercise-induced late asthmatic reactions with neutrophil chemotactic activity. *N Engl J Med* 308:1502–1505, 1983.
49. Lemanske, R.F., and Henke, K.G. Exercise-induced asthma. *In* Gisolfi, C.V., and Lamb, D.R. (Eds.), *Perspectives in Exercise Science and Sports Medicine. Vol. 2. Youth, Exercise and Sport.* Carmel, IN, Benchmark Press, 1989, pp. 465–511.

50. MacDonald, M.J. Postexercise late onset hypoglycemia in insulin dependent diabetic patients. *Diabetes Care* 10:584–588, 1978.

51. Maehlum, S., and Hemansen, L. Muscle glycogen concentrations during recovery after prolonged severe exercise in fasting subjects. *Scand J Clin Lab Invest* 38:557–560, 1978.

52. Matthys, D.M. The clinical value of exercise testing on treadmill in children after surgical correction of congenital heart disease. *In* Oseid, S., and Carlsen, K. (Eds.), *International Series on Sport Sciences. Vol. 19. Children and Exercise XIII.* Champaign, IL, Human Kinetics, 1989.

53. McFadden, E.R. Exercise-induced asthma. Assessment of current etiologic concepts. *Chest* 91:151S–157S, 1987.

54. McNamara, D.G., Bricker, J.T., Galioto, F.M., et al. Cardiovascular abnormalities regarding eligibility for competition—Task Force I: Congenital heart disease. *J Am Coll Cardiol* 6:1200–1208, 1985.

55. Mitchell, T.H., Abraham, G., Schiffrin, A., et al. Hyperglycemia after intense exercise in IDDM subjects during continuous subcutaneous insulin infusion. *Diabetes Care* 11:311–317, 1988.

56. National Heart, Lung and Blood Institute. Report of the second task force on blood pressure control in children—1987. *Pediatrics* 79:1–25, 1987.

57. Newacheck, P.W., Budetti, P.P., and McManus, P. Trends in childhood disability. *Am J Pub Health* 74:232–236, 1984.

58. Nudel, D.B., Gootman, N., Brunson, S.C., et al. Exercise performance of hypertensive adolescents. *Pediatrics* 65:1073–1078, 1980.

59. Oscai, L.B. Exercise and obesity: Emphasis on animal models. *In* Gisolfi, C.V., and Lamb, D.R. (Eds.), *Perspectives in Exercise Science and Sports Medicine. Vol. 2. Youth Exercise and Sport.* Carmel, IN, Benchmark Press, 1989, pp. 273–292.

60. Panico, S., Celentano, E., Krogh, V., et al. Physical activity and its relationship to blood pressure in school children. *J Chron Dis* 40:925–930, 1987.

61. Patel, K.R. Terfenadine in exercise-induced asthma. *Br Med J* 288:1496–1497, 1984.

62. Robbins, D.C., and Carleton, S. Managing the diabetic athlete. *Physician Sports Med* 17:45–54, 1989.

63. Rocchini, A.P. Childhood hypertension: Etiology, diagnosis, and treatment. *Pediatr Clin North Am* 31(6):1259–1273, 1984.

64. Rocchini, A.P., Katch, V., Schork, A., et al. Insulin and blood pressure during weight loss in obese adolescents. *Hypertension* 10:267–273, 1987.

65. Rosenthal, R.R., Campbell, J., and Norman, P.S. The protective effects of inhaled terbutaline and isoproterenol on exercise-induced bronchospasm. *Am Rev Resp Dis* 119 (Suppl):79–83, 1979.

66. Serjeant, G.R. *Sickle Cell Disease.* Oxford, Oxford University Press, 1985.

67. Schieken, R.M., Clarke, W.R., and Lauer, R.M. The cardiovascular responses to exercise in children across the blood pressure distribution: The Muscatine Study. *Hypertension* 5:71–78, 1983.

68. Schoeffel, R.E., Anderson, S.D., Gillam, I., et al. Multiple exercise and histamine challenges in asthmatic patients. *Thorax* 35:164–170, 1980.

69. Silverman, M., Konig, P., and Godfrey, S. Use of serial exercise tests to assess the efficacy and duration of action of drugs for asthma. *Thorax* 28:574–578, 1973.

70. Stirling, D.R., Cotton, D.J., Graham, B.L., et al. Characteristics of airway tone during exercise in patients with asthma. *J Appl Physiol* 54:934–942, 1983.

71. Stratton, R., Wilson, D.P., Endres, R.K., et al. Improved glycemic control after supervised eight week exercise program in insulin-dependent diabetic adolescents. *Diabetes Care* 10:589–593, 1987.

72. Strong, W.B., Miller, M.D., Striplin, M., et al. Blood pressure response to isometric and dynamic exercise in healthy black children. *Am J Dis Child* 132:587–591, 1978.

73. Sutton, J.R., and Farrell, P.A. Endocrine responses to prolonged exercise. *In* Lamb, D.R., and Murray, R. (Eds.), *Perspectives in Exercise Science and Sports Medicine. Vol. 1. Prolonged Exercise.* Indianapolis, Benchmark Press, 1988, pp. 153–212.

74. Szentagothai, K., Gyene, I., Szocska, M., et al. Physical exercise program for children with bronchial asthma. *Pediatr Pulmonol* 3:166–172, 1987.

75. Tunstall-Pedoe, D. Exercise and sudden death. *Br J Sports Med* 12:215–219, 1979.

76. Wallberg-Henriksson, H., Gunnarson, R., Henriksson, J., et al. Increased peripheral insulin sensitivity and muscle oxidative enzymes but unchanged blood glucose control in type 1 diabetics after physical training. *Diabetes* 31:1044–1050, 1982.

77. Wong, H.O., Kasser, I.S., and Bruce, L.A. Impaired maximal exercise performance with hypertensive cardiovascular diseases. *Circulation* 39:633–638, 1969.

78. Zinman, B., Zuniga-Guajardo, S., and Kelly, D. Comparison of the acute and long term effects of exercise on glucose control in type 1 diabetes. *Diabetes Care* 7:515–519, 1984.

Suggested Reading

1. Alpert, B.S., Dover, V., Strong, W.B., et al. Longitudinal exercise hemodynamics in children with sickle cell anemia. *Am J Dis Child* 138:1021–1024, 1984.

2. American Academy of Pediatrics Committee on Children with Handicaps and Committee on Sports Medicine. Sports and the child with epilepsy. *Pediatrics* 72:884–885, 1983.

3. American Academy of Pediatrics Committee on Sports Medicine. Participation in competitive sports. *Pediatrics* 81:737–739, 1988.

4. American Academy of Pediatrics Committee on Sports Medicine. Strength training, weight and power lifting and body building by children and adolescents. *Pediatrics* 86:801–803, 1990.

5. Braden, D.S., and Strong, W.B. Cardiovascular responses and adaptations to exercise in childhood. *In* Gisolfi, C.V., and Lamb, D.R. (Eds.), *Perspectives in Exercise Science and Sports Medicine. Vol. 2. Youth, Exercise and Sport.* Carmel, IN, Benchmark Press, 1989, pp. 293–333.

6. Horton, E.S. Exercise and diabetes in youth. *In* Gisolfi, C.V., and Lamb, D.R. (Eds.), *Perspectives in Exercise Science and Sports Medicine. Vol. 2. Youth, Exercise and Sport.* Carmel, IN, Benchmark Press, 1989, pp. 539–574.

7. Kark, J.A., Posey, D.M., Schumacher, H.R., et al. Sickle-cell trait as a risk factor for sudden death in physical training. *N Engl J Med* 317:781–787, 1987.

8. Lauer, R.M., Burns, T.L., Mahoney, L.T., et al. Blood pressure in children. *In* Gisolfi, C.V., and Lamb, D.R. (Eds.), *Perspectives in Exercise Science and Sports Medicine. Vol. 2. Youth, Exercise and Sport.* Carmel, IN, Benchmark Press, 1989, pp. 431–463.

9. Lemanske, R.F., and Henke, K.G. Exercise-induced asthma. *In* Gisolfi, C.V., and Lamb, D.R. (Eds.), *Perspectives in Exercise Science and Sports Medicine. Vol. 2. Youth, Exercise and Sport.* Carmel, IN, Benchmark Press, 1989, pp. 465–511.

10. Newacheck P.W., Budetti P.P., McManus P. Trends in childhood disability. *Am J Pub Health* 74:232–236, 1984.

11. Oscai, L.B. Exercise and obesity: Emphasis on animal models. *In* Gisolfi, C.V., and Lamb, D.R. (Eds.), *Perspectives in Exercise Science and Sports Medicine. Vol. 2. Youth, Exercise and Sport.* Carmel, IN, Benchmark Press, 1989, pp. 273–292.

CHAPTER SIX

THE DISABLED ATHLETE

Frank M. Chang, M.D.

ABILITY VS. DISABILITY

An *athlete* is an individual who uses his body and motor skills to compete in exercises, sports, or games requiring physical strength, agility, and stamina. The desire to compete has been present since the evolution of mankind, and athletic competition has been well documented for centuries in all known cultures.

An individual who is either born disabled or becomes disabled may still have an inherent desire to compete in athletics. Some disabled individuals have a strong desire to participate to prove something to themselves and others. We can assist these potential athletes to achieve their goals by facilitating and encouraging them to participate and also by educating parents, coaches, and the children themselves to prevent potential injuries. Stimulating a disabled child to participate and then watching him or her succeed is a very gratifying and emotional experience (Fig. 6–1). The overall sense of accomplishment and the rewards are great for a successful disabled athlete [15].

The spectrum of disabilities is very broad and may have a minimal to profound impact on any athletic endeavor depending on the specific disability involved. An amputee has an obvious mechanical handicap, whereas a child with impaired sensory integration may appear normal to the untrained observer. Classification of the diverse categories of disabilities is important so that competition occurs on an equal level. Almost all sports can be adapted by modifying the rules of the sport or by using adaptive equipment to allow the disabled athlete to participate. Examples include Alpine ski racing, swimming, golf, wheelchair basketball, wheelchair tennis, wheelchair track, and even rock climbing for the visually impaired.

CLASSIFICATION OF DISABILITIES

The classification of disabilities varies according to the perspective of the organization responsible for the classification. Similar disabilities must be organized and grouped so that individuals are competing on an equal basis. From an organizational perspective, it is advantageous to group as many similar individuals together as possible. They can then be organized into a league or competition comprising large enough groups of athletes to create meaningful competition. For example, if only individuals with a major fibular hemimelia and a Boyd or Syme amputation were included in a group, there would be inadequate participants for meaningful competition. By grouping these individuals with all other participants with a below-knee amputation, the competitors are functionally equivalent and there are enough of them to compete.

Classification begins by dividing disabilities into very broad categories—e.g., neuromuscular defects, amputees, Down's syndrome, orthopedic deformities, and physical impairments such as hearing loss or visual impairment. Each broad category is then further subdivided into categories to equalize the various differences. For example, amputees can be further classified into various upper and lower extremity levels, e.g., above-knee, below-knee, below-ankle, and so on. The neuromuscular category is further subdivided into diseases such as cerebral palsy, meningomyelocele, spinal cord injury, head injury, muscular dystrophies, and so on. Meningomyelocele and spinal cord injury can be combined and then subdivided into different spinal cord levels (e.g., cervical, thoracic, lumbosacral) or into specific levels such as T10 or L3. Cerebral palsy and head injuries can be grouped together and then categorized into hemiplegics, diplegics, quadriplegics, and so on or into ambulatory and wheelchair dependent. The ambulatory group can then be subdivided into those with or without walking aids, again depending on the type of competition and the size of the group competing.

The classification must also reflect the nature of the sport under consideration. For example, although arm swing affects cadence and balance, it is unnecessary to subdivide upper extremity amputation levels for running

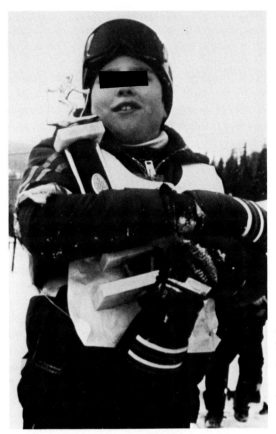

FIGURE 6–1
Disabled skier with cerebral palsy proudly clutches his trophy after winning a ski race.

sports. Conversely, the level of the lower extremity amputation (e.g., above-knee vs. below-knee) significantly affects performance in any sport requiring ambulatory skills but makes relatively little difference in wheelchair sporting competitions.

The use of prostheses, wheelchairs, and other adaptive equipment must be clearly defined to prevent any individual or group from receiving an advantage or disadvantage. For example, in national and international dis-

abled Alpine skiing competition, below-knee (BK) amputees must ski with their prosthesis and both skis regardless of the stump length. An above-knee (AK) amputee must ski three-track, regardless of the level of amputation from knee disarticulation to hip disarticulation. Three-track skiing is skiing with a ski on one leg and two short skis on outriggers supported by the upper extremities [45].

The classification process must be consistent and fair. In most situations the classification is obvious and easy to verify. Amputees fit this category. Other situations require physician input and documentation. A recent situation occurred at the United States National Disabled Skiing Championships, where athletes were competing for national ranking prior to the international competitions. An allegedly blind skier had been doing exceptionally well locally and was extremely competitive in the national competition. Some of the judges and other race officials noted discrepancies in the stated visual impairment, and after further investigation the competitor was disqualified.

Specific organizations have developed classification systems. Most of these organizations are advocate groups for specific disabilities, e.g., the cerebral palsy–based classification developed by the National Association of Sports for Cerebral Palsy (NASCP) [44]. The amputee-based classification system, developed by the United States Amputee Athletic Association, is based on level of amputation, above or below the knee or elbow, and various combinations of these four situations. The National Wheelchair Athletic Association (NWAA) supports its junior division for children 6 to 18 years old divided into four age groups and three neurologic impairment levels (Table 6–1). Other classification systems have been developed by organizations responsible for organizing various competitions (e.g., the NASCP classification modified by the International Sports Organization for the Disabled [ISOD] for winter sports). A basic and functional classification system is given in Table 6–2.

TABLE 6–1
NWAA Junior Medical Classification System

| Age Group | Disability Group | | |
	Class I	*Class II*	*Class III*
A (6–8 years)	NWAA adult classes IA–IC	NWAA adult classes II and III	NWAA adult classes IV–VI
B (9–12 years)			
C (13–15 years)		Thoracic level impairment (T1–T10)	Impairment below T10 level Includes amputees
D (16–18 years)	Cervical spinal level impairment (C1–C7)		

NWAA junior medical classification considers age and neurologic impairment level.
Each class defined by a specific neurologic impairment level is subdivided into four age groups.

TABLE 6–2
Basic Classification of Disabilities

I. Amputations
   A. Upper extremity
   B. Lower extremity, above knee (AK)
   C. Lower extremity, below knee (BK)
   D. Multiple extremities

II. Cerebral palsy and head injuries
   A. Ambulatory
      1. Without walking aids
      2. With walking aids
   B. Wheelchair

III. Spinal cord disruption (meningomyelocele and spinal cord injuries)
   A. Cervical
   B. High thoracic (T1–T5)
   C. Low thoracolumbar (T6–L3)
   D. Lumbosacral (L4–sacral)

IV. Neuromuscular disorders
   A. Muscular dystrophy
   B. Spinal muscular atrophy
   C. Charcot-Marie-Tooth syndrome
   D. Ataxia

V. Others with disease-specific disabilities
   A. Osteogenesis imperfecta
   B. Arthrogryposis
   C. Juvenile rheumatoid arthritis
   D. Hemophilia
   E. Skeletal dysplasia
   F. Down's syndrome

INJURIES IN THE DISABLED ATHLETE

The physician need not be intimidated by the disabled athlete. Injuries are usually the same in disabled children as in able-bodied children. When initially assessing a disabled child with an injury, either on the field or in the office, temporarily ignore the disability and evaluate the patient using your standard routine. The differential diagnosis is essentially the same, disabled or not. Talk to the child to obtain an accurate history. Listen to the child's perception of the symptoms at the time of and subsequent to the injury. If there is a history of an acute injury, the child can usually point to an area of tenderness that localizes the injured structure. Obtaining an accurate history from a younger child or a child with an intellectual impairment such as cerebral palsy or Down's syndrome is more of a challenge, and the practitioner must frequently rely on a history obtained from parents, siblings, coaches, and day care personnel. If there is no acute episode of trauma, the history may reveal that the child is suffering from an overuse syndrome. In this situation, a detailed history of all activities including organized sports, running, physical education, and play must be obtained. If the child is involved in sports, then the frequency of participation, training, practices, the shoes worn, and the temporal association of symptoms are all pertinent aspects of the history. The use of any ambulatory aids, adaptive equipment, or orthotics is also pertinent. Be sure to question both of the parents and especially the child. Do not forget to rule out infectious, neoplastic, or rheumatologic causes and other processes that involve children such as Legg-Calvé-Perthes disease or discitis. Do a thorough physical examination of at least the entire symptomatic extremity as well as the pelvis and spine if appropriate. As in an able-bodied child, the injured structure is almost always tender to palpation and painful to manipulation except in a child with a sensory deficit. Especially do not forget to examine the ipsilateral hip of a symptomatic knee or thigh because referred knee or anterior thigh pain is common in children with hip pathology due to referred pain.

The multiply disabled child, such as one with a high-level myelomeningocele with or without shunted hydrocephalus, is more likely to have an acute injury than an overuse injury. The multiply disabled child is usually not as active as an able-bodied child because of an osteopenic skeleton, weaker muscles, and less endurance. The evaluation remains the same because the anatomic structures are the same in a disabled child unless there is a congenital absence or duplication of parts. In a child with congenital absence of a structure, recognize that whichever skeletal element is absent or deficient, the attached muscular counterparts are usually also absent or deficient.

Skin and overlying soft tissue lesions should be appreciated. Acute injuries include contusions, abrasions, lacerations, and crush injuries. The skin is also vulnerable to sunburn and other thermal injuries. Children with sensory deficits are especially susceptible to these soft tissue injuries and are usually unaware of an injury. Once the protective skin layer has been damaged, the risk of cellulitis and deep infection increases.

Ligament Sprains

Ligamentous sprains and muscular strains are confirmed with accurate physical diagnosis. Injuries to ligaments are less common in children, first because children are more flexible, so the ligaments have more elasticity, and second, the ligaments are generally stronger than the adjacent epiphyseal plates, so the epiphyseal plate is more likely to fail, resulting in an epiphyseal fracture. Ligaments can be torn, especially in adolescent and young adult athletes. Disabled adolescent and young adult athletes with muscular weakness resulting from myelodysplasia or muscular dystrophy are especially vulnerable to sprains because they lack the extra protection normally provided by muscular control. Classification of ligamentous injury (grades 1 to 3) is the same, indicating the severity of the injury.

Treatment of sprains depends on the location and severity of the sprain. Grade 1 sprains are iced and splinted. The joint should be protected until the ligament has healed sufficiently, usually for 3 to 6 weeks. Grade 2 sprains are more severe and take longer to heal. The joint is also at higher risk for further injury because the ligament has been significantly weakened. Grade 3 injuries, which involve total disruption, usually require longer periods of immobilization, functional bracing for appropriate joints, and rehabilitation. Some grade 3 injuries require surgical reconstruction. Ligaments such as the anterior cruciate ligament (ACL) pose an additional dilemma. Reconstruction of the ACL is controversial in a skeletally immature patient because currently popular reconstructive procedures involve crossing the distal femoral physis and the proximal tibial physis, which risks growth arrest. At least one-third of anterior cruciate–deficient knees are asymptomatic, and another third function well with rehabilitation and bracing. If ACL reconstruction is necessary, the procedure should be delayed until skeletal maturity is reached, or else a technique should be used that avoids physeal damage.

Judgment must be used regarding continued competition following ligament injuries. The athlete usually wants to return to competition as soon as possible and definitely as the pain subsides. Some joints, such as those in a finger, may not be critical to performance of the sport and may be protected adequately to enable the athlete to return to competition prior to complete healing. A severe knee sprain is much more limiting and requires complete treatment and rehabilitation before competition is resumed.

Muscle Strains

Muscle strains are common in disabled children. Although children's muscles are more flexible than those of adults, the longitudinal growth of the skeleton is continuous, and thus the muscles must constantly stretch to maintain relative balance. During a ''growth spurt'' the muscles are ''relatively'' tight. Because disabled children are generally less active, they encounter fewer opportunities with activities of daily living for the muscles to stretch. Joint contractures also limit muscle excursion. Many neuromuscular conditions cause muscle imbalance, resulting in tighter groups of muscles that are prone to injury. We can help prevent these injuries by educating parents, coaches, and trainers. These individuals should encourage their athletes to stretch the muscles routinely to prevent muscle strains, especially after a warm-up but before participation in practices and competition. Muscle strains are also classified into three

grades—grade 1, a mild stretch tearing only a few fibers; grade 2, an intermediate tearing of muscle fibers; and grade 3, severe strain with complete disruption. Grade 3 strains are rare in children except when a muscle pulls off its bony apophysis, usually about the pelvis. The diagnosis is made by the history and physical examination. The location of tenderness and pain when the individual muscle is stressed against resistance confirms the diagnosis. A gap may be palpable between the muscle ends or between the bony fragment and its bed. Roentgenograms confirm an avulsion injury if the attached bony apophysis is ossified. In the insensate child, local swelling, warmth, and ecchymosis may be the only physical signs. Most muscle strains resolve after icing, splinting, and resting for an appropriate length of time.

Fractures

The diagnosis of fractures in disabled children is essentially the same as that in able-bodied children. In children the epiphyses are more vulnerable to injury and more difficult to diagnose radiographically. The Salter-Harris classification [50] can be used for prognosis and treatment. Physical examination, coupled with a high index of suspicion, is the key to diagnosis of an epiphyseal fracture. The entire epiphysis is tender circumferentially. This is easily differentiated from a ligament sprain, which is more tender over the joint crossed by the ligament and only on the side of the joint where the injured ligament is located. Diagnosis is obviously more difficult if the child has sensory loss, problems either in perceiving or interpreting pain, or difficulty in communicating effectively. In the insensate patient, a fracture is more difficult to diagnose because pain and tenderness are absent.

Children with meningomyelocele or spinal cord injuries are more likely to sustain fractures. Because these fractures may occur with minimal trauma, a history of significant trauma is often absent. The location of the fracture is typically metaphyseal, and the fracture may be misinterpreted as an infection [43] of the bone or adjacent joint. Fractures frequently present with erythema, swelling, and warmth near a joint. There is often an associated low-grade fever. Clinical instability, x-rays, appropriate laboratory studies, and a high index of suspicion confirm the correct diagnosis and avoid an embarrassing misdiagnosis.

Fractures in disabled children, as in able-bodied children, produce pain, swelling, deformity, and ecchymosis. These physical findings are less evident if the involved bone is covered by more soft tissue. If the bones are unstable, there will be abnormal motion, crepitus, and severe pain with any motion of the entire injured extremity. Appropriate treatment usually entails reduction and immobilization. Surgery is rarely indicated, except in special circumstances, such as in displaced Salter III and IV epiphyseal fractures and displaced fractures around the elbow or hip.

Overuse Syndromes

Overuse syndromes may involve almost any part under chronic stress. The bones, tendons, skin, and bursae are the most common structures involved. A full discussion of overuse syndromes is found in Chapter 8. Overuse is a relative term. Overuse for a disabled child may be the normal amount of activity for an able-bodied sibling. Neither the parents nor the child may realize that the child is overdoing it.

Stress fractures are more common in the lower extremities and are likely to occur just proximal to a brace or prosthesis. In children with normal growth and development, the additional weight and activity produce increasing forces in the skeleton. The response to the increased forces is an increase in bone strength via Wolff's law. When the stress forces increase at an accelerated rate (e.g., in a child starting a new sport and playing for hours without an adequate pretraining program), an overuse stress fracture results. The bone involved is usually tender with little associated swelling, deformity, or discoloration of the surrounding soft tissues. Radiographs are frequently normal initially but later show evidence of healing with sclerosis and endosteal, cortical, or periosteal reaction. Technetium bone scans demonstrate increased activity at the stress fracture site but are nonspecific.

Common overuse problems, such as Osgood-Schlatter disease or Sever's disease, are exacerbated by growth and associated contracted muscles. Sever's disease is overuse of the calcaneal tuberosity. Children typically present with heel pain and a history of increased running or jumping associated with sport participation. The diagnosis is made by the typical history, location of the symptoms and tenderness about the calcaneal tuberosity, frequently associated tight tendo-achilles, and normal x-rays. Osgood-Schlatter disease is an overuse syndrome involving the anterior tibial tubercle associated with increased quadriceps activity and rapid growth of the distal femur and proximal tibia (see Chap. 8).

Disabled children have unique types of overuse syndromes. The locations depend on the type of disability. Children with neuromuscular diseases, such as cerebral palsy, have muscle imbalances that create excessive stress on the musculotendinous unit. Spinal cord patients and children with meningomyelocele are prone to blisters and pressure sores. In children with congenital deformities or growth-related deformities, such as genu valgus or varus, excessive mechanical stresses are placed on the bones and related joints.

Compartment syndromes are rare in children. The deep posterior compartment of the leg is the most common location. Although the problem is rare, children who lack sensation in the lower extremities or lack the ability to communicate effectively cannot recognize or communicate the key symptom, pain. One must first consider the possibility, and second, evaluate it further if it is suspected. Intercompartment pressures must be measured for those children at risk.

Summary

The evaluation technique used for evaluating a disabled or handicapped child is generally the same as that used for any other child. Start with a history from both the child and the parents. During the physical examination look for specific problems related to the disease process such as weakness or muscle imbalance, deformity of the skeleton, the presence of braces or prosthesis, sensation aberrancies, and the usual clinical findings associated with musculoskeletal injuries or syndromes. Correlate all these findings to make a diagnosis or orient the appropriate x-rays or laboratory studies to confirm your diagnosis.

SPECIAL CONSIDERATIONS FOR THE DISABLED ATHLETE

Skin Sensitivity

There are two special areas of concern in regard to skin sensitivity. The first area is the child's awareness of skin sensibility, and the second is the additional risk present at the interface of the skin and an orthotic or prosthetic device or a mobility aid, such as a wheelchair or crutches.

Sensibility is a problem for children in general. Children do not seem to have the same regard for their body parts as do adults. In disabled children this problem is magnified. Children with intellectual and cognitive limitations, such as those with Down's syndrome or cerebral palsy, are even less aware of their bodies. Children with spina bifida or spinal cord injuries have impaired or absent sensation below the neurologic level affected. Although congenital insensitivity to pain is a rare diagnosis, these children are oblivious to pain.

Shoes, orthotics, and wheelchairs can all cause excessive localized pressure leading to skin irritation, blisters, skin breakdown, soft tissue infections, and osteomyelitis. Disabled children should be educated to become aware of their skin and its interface with their braces, chairs, and footwear. Coaches, physical education instructors, and parents also should be aware of the potential problems and check the skin periodically for erythema, calluses, blisters, and so on. Even if the child has never previously had problems with braces, the added stress of competitive sports can cause excessive skin pressure. In addition, children are constantly growing. With growth, the fit of the braces will change, which will eventually lead to altered pressure sites.

Children wearing prosthetic limbs are also at increased risk. In children with prosthetic lower limbs, the weight-bearing forces must be transferred to the skeleton through the skin and underlying soft tissues. It is more difficult for the prosthetist to transfer these forces successfully in some amputee levels than in others. In the child with a well-done Boyd or Syme amputation, the stumps are designed to be end-bearing. There is a large surface area within the BK prosthesis that distributes the pressure forces, but more important, the heel pad, the organ intended to transmit weight-bearing forces to the skeleton, has been preserved. The heel pad, a very specialized structure, acts as a hydraulic cushion [13], absorbing and dissipating energy or force and transferring the weight-bearing forces. For any lower extremity amputation above the level of the ankle, the skin and soft tissues transferring the weight-bearing forces are more susceptible to breakdown and pressure necrosis.

An athlete with a high BK amputation is at a disadvantage. In most competitions the athlete is grouped, for athletic classification purposes, with other BK amputees. Boyd and Syme amputees externally look the same. Both have a prosthesis that begins below the knee that is connected to a prosthetic foot. The child with the Boyd amputation is bearing weight through the heel pad and into the calcaneus, which approximates the normal situation. The child with a high BK stump is bearing some weight through the skin and whatever soft tissues the surgeon could find to cover the stump, and the remaining pressure is distributed by friction contact to the skin of the lower leg. For day-to-day normal activities both children may do equally well. But in the arena of competitive sports, the high BK amputee is at a disadvantage, and the added stress to the end-bearing skin interface may eventually provoke skin breakdown. In addition, children must deal with stump overgrowth.

Deformities of the Extremities

Deformities need not limit a child's participation in most sports. Psychologically, many children with deformities do not consider themselves disabled. Children with minor deformities often participate and compete with able-bodied children, especially in local neighborhood and "sandlot" type games. As the organization and the competition increase in a given sport, the deformities and disabilities may become a relatively greater handicap. At some point, the child or the team may decide that the continued participation of the disabled

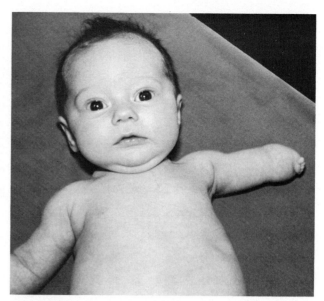

FIGURE 6–2
This child was born with a congenital terminal below-elbow amputation.

child is a handicap for the entire team and not just for the disabled individual.

Type of deformity is an important factor. Deformities can be classified into four groups: congenital, acquired, developmental, and neuromuscular. When considering participation in sports, it is also useful to further subdivide the deformities into upper extremity and lower extremity disabilities.

Congenital deformities, present at birth, imply that the deformity occurred during fetal development. The most dramatic and distressing to parents is a child born missing some significant parts. The missing part can be terminal (at the end of an extremity) or intercalary (somewhere in the middle of a segment). An example of a terminal deficiency is illustrated in Figure 6–2. A more severe example is illustrated (Fig. 6–3) in a child with

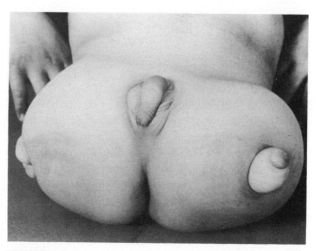

FIGURE 6–3
This child was born with congenital bilateral lower extremity terminal deficiencies, or congenital above-knee (AK) amputations.

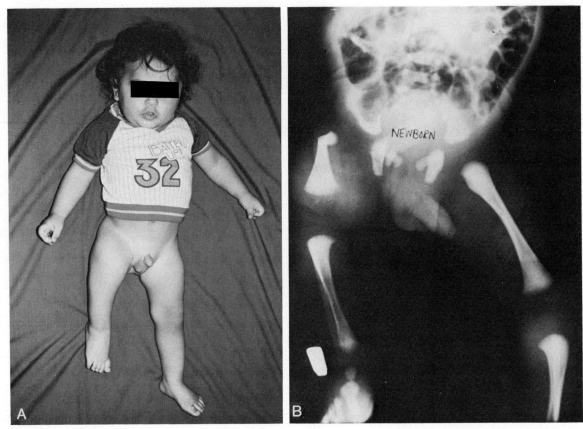

FIGURE 6–4

A, This child was born with an intercalary deficiency of more than half of the proximal femur (proximal femoral focal deficiency [PFFD]). *B,* Note deficiency of right proximal femur.

bilateral lower limb terminal deficiencies. The intercalary deficiency illustrated in Figure 6–4 is a proximal femoral focal deficiency (PFFD). Problems associated with PFFD depend on the type of PFFD involved but may include limb length discrepancy, hip instability, and knee deformity.

The treatment goal for a terminal deficiency or amputation is to maximize function by providing adequate skin and soft tissue coverage at the distal stump and to fit the child with an appropriate prosthesis. The technology associated with prostheses has continued to evolve and improve. Now we can offer the child more than just an unsightly "wooden leg." Very sophisticated, lightweight, cosmetically attractive materials, "high-tech" joints, and specialized terminal devices are now available. There are several different energy-storing feet, called "sports feet," that allow children to jump higher and run faster than the older style of static prosthesis. Specialized lower limbs designed exclusively for swimming are also available. Many specialized upper extremity terminal devices are available for specific sports. A terminal device may be designed to attach to a ski pole (Fig. 6–5).

Treatment for an intercalary deficiency is more chal-

lenging. The goal is again to optimize function. In the lower extremity, the foot is frequently amputated to facilitate prosthetic fitting, as illustrated in Figure 6–6, a case of fibular hemimelia. When indicated, this operation is performed at about 1 year of age so that prosthetic fitting can coincide with independent ambulation. The prosthesis is used to replace foot function and compensate for the difference in limb lengths. In fibular hemimelia the foot is frequently abnormal, missing the lateral rays, and in severe cases the ankle mortise is deficient laterally [2, 19, 25]. In PFFD the foot is usually normal. The normal foot is also usually amputated in this situation to facilitate prosthetic fitting; otherwise, a nonstandard prosthetic fitting would be necessary (Fig. 6–7). When athletic performance is considered, an alternative is a Van Nes "turn-around procedure" [56]. This procedure rotates the lower extremity 180 degrees and shortens it appropriately, allowing the ankle joint to substitute as an active knee joint (Fig. 6–8). This results functionally in a BK amputation that is athletically much stronger than an AK amputation owing to the active control of the prosthesis at the "knee."

In the upper extremity a similar intercalary deformity might require only therapy to improve the mobility of

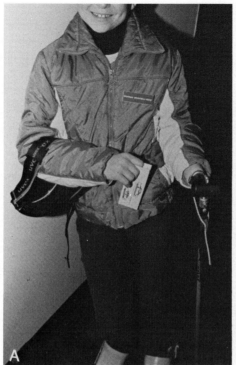 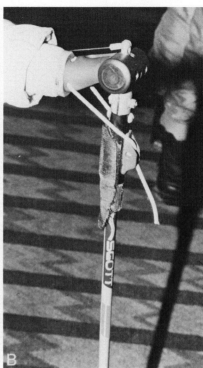

FIGURE 6-5
A and *B*, This child is wearing a below-elbow prosthesis with a Radocy modified terminal device designed to be attached to a ski pole.

the joints. The approach to upper extremity deformities is different from that for lower extremity deformities. Lower extremity prosthetics provide an effective replacement for the absent or deficient limb. At the time of this writing, hand function cannot be satisfactorily replaced prosthetically because sensibility is a primary function of the hand that cannot be replaced. Equal upper extremity length is not nearly as important for hand function, so little attempt is made to equalize upper limb length discrepancies unless they are severe. If sensation and some functional grasp are present, the hand should be preserved.

With newer surgical techniques, deformities that once demanded amputation and prosthetic use for impaired function may now be managed without ablative methods. Significant advances in limb lengthening techniques using distraction callotasis by ring or cantilever devices have been made in North America [46], Europe [23, 56, 57], and Asia [34, 35]. Management of acquired and especially congenital defects is changing as experience grows in the biology and physiology of limb lengthening. Indications for limbs previously thought to be too short to lengthen are now being reevaluated with renewed interest in using these newer techniques.

Congenital duplications occur as well as deficiencies. Duplicated toes or fingers are the most common (Fig. 6-9), and these can be easily removed if they interfere with function or are cosmetically displeasing to the patient. The problems most likely to affect the athlete are prob-

lems related to shoewear, which require modification of the shoe or surgical reconstruction of the foot. Timing of the surgery is usually not critical.

A classic example of failure of segmentation is a simple syndactyly (Fig. 6-10). In the foot the problem is mostly cosmetic. In the hand the deformity is more apparent and functionally disabling, so the fingers are usually separated surgically.

Acquired deformities can be either therapeutic or traumatic. An example of a therapeutic deformity is an amputation (Fig. 6-11) or surgical excision in a child with osteosarcoma using limb salvage techniques for reconstruction (Fig. 6-12). Traumatic amputations may be either primary or secondary. A primary amputation occurs at the time of the injury. A secondary amputation may be necessary if the surviving part is no longer viable or if function would be improved if the part were removed.

Developmental and neuromuscular deformities are grouped together for the purpose of this discussion. Developmental deformities are typically angular or rotational deformities that gradually evolve over time owing to a growth disturbance such as Blount's disease (Fig. 6-13), bone dysplasia, or metabolic disease. Children with neuromuscular imbalance such as that due to cerebral palsy begin with normal skeletal elements that gradually become deformed during growth (Fig. 6-14) owing to the abnormally balanced forces. The alteration of the normal balance of muscle forces across the skeleton

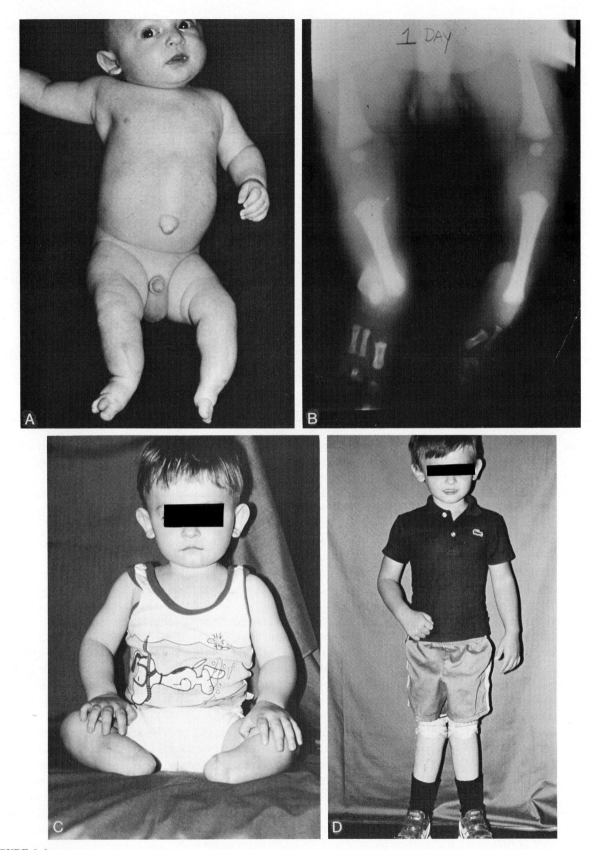

FIGURE 6–6
A, This child was born with bilateral fibular hemimelia. *B,* Note absent fibulas, short tibias, and deformed feet with absent lateral rays. *C,* Postoperative photograph following bilateral Boyd amputation to facilitate prosthetic fitting. *D,* Standing with bilateral below-knee (BK) prosthesis.

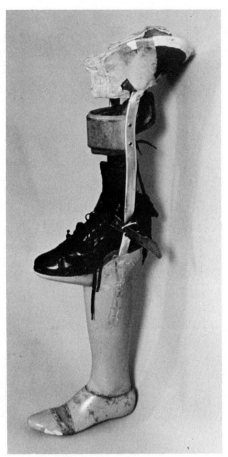

FIGURE 6–7
Nonstandard prosthesis is cosmetically and functionally less desirable than a foot amputation with a more conventional prosthesis.

influences the growing bones and produces angular or rotational deformities, shortening, joint deformities, or a combination of any of the four.

Growth disturbances have many causes, including (1) bone dysplasia (Fig. 6–15); (2) traumatic causes (Fig. 6–16), producing damage to the epiphyseal growth cartilage; (3) acquired conditions, such as an infection that damages the epiphyseal plate (Fig. 6–17); and (4) idiopathic conditions (Fig. 6–18). Traumatic or acquired epiphyseal dysfunction may result in angular deformity, shortening, or both (Fig. 6–19).

The clinical significance of these deformities varies. Angular deformities in the lower extremity concentrate abnormal forces across the adjacent joints, increasing the risk for injury and progressive degeneration. The knee and ankle are the joints most susceptible to sprains and progressive degenerative arthritis. Contrarily, rotatory deformities such as femoral anteversion or tibial torsion do not increase the risk for injuries or joint degeneration. Sequelae from limb length inequality depend on the severity of the disorder. Mild limb length inequalities of less than 2 cm are rarely symptomatic. Larger limb length discrepancies, especially when combined with neuromuscular imbalance, may result in pelvic obliquity and progressive spinal deformity, justifying limb length equalization procedures.

Loss of Coordination, Motor Power, and Endurance

Lack of coordination is a significant disadvantage in many sports. Hand-to-eye and foot-to-eye coordination are very important in most sports. Running and jumping are also affected. Neuromuscular conditions affecting the central motor system such as cerebral palsy, meningomyelocele, and head injuries are most likely to affect coordination. This situation not only affects performance but also increases the risk for injury. Children with deficient balance should wear protective head gear to prevent potential head injuries. More severely involved children may lack adequate sitting balance or head control. Special adaptations to wheelchairs are necessary to allow participation and prevent injuries. In addition to coordination defects, mentation may be affected, leading to impaired judgment.

Many disabilities affect motor power and control, especially the neuromuscular disabilities. If children are grouped according to similar levels of disability, competition can be fair.

Endurance is certainly a problem in disabled children. Most children with physical disabilities are not as physically active as able-bodied children. When they decide to participate in a sport, they need to build endurance gradually. If the buildup is too rapid, overuse syndromes may result. When endurance is inadequate and is exceeded in sports, the child becomes fatigued, increasing the risk of injury and decreasing the level of performance.

Sphincter Control

Sphincter control is a problem in children with neuromuscular disabilities, especially spina bifida and spinal cord injuries. Frequently these children are self-conscious of the social stigma, such as the odors and the different bowel and bladder routines they must practice. During participation in sports or athletic competition, the last thing on a child's mind is the status of the bowels or bladder, especially if sensation is lacking. As the bladder becomes distended, reflux can occur that will eventually result in permanent renal damage. The bladder is typically emptied on a regular schedule, frequently with assistance by parents. Most children can eventually become independent with these skills. These children and the supervising adults must be made aware of time and schedules and the proper techniques used for bowel and bladder management.

Text continued on page 63

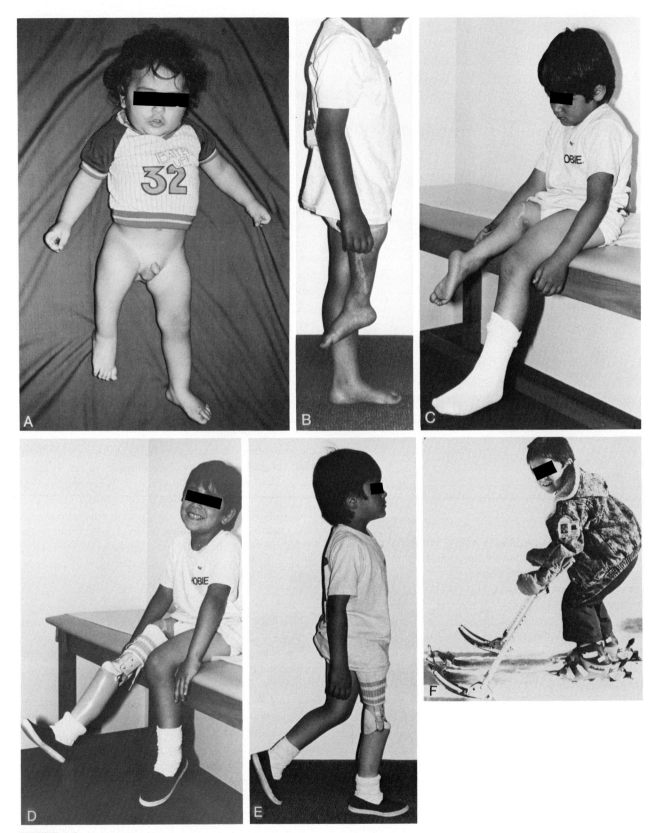

FIGURE 6–8

A, PFFD preoperatively. *B*, Postoperative view following Van Nes turn-around procedure. *C*, Active knee extension. *D*, Active knee extension with prosthesis. *E*, Ambulation with modified BK prosthesis. *F*, Skiing.

FIGURE 6–9
Polydactyly, congenital duplicated thumb.

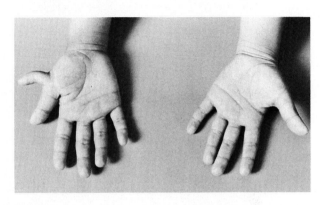

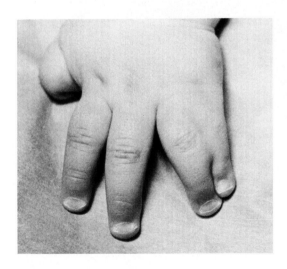

FIGURE 6–10
Syndactyly of fourth and fifth digits.

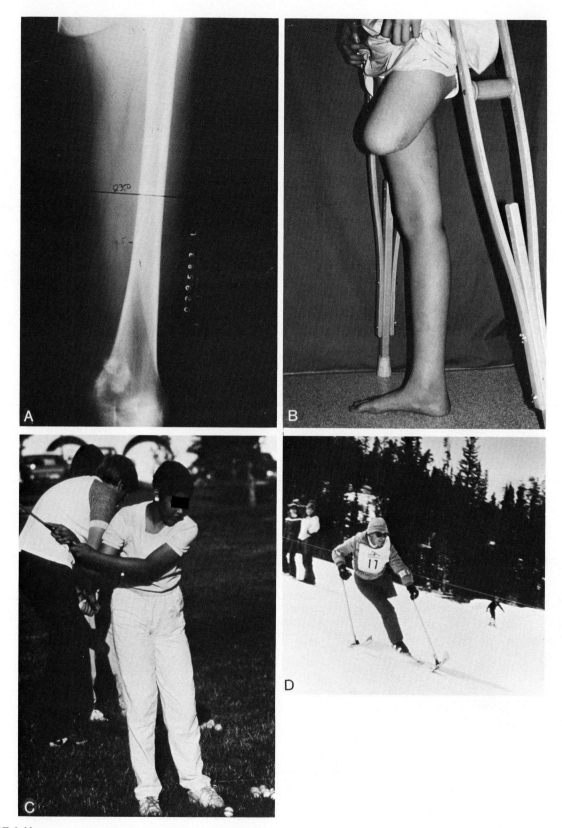

FIGURE 6–11
A, Osteosarcoma of the distal femur with preoperative amputation level marked on radiograph. *B*, Postoperative AK amputation. *C*, Playing golf with an AK prosthesis. *D*, Skiing three-track without a prosthesis.

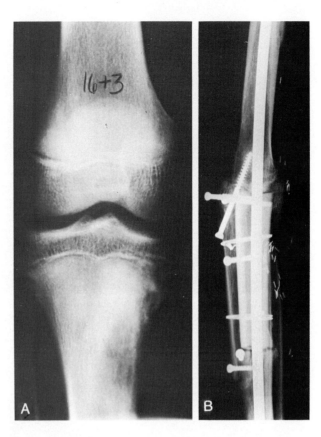

FIGURE 6–12
A, Osteosarcoma of the proximal medial tibial metaphysis. *B,* Postoperative radiograph: resection arthrodesis with intercalary allograft augmented with ipsilateral vascularized fibula.

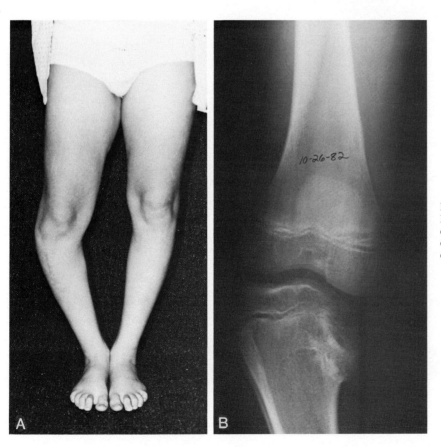

FIGURE 6–13
Blount's disease. *A,* Note severe genu varus deformity that is recurring after a previous osteotomy. *B,* Same patient demonstrating dysplastic lateral tibial plateau.

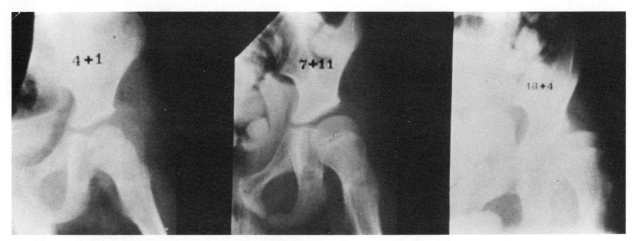

FIGURE 6–14
A child with spastic cerebral palsy who shows progressive neuromuscular hip subluxation with growth.

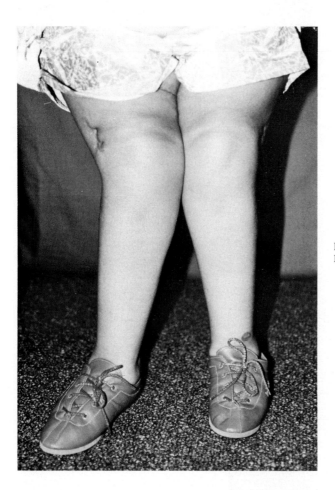

FIGURE 6–15
Metatrophic dwarfism with obvious genu valgus.

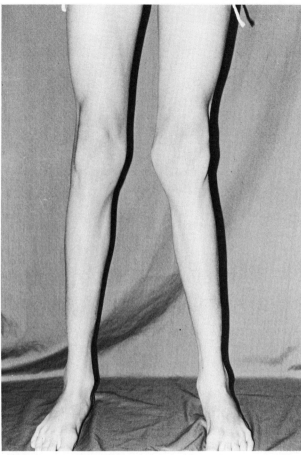

FIGURE 6–16
This patient suffered a Salter-Harris type III fracture of the lateral femoral condyle that resulted in growth arrest and produced femoral shortening and genu valgus.

If an adequate bowel program is not established, constipation can result in impaction, and incontinence can result in odors and skin breakdown. Children and their families must be educated about proper diet, stool sof-

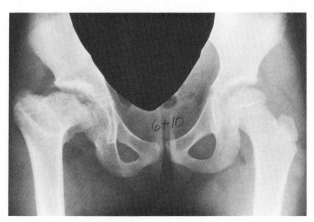

FIGURE 6–17
Septic arthritis with delayed diagnosis as an infant resulted in destruction of the femoral head and growth disturbance, leading to shortening and coxa vara.

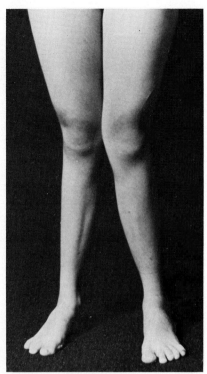

FIGURE 6–18
Nine-year-old girl with idiopathic genu valgus that does not fit the normal physiologic spontaneous correction pattern.

teners, and the importance of maintaining a regular schedule. Peer and social pressures can affect diet and disrupt regular schedules.

PARTICIPATION GUIDELINES BASED ON DISABILITIES

Generalized participation guidelines in various sports for disabled athletes are difficult to establish. Participation guidelines must be individualized. Both the characteristics of the sport and the child's disability should be considered in making a rational decision to participate in a specific sport. A child may want very much to participate in a specific sport, but the parents may be apprehensive and protective.

The Winter Park Seminar on Sports and Recreational Programs for the Child and Young Adult with Physical Disability [54] developed a "participation possibility chart," which includes the major physical disabilities and the most common sporting activities (Table 6–3). Activities are described as recommended, individualized, adapted, not recommended, or no notation if insufficient information is available. *Individualized* means that, although the activity may be clearly inappropriate for some children with certain disabilities, it may well be possible for others in the same category to participate and the activity is not contraindicated for all. Physician

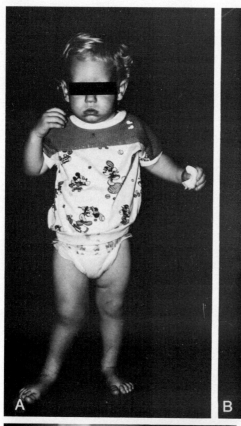
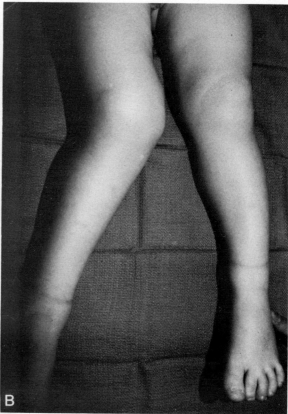
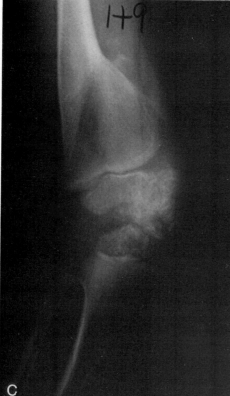

FIGURE 6–19
A, Epiphysealis hemimelia congenita producing genu valgus and limb length inequality. *B,* Note the large cartilaginous lesion deforming the medial femoral condyle. *C,* Radiographic view of this malformation.

TABLE 6–3
Participation Possibility Chart

	Individual Sports																									Team Sports											
	Archery	Bicycling	Tricycling	Bowling	Canoeing/Kayaking	Diving	Fencing	Field events[a]	Fishing	Golf	Horseback riding	Rifle shooting	Sailing	Scuba Diving	Skating: Roller & ice	Skiing: Downhill	Skiing: Cross-country	Swimming	Table tennis	Tennis	Tennis: Wheelchair	Track	Track: Wheelchair	Weight lifting	Wheelchair polling	Baseball	Softball	Basketball	Basketball: Wheelchair	Football: Tackle	Football: Touch	Football: Wheelchair	Ice hockey	Sledge hockey	Soccer	Soccer: Wheelchair	Volleyball
Amputations																																					
Upper extremity	RA	R	R	R	RA	R	R	R	R	RA	RA	RA	R	R	R	R	R	R	R	R		R		R		RA	R	R		R	R		R		R		R
Lower extremity AK	R	R	R	RA	RA	R	I	R	R	RA	R	RA	R	R	R	RA	RA	R	R	R	R	R	R	R	R	RA	RA	R	R	I	I	R		R	I	R	R
Lower extremity BK	R	R	R	R	R	R	R	R	R	R	R	R	R	R	R	R	R	R	R	R	R	R	R	R	R	R	R	R	R	R	R	R	R	R	R	R	R
Cerebral palsy																																					
Ambulatory	R	R	R	R	R	R	R	R	R	R	R	R	R	R	R	R	R	R	R	R		R		R		R	R	R		R	R		R		R		R
Wheelchair	R	I	I	R	I		I		R			R	R	R				R	R	R	R		R	R	R			I	R			R				R	
Spinal cord disruption																																					
Cervical	RA	I	RA	R	IA		RA	I	R	RA	X	RA	R	R		IA	IA	R	RA		IA		R	R	I	RA	RA	I				I					IA
High thoracic: T1–T5	R	I	R	R	R		RA	R	R	RA	I	R	R	R		IA	IA	R	R	R	R	R	R	R	R	RA	RA	R	R		R	R		R	R	R	RA
Low thoracolumbar: T6–L3	R	R	R	R	R		RA	R	R	RA	R	R	R	R		RA	RA	R	R	R	R	R	R	R	R	RA	RA	R	R		R	R		R	R	R	RA
Lumbosacral: L4–Sacral	R	R	R	R	R	R	R	R	R	R	R	R	R	R			R	R	R	R		R		R	R	R	R	R	R	R	R	R			R	R	R
Neuromuscular disorders																																					
Muscular dystrophy	RA	I	R	R	I		R	R	R	R	R	RA	R					R	R	R				R	R											R	
Spinal muscular atrophy	R	R	R	R	R		R	R	R	R	R	RA	R					R	R	R				R	X				R			R				R	
Charcot-Marie-Tooth syndrome	R	R	R	R	R		R	R	R	R	R	R	R		R		R	R	R	R		R	R	R	R			R		R	R	R			R	R	R
Ataxias	R	R	R	R	R	R	R	R	R	R	R	R	R	R		R	R	R	R	R		R		R				R	R				R		R		
Others																																					
Osteogenesis imperfecta	R	R	R	R	R	R	R	R	R	R	R	R	R	R	R		R	R	R	R	R	R	R	R	R			R	R	X	R		X	X	X	X	
Arthrogryposis	R	I	I	R	R	R	I	R	R	R	I	X	R	R			R	R	R	R		R	X	R	X			R	R	X	R		X	X	X	R	R
Juvenile rheumatoid arthritis	RA	I	I	RA	R	R	R	R	R	R	R	R	R	R			R	R	R	R	I		I	I	R			R			I	R			I		
Hemophilia	RA	R	R	R	R	R	R	R	R	R	R	R	R	R			R	R	R	R	R	R	R	R	R	R	R	R	R	X	R	R	X	I	R	R	R
Skeletal dysplasias	R	R	R	R	R	R	R	R	R	R	R	R	R	R	R	RA	R	R	R	R		R		R		R	R	R			R		R		R		

[a] Clubthrow, discus, javelin, shot put. *Abbreviations:* R, recommended; X, not recommended; A, adapted; I, individualized; Blank, no information or not applicable.

judgment and knowledge of the patient are important. *Adapted* means that in almost all cases adaptations of equipment or rules are necessary. *Not recommended* is self-explanatory and suggests that the activity is not safe and the risk of participation in it outweighs its benefits.

Amputations

As described earlier, amputations may be congenital or acquired. Congenital amputations present at birth are either intercalary or terminal. These groups are further subdivided into transverse or longitudinal defects. Proximal femoral focal deficiency (PFFD) is an example of an intercalary transverse deficiency because the proximal femur fails to form (Fig. 6–4). A terminal transverse congenital wrist amputation describes an absent hand (see Fig. 6–2). A fibular hemimelia may be either terminal longitudinal or intercalary longitudinal, depending on the absence or presence of the lateral rays of the foot. Acquired amputations may be either traumatic or therapeutic, for example, when a part may have to be removed owing to a malignancy or vascular insufficiency. A congenital intercalary amputation may be compounded electively by a terminal acquired amputation to improve prosthetic fitting. This occurs commonly in children with fibular hemimelia (see Fig. 6–6).

Amputations are further classified by the functional level remaining. Examples in the lower extremity are ankle, below-knee, above-knee, and hip disarticulation. Examples of upper extremity amputations are wrist, below-elbow, above-elbow, and shoulder disarticulation. Determining the proper functional level is important because it helps to ensure that athletes will compete against others with similar abilities. To illustrate this further, we can again look at the previous example of a PFFD in which a Van Nes "turn-around" procedure was performed instead of a terminal amputation (see Fig. 6–8). The ankle joint was substituted for the knee joint. This procedure allows this patient to function as a BK amputee instead of an AK amputee. In sports, the presence of an active knee joint provides a competitive advantage. This fact must be weighed against the potential cosmetic disadvantages.

Children with congenital deficiencies of the lower extremities usually also lack the corresponding muscles and associated soft tissues [37]. In addition, they may also lack other soft tissue structures that are not as obvious. Children with congenital short femurs (PFFD) usually also have an associated anterior cruciate–deficient knee [8, 37], manifested by positive drawer and Lachman signs. This condition should be understood so that it will not be mistaken for an acute rupture of the ACL. Many of these patients are fitted with a BK prosthesis. The rigid prosthesis has less flexibility and elas-

ticity than a normal lower leg, which also increases the risk of injury to the remaining knee ligaments. When participating in sports that carry significant potential for knee injuries, a second prosthesis with medial and lateral hinges and a thigh lacer for additional support and suspension should be prescribed to protect the knee.

Stump overgrowth is a constant problem in children with amputations [3, 4, 5, 53] (Fig. 6–20). Such overgrowth occurs most frequently in the fibula followed by the tibia, humerus, radius, ulna, and femur [3, 4]. During this process the bone grows through whatever soft tissues the surgeon left to cushion the end of the stump. As the child runs and jumps during athletic competition or during normal play, the skin is at high risk for breakdown. To prevent this, the child, family, coaches, physical education teachers, and anyone else supervising the child should be made aware of the potential problem. If the end of the stump begins to feel more bony, or if erythema and skin irritation begin, the child should be evaluated for stump overgrowth. The overgrown stump should be revised surgically to prevent potential complications. In a young child several stump revisions may be necessary at 2- to 3-year intervals [43] prior to skeletal maturity.

In children the criteria for amputation levels are different from those in adults, particularly at the knee and elbow, where in adults typically an amputation above the level of the joint facilitates placement of the prosthetic joint at the proper anatomic level. In a growing child the amputation should be a joint disarticulation if at all possible. Despite creating a more difficult and less cosmetic prosthetic fitting, because the prosthetic joint must be placed distal to the proper anatomic level, a joint disarticulation has distinct advantages. Joint disarticulation minimizes stump overgrowth and establishes an end-bearing stump. In addition to decreased stump complications, the remaining extremity will reach its full potential length, and the distal growth plate will be preserved. At skeletal maturity the amputation can be revised to allow better cosmetic placement of the involved prosthetic joint. If the epiphysis is sacrificed in a young child at the time of amputation, the potential growth from the epiphysis is lost, and with continued growth the stump will become relatively shorter and shorter. At skeletal maturity the functional use of the prosthesis may be compromised owing to inadequate length for suspension or control.

Interestingly, if the amputation is done through a joint and the physeal cartilage is left intact, the problem of stump overgrowth does not occur. Marquardt has shown that stump overgrowth can also be prevented by "capping" the end of a long bone diaphyseal stump with a viable autogenous epiphyseal plate [41, 42]. If the amputated stump has an epiphysis, this epiphysis can be used. For example, an AK amputation for a malignant

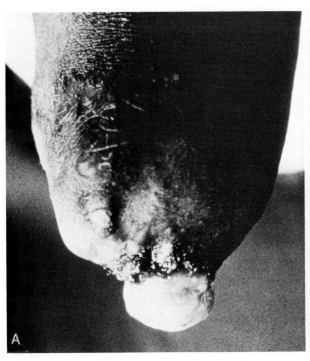

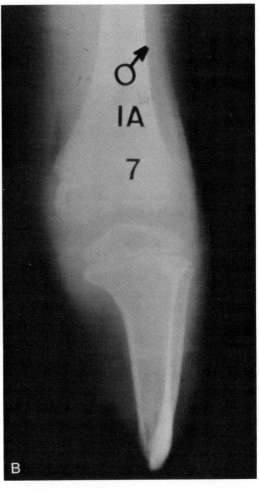

FIGURE 6–20
A and *B,* Stump overgrowth. The tibia has grown right through the skin and soft tissues.

tumor of the distal femoral metaphysis could be capped with the healthy amputated distal tibial epiphysis. When a healthy epiphyseal autograft is not available, a portion of the iliac apophysis can be substituted to accomplish the same result.

Cerebral Palsy

Cerebral palsy is defined as a nonprogressive central nervous system deficiency that is present during early childhood. A deficiency or insult involving the cerebral cortex results in spasticity, of the cerebellum in ataxia, and of the extrapyramidal tracts with involvement of the basal ganglia in athetosis. In the mixed type most commonly spasticity and athetosis are combined. The disease is further classified by anatomic involvement. Most common patterns include:

1. Monoplegia: one extremity is involved, usually a lower extremity
2. Hemiplegia: one upper and one lower ipsilateral extremity are involved

3. Paraplegia: both lower extremities are involved
4. Diplegia: all four extremities are involved, but the upper extremities are significantly less involved than the lower
5. Triplegia: three extremities are involved, usually sparing one upper extremity
6. Quadriplegia: all four extremities are significantly involved
7. Pentaplegia: a term sometimes used to suggest that the head is also significantly involved as well as all four extremities. Pentaplegic children are usually unable to participate in sports.

Children with cerebral palsy are susceptible to muscle strains and overuse syndromes. The risk of muscle strains is increased owing to the tightness of the muscles. Because these children are frequently less active, the muscles do not have the opportunity to stretch on a regular or frequent basis. "Muscle imbalance" magnifies the problem, which also results in tightness and contractures of major muscle groups. The spastic muscles are usually an agonistic group of muscles. For example, the triceps surae group of muscles attached to the

Achilles tendon is frequently spastic, overactive, and tight compared to the antagonistic ankle dorsiflexors. Because the bones are usually of normal strength, the risk of fractures is not increased.

The tight contracted muscles do result in joint stress. Patellar overload is common and frequently evolves into true chondromalacia. Both growth and spasticity result in progressive tightening of the hamstrings and quadriceps muscles. This causes a shortened stride length and increased pressure across the patellofemoral joint. In more severe cases, the tight hamstrings produce a crouched or flexed knee gait. If it is allowed to persist, proximal migration of the patella occurs. The increased pressure gradually results in increased wear and damage to the articular surface of the patella. The symptoms are the same as those seen in able-bodied children with patellar overload symptoms (see Chap. 18), but the problem is accentuated and is more refractory to treatment. In addition, the tension on the quadriceps mechanism can produce a syndrome similar to the ''jumper's knee'' seen in adolescents [14]. The constant pull of the patellar tendon results in fragmentation of the lower pole of the patella radiographically and causes pain and tenderness clinically.

Muscle tightness and imbalance across the hip joint gradually affect the normal development of the hip. In more severe cases the hip joint subluxes and eventually dislocates (see Fig. 6–14). In less severe cases the children may still develop coxa valga and acetabular dysplasia. Acetabular dysplasia may become symptomatic as the joint undergoes degenerative arthritic changes. As these changes occur, increased activity such as running and jumping will result in hip pain.

Inadequate motor control and lack of coordination are more significant problems for children with cerebral palsy who participate in sports than is their susceptibility to injuries. Impairment of hand-to-eye coordination results in difficulty with controlling gear such as rackets, bats, or golf clubs. Difficulty in catching and throwing and perceptual problems such as judging the speed of a ball are all hindrances but not unsurmountable obstacles. Running with speed is more difficult. These deficiencies in coordination can be improved to some extent with practice.

Children with head injuries are functionally very similar to children with cerebral palsy. Head-injured children have the potential for improvement in neurologic function as the injured tissue recovers. Visual field defects, which are present in some children with head injuries, increase the potential for injuries and can cause problems if an object such as a ball passes through the child's ''blind spot.''

Overall, children with spastic monoplegia, diplegia, or hemiplegia and children with athetosis can function relatively well and enjoy participating in sports.

Meningomyelocele

Meningomyelocele is the most severe congenital deformity compatible with life. The abnormal spinal canal development results in a damaged spinal cord that is inadequately protected. The patient lacks motor power and sensation below the involved level. In addition to motor and sensory deficits, bowel and bladder functions are impaired. Hydrocephalus, which is frequently associated, increases the risk of impaired cerebral function and mentation and damage to the motor cerebral cortex. The resulting damage produces spasticity above the level of spinal cord dysfunction. Care should be provided by a team of physicians, including a pediatrician, neurosurgeon, orthopedic surgeon, urologist, and physiatrist.

Participation in sports depends on several factors, the two most important being the functional level of the spinal cord and the severity of hydrocephalus. Hydrocephalus determines the severity of mental retardation and spasticity. The functional level of the spinal cord determines the motor function of the lower extremities. Classification of children with meningomyelocele is based on the functional level, i.e., the lowest nerve root level that is functioning. For example, if the ankle can be dorsiflexed actively but cannot be plantar flexed actively, the patient is functioning at the L5 level, or the fifth lumbar nerve root is functioning but nothing below that level. The sensory level usually corresponds to the motor level. The involvement may be asymmetrical. Usually the two sides are within one nerve root level of each other but we do see children with some spotty function below the primary level. Children with low lumbar and sacral level function can function almost normally. Patients with low lumbar level function require orthotics to stabilize the foot and ankle. Children with midlumbar level function also may require braces to stabilize the knee. Patients with higher level lesions function best in a seated position. Children with midlumbar level lesions perform athletic activities better in a wheelchair than when they are ambulatory in braces.

Another concern is lack of sensation. Children wearing braces who participate in sports may develop pressure sores and skin breakdown. Children sitting in wheelchairs for prolonged periods of time are also susceptible to pressure sores and skin breakdown from the seat of the wheelchair. Individuals with normal sensation experience discomfort as the pressure increases or as the tissues begin to become ischemic. They reflexly shift their position to relieve the increasing pressure. Children without adequate sensation do not have these protective mechanisms to guard the skin and underlying soft tissues. To avoid these problems, children, parents, and coaches must be educated to check the skin frequently visually until the skin pressure tolerances can be determined. The children must be taught to shift their weight frequently and to use their upper extremities to lift themselves off their seats. To decrease excessive pressure while sitting in the wheelchair, specially designed cushioned seats are available to distribute the weight evenly and dissipate pressure.

Children with meningomyelocele are more susceptible to fractures secondary to osteopenia. Fractures are more difficult to diagnose. Due to altered or absent sensation there is no associated pain. Because the injured area may appear locally inflamed, a fracture can easily be mistaken for an infection with swelling, erythema, increased local temperature, and low-grade fever. Immobilization of a fractured extremity results in the bone becoming even more osteoporotic and susceptible to refracture when immobilization ends. Gradual and progressive weight bearing after a fracture or recent operation and the use of functional braces can help to prevent a refracture. Limiting the time of immobilization and nonweight bearing will decrease the incidence of refracture.

Children with meningomyelocele are also susceptible to muscle strains. Muscles at the lowest spinal functioning level usually have less than 100% of normal strength. Because children with spinal defects are less active, their overall motor power is not as well developed. Finally, because of muscle imbalance, some muscles are tighter than normal and are prone to strains caused by decreased flexibility.

Children with meningomyelocele are able to participate in sports similar to those suitable for a patient with a spinal cord injury. The one major difference relates to hydrocephalus. Hydrocephalus may result in intellectual compromise with implications for competitive sports ranging from not having the drive to compete and not understanding the rules of the sport to perceptual problems that can affect performance. Children with severe hydrocephalus should wear adequate head protection to prevent head injury and shunt damage.

Spinal Cord Injuries

Spinal cord injuries in children, although uncommon, account for 13% to 15% of all spinal cord injuries, with boys predominating 2:1 [33, 36]. Spinal cord injuries are typically traumatic and are associated with spinal fractures. Young children under 10 years of age, because of their generalized ligamentous laxity, may present with spinal cord injuries without associated fractures. Leventhal demonstrated, in an infant's spine, that the spinal canal can be stretched 2 inches, but the cervical cord can be stretched only 1/4 inch [40]. This ligamentous laxity may allow enough motion to damage the cord [6, 9, 10, 28, 32, 36, 38].

In many respects the problems experienced with spinal cord injury are similar to those seen with menin-

gomyelocele. Differences include the absence of hydrocephalus or intellectual deficit unless a head injury is associated, the less common presence of mixed levels of dysfunction, and the possible presence of cervical levels of dysfunction. Spinal cord injuries, except in special circumstances such as Brown-Séquard lesions, are typically transverse lesions with symmetrical involvement. Spinal cord injuries can involve the cervical spinal levels, which compromise upper extremity function.

Thermal regulation is a problem in patients with spinal cord injuries, especially in the higher level lesions. Children with spinal cord injuries above T8 cannot maintain normal body temperatures [31] because constant body temperature depends on heat dissipation and heat production. Both heat production mechanisms such as shivering and heat dissipation mechanisms such as perspiration are absent below the level of the spinal cord injury. The higher the neurologic level of the injury, the more difficult it is for the individual to compensate for changes in ambient temperature. Children with meningomyelocele have similar problems with thermal regulation. Precautions must be taken when these children participate in winter sports, and they must be closely observed in very warm environments. In a survey of competitors at the 1990 USA Junior National Wheelchair Games, almost half (49%) of the track participants listed hyperthermia as a problem, and 9% of those competing in swimming listed hypothermia [58] as a concern.

Down's Syndrome

Children with Down's syndrome seem to love sports and can be very competitive. Most of the orthopedic problems in children with Down's syndrome occur because the chromosomal abnormality results in a defect in production of normal collagen. The abnormal collagen produced results in generalized ligamentous laxity and decreased muscle tone. Ligamentous laxity causes hyperflexibility of the joints and related problems such as flexible flat feet and joint instability with associated subluxations and dislocations. Judgment may also be impaired by intellectual compromise, which is compounded by the fact that children with Down's syndrome frequently do not complain about discomfort or pain and may continue to participate despite the presence of symptoms.

Atlantoaxial subluxation is potentially the most devastating problem in the athlete with Down's syndrome. The radiologic incidence of this instability in this population is approximately 15%. The subluxation is due to laxity of the annular ligament of C1 and is magnified by the generalized hypotonia. The space available for the spinal cord (SAC) consequently diminishes (Fig. 6–21).

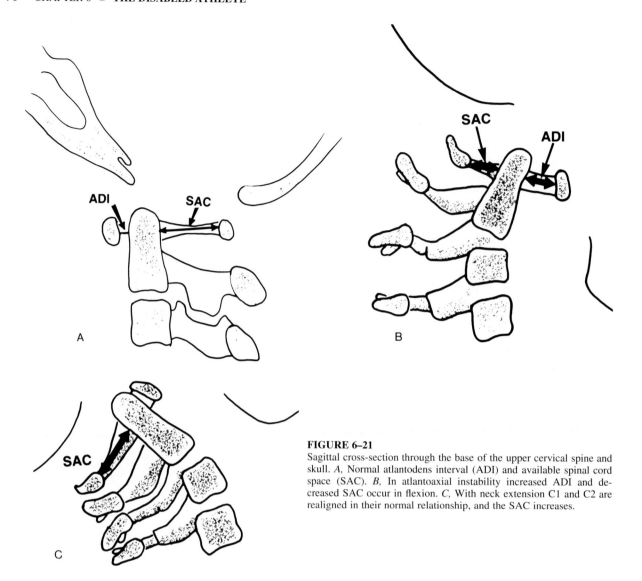

FIGURE 6–21
Sagittal cross-section through the base of the upper cervical spine and skull. *A,* Normal atlantodens interval (ADI) and available spinal cord space (SAC). *B,* In atlantoaxial instability increased ADI and decreased SAC occur in flexion. *C,* With neck extension C1 and C2 are realigned in their normal relationship, and the SAC increases.

Excessive motion at this level can result in permanent damage to the spinal cord. If the motor tracks are injured, the patient is left quadriplegic or quadriparetic with respiratory compromise.

There have been sporadic reports of symptomatic atlantoaxial instability in Down's syndrome children since 1965. Since 1983 the Special Olympics has required screening for atlantoaxial instability in athletes with Down's syndrome prior to participation in any sport placing excessive stress on the head or neck (gymnastics, diving, pentathlon, butterfly stroke in swimming, diving start in swimming, high jump, and warm-up exercises that place undue stress on the head and neck muscles) [51, 52]. This requirement has made families and the medical community much more aware of the existence of the problem. Many school districts now also require screening prior to participation of these children in physical education classes. The American Academy of Pediatrics issued a policy statement in 1984 after carefully analyzing the data and statistics reported in the literature [1]:

1. All children with Down's syndrome who wish to participate in sports that involve possible trauma to the head and neck should have lateral-view roentgenograms of the cervical region in neutral, flexion, and extension positions within the patient's tolerance before beginning training or competition. This recommendation applies to all participants in the high-risk sports who have not previously had normal findings on cervical roentgenograms.

Some physicians may prefer to screen all patients with Down's syndrome routinely at 5 to 6 years of age to rule out atlantoaxial instability.

2. When the distance between the odontoid process of the axis and the anterior arch of the atlas exceeds 4.5 mm or the odontoid is abnormal, there should be restrictions on sports that involve trauma to the head and neck, and the patient should be followed up at regular intervals.

3. At the present time, repeated roentgenograms are not indicated for those who have previously had normal findings.

Indications for repeated roentgenograms will be defined by research.

4. Persons with atlantoaxial subluxations or dislocations and neurologic signs or symptoms should be restricted in all strenuous activities, and operative stabilization of the cervical spine considered.

5. Persons with Down's syndrome who have no evidence of atlantoaxial instability may participate in all sports. Follow-up is not required unless musculoskeletal or neurologic signs or symptoms develop.

Atlantoaxial subluxation is screened by lateral cervical spine x-rays in maximum flexion and extension. The flexion and extension views are compared to assess the atlantodens interval (ADI) (Fig. 6–22). The ADI is nor-

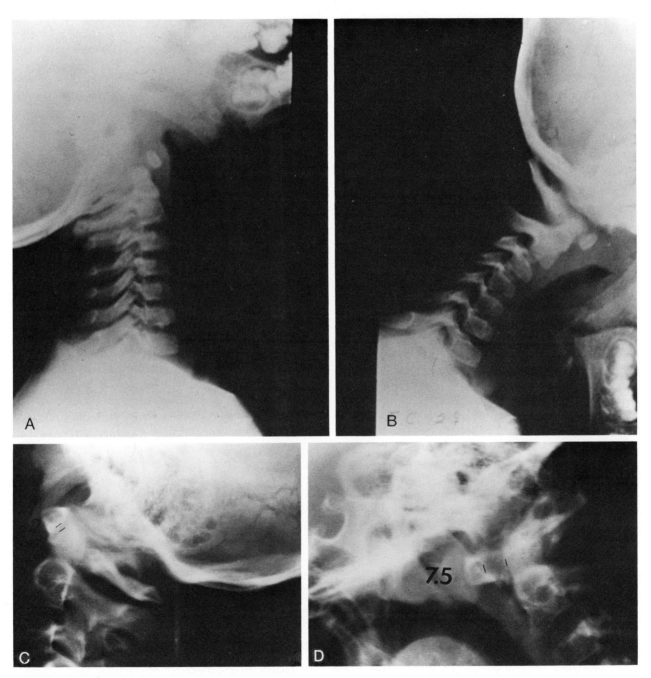

FIGURE 6–22
Lateral cervical flexion-extension radiographs. *A*, Normal extension. *B*, Normal flexion. *C*, Extension measures a normal 2 mm in an abnormal patient with Down's syndrome and atlantoaxial instability. *D*, Same patient as in *C* now demonstrates laxity in flexion with an abnormal 7.5 mm.

mally less than 2.5 mm, but the highest value acceptable is 4.5 mm in a child with Down's syndrome. In an asymptomatic child with an ADI greater than 4.5 mm, activities that will increase the risk to the cervical spine should be restricted. Such sports include tumbling, gymnastics, diving, soccer, high jumping, football, and skiing. If the ADI is excessive (greater than 6.0 mm) or if the child has neurologic symptoms, the child is a candidate for cervical surgical stabilization. Screening should be done before the child is enrolled in any high-risk activities, at the onset of school, or if neurologic symptoms are present. Subsequent screening is becoming better defined. Although some physicians still recommend follow-up screening at 3- to 5-year intervals until skeletal maturity is reached, there is no evidence in the literature to support this practice. Pueschel and Scola [47] reported on 404 patients, 95 of whom were followed longitudinally; none showed any progression of the ADI. The time of highest risk is statistically between 5 and 10 years of age. Neurologic symptoms include neck pain, stiff neck, torticollis, progressive weakness or change in sensation in any extremity, decreasing endurance, loss of bowel or bladder control or a change in bowel habits, increased clumsiness, or change in gait pattern.

An analogous problem can occur between C1 and the occiput, but the parameters for measurement and the norms for Down's syndrome are less well defined. French and colleagues recommend that all children with Down's syndrome be restricted from high-risk sports such as tumbling, trampoline, and gymnastics [26]. They found a 3% incidence of upper cervical ossicles, which they postulated were acquired in origin because half the patients in the study group had previously documented normal radiographs. The ossicles are thought to be avulsion fractures of the dens, pulled off by the alar ligaments.

Two other joints may cause problems in children with Down's syndrome. The patellofemoral joint may be unstable and may become chronically subluxated or dislocated, and occasionally the hip joint may become unstable. Patellofemoral joint laxity can intensify any anatomic abnormalities such as genu valgus, patella alta, or a hypoplastic medial femoral condyle, resulting in instability. Recurrent subluxations may not produce complaints in a child with Down's syndrome. A dislocation may produce more pain and swelling, but even with an acute dislocation the child with Down's syndrome may complain very little. Treatment is more difficult because, in addition to ligamentous laxity, the children are also relatively hypotonic. Conservative measures frequently fail. Surgical realignment of the extensor mechanism may be necessary on rare occasions (see Chap. 18).

Hip instability is an even more difficult problem to treat. Excessive joint laxity can result in a distended hip capsule, which allows the hip to dislocate. Parents describe audible clunking or popping sounds, with usually very little evidence of symptoms. Some children with Down's syndrome may even actively dislocate the hip to gain attention or for self-stimulation. This problem is similar to the individual with voluntary shoulder dislocation. Conservative measures such as temporary casting or prolonged abduction bracing produce inconsistent results. Even surgical correction with a femoral or pelvic osteotomy combined with capsulorrhaphy and prolonged postoperative casting do not always ensure permanent hip stability. Although hip damage and eventual degenerative changes do occur, the natural history of this problem is not well documented. The instability does seem to diminish somewhat with progressive growth and development.

Flexible flatfeet are normally present in children with Down's syndrome. Most are asymptomatic. If planovalgus deformities are symptomatic, a UCBL (University of California Berkeley Labs) orthosis helps to minimize symptoms and excessive shoewear.

Hearing Impaired

Children with a hearing impairment are not predisposed to any specific injuries and can participate in all sports. They are at a disadvantage and will have difficulty in participating in some sports. Communication with other participants is compromised. Not only can they not hear someone giving instructions, but often speech is also impaired. Further, they lack the ability to receive auditory cues or to hear other players who are trying to get their attention verbally. Because they do not have any visible physical disability, these children tend to play with other able-bodied individuals, leaving them at some disadvantage. Since the inner ear is connected to the vestibular apparatus, balance may be affected.

Hearing aids are useful for some children. Lip reading and signing will facilitate communications but have obvious disadvantages during the heat of competition, especially in sports involving other team members or other competitors. For hearing impaired children to experience maximum success in sports, individual activities such as tennis, skiing, and running, in which the need for communication is minimal, may be chosen.

Visually Impaired

Participation without eyesight in sports is at best a difficult situation. Occasionally auditory cues can be substituted during some sports such as skiing. Special

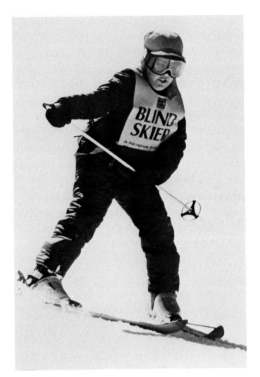

FIGURE 6–23
A blind skier.

programs have been developed at a few ski resorts (Fig. 6–23). As the proficiency and skills of the skier increase, the individual can ski faster and on more difficult terrain. Other sports have been successfully adapted in recent years. Rock climbing, speed skating, tandem cycling, and competitive swimming are all gaining popularity with visually impaired athletes.

Children with head injuries may have a limitation in the visual field depending on the anatomic location of the lesion. Awareness of the location of the visual field defect is important for safety and for choosing a sport that will not be significantly affected by the child's "blind spot."

SPECIAL OLYMPICS

The Special Olympics is an international program that promotes physical fitness and athletic competition for mentally impaired children and adults [52]. It features competition in various sports similar to the Olympic summer and winter games. Participants compete in different divisions based on age and ability. Local and regional competitions are held annually. Winners of the regional competitions can go on to compete nationally, and every 4 years an international competition is held equivalent to the Olympic games. The psychosocial rewards are gratifying for participants. Children and adults with almost any disability may participate. Children with

Down's syndrome must be screened for cervical instability prior to participating in some sports.

ADAPTIVE EQUIPMENT

Children with disabilities should be given the opportunity and encouraged to participate in sports. Depending on the disability and the sport, various types of adaptive equipment can be used to enhance their participation, performance, and enjoyment. Some equipment may be as simple as the ankle foot orthosis (AFO) that the child uses every day to stabilize the ankle. At the other end of the spectrum, very specialized devices are now available that facilitate athletic performance. A child who is a wheelchair ambulator and has a very functional chair for daily use may obtain a low-profile, lightweight sports wheelchair to participate in competitive sports. Specialized upper extremity prostheses are available with interchangeable terminal devices that are adapted to hold bats, rackets, and even ski poles (see Fig. 6–5). Technology has also provided specialized energy-storing feet and lighter and stronger materials that enhance athletic performance as well as daily use by those who use lower limb prostheses.

The wheelchair-dependent child has many opportunities to participate in athletic competition. In the early 1980s the NWAA created a junior division for children 6 to 18 years old. Three groups of athletes were defined based on the level of spinal cord function; these were subdivided further into four age groups (see Table 6–2). Injuries are common in these athletes. Ninety-seven percent of participants reported injuries in track competitions at the 1990 Junior Wheelchair National competition [59]. The majority of the reported injuries were soft tissue injuries: blisters 77%, wheelburns 71%, bruising 41%, abrasions 38%, shoulder soft tissue injuries (including sprains, strains, and tendinitis) 19%, pressure sores 14%, wrist soft tissue injuries 11%, and elbow soft tissue injuries 7%. Fractures occurred in 6%, bladder infections in 22%, and 49% reported problems with overheating or hyperthermia in the same group of children. These problems can be minimized with awareness, vigilance, appropriate protective equipment, clothing, padding, and improved training programs.

At the Children's Hospital in Denver, Colorado, we have had the unique experience of developing a very sophisticated and successful ski and sports program for children with many different types of disabilities. In the ski program each child is evaluated individually to determine what adaptive equipment will optimize his or her performance. Depending on the specific disability involved, the child is placed in one of four skier categories. Major skier categories include:

1. Three track: One ski and two outriggers
   a. AK and higher amputees
   b. Severely deformed, damaged, weakened, or fragile single lower extremity
   c. BK amputee with less than a 4-inch stump
   d. Post polio (monoplegia)
2. Four track: Two skis and two outriggers
   a. Mid- to low lumbar level spina bifida
   b. Moderate to severe cerebral palsy
3. Two track: Two skis with one, two, or no poles
   a. Upper extremity amputee, unilateral or bilateral
   b. Spastic diplegic or triplegic cerebral palsy
   c. BK amputee with 4-inch or longer stump
4. Sit skier: Sitting in some modification of a sled device

   a. High lumbar or thoracic level spina bifida or spinal cord injury
   b. Any child dependent on a wheelchair

The child's stance is analyzed. If there is a limb length discrepancy, lifts are incorporated between the ski and the binding (Fig. 6–24). If the child cannot achieve a balanced posture with his weight balanced over his feet or slightly forward, heel lifts are incorporated into the ski boot, or the binding and the entire foot plate are canted forward in the more severe cases. The presence of deformed lower limbs (varus or valgus) can also be compensated by canting the foot plate appropriately. If the child has compromised balance, weakness in the lower extremities, or difficulty in controlling his legs

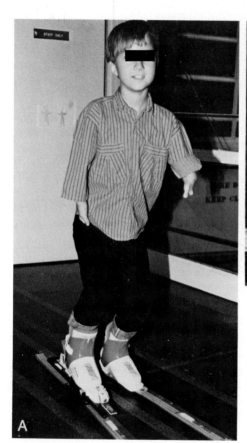

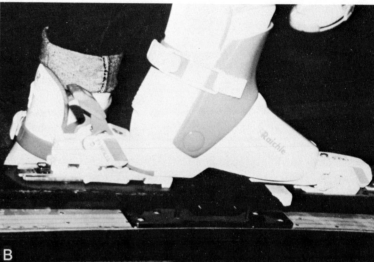

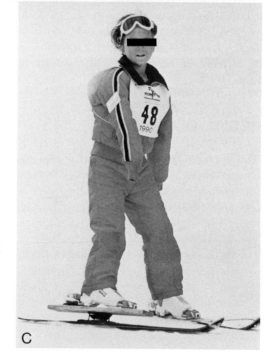

FIGURE 6–24
A, Preseason ski fitting using platform to equalize limb lengths. *B,* Binding and boot attached to platform. *C,* Skiing on the platform fitted to the right ski.

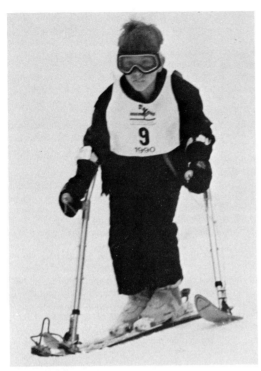

FIGURE 6–25
Child skiing with ski bra attached to tips of skis.

and feet, a ski bra is used (Fig. 6–25). A ski bra provides a more stable platform. As the child's skills improve, a bungie cord replaces the ski bra. A bungie cord is elastic, providing some stability but more flexibility. Finally, as the child becomes more proficient and confident, the bungie is removed, and the child is allowed independent control of both skis.

We feel that this program allows children to participate in sports that enhance many aspects of their lives. Skiing improves strength, endurance, balance, motivation, self-image, and self-confidence. I truly believe that the handicapped ski program changes the lives of these children in a positive way and ultimately helps them to cope in a world of adults without handicaps.

Alpine skiing may not be appropriate for your area, but involving your disabled patients in a sports program certainly is. Participation in sports is safe, healthy, rewarding, exciting, and gratifying for both patients and their families. Physicians can help and encourage them to become involved.

References

1. Academy of Pediatrics, Committee on Sports Medicine. Atlantoaxial instability in Down syndrome *Pediatrics* 74:152–154, 1984.
2. Achterman, C.A., and Kalamchi, A. Congenital deficiency of the fibula. *J Bone Joint Surg* 61B:133–137, 1979.
3. Aitken, G.T. Overgrowth of the amputation stump. ICIB 1:1, 1962.
4. Aitken, G.T. The child amputee. *Orthop Clin North Am* 3:447, 1972.
5. Aitken, G.T., and Franz, C.H. The juvenile amputee. *J Bone Joint Surg* 35A:659, 1953.
6. American Academy of Orthopaedic Surgeons. Critical needs of the child with long term orthopaedic impairment. Conference report. Park Ridge, IL, American Academy of Orthopaedic Surgeons, 1984.
7. Babcock, J.L. Spinal injuries in children. *Pediatr Clin North Am* 22:487–500, 1975.
8. Bennet, G.C., Rank, M., Roye, D.P., et al. Dislocation of the hip in trisomy 21. *J Bone Joint Surgery* 64B:289, 1972.
9. Bevan-Thomas, W.H., and Millar, E.A. A review of proximal focal deficiencies. *J Bone Joint Surg* 49A:1378, 1967.
10. Burke, D.C. Spinal cord trauma in children. *Paraplegia* 9:1–14, 1971.
11. Burke, D.C. Traumatic spinal paralysis in children. *Paraplegia* 11:268–276, 1974.
12. Bleck, E.E. *Orthopaedic Management of Cerebral Palsy.* Philadelphia, W.B. Saunders, 1987.
13. Bleck, E.E., and Nagel, D.A. *Physically Handicapped Children, A Medical Atlas for Teachers.* New York, Grune & Stratton, 1982.
14. Blum, C.E., and Kalamchi, A. Boyd amputations in children. *Clin Orthop* 165:138, 1982.
15. Cahuzac, M., Nichil, J., Olle, R., et al. Les fractures de fatigue de la rotule chez l'infirme moteur d'origine cerebrale. *Rev Chir Orthop* 65:87–90, 1979.
16. Chang, F.M., and Chang, N.S. They're reaching the highest mountain. *Sport Care Fitness* 2:43, 1989.
17. Chang, F.M. Gait analysis and intoeing. *Instruct Course Lect* 37:107, 1988.
18. Clark, M.W. Competitive sports for the disabled. *Am J Sports Med* 8(5):366, 1980.
19. Committee on Physical Fitness, Recreation, and Sports Medicine. Athletic activities by children with skeletal abnormalities. *Pediatrics* 51(5):949, 1973.
20. Coventry, M.D., and Johnson, E.W. Congenital absence of the fibula. *J Bone Joint Surg* 34A:941–955, 1952.
21. Curtis, K.A. *Injuries in Wheelchair Athletes.* Sports and recreational programs for the child and young adult. Proceedings of the Winter Park seminar. Park Ridge, IL, American Academy of Orthopaedic Surgeons, 1983.
22. Davidson, R.G. Atlantoaxial instability in individuals with Down syndrome: A fresh look at the evidence. *Pediatrics* 81:857–865, 1988.
23. DeBastiani, G., Aldefheri, R., Renzi-Brivo, L., et al. Limb lengthening by callus distraction (callotasis). *J Pediatr Orthop* 7:129, 1987.
24. Diamond, L.S., Lynne, D., and Sigman, B. Orthopedic disorders in patients with Down's syndrome. *Orthop Clin North Am* 12:57–71, 1981.
25. Farmer, A.W., and Laurin, C.A. Congenital absence of the fibula. *J Bone Joint Surg* 42A:1–12, 1960.
26. French, H.G., Burke, S.W., Roberts, J.M., et al. Upper cervical ossicles in Down syndrome. *J Pediatr Orthop* 7:69–71, 1987.
27. Giblin, P.E., and Micheli, L.J. Management of atlantoaxial subluxation with neurologic involvement in Down syndrome: A report of two cases and review of the literature. *Clin Orthop* 140:66–71, 1979.
28. Glasauer, F.E., and Cares, H.L. Traumatic paraplegia in infancy. *JAMA* 219:38–41, 1972.
29. Goldberg, M.J. *The Dysmorphic Child, An Orthopedic Perspective.* New York, Raven Press, 1987.
30. Gore, D.R. Recurrent dislocation of the hip in a child with Down's syndrome. *J Bone Joint Surg* 63A:823, 1981.
31. Guttmann, L., Silva, J., and Wyndham, C.H. Thermoregulation in spinal man. *J Physiol* (Lond.) 142:406, 1958.
32. Hachen, H.J. Spinal cord injury in children and adolescents: Diagnostic pitfalls and therapeutic considerations in the acute stage. *Paraplegia* 15:55–64, 1978.
33. Horal, J., Nachemson, A., and Scheller, S. Clinical and radiologi-

cal long term follow-up of vertebral fractures in children. *Acta Orthop Scand* 43:491–503, 1972.

34. Ilizarov, G.A., and Deviatov, A.A. Operative elongation of the leg with simultaneous correction of the deformities. *Orthop Travmatol Protez* 30:32, 1969.

35. Ilizarov, G.A., and Trohova, V.G. Operative elongation of the femur. *Orthop Travmatol Protez* 34:51, 1973.

36. Kewalramani, L.S., and Tori, J.A. Spinal cord trauma in children: Neurologic patterns, radiographic features, and pathomechanics of injury. *Spine* 5:11–18, 1980.

37. Kalamchi, A. *Congenital Lower Limb Deficiencies.* New York, Springer-Verlag, 1989.

38. Lancourt, J.E., Dickson, J.H., and Carter, R.E. Paralytic spinal deformity following traumatic spinal cord injury in children and adolescents. *J Bone Joint Surg* 63A:47–53, 1981.

39. Lawhon, S.M. Orthopaedic aspects of Down's syndrome. *Contemp Orthop* 20(4):395, 1990.

40. Leventhal, H.R. Birth injuries to the spinal cord. *J Pediatr* 56:447–453, 1960.

41. Marquardt, E. The multiple limb-deficient child. *In* American Academy of Orthopedic Surgeons, *Atlas of Limb Prosthetics.* St. Louis, C.V. Mosby, 1981, pp. 27–75.

42. Marquardt, E., and Correll, J. Amputation and prosthesis for the lower limb. *Int Orthop* 8:139, 1984.

43. Morrissy, R.T. *Lovell and Winter's Pediatric Orthopaedics.* Philadelphia, J.B. Lippincott, 1990.

44. National Association of Sports for Cerebral Palsy. *Classification and Sports Rules Manual.* New York, United Cerebral Palsy Associations, 1982.

45. O'Leary, H. *Bold Tracks, Skiing for the Disabled.* Evergreen, CO, Cordillera, 1987.

46. Paley, D. Current techniques of limb lengthening. *J Pediatr Orthop* 8:73, 1988.

47. Pueschel, S.M., and Scola, F.H. Atlantoaxial instability in individuals with Down syndrome: Epidemiologic, radiographic, and clinical studies. *Pediatrics* 80:555–560, 1987.

48. Rang, M. Dislocation of the hip in Down's syndrome. *J Bone Joint Surg* 54B:770, 1972.

49. Salenius, P., and Vannka, E. The development of the tibio-femoral angle in children. *J Bone and Joint Surg* 57:259, 1975.

50. Salter, R.B., and Harris, W.R. Injuries involving the epiphyseal plate. *J Bone Joint Surg* 45:587, 1963.

51. Special Olympics Bulletin. *Participation by Individuals with Down's Syndrome Who Suffer from Atlantoaxial Dislocation Condition.* Washington, D.C., Special Olympics, March 31, 1983.

52. *Special Olympics Rule Book.* Special Olympics International, New York, 1992.

53. Speer, D.P. The pathogenesis of amputation stump overgrowth. *Clin Orthop* 159:294, 1981.

54. *Sports and Recreational Programs for the Child and Young Adult with Physical Disability.* Proceedings of the Winter Park Seminar. Park Ridge, IL, American Academy of Orthopaedic Surgeons, 1983.

55. Tachdjian, M.O. *Pediatric Orthopedics.* Philadelphia, W.B. Saunders Co., 1990.

56. Van Nes, C.P. Rotation-plasty for congenital defects of the femur. Making use of the ankle of the shortened limb to control the knee joint of a prosthesis. *J Bone Joint Surg* 32B:12, 1950.

57. Wagner, H. Operative lengthening of the femur. *Clin Orthop* 136:125, 1978.

58. Wagner, H. Surgical lengthening of the femur. Report of 58 cases. *Ann Chir* 43:263, 1980.

59. Wilson, P.E., and Washington, R.L. Pediatric wheelchair athletics: Sports injuries and prevention. Unpublished data, 1991.

PSYCHOLOGICAL ASPECTS OF SPORT

Frances L. Geigle-Bentz, Ph.D.
Brandon G. Bentz, M.D.

Societal awareness of the need for and benefits of physical fitness has grown in recent years into a full-scale obsession. This awareness, along with a desire to deter disease through personal prevention, has created an explosion of athletic participants at every level from the recreational athlete to the avid competitor. Increased athletic participation has sparked a need to understand the benefits and detriments that accompany this activity. The greatest focus of investigation has been on the physiologic advantages and disadvantages brought about by sports participation. Recently, society has paid more attention to the psychological contributions of physical exertion. A complete understanding of the effects of participation in sports and physical fitness must include aspects of cognitive, social, and psychological health along with the physiologic aspects.

Children's unique experiences in sports and physical fitness require special approaches, especially since the societal realization of physical fitness benefits has brought about increasing pressure on children to participate in a wide variety of sports at younger ages. These special approaches, due to unusual age- and sport-related stressors, are best handled by individuals equipped to treat youth developmentally from cognitive, social, and psychological standpoints, such as sports psychologists or behavioral scientists.

Sports psychology is a rather new field in the United States. The use of sports psychologists has gained little acceptance among many athletes because, first, the validity of cognitive, social, and psychological effects is questioned and second, skepticism exists about the influence of the psychological expert. In addition, the child athlete is seen as participating in sports for recreational purposes, and therefore the psychological implications seem less important to the sports lay person. As a result, the importance of psychological issues has had little impact.

Despite a move in recent years toward administration of health care by a team of providers, the physician remains the primary health care provider for virtually all ailments. Although the psychological or behavioral specialist may have a greater understanding of the cognitive, social, or psychological problems faced by these youths, it is the physician who occupies the initial, if not central, position in the treatment of these problems. Consequently, it is the physician who has the opportunity to identify the psychological issues affecting the child athlete and organize as well as coordinate the intervention. Therefore, the physician must understand the psychological issues facing young people in sports and recognize their symptoms. An understanding of the motivational reasons for participation in sports, the implications of parental, coach, and peer pressures, performance anxiety, winning-losing attitudes along with the associated guilt, the effect of sports injuries on psychological health, and each child's unique disposition potentiates accurate interventions.

A repertoire of sound and basic approaches enables the practitioner to address many problems seen in the office. Such approaches may include goal-setting, imagery, and self-affirmation techniques. The practitioner will find that these and other avenues are not only easy but very effective. Should the practitioner find that a particular problem is beyond his or her professional expertise, a referral to a psychological specialist may be the most prudent action.

With a basic understanding of some psychological issues and a few methods of intervention, the practitioner will be better prepared to observe a broader spectrum of problems, coordinate treatment, and thus facilitate enhanced enjoyment and motivation to participate in sports, a greater sense of accomplishment, and enhanced self-esteem and self-confidence in the young athlete. Practitioners will further promote health by decreasing cognitive, social, psychological, and physiologic disease.

There is little research available about young people's involvement in athletics, especially from a psychological standpoint. Therefore, attempts are frequently made to apply research in adult athletes whenever necessary and wherever applicable to the young athlete. Although many of the issues addressed in this chapter are at times supported by studies of the adult in sports, children are not little adults and require a unique sensitivity to their needs as young individuals [153].

MOTIVATION AND REWARDS FOR PARTICIPATING IN SPORT

Young people are motivated to participate in sport activities for many different reasons, each carrying its own psychological impact. Research has found that youngsters participate in sports primarily for fun and enjoyment. Enjoyment is defined as excitement, personal achievement, performing and improving the specific sport skills, and positively comparing oneself to others in the sport activity. Fun is the feeling of happiness, being friendly and cheery as opposed to feeling sad and angry. Some children view being part of a team and having friends as important, but second to fun, whereas winning, rewards, and pleasing others are viewed as less important [186]. The need to win is far less important to children than is often assumed by adults, although winning can be a part of the broad concept of fun.

Rewards and accomplishments are important to older youth. Teens in some studies believe that participation in sports enhances one or more of the following parameters: (1) teaches the value of mastery and cooperation, (2) gives people a lifelong physical activity, (3) helps to make athletes good citizens, (4) develops competitive skills, (5) helps individuals obtain a career of status, (6) enhances self-esteem, and (7) develops good social skills that facilitate getting ahead and elevating social status [49].

It appears that young people have real reasons for sport participation, but more research is needed in this area. Based on the limited information available, it seems that children and youth participate in sports to have fun and that, at a certain point in their development, they also expect some benefits and rewards to accrue from their participation in sports.

BENEFICIAL AND DETRIMENTAL EFFECTS OF SPORT ACTIVITIES

There is evidence that participation in normal (as opposed to intense) sports activity can facilitate growth in a variety of ways for the athlete [172]. Generally, normal physical activity or training enhances the functional capabilities of youth. Physical involvement is perceived to be an effective tool in the development of certain psychosocial aspects of developing youth. Such traits as character development, social adjustment, positive personality traits and attitudes, emotional control, sportsman-like behavior, leadership skills, empathy for others, cooperation, self-discipline, self-confidence, initiative, courage, loyalty, and self-expression have all been related to sport and its benefits [77, 108, 109, 172]. It is believed that children, and boys in particular, who participate in sports enjoy greater social status than do their nonparticipating peers. Some studies characterize athletes as more outgoing and socially well adjusted than nonathletes [172]. Evidence indicates that competitive and cooperative behaviors begin at 3 to 4 years of age and that such survival skills can be developed through normal sport experience [35]. Generally, evidence points to the fact that young people who participate in normal sport display both physiologic and psychological benefits.

However, some problems are associated with intense and stressful sport activity, and some symptoms appear in normal sport conditions as well. For example, youth who are categorized as elite level participants and are involved in intense competitive activity have a higher potential for burnout than those who participate on a less competitive basis [59, 62]. Increasing data indicate that alarmingly high and increasing numbers of children are dropping out of all types of sport involvement [129].

Several criticisms related to specific problems in the normal psychological development of youngsters have been leveled against competitive sports programs for young athletes. Certain maladies are brought about by the undue pressure and emotional stress placed on children by overzealous adult leaders and the extreme emphasis placed by adults on winning. These stressors can cause unhealthy competitive attitudes that can result in serious interpersonally antisocial behavior [29, 43, 124, 130, 172]. When youngsters are threatened with elimination or are left out of play [199], they often respond with negative stressed states of anxiety and with increased physical strain [153]. These few examples alone reemphasize the need for parents, coaches, and sport practitioners to understand the psychological aspects of sport involvement and its implications for children and youth.

SPORTS ACTIVITY AND STRESS

Stress is a behavioral response to an environmental stimulus. Stress can be positive and beneficial, as in excitation and activation, or negative and detrimental, as in tension and anxiety [62]. This conceptualization of stress was first used popularly by Hans Selye in 1936. Since that time the word strain has been used as well to indicate the physiologic effects imposed by an event or trauma on an individual [35, 166].

Stress is displayed through a variety of responses and symptoms. Responses appear in the following three fashions: acute (reaction to a specific incident), delayed, and cumulative (response to the buildup of stress as in burnout). To be more specific, acute stress reactions are displayed through some of the following physical signs and symptoms: fatigue, nausea, muscle tremors, twitches, shock symptoms, profuse sweating, chills, dizziness, and gastrointestinal upset. In acute stress cognitive responses may include memory loss, anomia, difficulty in decision making and problem solving, confusion of trivial with major items, concentration problems, shortened attention span, and calculation difficulties. Emotional symptoms of acute stress reaction may be displayed by anxiety, fear, grief, depression, hopelessness, irritability, anger, and signs of being overwhelmed. Characteristics of delayed stress may appear as fears of stressor repetition, the above forms of physical and emotional symptoms, and even intrusive images. Cumulative stress, or burnout, is usually noted as a state of fatigue or frustration resulting from disappointment and excessive exposure to stress over a period of time. Physical and emotional exhaustion, apathy, and deterioration in performance characterize this stress response.

It is clear that stress can be present in the world of sports for the young athlete. Demands placed on athletes such as peer, parent, and coach pressure, performance anxiety, fear of injury, pressure to win, identity crises, time management problems, and even social isolation due to practice, travel, and competition cause athletes to feel and react as though they are in a state of negative stress. Some studies indicate that athletes under sport-related stress display more developmental conflicts and psychopathologic syndromes than do their nonathletic peers [151].

Because of the increased numbers of children and youth in competitive sport [179], the growing number of dropouts from youth athletics, the concern about burnout among elite athletes, the possible psychological and physical detriments associated with negative stress in athletics, and the real lack of clear understanding gained by overwhelming sound evidence, the desire to understand the psychological principles governing sport stress has increased significantly during the past 10 years [129]. The increased interest and activity in this area have intensified owing to a sense that not only can there be gains in sport through answers to the above problems, but also research and understanding in sport and exercise can help contribute to the prevention of disease and promotion of health overall [45].

THE STRESSORS OF SPORT ACTIVITY FOR CHILDREN AND YOUTH

To repeat and emphasize, among the many stressful situations for children and youth in sports, some particular aspects demand close attention. First, the presence of pressure from parents, coaches, and peers and even organizational pressures introduce factors that cause children and youth to behave in a stressed manner. Second, performance causes anxiety behaviors for many athletes and is a source of great concern for interested adults. Third, stress is frequently caused by the pressure to win and guilt when losses occur. Last, injury itself can be a source of tremendous stress, including the fear of injury and the fear of returning to normal sport activity from an injured state.

The physiologic and psychological changes that children go through occur so rapidly that it is extremely difficult to formulate a common theory as well as approaches for educators, trainers, parents, and coaches to enable them to understand and treat children's psychosocial difficulties. Owing to this complexity, a developmental approach seems most advantageous for use in sports psychology. This approach emphasizes the psychological and behavioral characteristics of children at different age levels and facilitates the examination of children from a social, cognitive, and psychological perspective [50].

Developmental Considerations

Practitioners usually find Erik Erikson's description of developmental stages useful. Briefly, Erikson describes the child from 4 to 6 years of age as in a stage of psychosocial development in which the child experiences an increased identification with parents, increased motor control and language development, and an expanding imagination. Play is essential for the resolution of internal crises and the management of inner conflicts during this period. If adult figures give punitive or unsupportive treatment, guilt develops [57]. This guilt may become very detrimental to the child's entire development should it not be resolved. Simply speaking, at this time in a child's life, play, with adult encouragement and support and without punishment, is the most helpful contribution to development.

The child between the ages of 6 and 11 years, the latency period, begins to solidify the ego through learning. The child feels that she or he is what she or he learns and masters. A healthy ego is based on perceived competence in certain basic skills. Early failures produce feelings of inadequacy and inferiority [57]. Once again, inadequacy and inferiority that are left unresolved can bring about detrimental effects on the child's overall development. In this stage it is important for young people to set goals, small ones if necessary, and to accomplish these goals with a sense of success.

With the onset of adolescence and throughout this developmental period, confusion reigns for both the child and the concerned adult. From approximately 12 to 21 years of age, youth seek identity. This period of confusion and uncertainty is one of social turmoil and search for stability and continuity in life [57]. The adolescent begins the process of separating himself from family and assuming independence, learning to manage intimacy, developing values, and recognizing career goals. Feelings of dependency are overcome as athletic, social, and academic demands take on greater importance [151].

The value of this developmental information has become increasingly apparent in recent years. For the early adolescent, high school–aged athletes are some of the most admired individuals in that stage's social milieu. The early adolescent's athletic ability qualifies the athlete for acceptance by peers, support from the family, and support from the community. Moving into the latter years of this developmental stage, the adolescent may find himself in an environment less supportive of psychosocial needs. Increased pressure to perform and more demands to practice are placed on the adolescent athlete. Adolescents who cannot perform up to these increased expectations in the latter part of this stage may experience self-doubt [151], internal conflict, and stress that are frequently difficult to understand by the athlete himself or to observe by the interested adult.

To maximize youth involvement at all stages of sport, developmental issues must play a part in the administration of health care. Additionally, developmental issues within particular stages must be addressed. Read [153] has suggested that the attempt should be made not to develop children for sport activities but to develop sport activities for children.

Pressures: Parent, Coach, Peer, Organization

Recent evidence relating to youth participation in sports appears to show certain consistent sociologic and psychological effects that in some instances may produce detrimental results. Some of the most striking negative effects result from pressures placed on the athlete by parents, coaches, and peers. Frequently, these pressures coalesce to form a fourth negative psychological influence, the effects of the entire sporting organization on the potentially positive learning experiences inherent in games and sports. In light of the fact that organized

sports have been around for a long time, as for example, Little League baseball, which was organized in 1936 in Williamsport, PA, an entire generation of youth have participated in sports without a great deal of psychological support and knowledge.

The first three pressures (parents, coaches, and peers) seem to exert a dynamic influence on the psychological health of young athletes. In a variety of sports, several investigators, including Loy and associates [118], Greendorfer and Lewko [73], Snyder and Spreitzer [175], and Higginson [87], found that the impact of parent, coach, and peer pressure changed across a child's athletic lifespan. The predominant socializing influence in the early years of both male and female athletes was the parents. Later, the major socializing agents shifted to peers, coaches, and teachers as parents assumed a less influential role. As major socializing agents, these three groups can be sources of dysfunction due to many types of pressures placed on athletes.

Parents. As an early socializing agent, parents' influence is displayed in a study by Pease and Anderson [146]. Children's attitudes toward such values as the importance of winning were fixed by 10 to 12 years of age. Parents have the greatest influence on the young athlete during these early years of life. It is logical to conclude that parental influence is the most important factor in shaping these values in the child athlete. Furthermore, Pease and Anderson found that these values change little after 10 to 12 years of age. Therefore, parental influence is a long-term determinant of values.

The nature of parental influence depends not only on the kind of influencing pressures exerted but also on the degree of influence. Balazo [7] found that in 24 female Olympic athletes *both* parents were highly supportive of the athlete's efforts from an early age. Snyder and Spreitzer [173] found that sport-centered practices supported by the entire family were very predictive of both male and female athletic participation in competitive sports. But as Devereux [44] comments, a parent who puts the accomplishments of the child before everything else does a grave disservice to the parent, the sport, and especially the child.

For example, evidence has demonstrated that parental influence can be too enthusiastic, conveying values that ultimately destroy the very athletic appetite that parents wish to nurture. Adults interested in organized children's sports have frequently observed parents whose main interest is to maximize the performance and benefits of their child at all costs. The parent does this by going to any length of sacrifice to further the child's progress. These actions can produce a negative reaction by the child to the point of avoiding activity and refusing to participate in the sport.

The beneficial effects of parent and child interactions were studied experimentally by McClelland [131] and

Sears and associates [165]. McClelland observed that parents who encouraged, joked, made suggestions, and generally supported their child's performance appeared to motivate their children to perform better while positively affecting character development. Sears and colleagues showed that children of relaxed, supportive parents were more self-confident, honest, and mature. In conclusion parental pressures have an impact, are a source of excitation, and can exert a positive or negative effect on the development of athletic values.

Coach. As an athlete continues to mature, the most significant socializing pressure ceases to be the parent and becomes the coach. The coach's influence is not so much on the development of attitudes toward winning and participation but on the player's self-esteem and self-perception. The coaching techniques utilized by the coach are crucial factors in the way an individual player views himself or herself in the sport and ultimately in society [167].

Coaching techniques are multifaceted behaviors that are difficult to classify and examine. One of the primary mechanisms by which coaches go about teaching the techniques of a given sport is the use of positive and negative reinforcements. These reinforcements provide feedback to the player on the efficacy of his or her athletic performance. They are also used to shape and develop desired behaviors within and outside sports contexts. When used unwisely, these reinforcements can produce negative, debilitating outcomes that impede the progress and performance of a given athlete [167].

Reinforcement is, however, a very broad concept. Therefore, Smith and associates [171] developed a group of categories, termed the Coaching Behavior Assessment System (CBAS), which is used to qualify and study coaching behaviors. Included among these categories are such behaviors as reinforcement, nonreinforcement, encouragement, and technical instruction in both general and mistake-contingent contexts, punishments, punitive technical instructions, organization, and others.

Not only is it important to identify the specific coaching behaviors, it is also essential to understand the effects of these behaviors. Smith and colleagues found that there were important age differences in the athletes' reaction to coaching behaviors. The youngest children paid attention predominantly to variations of negative behavior, children of intermediate ages responded to positive and supportive behaviors, and senior athletes responded to technically instructional and organizational behaviors. Additionally, a positive relationship was found between technical instructions, including encouragement in both general and mistake-contingent contexts, and the positive attitudes of players toward the coach. Punishment and punitive technical instructions were associated with negative feelings toward the coach. Although positive or negative feelings toward the coach may not be the most

essential factor in sports, it is valid to state that most athletes respond better in any situation if they feel positive rather than negative toward the coach.

What is ultimately of greatest importance is the athlete's self-concept and self-esteem. Smith and his colleagues found a highly significant correlation between supportive reinforcement and positive general self-esteem. Sinclair and Vealey [167] found that gains in self-confidence were highly associated with immediate feedback provided by coaches. Furthermore, athletes for whom coaches had high expectations were given more immediate feedback than athletes from whom little or no performance was expected. Additionally, Anshel and Hoosima [5] found that performance stability was more consistent when athletes were exposed to positive rather than negative feedback. To encapsulate, athletes feel good about themselves and do well when feedback from the coach is immediate and supportive.

Peers. Due to the nature of sports activity, athletes experience social relationships that are very complex. For example, the athlete must both compete and cooperate with teammates at various times and in various ways. On the one hand, an athlete may find that he or she feels more integrated into a team if several friendships are fostered within the team. On the other hand, the outstanding athlete may rise above the athletic performances of his or her peers, and this can create jealousy and resentment, even loneliness. The choice of whether or not to pursue an outstanding level of performance may be largely dependent on the interplay between the athlete's need to achieve personal recognition and the need for social acceptance. The successful athlete may find that he or she must reject his friends to become outstanding among his or her peers. The average athlete may find the social gratification of friendship more rewarding than the infrequent rewards of success. Even the gifted athlete may desire the social rewards more at times and may judiciously lose from time to time to thwart the jealousy of his or her friends. These peer pressures or stressors express themselves through overt observable behaviors [87].

Members of athletic teams tend to like one another more when they are experiencing success. A successful season makes members more prone to do things together outside the context of sports. As a consequence of this friendliness among team members, there may be reluctance to criticize teammates for poor performance, or athletes may adjust their style of play to convey friendship behaviors. This interteam bonding brings about a unique and sometimes difficult quality to identify, that of group cohesion, a team feeling a oneness that is a positive experience yet at the same time a personal stressor, especially in its development and maintenance.

Cohesion essentially reflects the reason why groups of people form and stay together. Group cohesion can be best understood by looking at certain variables. These variables may be divided into categories such as the personalities and needs of individual members, individual abilities, group size, and the task at hand. In addition, there are dynamic qualities that vary over time, such as feelings of group success and failure, stresses imposed by the group on each individual, the clarity and acceptability of group goals, and the type and quality of the leadership. Factors such as homogeneity of the group favor cohesion [53]. High coach or player turnover tends to reduce group cohesion [55]. A group cohesive quality is identified by such behaviors as the ability of individuals on the team to anticipate each other's movements and the timing of one member's actions to maximize another's actions [33]. Group cohesion has been shown to be easier to achieve in winning teams, whereas losing tends to destroy team cohesion [6, 147]. Findings indicate that regardless of whatever individual qualities each team member brings to the task, the quality of the group as a whole, that cohesive quality, is the most important factor in team success. Overall, peer and group interactions are complex and multifaceted components that influence the individual personally, socially, and athletically and also influence the team as a whole.

The above pressures from parents, coaches, and peers are all stressors, but they become detrimental or negative only if they are overzealously applied. In addition, Devereux [43] points out that these pressures frequently coalesce into an organized sports environment that can suppress the normal learning experiences that informal game playing can provide. Devereux believes that today's game culture has lost these crucial developmental experiences owing to excessive adult supervision and control. Devereux believes that important educational experiences fostered by play and games are eliminated by rigid and organized sport activities. Children's games and play activities represent miniature safe models of a wide variety of cultural and social situations and concerns. Children can experiment with different personal styles and can more easily practice anxiety management in less rigid experiences [148]. The famed Jean Piaget [149] noted that social rules to developing children originally appear to be part of an external situation that is defined and reinforced by powerful adults. In the early stages of development, children attempt to avoid punishment and maintain the good will of their parents through obedience to these rules, and they do so especially in the rigid context of formal game. Informal games and play with peers offer a unique opportunity for young people to internalize social rules and formulate their own personal guidelines. Parsons and Bales [143] theorized that when an equality of power is perceived by the child as existing between the athlete and his or her peers, the perception allows the child to develop social relationships guided by relative universalistic principles and

rules that are equally followed by all participants. What rigid, formal, and organized sports have done is to remove the social opportunities for incidental learning that occur through spontaneous, self-organized, and self-regulated children's games.

Whether parents push too hard or not hard enough, whether parents create appropriate values, whether the coach fosters a positive self-esteem or destroys it, whether the athlete's peers participate constructively or destructively, and whether the child has enough informal game playing experiences to facilitate social growth may not be things that practitioners can control or even observe. Nevertheless, knowledge of these psychological effects can allow the practitioner perhaps to intervene, helping young athletes to cope with problems that have become burdensome and negatively stressful.

Performance Anxiety

Anxiety is frequently defined as an emotional state consisting of feelings such as worry, apprehension, nervousness, and tension combined with an arousal of the autonomic nervous system [177]. Anxiety is an unpleasant reaction, which, if persistent, can lead to such stress-related disorders as insomnia and headaches [178]. Chronically high levels of anxiety can interfere with the performance and enjoyment of almost any aspect of sports participation [126]. Although anxiety reactions occur infrequently in youth sports, there is a need to address the problem.

There is a belief that performance anxiety is ultimately related to perceptions of competence and motives for participation in sports. Harter [84, 85] proposed a theory about anxiety, expanding on former thoughts. Competence motivation theory suggests that individuals possess an innate desire to feel and express competence and control in any achievement-oriented situation. A positive result is associated with successful mastery of a particular experience. This positive response or mastery results in reinforcement of the "competence motive." An athlete who perceives the lack of requisite competence for mastery or the lack of adequate situational control experiences a negative effect, which takes the form of performance anxiety. This performance anxiety weakens the competence motive and feelings of competence.

Anxiety is a complex phenomenon, and, despite much study in the last few decades, it is a condition that still defies clear understanding and treatment. Conceptualization and measurement of anxiety have been enormously aided and advanced by Spielberger's study [176], which divides the general anxiety response into two types: state anxiety (A-state) designates an individual's reaction to a perceived situational threat, whereas trait anxiety (A-trait) is related to personal anxiety characteristics that remain constant throughout many different situations. Building on these thoughts and theories, a growing body of anxiety research specifically related to sports has developed in the form of competitive trait anxiety and competitive state anxiety [176].

Competitive trait anxiety is a "construct that describes individual differences in the tendency to perceive competitive situations as threatening" [126]. High levels of competitive trait anxiety occur when athletes perceive that they do not have the basic requisites needed for success in the competitive task. In one study, boys who experienced frequent physical competitive trait anxiety symptoms were found to have lower self-esteem, felt greater upset following a poor performance, and preferred to avoid sport competition and the anxiety related to possible negative results [112]. Cognitive competitive trait anxiety symptoms were more likely to occur in the presence of perceptions of parental or coach shame and upset, greater negative adult evaluation, and conditions of general parental pressure. It was found by Lewthwaite and Scanlan [112] that individuals with high competitive trait anxiety tended to avoid stress-inducing events.

The second division of general anxiety in the sport context is competitive state anxiety. Davidson and Schwartz [39] and Liebert and Morris [113] utilized a multidimensional view of state anxiety that separated the mental or cognitive component from the physical or somatic part. The cognitive component of state anxiety was defined by negative thoughts, difficulty with concentration, and disbursed attention, whereas the physical component encompassed strong body signs of anxiety such as autonomic arousal. Cues to somatic state anxiety are thought to be of short duration and include conditioned responses to environmental stimuli such as the locker room, the stadium, or fans. Many times these cues remain unchanged throughout a season, and therefore somatic anxiety shows a characteristic and consistent pattern prior to competition, with rising anxiety as competition draws near, peaking as competition begins, and then rapidly falling off after the onset of competition [21]. Cognitive state anxiety is believed to arise when personal expectations of success become negative. This type of anxiety accounts for the worry athletes experience several days before competition. This worry remains constant up to and during competition unless changes in expectations occur.

Research has consistently shown an inverted-U relationship between performance and general state anxiety. This research has demonstrated that optimal amounts of anxiety actually enhance performance through the attainment of optimal physiologic readiness, but increasing or decreasing anxiety beyond this optimal level causes performance to fall off [107].

To repeat, the literature on anxiety indicates that performance is affected by anxiety. The relationship is very complex and multifaceted but is undeniably important. Therefore, it is worth serious continuous investigation by practitioners involved in the treatment and care of young athletes.

Winning and Losing

Green Bay Packers coach Vincent Lombardi once said that "winning isn't everything, it's the only thing." This statement typifies a societal value. Leonard [111] pointed out that many scholars believe that a society's basic social structure is characterized by its sports and games. Today we are witnessing the end of a social structure based on honor and a movement toward one of winning above all else. Competition need not be detrimental if it is put in proper perspective: "Like a little salt, it adds zest to the game and life itself." But competition produces more losers than winners. Losing can become a habit and can therefore affect self-worth and self-esteem, especially if winning is valued above all else. Losing is an undesirable state to be in, a state of stress, of disequilibrium—an unhealthy state.

Many parents do not appear to question the impact of the "winning above all" value on a child's development because this value is often imparted indirectly and appears to be a cultural norm in American society. Competition and the importance of winning are taught to children at a very young age [146]. As was stated earlier in this chapter, it is parents who have the greatest influence on their children in the very early years of athletic development. This is the time in which youngsters' attitudes toward participation and winning in competition begin to take form. Piaget stated that competitive behavior begins about the time youngsters start to understand the rules that govern winning and losing, to perceive success and failure, and to compare their efforts with others'. Piaget believed that this development begins around 4 to 5 years of age. In support of these hypotheses, Greenberg [72] found that children before the age of 3 showed no competitive behavior, whereas by the age of 5, 10% of surveyed youngsters exhibited some type of competitive response. The findings seem to indicate that competitive behavior is a learned characteristic [72]. Competitive behavior in youngsters has subsequently been characterized as the ability to conceptualize (1) something worth striving for, (2) the realization that the "self" has an opportunity to acquire that something, and (3) the realization that another individual is also striving to acquire the same goal.

White [191] explored competitive development from another perspective. In the early stages children begin to explore their environment, learning autonomy by relying on themselves as individuals. Subsequently, they pay increasing attention to the acquisition and mastery of motor skills, fostering self-esteem and assertiveness. Following the mastery of skills, children begin to impersonate adult behaviors, bringing about a knowledge of power roles and their perceived importance in competition and winning. Finally, in the later stages, peer groups begin to take on an increasing degree of importance. Evaluations of performance in competitive situations from both peers and oneself serve to reinforce competitive behaviors positively or negatively. A positive evaluation encourages the development of a competitive mind set, open to feedback and growth, whereas negative evaluations tend to enforce a passive attitude, reducing the exposure. Scanlan [161] noted that with continuous positive evaluations, a child becomes an ''evaulation seeker,'' continuously displaying behavior that can be considered competitive.

Coaches are involved in the development of winning or losing attitudes. Chaumeton and Duda [29] found significant variations among coaching behaviors in competitive environments. Winning had increased significance for coaches with higher levels of competition, reinforcing the competitive attitudes already established by the young athlete's parents early in life.

Competition, the increased significance of winning, and the development of winning or losing attitudes affect young people in many ways. Generally, the more important winning is, the greater the chance that a loss will be attributed to something or someone other than the individual [154]. In addition, members of successful teams attribute winning to more controllable and stable factors than do unsuccessful groups. Individuals who evaluate their accomplishments of a task, regardless of the outcome, with more positive attitudes tend generally to perform better than individuals who evaluate outcomes with a negative bias [80]. The fun of participation can bring about a positive effect that in turn potentiates self-evaluation with a positive attitude, thus bringing about better performance [186]. Hardy and Silva [82] found that athletes who are tense, frustrated, apprehensive, submissive, and humble are more fearful of the consequences of success than those who are relaxed, unfrustrated, self-assured, assertive, venturesome, and controlled. Guilt, with all of its negative feelings and stressors, naturally follows for the athlete who feels the essential importance of winning and the practical effects of a loss. This situation can leave a young person feeling helpless and unduly stressed.

Winning is not everything! The feeling that winning is a desired goal, to be attained at all costs, can be very detrimental. As Burke and Kleiber point out [19], it is more constructive to promote cooperation through the forming and maintaining of children's self-made games. Competition, winning, and losing are real-life events, and young people need opportunities to experience these normal happenings. What may be most essential and fruitful is to allow children to learn from the experience and to minimize the potential harm.

Injury

Despite an estimated 3.3 million injuries that occur every year, minimal investigation has been done on the psychology of athletic injury [103]. This fact again highlights the desperate need for research and treatment strategies aimed at addressing the psychological implications that may accompany athletic injury. The psychology of athletic injury must be examined from two perspectives. On the one hand, there is evidence that a psychological predisposition to athletic injury may exist, and this should be dealt with if the opportunity for diagnosis occurs. On the other hand, an athlete who has a debilitating injury can undergo psychophysiologic responses that, if untreated, can impair or prevent successful rehabilitation and reentry into sports.

If the sport practitioner has an opportunity to evaluate an athlete's preinjury psychological state, a thorough history and physical examination can reveal predisposing factors. The major emphasis of recent research into predisposing factors has been on the relationship between stress and injury. Initially, Holmes and Rahe [89] found that individuals with high life stress, which is defined generally as a life filled with major changes, seem to be at greater risk of disease than individuals with low levels of stress. The relationship between stress and injury or accident has been confirmed by Stuart and Brown [180].

More specifically, in analyzing the life stress–accident relationship to athletic injuries in football players, an early study discovered that high life stress players have a greater probability of incurring injury than low life stress players [88]. A modified version of the life stress scale of Holmes and Rahe was developed for athletes and sport. This social and athletic readjustment rating scale (SARRS) reestablished the original conclusions of Holmes and Rahe [11, 30, 37, 89]. Although all of the initial research on the relationship between life stressors and injury was done on football players, Lysens and associates [121] and Kerr and Minden [99] found a clear correlation between high life stress individuals and the predisposition toward injury in physical education students and gymnasts.

Certain objections have been made to Holmes and Rahe's research assumption that all major life changes are stressful and deleterious to an individual's health. Other researchers have shown that only negative life events are related to negative outcomes [81, 145, 184]. In addition, most of the research to date has paid little attention to the complexity of life stressors, the individuals affected, or the physiologic and psychological outcomes for each individual or stressor. A working model was proposed by Williams and Andersen [193]. The benefits of this model are that it not only proposes certain stressful life events but also sheds light on other aspects of stress and psychosocial factors that may influence the occurrence of injury. Additionally, this model suggests that some physiologic mechanisms are theoretically responsible for mediating these stressors, and finally, it suggests several specific interventions that can be taken by the practitioner [3].

At the center of this model is the stress response, which is mediated primarily through physiologic or attentional responses that are requisite for the specific sports task. Individuals with high life stress may exhibit a response that brings about increased general muscle tension leading to rapid muscle fatigue, a narrowing of the visual field that does not allow the individual to attend to the stimuli necessary to avoid athletic injury, and a heightened distractibility that demands more attention to extraneous stimuli. These stress responses can be modified by many factors. One's cognitive appraisal of the demands of the task, the resources at hand, and the consequences of the task achievement can have either a positive or negative influence on the stress response. The individual's personality, such as his or her competitive trait anxiety or achievement motivation, can also influence the response. Additionally, the individual's history of stress including life stressors, daily hassles, and previous injury stressors all influence the response. Finally, the individual's coping resources, such as support systems and stress management skills, may have a bearing on this stress reaction.

If the practitioner believes that a particular athlete is at high risk for psychogenerated sports injury, a number of interventions can be used to prevent injurious outcomes. Through such interventions as relaxation skills, imagery, and desensitization, to name a few, the psychological implications can be managed. Some of these techniques will be discussed later in this chapter. Although the practitioner may find occasion to use a preventive approach to sports injuries, most psychological treatments that are implemented are usually of the postinjury type. The timing is primarily due to the tendency to seek assistance only after an injury or disease has occurred.

Early in the development of theory about the relationship between injury and psychology, psychiatrist Kübler-Ross [105] determined that terminally ill patients go through stages of denial, anger, bargaining, depression, and acceptance. From this work, Kübler-Ross hypothesized that the injured athlete also goes through a similar grief cycle, but the athlete should be considered as having unique characteristics that cannot be generalized from other patient populations.

Little [115] found that 72.5% of athletes with neuroses experienced some sort of physical illness or injury prior to the development of their psychological symptoms, whereas only 10.9% of nonathletes experienced similar maladies. Furthermore, despite the finding that the athletic population was more extroverted and vigorous than nonathletes, the prognosis for recovery from injury among athletes was much poorer than among nonathletes. Little concluded that a preoccupation with fitness and sports placed the athlete in a vulnerable position that predisposed him or her to neuroses as a result of mandatory exercise deprivation.

Smith and colleagues [169] examined the presence, type, magnitude, and time course of the emotional responses that occurred throughout the entire injury process from onset to return to participation in sports. Using an Emotional Response to Injury Questionnaire (ERIQ) and the Profile of Mood States (POMS) evaluation, levels of frustration, depression, and anger were studied. Denial was found to be absent, and global mood disturbances were found instead of the stages postulated by Kübler-Ross. The severity of the injury, the perception of recovery, and the loss of athletic fulfillment were found to be the probable bases for the mood disturbances. In contrast to Smith's results, Weiss and Troxel [188] found that disbelief, rage, depression, tension, fatigue, and somatic complaints were commonly associated with injury. Chan and Grossman [28] found elevated levels of depression, anxiety, and confusion and lower self-esteem in "prevented runners." In addition, Morgan [135] found that prevented runners scored higher on a negative mood scale of depression, tension, and confusion than continuing runners. Morgan attributed this to loss of a coping strategy for those who used physical exertion as a stress management technique.

Although none of these studies were conducted with "elite" athletes, knowledge of these emotional responses following injury in athletes provides the practitioner with some understanding of why certain athletes choose to resume physical activity or sport contrary to the recommendations of their coaches and physicians [45]. These athletes may find that coping with the physical discomfort of the injury is easier than coping with the emotional discomfort experienced in the absence of exercise. Nonetheless, the emotional response to injury is influenced by many personality factors, history of stressors, predisposing psychological influences, and normal coping skills.

Tunks and Bellissimo [183] organized normal coping skills into three categories: (1) the appraisal-focused coping strategy in which the athlete attempts to understand and find meaning in a crisis; (2) the problem-focused strategy in which the athlete confronts the reality of a crisis by dealing with the tangible consequences through constructing a more gratifying situation; and (3) the emotion-focused strategy in which the athlete aims to cope with the feelings brought about by the crisis and to maintain an effective balance.

Carmen and colleagues [24] and Pierce [150] both noted that noninjured athletes seem to prefer physical exertion to verbalization as a normal means of coping with stress. Scanlan and associates [162] found that 23% of the elite figure skaters they interviewed believed that skating was an adequate means of coping with stressors. The development of neuroses in athletes following an injury may be due to deprivation of a perceived normal method of coping [115, 116].

Wiese and Weiss [192] proposed a four-stage model of injury rehabilitation. The first stage is simply the state of recognition, the "actual injury" that is a stressor itself. Second, the athlete appraises the situation that caused the injury. The injury may be ascribed to such things as self, equipment failure, opponents or teammates, the inherent risk of the sport, or a coaching error. Also, the injury may be appraised with regard to its severity and impact on the athlete's future goals. These factors influence the emotional response, which is the third stage. This stage may influence such factors as the immune response, which can be counterproductive to the healing process. The psychological (coping techniques) and physiologic consequences of injury finally follow in the last stage.

Injury is very important in the life of an athlete. Thus, the prevention and care of injuries must bring together every possible resource available to hasten the participants' reentry into athletics. This care must address the psychological implications because neglect of these factors can slow recovery and increase the likelihood of recurrence.

MANAGEMENT TECHNIQUES

Although research on management techniques in sports for youth is limited, the management of sport-related issues from a psychological standpoint demands that serious consideration be given to developmental issues. Understanding of development includes physical, intellectual, social, and psychological perspectives. Although both developmental issues and management techniques have been briefly addressed in this chapter, it is suggested that a more thorough review of both these subjects may be undertaken by the reader, using references given at the end of the chapter.

With regard to management techniques, the most basic, simple, and easy methods are usually the most effective. Common sense is, in addition, an excellent guide. If basic nonintrusive techniques and common sense do not have an observable effect, expert advice is always available. The following suggested management aids are a few of the many that exist and are meant to be only examples of possible approaches. Many of these aids overlap and can be used with individuals or with groups or teams to deal with motivation and fun, performance anxiety, parent, coach, and peer pressures, team organization, winning and losing, and injuries.

Management techniques can be divided into several categories. First, recognizing and dealing with stress while facilitating concentration and control require relaxation, anxiety management, and attention control techniques. Second, techniques helpful in improving practice and activating an athlete include imagery, motivation, and the psych-up pep talk. Third, young people need positive attitudes and definite objectives to potentiate success. This can be accomplished through the techniques of goal setting, self-esteem and confidence building, and the use of rewards and reinforcements. Last, there are many general issues that need to be addressed such as persistence, toughness and aggression, and competition and cooperation. Injury, burnout, and dropping out are areas of concern, but suggested interventions for these involve all of the above techniques. Expert counseling is always available should basic techniques and common sense fail.

Dealing with Stress, Anxiety, and Control

The following techniques are most effective if basic and simple, since they are generally needed by athletes at one point or another.

Stress Anticipation, Stress Management, and Relaxation Techniques

Anticipating stress before an athletic event means that one does the job of worrying prior to the event. Anticipation can prove to be one of the most useful stress management techniques if the athlete understands the physiologic and cognitive components of the stressor and can effectively use techniques to control the impact. Effective techniques include cognitively going through the details of the athletic experience, practicing feedback, increasing real situational awareness, and shifting control from external to internal cues [64].

The first step toward managing stress is recognition by the athlete that she or he is experiencing stress. Symptoms can be observed physiologically, psychologically, or behaviorally. Physiologic symptoms include increased heart rate, sweating, pupil dilation, increased muscle tension, "cotton mouth," and frequent urination.

Psychological changes include worry, feelings of being overwhelmed, inability to make decisions, confusion, inability to concentrate, out of control feelings, or feeling "different." Behavioral manifestations of stress may be rapid talking, nail biting, foot tapping, muscle twitching, pacing, scowling, increased blinking, yawning, trembling, or a broken voice [127].

Simply stated, the practitioner of sports medicine can do many things to lessen stress and reduce uncertainty through answering any questions the athlete may have about stressors or management techniques, removing hazards that may produce anxiety such as poor equipment, eliminating surprise, avoiding humiliation, being consistent, letting the athlete know that the contributions he or she makes are a valuable asset to the team, diminishing the importance of the activity for the athlete by diminishing the vital importance of winning without displaying disinterest, and downplaying or eliminating practice or recognition awards and elite groups. All of the above may be avenues for consideration [127].

One of the most beneficial ways of reducing stress is the use of relaxation techniques. Relaxation imaging, progressive relaxation training, and biofeedback relaxation are but a few of these techniques. Elimination of negative self-talk by using symptomatic desensitization techniques and "thought-stopping" is a viable approach in the management of cognitive stress [127]. Relaxation basically involves the following three steps in the management of stress: (1) self-observation, helping the athlete get to know himself, (2) elimination of maladaptive thoughts and beliefs (thought-stopping), and (3) cognitive development of new behaviors (relaxation imaging) [179].

Stress and Anxiety Management

Anxiety and its symptoms were discussed earlier in this chapter in the section on stress and performance anxiety. Practitioners may find that one technique that is helpful in controlling anxiety is stress inoculation training [122]. The three-phase technique is made up of five to seven sessions, each approximately 45 minutes in duration. The first contact with the athlete is an educational one in which the athlete is given information about stress, how it occurs, and the relationship between stress and performance. The participant is encouraged to describe his or her feelings and experiences during any period of the athletic performance. Each session that follows this initial encounter teaches the athlete how to relax progressively, rehearse mentally, visualize anxiety-provoking situations, and make positive self-remarks. In these sessions the athlete cognitively experiences situations that provoke increasing anxiety. An intentional attempt is made to intensify subsequent encounters. Thus,

through simulated experiences, the athlete develops the ability to cope with his or her anxiety.

The three phases of stress inoculation are the education phase, in which the athlete learns about the impairment; the rehearsal phase, in which the athlete learns to use coping skills appropriate to the particular problem and to develop coping self-statements, visualizations, and mental exercises; and the last phase, in which the athlete has an opportunity to practice these coping skills in gradually more stressful situations. Normally, such interventions are best accomplished with the guidance of a skilled behavioral scientist.

Attention Control

The ability to concentrate and prevent inappropriate distractions is essential for an athlete. Little research on attention control exists, but it appears that an attention disruption or loss of control can be easily counteracted using concentration and association techniques. Loss of control is recognized by increased levels of arousal and a change in the normal ability to focus or attend. Other signs may include increased muscle tension, changes in breathing, twitching movements in or around the face, increased jaw muscle tension, and extraneous behaviors such as yawning, stretching, laughing, or crying.

To facilitate attention control it is important not to overload the athlete with information. One or two pieces of constructive advice, spoken slowly, provide structure and clear direction. For example, asking the athlete to repeat what has been verbalized and making eye contact enable the athlete to focus on listening. During a performance, encouraging the athlete to focus his or her attention on a few specific critical cues such as steps in the movement or a location in the arena gives some structure. Distracting the athlete from the event during breaks reduces possible anxiety that may be the result of ongoing attention control problems. Most of all, reassuring the athlete that his feelings are normal and that they will pass is extremely beneficial [138]. The centering procedure is a training exercise that can be practiced physically and mentally and is especially effective in gaining attention control. The procedure is more complex than other procedures but after a few practice sessions it can become incorporated into a repertoire of behaviors that is available to the athlete should concentration become a problem during performance [138].

Practice and Activation

To prepare for a performance and to "psych-up" for the actual event, mental exercises such as the following are effective.

Imagery

Imagery is cognitively experiencing a situation in the absence of external stimuli. In other words, imagery simulates a real-life experience through mental exercise [127]. Imagery is used to help athletes practice motor skills, rehearse strategies, and acquire psychological dexterity. Imagery helps the athlete develop a mental framework through a three-part program of sensory awareness with vivid training and practice control. A facilitator or practitioner can aid in the development of this technique by providing an environment without distractions.

Most important to success with imagery is accurate and systematic practice of the technique. Mental accuracy, even with the use of guided instruction on videotape, helps, and sight, sound, touch, smell, and taste stimulation intensifies sensory awareness and the vividness of the experience [127].

Motivation, Activation, and Psych-Up

Motivating an athlete requires an understanding of the individual and a knowledge of the techniques that are most effective in certain situations. Motivation is an interactive process between the motivator and the athlete. Some athletes are intrinsically motivated, whereas others are extrinsically motivated. In almost all cases, positive reinforcement accomplished by catching the athlete doing something right and reinforcing the behavior through praise or encouragement motivates and activates the athlete.

Reinforcement should be given as soon as possible after the event and should be as clear and specific as possible. It should be given continuously during the initial learning phases and intermittently once skill has been developed in order to maximize the effect. Positive reinforcement should not be given for undesirable behaviors, and punishment should be avoided if possible. The practitioner should control the sport environment to reduce stress and chaos while exciting, arousing, or activating the athlete. Generally most exciting for an athlete is goal setting. Athletes are automatically motivated when they are involved in setting goals for practice or performance.

Sport practitioners can "psych-up" athletes through the pep talk. The purpose of such an experience is to motivate athletes to want to win. The pep talk is no more than a last-minute effort to maximize psychological and physiologic readiness. The best motivation is guidance, direction, support, and excitation of the athlete throughout preparation in a constant and devoted manner, even during times when results are not optimum [23].

Building Positive Attitudes and Objectives for Success

If success occurs and self-esteem is enhanced, the athlete grows. Success is potentiated through techniques of goal setting, confidence building, and, as stated before, reinforcement.

Goal Setting

The satisfaction generated by collaborative team goal setting in sports cannot be understated. Studies support the idea that young people are capable of setting performance standards and that they will use these standards to evaluate their own performance [90]. This is particularly true if long-term goals are reduced to a series of achievable, intermediate, and short-term goals.

Two types of goals can be utilized—product and process. Product goals define an end result to be achieved through performance of the athletic task, whereas process goals define the steps in the performance that the participant will take in preparing or actually performing the task. These goals should specify measurable milestones that are achievable, realistic, and worthwhile to the performer. The availability of feedback is necessary to provide a means of evaluating progress. Most important, the athlete must accept and be committed to the defined goals for the process to work [83]. Use of this technique will help the practitioner to circumvent the onset or development of burnout and performance anxiety as well as facilitate a sense of accomplishment.

Self-Esteem and Confidence Building

Self-confidence is always enhanced when an athlete has realistic expectations about achieving success, not necessarily when he believes that he or she will win. Self-confidence is based on a person's feelings of self-worth and self-esteem. Athletes who feel successful become more self-confident, gain greater self-esteem, and feel more worthy, making them more motivated. On the other hand, athletes who experience initial failure become insecure and feel less worthy. A mistake does not destroy a self-confident athlete, but insecure athletes fear the anxiety brought on by a mistake or failure so intensely that they are easily intimidated and act timidly, increasing the possibility of failure. A spiraling exposure ensues from negative expectations to failure to insecurity to further negative expectations, failure, and more insecurity.

Self-fulfilling prophecies need not be negative. Positive yet realistic expectations can potentiate positive results. A technique used to encourage athletes is the use of affirmation techniques such as "I can, I will" statements. These statements aid in the self-affirmation that athletes may need to form a stable basis for self-esteem. Self-affirmation can generate self-confidence. Wholesome self-confidence in athletes is also facilitated through learning the techniques and tactics of the sport well. In addition, positive feedback about the athlete's self-worth apart from the sport is affirming and generally aids in the overall result—confidence [127].

Reward and Reinforcement

Although reinforcement and reward were addressed earlier in the chapter, it is important to address briefly the division between intrinsic and extrinsic rewards. If an athlete performs in order to feel delight or joy, he is seeking intrinsic or internal rewards. On the other hand, if he performs to gain recognition and rewards from others, he needs extrinsic and external reinforcements. It is only when an athlete perceives success and reinforcement that he will feel fulfilled and have fun [23].

It is helpful to identify the reinforcements that appear to be best for each young athlete. However, it is the immediate and personal feedback, rather than the external rewards of status or winning, that conveys the quality that is of primary importance to young athletes—the growth of self-esteem and self-worth [23].

Individual and Group Issues

Unique and sometimes conflicting issues exist in athletics such as the need to be tough in an environment that encourages aggressive behavior and the need to compete and cooperate at the same time.

Toughness and Aggression

Great athletes are thought to have a strong will to win. The will to survive and the need to be tough at all times are present in all living organisms. Sport participation may be similar to life in that many athletes describe sport involvement as survival, persistence, total concentration, commitment, motivation [23], and even aggression [46].

In attempting to understand and manage aggression, it is necessary to determine which athletes are likely to be aggressive in competition, ascertain the requirements of the sport and the content of the behavior that constitutes excessive aggression, predict situations that will likely

cause team aggression, and be able to calm an overly aggressive athlete or the team as a whole.

A number of factors may heighten the probability of an aggressive act. These factors include an unfit player; a player with a hostile group of spectators; a losing team; a loss by a close score; competition between two teams that are close in rank or standing; competition between teams that are very different (racially, ethnically, or politically); a competitive situation that has a history of hostility; and an aggressive act by one individual that goes undisciplined or brings about an unfair advantage [35]. Recognizing these factors and dealing with them before an aggressive act occurs teaches discipline and good sportsmanship to young athletes.

Competition and Cooperation

Competitive and cooperative behaviors are present in practice as well as actual performance situations and may bring about anxiety that can be self-defeating. It is important to note individual differences in practice situations prior to competition. Helping athletes to realize appropriate sportsman-like values and attitudes toward success is usually more easily accomplished than demanding competitive behavior from them in a nondestructive cooperative manner.

If the stress aroused during intersquad competition becomes too great, it is important to direct the athlete to an unstructured fun program during a particular practice. If the stress of a forthcoming competition is inordinate, it will help to lessen the threat of losing, encourage the athlete to see the rivals in human terms, or try to put the forthcoming competition into a proper, gamesman-like perspective [35]. Above all, it is essential to develop not only competitive athletes for sport activity but also cooperative citizens for a future society.

Injury, Burnout, and Counseling

If the sample strategies given earlier, including counseling as an alternative, are used by leaders in youth sports, the problems of prevention and treatment of injury, burnout, and dropout, and psychosocial issues will be more clearly understood, and sporting activities will be a joy, a pleasure, and a growing experience for children and adolescents.

CONCLUSION

Educational philosophers and leaders such as Socrates, Aristotle, Comenius, John Locke, and John Dewey advocated play and sporting activity as an important educational experience for children. As Lawther states, children's physical activity and sport loses much of its meaningful pleasure, educational and recreational value, mental health value, and skill-attainment value if it becomes an obligation, without joy or fun. Our job is to ensure that the value of fun endures and that the benefits are experienced by children and youth today and always [179].

References

1. Abernethy, B. Expert-novice differences in perception: How expert does the expert have to be? *Can J Sport Sci* 14(1):27–30, 1989.
2. Alberts, M. E. Parental interference. *Iowa Med* 76(7):324, 1986.
3. Andersen, M. B., and Williams, J. M. A model of stress and athletic injury: Prediction and prevention. *J Sport Exerc Psychol* 10:294–306, 1988.
4. Andersen, M. B., and Williams, J. M. Gender and sport competition anxiety: A re-examination. *Res Q Exerc Sport* 58:52–56, 1987.
5. Anshel, M. H., and Hoosima, D. E. The effect of positive and negative feedback of casual attributions and motor performance as a function of gender and athletic participation. *J Sport Behav* 12(3):119–130, 1989.
6. Arnold, G. Team Cohesiveness, Personality Traits, and Final League Standing of High School Varsity Basketball Teams. Thesis, Ithaca, NY, Ithaca College, 1972.
7. Balazo, E. K. Psycho-social study of outstanding female athletes. *Res Q* 46(3):267–274, 1975.
8. Bar-Eli, M. and Tenenbaum, G. Game standings and psychological crisis in sport: Theory and research. *Can J Sport Sci* 14(1):31–37, 1989.
9. Blais, M. R., and Vallerand R. J. Multimodel effects of electromyographic biofeedback: Looking at children's ability of control precompetitive anxiety. *J Sport Psychol* 8:283–303, 1986.
10. Blinde, E. M., and Greendorfer, S. L. Structural and philosophical differences in women's intercollegiate sport programs and the sport experience of athletes. *J Sport Behav* 10(2):59–72, 1987.
11. Bramwell, S. T., Masuda, M., Wagner, N. N., et al. Psychological factors in athletic injuries: Development and application of the social and athletic readjustment rating scale (SAARS). *J Hum Stress* 1:6–20, 1975.
12. Brand, H. J., Hanekom, J. D. M., and Scheepers, D. Internal consistency of the sport competition anxiety test. *Perceptual Motor Skills* 67:441–442, 1988.
13. Bredemeier, B. J., Weiss, M. R., Shields, D. L., et al. The relationship of sport involvement with children's moral reasoning and aggression tendencies. *J Sport Psychol* 8:304–318, 1986.
14. Brodie, D. A., Lamb, K. L., and Roberts, K. Body composition and self-perceived health and fitness among indoor sports participants. *Ergonomics* 31(11):1551–1557, 1988.
15. Brody, E. B., Hatfield, B. D., and Spalding, T. W. Generalization of self-efficacy to a continuum of stressors upon mastery of a high-risk sport skill. *J Sport Exerc Psychol* 10:32–44, 1988.
16. Brustad, R. J. Affective outcomes in competitive youth sports: The influence of intrapersonal and socialization factors. *J Sport Exerc Psychol* 10:307–321, 1988.
17. Brustad, R. J., and Weiss, M. R. Competence perceptions and sources of worry in high, medium, and low competitive trait-anxious young athletes. *J Sport Psychol* 9:97–105, 1987.
18. Buhler, C. Die ersten sozialen Verhaltensweisen des Kindes in soziologischen und psychologischen Studien des ersten Lebensjahrcs. *Quell N Stud Z Jugendk* V:1–102, 1927.
19. Burke, E. J., and Kleiber, E. Psychological and physical implications of highly competitive sports for children. *In* Straub, W. F. (Ed.), *Sports Psychology; An Analysis of Athlete Behavior.* Ithaca, NY, Mouvement Publications, 1980.
20. Burke, E. J., and Kleiber, E. Psychological and physical implications of highly competitive sports for children. *Physical Educator* 33:63–70, 1976.
21. Burton, D. Do anxious swimmers swim slower? Reexamining the elusive anxiety-performance relationship. *J Sport Exerc Psychol* 10:45–61, 1988.
22. Burton, D., and Martens, R. Pinned by their own goals: An exploratory investigation into why kids drop out of wrestling. *J Sport Psychol* 8:183–197, 1986.
23. Butt, D. S. *Psychology of Sport: The Behavior, Motivation, Personality, and Performance of Athletes.* Malabar, FL, Robert E. Krieger, 1982.
24. Carmen, L., Zerman, J. L., and Blaine, G. B. The use of the Harvard psychiatric service by athletes and non-athletes. *Ment Hyg* 52, 1968.
25. Carron, A. V. *Social Psychology of Sport: An Experimental Approach.* London, Ontario, Mouvement Publications, 1981.
26. Caruso, C. M., Dzewaltowski, D. A., Gill D. L., et al. Psychological and physiological changes in competitive state anxiety during noncompetitive and competitive success and failure. *J Sport Exerc Psychol* 12:6–20, 1990.
27. Cassmen, M. H., and Haskett, T. P. Psychiatric consultations in a coronary care unit. *Ann Intern Med* 75:9–14, 1971.
28. Chan, C. S., and Grossman, H. Y. Psychological effects of running loss on consistent runners. *Perceptual Motor Skills* 66:875–883, 1988.
29. Chaumeton, N. R., and Duda, J. L. Is it how you play the game or whether you win or lose?: The effect of competitive level and situation on coaching behaviors. *J Sport Behav* 11(3):157–174, 1988.
30. Coddington, R. D., and Troxell, J. R. The effects of emotional factors on football injury rates: A pilot study. *J Hum Stress* 6:3–5, 1980.
31. Comrey, A. Group performance in manual dexterity task. *J Appl Psychol* 37:207, 1953.
32. Comrey, A., and Deskin, G. Group manual dexterity in women. *J Appl Psychol* 38:178, 1954.
33. Comrey, A., and Deskin, G. Further results in group manual dexterity. *J Appl Psychol* 39:354–356, 1955.
34. Comrey, A., and Staats, C. K. Group performance in cognitive task. *J Appl Psychol* 39:354–356, 1955.
35. Cratty, B. J. *Social Psychology in Athletics.* Englewood Cliffs, NJ, Prentice-Hall, 1981.
36. Crocker, P. R. Alderman, E., Rikk, B., et al. Cognitive-affective stress management training with affect, cognition, and performance. *J Sport Exerc Psychol* 10:448–460, 1988.
37. Cryan, P. O., and Alles, E. F. The relationship between stress and football injuries. *J Sports Med Phys Fitness* 23:52–58, 1983.
38. Csizma, K. A., Wittig, A. F., and Schurr, K. T. Sport stereotypes and gender. *J Sport Exerc Psychol* 10:62–74, 1988.
39. Davidson, R. J., and Schwartz, G. E. The psychobiology of relaxation and related states: A multi-process theory. *In* Mostofsky, D. I. (Ed.), *Behavior Control and Modification of Physiological Activity.* Englewood Cliffs, NJ, Prentice Hall, 1976, pp. 399–442.
40. Deakin, J. M., Starkes, J. L., and Elliott, D. Feature integration of children during exercise. *J Sport Exerc Psychol* 10:248–261, 1988.
41. Demoja, C. A., and Demoja, G. Analysis of anxiety trend before a sport competition. *Perceptual Motor Skills* 62:406, 1986.
42. Dervin, D. A psychoanalysis of sports. *Psychoanal Rev* 72(2):277–299, 1985.
43. Devereux, E. C. Backyard versus Little League baseball: Some observations on the impoverishment of children's games in America. *In* Landers, D. (Ed.), *Social Problems in Athletics.* Urbana, IL, University of Illinois Press, 1976.
44. Devereux, E. C. Backyard versus Little League baseball: Some observations on the impoverishment of children's games in contemporary America. *In* Yiannakis, A. (Ed.), *Sports Sociology: Contemporary Themes* (2nd ed.). Dubuque, IA, Kendall/Hunt, 1979.
45. Dishman, R. K. Medical psychology in exercise and sport. *Med Clin North Am* 69(1):123–143, 1985.

46. Dollard, J., Doob, N., Mowrer, O., et al. *Frustration and Aggression.* New Haven, Yale University Press, 1939.
47. Dowell, L. J. Environmental factors of childhood competitive athletics. *Physical Educator* 28:17–21, 1971.
48. Drabik, J. Sexual dimorphism and sports results. *J Sports Med Phys Fitness* 28(3):287–292, 1988.
49. Duda, J. L. Relationship between task and ego orientation and the perceived purpose of sport among high school athletes. *J Sport Exerc Psychol* 11:318–335, 1989.
50. Duda, J. L. Toward a developmental theory of children's motivation in sport. *J Sport Psychol* 9:130–145, 1987.
51. Dunham, P., Jr. Coincidence—anticipation performance of adolescent baseball players and nonplayers. *Perceptual Motor Skills* 68:1151–1156, 1989.
52. Dunham, P., Jr., Dunham, T., and Dunham, T. A. Effect of practice procedure on skill acquisition. *Perceptual Motor Skills* 66:512–514, 1988.
53. Durkheim, E. *The Division of Labor in Society.* Simpson, G. (trans.). Glencoe, IL, Free Press, 1947.
54. Dwyer, J. J., and Carron, A. V. Personality status of wrestlers of varying abilities as measured by a sport specific version of a personality inventory. *Can J Appl Sports Sci* 19–30, 1985.
55. Eitzen, S. D. Group structure and group performance. *In* Straub, W. (Ed.), *Sports Psychology: An Analysis of Athlete Behavior.* Ithaca, NY, Mouvement Publications, 1980.
56. Enns, M. P., Drewnowski, A., and Grinker, J. A. Body composition, body size estimation, and attitudes towards eating in male college athletes. *Psychosom Med* 49(1):56–64, 1987.
57. Erikson, E. H. *Childhood and Society.* New York, W. W. Norton, 1963.
58. Erikson, E. H. *Identity, Youth and Crisis.* New York, W. W. Norton, 1968.
59. Ewing, M. E., Feltz, D. L., Schultz, T. D., et al. Psychological characteristics of competitive young hockey players. *In* Brown, E., and Branta, C. (Eds.), *Effects of Competitive Sports in Children and Youth: Proceedings from the 1985 CIC Symposium.* Champaign, IL, Human Kinetics, 1987.
60. Feltz, D. L. Path analysis of causal elements of Bandura's theory of self-efficacy and an anxiety based model of avoidance behavior. *J Personality Social Psychol* 42:764–781, 1982.
61. Feltz, D. L. Self-efficacy as a cognitive mediator of athletic performance. *In* Straub, W. F., and Williams, J. M. (Eds.), *Cognitive Sport Psychology.* New York, Sport Science Associates, 1984.
62. Feltz, D. L., and Ewing, M. E. Psychological characteristics of elite young athletes. *Med Sci Sports Exerc* 19(5):598–605, 1987.
63. Feltz, D. L., and Riessinger, C. A. Effects of in vivo emotive imagery and performance feedback on self-efficacy and muscular endurance. *J Sport Exerc Psychol* 12:132–143, 1990.
64. Fenz, W. D. Learning to anticipate stressful events. *J Sport Exerc Psychol* 10:223–228, 1988.
65. Gauron, E. F. The art of cognitive self-regulation. *Clin Sports Med* 5(1):91–101, 1986.
66. Gill, D. L., Dzewaltowski, D. A., and Deeter, T. E. The relationship of competitiveness and achievement orientation to participation in sport and nonsport activities. *J Sport Exerc Psychol* 10:139–150, 1988.
67. Glick, I. D., and Marcotte, D. B. Psychiatric aspects of basketball. *J Sports Med Phys Fitness* 29:104–112, 1989.
68. Gould, D., Petlichkoff, L., and Weinberg, R. S. Antecedents of temporal changes in and relationships between CSAI-2 subcomponents. *J Sports Psychol* 6:289–304, 1984.
69. Gould, D., Petlichkoff, L., Simmons, J., et al. The relationship between competitive state anxiety inventory-2 subscale scores and pistol shooting performance. *J Sports Psychol* 9:33–42, 1987.
70. Gould, D., Hodge, K., Peterson, K., et al. An exploratory examination of strategies used by elite coaches to enhance self-efficacy in athletes. *J Sport Exerc Psychol* 11:128–140, 1989.
71. Grant, R. W. *The Psychology of Sport: Facing One's True Opponent.* Jefferson, NC, McFarland & Co., 1952.
72. Greenberg, P. T. Competition in children: An experimental study. *Am J Psychol* 44:221–248, 1932.
73. Greendorfer, S. L., and Lewko, J. H. The role of family members in sports socialization of children. *Res Q* 49:146–152, 1978.
74. Greenspan, E. *Little Winners: Inside the World of the Child Sports Star.* Boston, Little, Brown, 1983.
75. Griffin, N. S., and Crawford, M. E. Measurement of movement confidence with a stunt movement confidence inventory. *J Sport Exerc Psychol* 11:26–40, 1989.
76. Hackford, D., and Spielberger, C. D. *Anxiety in Sports: An International Perspective.* New York, Hemisphere Publishing, 1989.
77. Hale, C. J. What research says about athletics for pre-high school age children. *J Health, Phys Ed Recreation* 30:19–21, 43, 1959.
78. Hall, H. K., Anthony, T. J., and Byrne, D. D. Goal setting in sport: Clarifying recent anomalies. *J Sport Exerc Psychol* 10:184–198, 1988.
79. Hall, H. K., Weinberg, R. S., and Jackson, A. Effects of goal specificity, goal difficulty, and information feedback on endurance performance. *J Sport Psychol* 9:43–54, 1987.
80. Halvari, H. Effects of achievement motives on wrestling ability, oxygen uptake, speed of movement, muscular strength, and technical performance. *Perceptual Motor Skills* 65:255–270, 1987.
81. Hardy, C. J., Prentice, W. E., Kirsanoff, M. T., et al. Life stress, social support, and athletic injury: In search of relationships. *In* Williams, J. M. (Ed.), *Applied Sport Psychology: Personal Growth To Peak Performance.* Palo Alto, Mayfield, 1987, pp. 185–207.
82. Hardy, C. J., and Silva, J. M., III. The relationship between selected psychological traits and fear of success in senior elite level wrestlers. *Can J Appl Sport Sci* 11(4):205–210, 1986.
83. Hardy, L., and Nelson, D. Self-regulation training in sport and work. *Ergonomics* 31(11):1573–1583, 1988.
84. Harter, S. Effectance motivation reconsidered: Toward a developmental model. *Hum Dev* 21:34–64, 1978.
85. Harter, S. A model of intrinsic mastery motivation in children: Individual differences and developmental change. *In* Collins A. (Ed.), *Minnesota Symposium on Child Psychology,* Vol. 14. Hillsdale, NJ, Lawrence Erlbaum Associates, 1981, pp. 215–255.
86. Hecker, J. E., and Kaczor, L. M. Application of imagery theory to sport psychology: Some preliminary findings. *J Sport Exerc Psychol* 10:363–373, 1988.
87. Higginson, D.C. The influence of socializing agents in the female sport-participation process. *Adolesence* 20(77):73–82, 1985.
88. Holmes, T. H. Psychological screening. *In Football Injuries*: Papers presented at a workshop sponsored by the Subcommittee on Athletic Injuries, Committee on the Skeletal System, Division of Medical Sciences, National Research Council, February, 1969. Washington, D.C., National Academy of Sciences, 1970, pp. 211–214.
89. Holmes, T. H., and Rahe, R. H. The social readjustment rating scale. *J Psychosom Res* 11:213–218, 1967.
90. Horn, T. S., and Hasbrook, C. A. Psychological characteristics and the criteria children use for self-evaluation. *J Sport Psychol* 9:208–221, 1987.
91. Howard, W. L., and Reardon, J. P. Changes in the self concept and athletic performance of weight lifters through a cognitive-hypnotic approach: An empirical study. *Am J Clin Hypnosis* 28(4):248–257, 1986.
92. Howe, B. L., and Robinson, D. W. Casual attribution and mood state relationships of soccer players in a sport achievement setting. *J Sport Behavior* 10(3):137–146, 1987.
93. Hughes, S. Implementing psychological skills training program in high school athletics. *J Sport Behav* 13(1):15–22, 1990.
94. Jackson, S. A., and Marsh, H. W. Athletic or antisocial? The female sport experience. *J Sport Psychol* 8:198–211, 1986.
95. Jones, J. G., and Cale, A. Precompetition temporal patterning of anxiety and self-confidence in males and females. *J Sport Behav* 12(2):183–195, 1989.
96. Jowdy, D. P., and Harris, D. V. Muscular responses during mental imagery as a function of motor skills level. *J Sport Exerc Psychol* 12:191–201, 1990.
97. Kane, M. J. The female athletic role as a status determinant within the social system of high school adolescents. *Adolescents* 23(90):253–264, 1988.
98. Kendall, G. Hrycaiko, D., Martin, G. L., et al. The effects of an

imagery, rehearsal, relaxation, and self-talk package on basketball game performance. *J Sport Exerc Psychol* 12:157–166, 1990.

99. Kerr, G., and Minden, H. Psychological factors related to the occurrence of athletic injuries. *J Sport Exerc Psychol* 10:167–173, 1988.

100. Kerr, J. H., and Cox, T. Effects of telic dominance and metamotivational state on squash task performance. *Perceptual Motor Skills* 67:171–174, 1988.

101. Klint, K. A., and Weiss, M. R. Perceived competence and motives for participating in youth sports: A test of Harter's competence motivation theory. *J Sport Psychol* 9:55–65, 1987.

102. Krane, V., and Williams, J. Performance and somatic anxiety, cognitive anxiety, and confidence changes prior to competition. *J Sport Behav* 10(1):47–56, 1987.

103. Kraus, J. F., and Conroy, F. Mortality and morbidity from injuries in sports and recreation. *Annu Rev Public Health* 5:163–192, 1984.

104. Krentz, E. W. Improving competitive performance with hypnotic suggestions and modified autogenic training: Case reports. *Am J Clin Hypnosis* 27(1):58–63, 1984.

105. Kübler-Ross, E. *On Death and Dying.* New York, Macmillan, 1969.

106. Lacy, A. C., and Goldston, P. D. Behavior analysis of male and female coaches in high school girls' basketball. *J Sport Behav* 13(1):29–39, 1990.

107. Landers, D. M., and Boutcher, S. H. Arousal-performance relationship, *In* Williams, J. M. (Ed.), *Applied Sports Psychology: Personal Growth to Peak Performance.* Palo Alto, Mayfield, 1986, pp. 163–184.

108. Larson, D. L., Spreitzer, E., and Snyder, E. E. An analysis of organized sports for children. *Physical Educator* 33:59–62, 1976.

109. Larson, D. L., and McMahan, R. O. The epiphyses of the childhood athlete. *JAMA* 196:607–612, 1966.

110. Lee, C. Psyching up for a muscular endurance task: Effects of image content on performance and mood state. *J Sport Exerc Psychol* 12:66–73, 1990.

111. Leonard, G. B. Winning isn't everything, it's nothing. *In* Yiannakis, A. (Ed.), *Sports Sociology: Contemporary Themes.* Dubuque, IA, Kendall/Hunt Publishing, 1976.

112. Lewthwaite, R., and Scanlan, T. K. Predictors of competitive trait anxiety in male youth sport participants. *Med Sci Sports Exerc* 21(2):221–229, 1989.

113. Liebert, R. M., and Morris, L. W. Cognitive and emotional components of test anxiety: A distinction and initial data. *Psychol Rep* 20:975–978, 1967.

114. Linder, D. E., Pillow, D. R., and Reno, R. R. Shrinking jocks: Derogation of athletes who consult a sports psychologist. *Sport Exerc Psychol* 11(3):270–280, 1989.

115. Little, J. C. The athletes' neurosis: A deprivation crisis. *Acta Psychiatr Scand* 45:187–197, 1969.

116. Little, J. C. Neurotic illness in fitness fanatics. *Psychiatr Ann* 9(3):148–152, 1979.

117. Longhurst, K., and Spink, K. S. Participation motivation of Australian children involved in organized sport. *Can J Sport Sci* 12(1):24–30, 1987.

118. Loy, J., McPherson, B. D., and Kenyon, G. *Sports and Social Systems.* Reading, MA, Addison Wesley, 1978.

119. Luginbuhl, J., and Bell, A. Casual attributions by athletes: Role of ego involvement. *J Sport Exerc Psychol* 11:399–407, 1989.

120. Lundholm, J. K., and Littrell, J. M. Desire for thinness among high school cheerleaders: Relationship to disordered eating and weight control behaviors. *Adolescence* 21(83):573–579, 1986.

121. Lysens, R., Auweele, Y. V., and Ostyn, M. The relationship between psychosocial factors and sports injuries. *J Sports Med Phys Fitness* 26:77–84, 1986.

122. Mace, R., and Carroll, D. Stress inoculation training to control anxiety in sport: Two case studies in squash. *Br J Sports Med* 20(3):115–117, 1986.

123. MacMahon, J. R. The psychological benefits of exercise and the treatment of delinquent adolescents. *Sports Med* 9(6):344–351, 1990.

124. Maehr, M. L. Continuing motivation: An analysis of a seldom considered educational outcome. *Rev Educ Res* 46:443–462, 1976.

125. Mallick, J. M., Whipple, T. W., and Huerta, E. Behavior and psychological traits of weight-conscious teenagers: A comparison of eating-disordered patients and high- and low-risk groups. *Adolescence* 22(85):157–168, 1987.

126. Martens, R. *Sports Competition Anxiety Test.* Champaign, IL, Human Kinetics, 1977.

127. Martens, R. *Coaches' Guide to Sport Psychology.* Champaign, IL, Human Kinetics, 1987.

128. Masters, K. S., and Lambert, M. The relations between cognitive coping strategies, reasons for running, injury, and performance of marathon runners. *J Sport Exerc Psychol* 11:161–170, 1989.

129. McAuley, E. Sport psychology in the eighties: Some current developments. *Med Sci Sports Exerc* 19(5):595–597, 1987.

130. McCarthy, J. J. Little League lunacy. *Nat Elementary Principal* 43:80–83, 1963.

131. McClelland, D. *The Achieving Society.* New York, Van Nostrand, 1961.

132. Meyers, M. C., Sterling, J., LeUnes, A. D., et al. Precompetitive mood state changes in collegiate rodeo athletes. *J Sport Behav* 13(2):114–121, 1990.

133. Miller, R. Effects of sports instruction on children's self-concept. *Perceptual Motor Skills* 68:239–242, 1989.

134. Miller, T. W., Vaughn, M. P., and Miller, J. M. Clinical issues and treatment strategies in stress-oriented athletes. *Sports Med* 9(6):370–379, 1990.

135. Morgan, W. P. Psychologic characteristics of the elite long distance runner. *Ann Acad Sci* 301:382–403, 1977.

136. Morris, L., David, D., and Hutchings, C. Cognitive and emotional components of anxiety: Literature review and revised worry-emotional scale. *J Educ Psychol* 73:541–555, 1981.

137. Murphy, S. M., Woolfolk, R. L., and Bundney, A. J. The effects of emotive imagery on strength performance. *J Sport Exerc Psychol* 10:334–345, 1988.

138. Nideffer, R. M. *The Ethics and Practice of Applied Sport Psychology.* Ithaca, NY, Mouvemer Publications, 1981.

139. Orlick, T. D., McNally, J., and O'Hara, T. Cooperative games: Systematic analysis and cooperative impact. *In* Smoll, F. (Ed.), *Psychological Perspectives in Youth Sports.* Seattle, Hemisphere Publishing, 1978.

140. Orlick, T. D. Family sports environment and early sports participation. Paper given at the Fourth Canadian Psycho-Motor Learning and Sports Psychology Symposium, Waterloo, Ontario, University of Waterloo, October, 1972.

141. Orlick, T. *Psyching for Sport: Mental Training for Athletes.* Champaign, IL, Leisure Press, 1986.

142. Paivio, A. Cognitive and motivational functions of imagery in human performance. *Can J Sport Sci* 10(4):225–285, 1985.

143. Parsons, T., and Bales, R. F. *Family, Socialization and Interaction Process.* Glencoe, IL, Free Press, 1955.

144. Passer, M. W. Fear of failure, fear of evaluation, perceived competence, and self-esteem in competitive trait anxious children. *J Sports Psychol* 5:172–188, 1983.

145. Passer, M. W., and Seese, M.D. Life stress and athletic injury: Examination of positive versus negative events and three moderator variables. *J Hum Stress* 9:11–16, 1983.

146. Pease, D. G., and Anderson, D. F. Longitudinal analysis of children's attitudes toward sport team involvement. *J Sports Behav* 9(1):3–10, 1986.

147. Petley, J. *The Cohesiveness of Successful and Less Successful Wrestling Teams* (research project). Ithaca, NY, Ithaca College, 1973.

148. Phillips, R. H. The nature and function of children's formal games. *Psychoan Q* 29:200–207, 1960.

149. Piaget, J. *The Moral Judgement of the Child.* New York, Harcourt, 1932.

150. Pierce, R. A. Athletes in psychotherapy: How many, How come? *J Am Coll Health Assoc* 17:244–249, 1969.

151. Pinkerton, R. S., Hinz, L. D., and Barrow, J. C. The college student-athlete: Psychological considerations and interventions. *J Coll Health* 37:218–226, 1989.

152. Raglin, J. S. Exercise and mental health: Beneficial and detrimental effects. *Sports Med* 9(6):323–329, 1990.
153. Read, M. Children in sport. *Sport Med* 232:1325–1328, 1988.
154. Roberts, G. C. Children's assignment of responsibility for winning and losing. *In* Smoll, F., and Smith, R. (Eds.), *Psychological Perspectives in Youth Sports.* Washington, D.C., Hemisphere, 1978.
155. Robinson, D. W., and Howe, B. L. Casual attribution and mood state relationships of soccer players in a sport achievement setting. *J Sport Behav* 10(3):137–146, 1987.
156. Rowley, S. Annotation of psychological effects of intensive training in young athletes. *J Child Psychol Psychiatr* 28(3):371–377, 1987.
157. Rucinski, A. Relationship of body image and dietary intake of competitive ice skaters. *J Am Diet Assoc* 89(1):98–100, 1989.
158. Rushall, B. S., and Wiznuk, K. Athletes' assessment of the coach: The coach evaluation questionnaire. *Can J Sport Sci* 10(3):157–161, 1985.
159. Rutherford, O. M., and Jones, D. A. The role of learning and coordination in strength training. *Eur J Appl Physiol* 55:100–105, 1986.
160. Salokun, S. O., and Toriola, A. L. Personality characteristics of sprinters, basketball, soccer, and field hockey players. *J Sports Med* 25:222–226, 1985.
161. Scanlan, T. K. Antecedents of competitiveness. *In* Magill, P. A., Ash, M. J., and Smoll, F. (eds.), *Children in Sports: A Contemporary Anthology.* Champaign, IL, Human Kinetics, 1978.
162. Scanlan, T. K., Stein, G. L., and Ravizza, K. An in-depth study of former elite figure skaters: Part II. Sources of enjoyment. *J Sports Exerc Psychol* 11:65–83, 1989.
163. Scanlan, T. K., and Lewthwaite, R. Social psychological aspects of competition for male youth sports participants. I. Predictors of competitive stress. *J Sports Psychol* 6:208–226, 1984.
164. Scanlan, T. K., and Lewthwaite, R. Social psychological aspects of competition for male youth sport participants. IV. Predictors of enjoyment. *J Sport Psychol* 8:25–35, 1986.
165. Sears, R. R., Rau, L., and Alpert, R. *Identification and Child Training.* Stanford, Stanford University Press, 1965.
166. Selye, H. *The Stress of Life.* New York, McGraw-Hill, 1978.
167. Sinclair, D. A., and Vealey, R. S. Effects of coaches' expectations and feedback on the self-perceptions of athletes. *J Sport Behav* 11(3):77–91, 1988.
168. Skubic, E. Studies of Little League and middle league baseball. *Res Q* 27:97–110, 1956.
169. Smith, A. M., Scott, S. G., O'Fallon, W., et al. The emotional responses of athletes to injury. *Mayo Clin Proc* 65:38–50, 1990.
170. Smith, A. M., Scott, S. G., and Wiese, D. M. The psychological effects of sports injuries. *Sports Med* 9(6):352–369, 1990.
171. Smith, R. E., Smoll, F. L., and Curtis, B. Coaching behaviors in Little League baseball. *In* Smoll, F. (Ed.), *Psychological Perspectives in Youth Sports.* Washington, D.C., Hemisphere Publishing, 1978.
172. Smoll, F. L., and Smith, R. E. *Psychological Perspectives in Youth Sports.* Washington, D.C., Hemisphere Publishing, 1978.
173. Snyder, D., and Spreitzer, E. A. Family influences and involvement in sport. *Res Q* 44(3):249–255, 1973.
174. Snyder, E. E., and Spreitzer, E. Correlates of sports participation among adolescent girls. *Res Q* 47:804–809, 1976a.
175. Snyder, E. E., and Spreitzer, E. Family influence and involvement in sports. *Res Q* 47:238–245, 1976b.
176. Spielberger, C. D. Theory and research on anxiety. *In* Spielberger, C. D. (Ed.), *Anxiety and Behavior.* New York, Academic Press, 1966, pp. 3–20.
177. Spielberger, C. D. Anxiety as an emotional state. *In* Spielberger, C. D. (Ed.), *Anxiety: Current Trends in Theory and Research,* Vol. 1. New York, Academic Press, 1972.
178. Stoyva, J. M., and Budzynski, T. H. Cultivated low arousal—An antistress response? *In* DiCara, L. V. (Ed.), *Recent Advances in Limbic and Autonomic Nervous Systems Research.* New York, Plenum, 1974, pp. 370–394.
179. Straub, W. F. *Sport Psychology: An Analysis of Athlete Behavior.* Ithaca, NY, Mouvement Publications, 1980.
180. Stuart, J. C., and Brown, B. M. The relationship of stress and coping ability to incidence of diseases and accidents. *J Psychosom Res* 25:255–260, 1981.
181. Taylor, J. Predicting athletic performance with self-confidence and somatic and cognitive anxiety as a function of motor and physiological requirements in six sports. *J Personality* 55(1):139–153, 1987.
182. Terry, P. C., and Howe, B. L. Coaching preferences of athletes. *Can J Appl Sport Sci* 9(4):188–193, 1984.
183. Tunks, T., and Bellissimo, A. Coping with the coping concept: A brief comment. *Pain* 34:171–174, 1988.
184. Vinokur, A., and Selzer, M. L. Desirable versus undesirable life events: Their relationship to stress and mental distress. *J Personality Soc Psychol* 32:329–337, 1975.
185. Wandzilak, T., Ansorge, C. J., and Potter, G. Comparison between selected practice and game behaviors of youth sport soccer coaches. *J Sport Behav* 11(2):78–88, 1988.
186. Wankel, L. M., and Sefton, J. M. A season-long investigation of fun in youth sports. *J Sport Exerc Psychol* 11:335–366, 1989.
187. Weinberg, R., Bruya, L., Garland, H., et al. Effect of goal difficulty and positive reinforcement on endurance performance. *J Sport Exerc Psychol* 12:144–156, 1990.
188. Weiss, M. R., and Troxel, R. K. Psychology of the injured athlete. *Athletic Training* 104–109, 1986.
189. Weiss, M. R., McAuley, E., Ebbeck, V., et al. Self-esteem and casual attributions for children's physical and social competence in sport. *J Sport Psychol* 12:21–36, 1990.
190. White, R. Motivation reconsidered: The concept of competence. *Psychol Rev* 66:297–323, 1959.
191. White, R. W. Competence and psychosexual stages of development. *In* Jones, M. R. (Ed.), *Nebraska Symposium on Motivation,* Vol. 8. Lincoln, University of Nebraska Press, 1960.
192. Wiese, D. M., and Weiss, M. R. Psychological rehabilitation and physical injury: Implications for the sports medicine team. *Sports Psychologist* 1:318–330, 1987.
193. Williams, J. M., and Andersen, M. B. The relationship between psychological factors and injury occurrence. *In* Heil, J. (Ed.), *Psychological Aspects of Sport Injury.* Symposium conducted at the meeting of the NASPSPA, Scottsdale, AZ, June, 1986.
194. Williams, J. M., Haggert, J., Tonymon, P., et al. Life stress and prediction of athletic injuries in volleyball, basketball, and cross-country running. *In* Unestahl, L. E., (Ed.), *Sports Psychology in Theory and Practice.* Orebro, Sweden, Veje Publishers, 1986.
195. Williams, J. M., Tonymon, P., and Wadsworth, W. A. Relationship of stress to injury in intercollegiate volleyball. *J Human Stress* 12:38–43, 1986.
196. Williams, J. M., and Parkhouse, B. L. Social learning theory as a foundation for examining sex bias in evaluation of coaches. *J Sport Exerc Psychol* 10:322–333, 1988.
197. Wine, J. D. Cognitive attentional theory of test anxiety. *In* Sarason, I. G. (Ed.), *Test Anxiety: Theory, Research and Applications.* Hillsdale, NJ, Erlbaum, 1980, pp. 349–385.
198. Winget, C. M., DeRoshia, C. W., and Holley, D.C. Circadian rhythms and athletic performance. *Med Sci Sports Exerc* 17(5):498–516, 1985.
199. Yiannakis, A., McIntyre, T., Melnick, M. J., et al. *Sport Psychology: Contemporary Themes.* Dubuque, IA, Hunt Publishing, 1979.

OVERUSE SYNDROMES

Carl L. Stanitski, M.D.

MUSCULOSKELETAL OVERUSE

Acute injury secondary to macro stress is one type of musculoskeletal problem generated by athletic endeavor. A recently recognized genre of sports-related musculoskeletal injury is due to overuse, i.e., conditions caused by unresolved submaximal stress in previously normal tissues.

Increased musculoskeletal stress is common in young athletes and reflects the escalating intensity of training and competition at younger and younger ages [6, 23, 25, 37, 46, 52, 54]. The duration of competitive and training seasons has been prolonged. Athletes often go directly from one sports season to the next or continue to participate in prolonged seasons without respite. Intense activity at "sports camps" adds to the musculoskeletal demands. In the current sports environment, a serious young athlete's training begins early in life and continues with increased intensity and duration as sports have become a year-round focused cycle of training and competition.

Stress injuries are an extension of the spectrum of physiologic adaptation that occurs in response to stimuli from normal use. Stress is essential for normal connective tissue homeostasis [7, 11, 12, 16, 18, 39, 48, 53, 57, 59–61]. Excessive use produces unresolved stress within previously normal tissues and leads to subsequent soft tissue and bone injuries [1–4, 9, 10, 13–15, 19, 21, 22, 31, 33–35, 43, 45, 49, 50, 58, 63, 64]. Superimposed on the stress effect is an inadequate time frame for resolution of stress and its effects. This time compression is seen in demand situations, a setting in which peers, parents, or coaches insist on and encourage efforts that are either too much, too soon, or both in the unconditioned or unprepared young athlete. Even in the extremely fit and capable athlete, too much effort can be demanded, and tissue failure and injury ensue.

In addition to the gravitational effects of weight bearing, muscle force including both concentric and eccentric loading is superimposed on the musculoskeletal lever system. The latter type of loading produces greater force than the former. Eccentric loading is extremely common in both upper and lower extremities during sports tasks.

Many stress-related injuries in the skeletally immature athlete are junctional problems occurring at bone–muscle, muscle–tendon, or tendon–bone interfaces. Clinically, they are commonly recognized conditions such as Osgood-Schlatter disease (Fig. 8–1), Sever's disease (Fig. 8–2) [28, 29, 36], and Little League elbow (Fig. 8–3) [21, 22, 31, 42], which are discussed elsewhere in

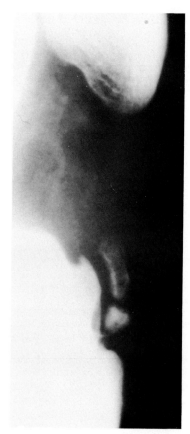

FIGURE 8–1
Changes due to Osgood-Schlatter disease in a symptomatic 13-year-old wrestler.

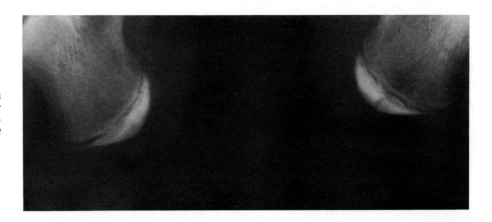

FIGURE 8–2
Radiographs of the calcanei of a symptomatic 10-year-old soccer player. The fragmentation of the calcaneal apophysis is normal and is *not* pathognomonic of Sever's disease.

this text. They may also occur in less common areas, e.g., at the medial or lateral malleoli (Fig. 8–4). These junctions are sites of force transmission and transition via tissues of varying mechanical properties, properties that change rapidly relative to phases of growth. Soft tissues and bone act as viscoelastic, heterotopic mechanical systems whose properties depend on the rate and direction of loading. The soft tissue stress response is a direct function of the properties of collagen [38].

Healing of acute soft tissue injury proceeds in an ordered three-phase manner [15, 20, 32, 62]. The initial phase lasts for approximately 2 weeks after the injury and is primarily an inflammatory response that begins within the first 48 hours. Primitive collagen formation starts at that time. In the second stage the newly formed collagen begins to be organized. Three to four weeks postinjury, the third phase begins, characterized by remodeling of the collagen matrix. Progressive collagen organization and maturation may continue for up to a year and is directed by stress demands.

Musculoskeletal fitness must be considered a goal, not an event. Fitness occurs through adaptation of the biologic system to graduated stress and is a stepwise process. Until the system adjusts to the stresses at one level, it cannot respond appropriately if demands are placed on it requiring a higher level of fitness. If this occurs, the system, be it soft tissue or bone, is overwhelmed (Fig. 8–5). Overuse injury occurs at two particular times during training. Overuse injuries are commonly seen in "underused" participants, and the first peak of injury occurs when previously unfit or partially conditioned athletes are placed in demand situations, e.g., preseason football or cross-country training. Musculoskeletal stresses in these settings are commonly limited by fatigue and cardiopulmonary reserve, the body exhibiting a built-in control system. When further demands are made, the system is overwhelmed, and overuse injury occurs. A second peak of injury occurs in the extremely fit athlete who through adaptation is closer to the ultimate innate breakdown boundary of the musculoskeletal system. The tissue reserve is depleted as efforts are made

to obtain the final bit of available adaptation. If progressive symptoms do not produce discontinuation of activities, tissue failure occurs, and a full-blown stress condition becomes manifest.

All young athletes are not equally prepared for sports demands. Natural selection based on ability and sport interest begins to occur at about the age of 9 to 10. Those children with a genetically limited kinesthetic sense feel like "motor morons" whose bodies simply will not do what is requested of them during sports, be they hand-eye or hand-foot tasks [8]. A transient period of uncoordination is commonly seen during the adolescent growth spurt. Blessedly, this condition passes, and more normal motor ability returns. In boys and girls with exaggerated growth, several years may pass before they "grow into their bodies." Because of this ungainliness, which is often coupled with limited strength and endurance, the child may be awkward in sports tasks, and overuse results because of limited sports-specific skills. Because of peer pressure, younger children often feel they must engage in sports even though they have limited talent or interest in such activity. Despite this feeling that sports participation is an important part of their social scheme, these less than willing (and able) participants (whom I term "atheloids'") are often prone to injury. These children need to be guided into a sport appropriate for them, often one of the nontraditional ones. If they continue to be forced into the more standard sport venues, overuse injuries commonly follow along with a lifelong disdain for sport activity.

Diagnosis

The primary diagnostic effort when dealing with stress injuries is to identify the factor or factors that have led to the symptoms. Broadly stated, these include anatomic, environmental, and training factors. The primary aid used to diagnose overuse injury is the patient's history. Overuse complaints usually produce a mechanical type of pain, i.e., one that increases with activity and

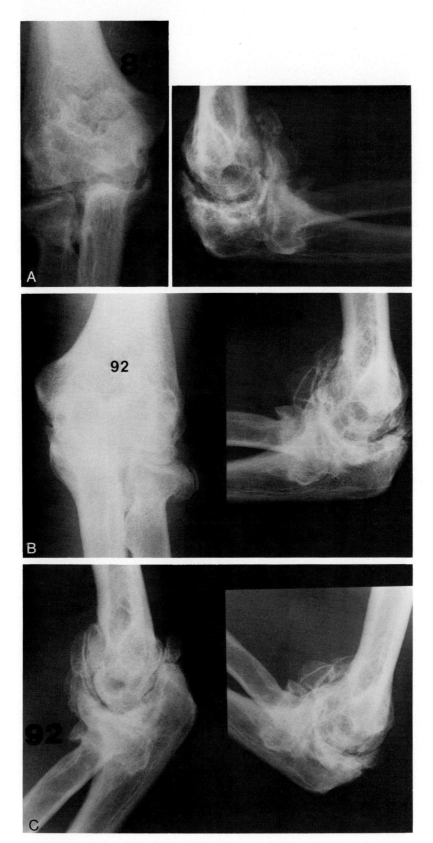

FIGURE 8–3
Serial radiographs of a 30-year-old man who was a high-level pitcher/catcher from the age of 9 to 22. *A*, Radiograph (1985) prior to loose body excision surgery. *B*, Radiograph 7 years later showing continued tricompartment DJD. *C*, Extension and flexion maximums. (Courtesy Greg Housner, M.D.)

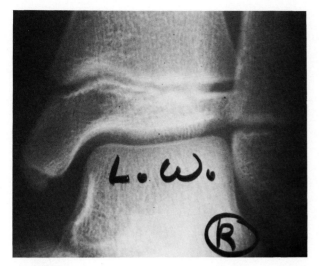

FIGURE 8–4
Symptomatic medial malleolar accessory ossification center in a 10-year-old hockey player.

diminishes with rest. It is helpful to characterize such discomfort into one of three levels based on pain relative to activity. Level I is pain that occurs only with strenuous sport activity; level II is pain with limited sports participation, and level III is pain with routine daily activity. Previous injury and treatment must also be considered to determine compliance with former treatment programs, which gives one a sense of patient commitment to improvement.

Environmental factors include equipment and playing surfaces. The equipment used by an athlete may have a significant role in the generation of overuse disorders. Inappropriately sized balls, racket grips or string tensions, swimming hand paddles, gymnastic dowel grips, inappropriately supervised strength training machines, and inadequate footwear are all sources of childhood and adolescent overuse injuries. Running laps in football cleats may not be the best practice, and running shoes should be substituted to reduce stress. In patients in running sports, footwear should be assessed by looking

for clues to excessive or unbalanced wear. Uneven running surfaces, rigid gymnasium floors, and unforgiving floor mats also generate unfriendly forces.

Inadequate or inappropriate sports-specific techniques cause excessive stresses. In younger athletes whose level of enthusiasm greatly surpasses their skill level, incorrect throwing, jumping, or running motions are sources of excessive submaximal trauma. This is particularly evident in Little League pitchers [4, 21, 49]. As sports tasks become more complex to accommodate a rise in sport skills (e.g., in gymnastics [56], training intensifies, and these increased demands may overwhelm a system that easily withstood lesser stresses [3, 13, 24, 34, 35, 43, 45].

An abnormal anatomic alignment due to a fixed or dynamic deformity may add to stress. Congenital or developmental conditions such as tarsal coalition (Fig. 8–6) or cavus feet can predispose the athlete to injury [17, 38, 41]. Because both circumstances affect the delicate lower extremity linkage, tibial and knee symptoms may be produced by improper foot mechanics.

The most common significant factor in the generation of overuse injuries is the training program. In noncontrolled systems, e.g., free play, acute injuries occur, but one sees very few stress injuries [64]. It is only when parental, peer, and coaching pressures make unreasonable demands that overload occurs. While taking the history one must look for rapid changes in frequency, magnitude, intensity, or duration of workouts, estimated at greater than 10% per week. Sudden demands for strength training (especially in previously unfit individuals) may produce symptoms of overuse. Cross-training can reduce overuse but can also be a source of injury if inappropriate strength training demands are required.

In the physical examination a multitude of parameters must be assessed in both the upper and lower extremities and the spine. Lower extremity mechanical alignment must be checked to rule out excessive ligamentous laxity and angular, rotatory, or longitudinal deformities (Fig. 8–7). The range of motion of all joints in the involved extremity and its mate is recorded. Generalized as well

FIGURE 8–5
Schematic diagram representing relationship of training effort, conditioning response, and tissue tolerance. Note inverse relationship between latter two factors.

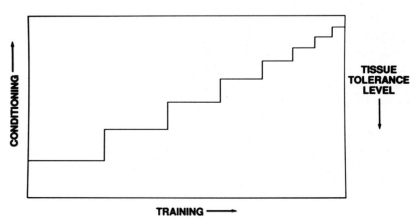
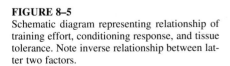

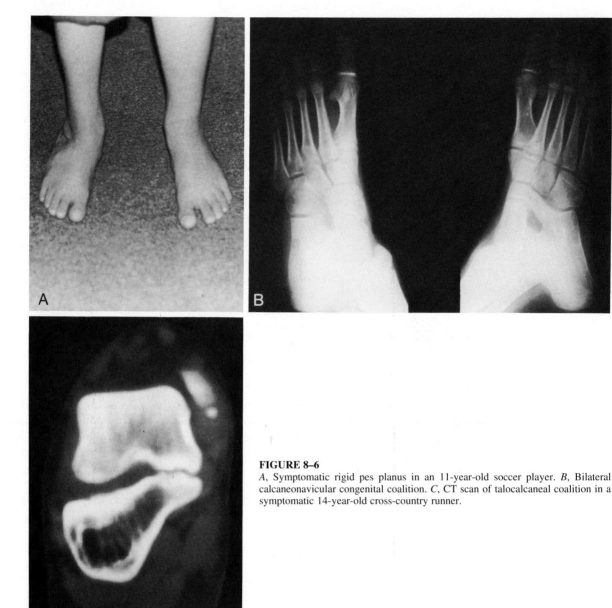

FIGURE 8–6
A, Symptomatic rigid pes planus in an 11-year-old soccer player. *B*, Bilateral calcaneonavicular congenital coalition. *C*, CT scan of talocalcaneal coalition in a symptomatic 14-year-old cross-country runner.

as regional flexibility must be assessed. It should be recognized that a "normal" range of motion may not be satisfactory for specific sport demands, such as in gymnastics or ballet. Anterior and posterior muscle group strength and flexibility balance in both upper and lower extremities should be assessed so that appropriate ratios can be restored if necessary. Objective isokinetic muscle strength testing allows such an evaluation. Focal tenderness and increased warmth and swelling are common manifestations of various "itises" (tendinitis, apophysitis, bursitis) as well as stress fractures.

Diagnostic studies are used as needed to assess overuse disorders. Routine roentgenograms may be unhelpful and at times are confusing. Technetium bone scanning may be more sensitive for the diagnosis of stress fractures. Single-photon emission computerized tomography (SPECT) bone scintigraphy may be useful to rule out otherwise image-negative spondylolysis. Magnetic resonance imaging is useful for the assessment of soft tissue thickening and swelling in locations that are not readily palpable.

Isokinetic strength testing by a variety of machines is helpful when done at functional rates, especially the rates demanded by a particular sport. In a cooperative patient, these tests provide objective measurements that can be used to document progression or regression during a rehabilitation program. Such demonstrative data can also be used to emphasize functional capability in

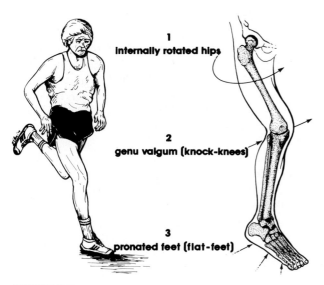

FIGURE 8–7
''Miserable malalignment'' is often a source of foot, ankle, knee, or hip symptoms.

TABLE 8–2
Running Injury Analysis: Six "S's"

Shoes	Wear status or pattern
Surface	Uneven topography
Speed	Too much, too soon
Stretching	Flexibility
Strength	Muscle group imbalance
Structure	Anatomic malalignment

appropriate for the young athlete may be required (Fig. 8–8).

''Relative rest'' is an emerging concept that needs to be incorporated into the rehabilitation effort. Such rest requires reduced duration, intensity, magnitude, and frequency of training to levels that do not produce symptoms. This program allows the athlete to continue training so that body image is maintained and the effects of disuse, underuse, or misuse are diminished. It is important for the athlete to understand that this is a transient period and that as recovery accelerates, a coincident increase in training magnitude, duration, and intensity will be allowed. Substitution of sports activities such as walking, running, swimming, or biking is helpful. Running in water while suspended by an inner tube or life

patients who are less than compliant with a rehabilitation program and can help to determine when return to full activity is possible.

Treatment

The treatment scheme used for overuse problems is a common one and consists of five phases (Table 8–1). These phases are not isolated but are often concurrent. The first phase is identification of the overuse factors. In lower extremity overuse conditions resulting from running, these factors may be broken down into the six S's (speed, shoes, surface, structure, strength, and stretching) (Table 8–2).

The second stage is modification of the offending factor or factors. A review of sports-specific mechanics (e.g., tennis stoke, pitching motion, or running stride) should be done, and the mechanics must be improved as part of the progressive program. Communication with the coach expedites this process. Elimination of inappropriate equipment or modification of equipment to a size

TABLE 8–1
Overuse Treatment Protocol

Identify risk factors
Modify offending factors
Institute pain control
Undertake progressive rehabilitation
Continue maintenance

Note: Phases are often concurrent (e.g., pain control and rehabilitation).

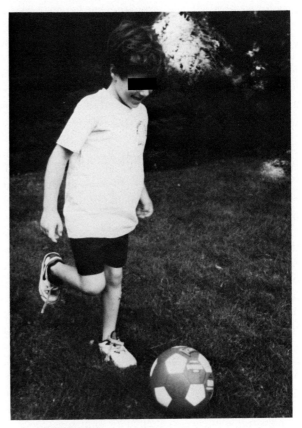

FIGURE 8–8
Soccer ball size appropriate for age group involved.

jacket allows the athlete to maintain continuous aerobic fitness. Strength training in the uninjured extremities allows maintenance of strength in those areas and prevents progressive atrophy. Parental and coaching education are essential during this phase to prevent repetition of incorrect or misdirected training techniques and demands.

The third phase is pain control once the appropriate diagnosis has been made. Pain medicine should not be allowed until the diagnosis has been made. The pain needs to be attenuated so that gradual, supervised rehabilitation is possible. Pain control can be done using a variety of physical modalities (e.g., contrast). Nonsteroidal anti-inflammatory medications or aspirin are helpful for mild pain control, but if started too early (i.e., within the first 48 hours), these medications may inhibit the acute inflammatory response that initiates healing [20, 32, 62].

The fourth phase is progression of functional activity with emphasis on restoration of full flexibility, endurance, and strength. This progressive program leads to the fifth phase, maintenance. This phase of the program must be emphasized to the athlete as a means of preventing new injuries or recurrence of previous injuries.

In both the lower and upper extremities, a baseline level of tensile, compressive, and rotatory stresses is needed to maintain normal soft tissue and bone formation and growth. The particular minimal activity necessary for such growth and maturation has not been specifically established. Limited data are available concerning musculoskeletal exercise tolerance in skeletally immature humans or animals [11, 12, 16, 53, 59, 62]. Previous laboratory studies of soft tissue and bone stress have included acute tests to failure, most commonly in tension and often performed at nonfunctional rates of loading in mature models (canine, lapin, etc.). On the other hand, sports most commonly produce cyclical loading interspersed with an occasional acute maximal load, but in an unpredictable direction. Few data exist about chronic cyclical loading of soft tissue and bone in mature animals, and almost none are available in immature specimens.

Repetitive systematic overload will cause hypertrophy in skeletally immature soft tissues and bone. This was demonstrated by Alekseev [5], who studied the extremities of ski racers aged 11 and 12. He found that these children had hands and feet that were significantly larger than those of similarly aged children not involved in such intense exercise. The greatest difference seemed to occur in the bones with the greatest load. Kato and Ishiko [26] postulated that repetitive heavy work would result in physeal injury, but they presented limited data to substantiate this claim. Long-term follow-up of people involved in impact-loading sports (e.g., running) did not demonstrate evidence of premature joint senescence or degenerative joint disease [27, 30, 51].

SUMMARY

The long-term effects of chronic submaximal stress in skeletally immature athletes are still unknown. A fine line exists between acceptable training loads and loads that produce either bony or soft tissue injury. Overuse problems of the musculoskeletal system have been only recently appreciated. Their incidence and prevalence rival those of acute injuries in pediatric and adolescent athletes, such acute injuries consisting primarily of contusions, abrasions, and sprains that are usually self-limiting and cause little time lost from training or competition. The effects of unresolved microtrauma need to be understood and appreciated so that appropriate guidance can be carried out. The most common etiologic factor in the production of overuse problems is training error, as manifest by either too much, too soon, or just too much. Training must be assessed as the initial step in diagnosis and treatment. A five-step management approach is recommended that includes factor identification, modification of offending agents, pain control, progressive rehabilitation, and maintenance programs. Such a plan will aid and speed symptom resolution and will diminish recurrent injury. Patient, parent, and coach education remains a significant component of management of overuse problems and focuses on training abuse and improper equipment.

STRESS FRACTURES

Bone is a viscoelastic, anisotropic tissue, that is, one whose properties depend on the direction and rate of loading [78, 79, 81, 91, 98, 118, 135, 144]. Ninety percent of the organic tissue of bone is collagen, which reflects much of its response to stress. Eighty percent of the cortical weight of bone is made up of calcium hydroxyapatite crystals, which must interact with the nonmineralized collagen. Optimal stress is stress that produces a balance between bone regeneration and bone resorption. Children are able to absorb greater degrees of deformation prior to fracture than adults. Elastic deformation is proportional to the stress applied. With further persistent force, plastic deformation occurs, which is permanent. Deformity occurs along slip lines with shear of the collagen and crystalline lattice structures. The collagen phase of bone resists tensile stress better than the mineral phase, which in turn resists compressive forces better than collagen. This complex interplay between muscle forces and organic and mineral matrix is reflected in Wolff's Law [144]—the response to deforming strain causes mechanically invoked remodeling. It is uncertain what specific trigger—chemical, physical, or a combination of these—causes the conversion of mechanical stresses and strains to the biologic response of bone [135]. Bony adaptation is a function of a number of loading cycles, cycle frequency, amount of strain, strain rate, and strain duration per cycle [78, 79, 98, 107]. Dietary factors (weight loss for body image, competitive weight) including eating disorders (anorexia, bulimia) and hormonal imbalances also play major roles in calcium homeostasis [89].

Bone exists in a soft tissue envelope, and muscle forces cause effects on bone. Stanitski and colleagues [140] hypothesized that highly concentrated eccentric and concentric muscle forces acted across specific bones and that the demands imposed by particular sports tasks enhanced the loading that occurred and were additive to the direct weight bearing load of the affected part. These authors believed that rhythmical, repetitive muscle action predisposed the bone to failure (Table 8–3). In a demand situation in which time was not available for normal bone repair, these relentless muscle forces provided sufficient unresolved submaximal trauma to cause a stress fracture. Nordin and Frankel [118] also suggested that muscle fatigue played a role in stress fracture production. As the muscle envelope becomes more fatigued, its stress attenuating capability becomes progressively more limited and more force is taken by the underlying bone, leading to subsequent stress fracture production. Li and associates [107] showed that the initial osteoclastic response to stress may outstrip new bone formation by a subsequent osteoblastic response. New loading regimens must last more than 2 weeks before bone responds with increased mineral content and increased strength [113]. These research findings in a non-weight bearing fowl model were clinically correlated in studies [137, 141] of military recruits, who modified their training in the third week and suffered one-third the rate of lower extremity stress fractures compared with a group that did not undergo such training modification during the critical third week. Military recruits

TABLE 8–3
Muscle Forces Leading to Stress Fracture

Increased muscle force
+
Change of remodeling rate
↓
Resorption and rarefaction
↓
Focal microfractures
↓
Periosteal/cortical/endosteal
Response (stress fracture)
↓
Linear fracture
(Stress fracture)
↓
Displaced fracture

[93, 137, 141] who participated in a conditioning program prior to vigorous activity also experienced significant decreases in stress fractures compared with nonpreconditioned Swiss recruits.

Only three animals sustain stress fractures on a regular basis: racing greyhounds [84], race horses [113, 120], and humans [68, 85, 97, 100, 109, 140, 143, 145]. All these animals are placed in situations in which repetitive musculoskeletal demands are made without sufficient time between training cycles or competition to allow restitution of subclinical bone injury.

Originally described in and commonly seen among military recruits [72, 93, 137, 141], stress fractures have become a significant source of sports disability. Stress fractures do occur in children and have a direct relationship to age (i.e., children have fewer fractures than adolescents, who have fewer than adults) [83, 90, 124, 140, 143, 145]. In a study of 368 stress fractures by Orava and colleagues [124], 9% of the fractures occurred in children less than 15 years of age, 32% in 16- to 19-year-olds, and 59% in those over 20 years. In a literature review, Yngve [145] found 113 reported fractures in children less than 14 years old. Multiple anatomic sites of stress fractures in pediatric and adolescent athletes have been reported in association with a wide variety of sport endeavors [65, 67, 70, 74, 82, 83, 86, 88, 101–106, 110, 112, 116, 117, 119, 121, 124, 125, 128, 129, 138, 140, 142, 145, 147]. These include various epiphyseal locations [75, 95, 146]. Epiphyseal distal femoral stress fractures reported by Godshall and colleagues [95] healed without complications or growth impairment following discontinuation of the offending activity. In both Yngve's and Orava's reviews [124, 145], the tibia was the most common site of fracture and had the same frequency of involvement as that seen in adults, i.e., approximately 50% of stress fractures. This frequency of involvement may occur because of the diminished bending strength of the tibia in the frontal plane.

Stanitski and colleagues [140] reported on 14 patients with 16 stress fractures of the tibia, femur, or humerus. Sports producing these injuries included diving, track, baseball, basketball, and tennis. In this series, 11 patients 16 years of age or younger had stress fractures in 13 bones. The tibia was involved in 11 of the 13 fractures (Fig. 8–9).

Standard radiograms are usually unhelpful because in the early phase many stress fractures are roentgenographically silent. Devas and others [85, 106, 133, 140, 145] emphasized the need to distinguish the periosteal reaction of stress fractures from that seen with bone malignancy (Fig. 8–10). Stress fractures may produce symptoms at sites of compromised bone architecture, drawing attention to the lesion (Fig. 8–11).

Technetium-99 bone scanning has proved extremely helpful in early diagnosis of stress fractures [69, 73, 92,

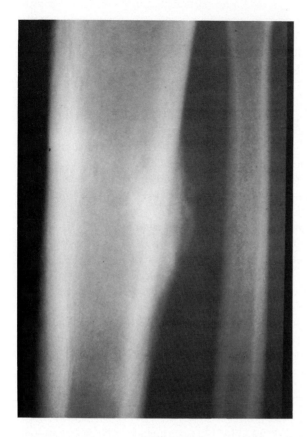

FIGURE 8–9
Proximal tibial stress fractures in a 13-year-old cross-country runner. Note periosteal and endosteal responses.

FIGURE 8–10
Distal femoral stress fracture in a 14-year-old soccer player, originally diagnosed as an osteogenic sarcoma.

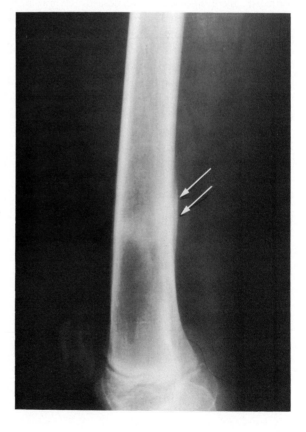

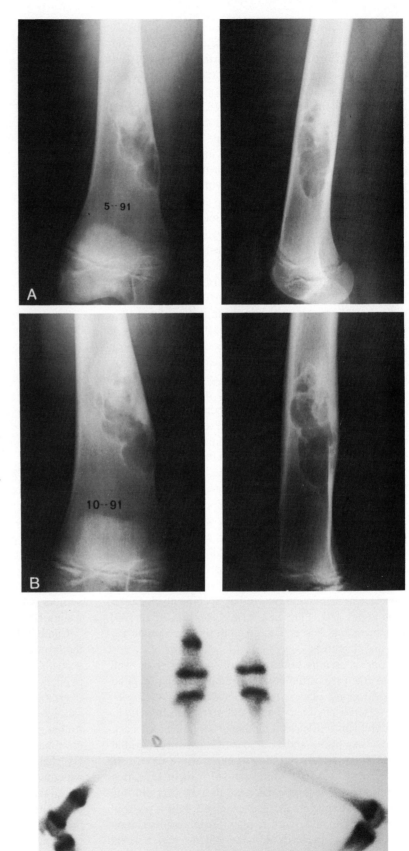

FIGURE 8–11
Femoral deformity with periosteal and cortical response from stress fractures at site of large nonossifying fibroma of the distal femur in a 13-year-old boy. *A*, Radiographs 3 months after onset of symptoms while playing baseball. *B*, Radiographs 5 months later. Pain was present when playing soccer. *C*, Marked increased uptake on bone scan at time of second radiograph.

132, 133, 136]. Technetium-99 scanning is positive about 12 to 15 days following the onset of stress fracture symptoms [73, 92, 133]. This corresponds well with experimental data demonstrating that training must continue for more than 2 weeks before bone is able to respond with increased strength [78, 91, 107]. Scintigraphic findings are not always focal and may vary widely. Diffuse uptake of the isotope may be seen (Fig. 8–12). Multifocal sites of uptake may also be noted, even within the same bone. On further questioning, a patient may relate a past history (within 3 to 6 months) of such symptoms in sites that are now asymptomatic but are still foci of increased bone turnover, as reflected by increased concentration of the nucleotide, which may persist for up to 12 to 16 months postinjury (Fig. 8–13).

In Devas' series [83] of stress fractures in children, 30 patients had proximal tibial fractures. Engh and colleagues [90] reported 11 children less than 12 years old with stress fractures, the majority in the proximal tibia. Rosen and associates [132] reported stress fractures in patients involved in running sports. At the time of assessments 46% of these athletes showed a multifocal ipsilateral stress area, the tibia being the most common site. Clement and colleagues [80] and Puranen [126] reported a medial stress tibial syndrome secondary to periostitis along the tibia due to repetitive submaximal stress, which produced a mechanically related pain brought on by athletic activity and reflected an augmented physiologic response to loading. Mubarek and Hargens [114] studied compartment pressures in 12 patients with stress fracture–type symptoms and found no evidence of compartment syndrome with this medial tibial stress disorder. The term "shin splints" is nonspecific and should be discarded. The differential diagnosis of exercise-induced leg pain should include stress fracture, tibial stress syndrome, compartment syndrome, muscle tear herniation, and other specifically localized pathologies [80, 111, 114, 115, 126, 127, 131, 139]. Treatment can then be addressed to the appropriate factors and diagnosis.

Upper extremity stress fractures may occur as well. Stress fractures of the upper extremity in high-level adolescent tennis players have been reported. A 13-year-old suffered an ulnar diaphyseal stress fracture in his nondominant arm caused by use of a two-handed backhand stroke [129], and a 15-year-old sustained a midhumeral stress fracture resulting from excessive service and overhead strokes [67]. Murakami [116] reported a stress fracture of the second metacarpal in a 16-year-old high school tennis player; the pain resolved with a program of rest and gradual return to play. Stress fractures about the elbow may occur in throwing athletes, e.g., baseball pitchers and javelin throwers [101, 104, 112, 119, 125]. Caine [76] and others [65, 77, 108, 128, 134, 146] emphasize the occurrence of distal radial epiphyseal stress

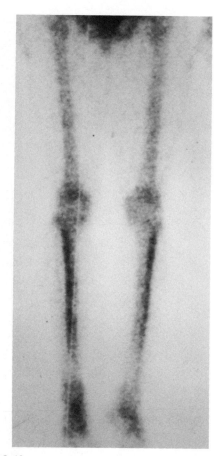

FIGURE 8–12
Diffuse tibial bilateral increased uptake in an 18-year-old hockey player.

fractures in gymnasts who use their upper extremities as weight-bearing columns. Stress fractures of the upper extremity demonstrate that these injuries may occur in nonweight-bearing bones that are subjected to high repetitive stresses or in particular sports that impose weight-bearing demands on the upper limbs.

Cahill and colleagues [75] reported stress fractures of the proximal humerus in six cases involving 11- and 12-year-old Little League pitchers. The presenting complaint was inability to pitch because of pain. These patients' symptoms resolved with diminution of activity followed by gradual resumption of throwing under controlled guidance. In studying the reaction to stress of the proximal humerus in skeletally immature baseball players, these authors noted abundant callus formation and widening of the proximal physeal humerus. They believed that these reactions were related to the stress fracture, which healed when the patients were removed from the pitching environment for a 6-week period.

Even in children, once a stress fracture becomes established, treatment is difficult, and there is a prolonged recovery period, especially in a tensile-type anterior midtibial stress fracture. Green and colleagues [96] re-

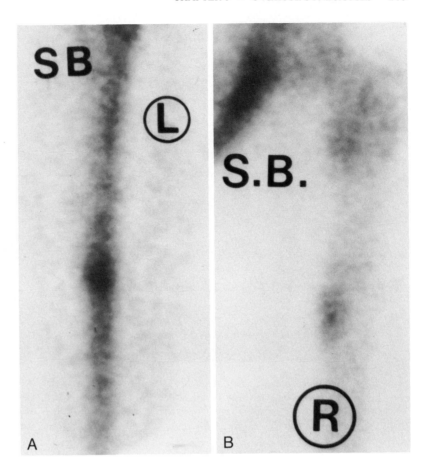

FIGURE 8–13
Increased uptake loci in both femurs in an 18-year-old cross-country runner. At the time, she had symptoms in her left leg. On further questioning, she recalled similar symptoms in the right leg 7 months previously.

ported increased difficulty in healing tibial stress fractures in children and young adults when the fracture was located in this zone. Five of six stress fractures seen by these authors progressed to complete fracture following initial presentation. Three of the patients were aged 10, 11, and 13 years. All stress fractures with this pattern went on to nonunion and required bone grafting. Because of the increased tensile stress across the anterior tibia as well as its marked cortical thickening, stress fractures in this location, which occur primarily in patients with lower extremity malalignment who are involved in jumping sports [71, 96, 122, 123, 130], produce excessive force at the site (Fig. 8–14). These fractures should be considered for debridement of the area and bone grafting if progressive rapid union is not obtained with the usual initial measures. Stress fractures of the tarsal navicular may be particularly resistant to treatment. Nonweight-bearing short-leg cast treatment may be necessary [66, 102, 136, 142].

Dickson and Kichline [87] advocated use of a pneumatic leg brace for management of tibial and fibular stress fractures. Thirteen female athletes with stress fractures of either the tibia or the fibula were treated with this technique, which allowed all 13 to return to sports and participate at a high level with few or no symptoms in a relatively short period of time. All fractures healed uneventfully. The pneumatic device seems to distribute the stress throughout the lower extremity soft tissue envelope in such a way that the fracture site stress is diminished and healing progresses.

Proper shoe orthotics may allow continued symptomless participation in athletes with metatarsal stress fractures by dissipating forces in an even manner across the foot and relatively unweighting the stress fracture.

In addition to inducing stress fractures in the lower extremity, repetitive impact loading may cause difficulty in the upper extremity in athletes, particularly in weight-bearing demand sports such as gymnastics. Roy and colleagues [70] noted distal radial epiphyseal roentgenographic changes due to stress in 21 high-performance gymnasts. Clinical and roentgenographic recovery required approximately 3 months following diminution of activity. These radial epiphyseal stress fractures were directly related to the level of competition, the higher incidence of stress-related injuries occurring among the higher level competitors. These authors suggested that factors that may aggravate or produce such stress injuries in gymnasts include soft mats (which aggravate wrist dorsiflexion), vaulting techniques, torsional forces on the forearm, wrist, and hand during tumbling, and increased numbers of repetitions of particularly demanding moves. They emphasize the need to educate gym-

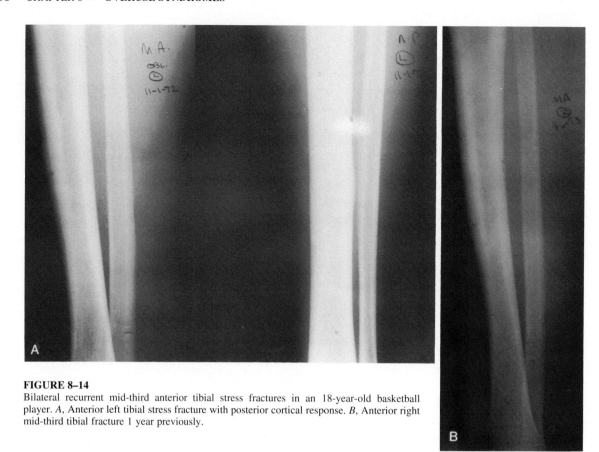

FIGURE 8–14
Bilateral recurrent mid-third anterior tibial stress fractures in an 18-year-old basketball player. *A*, Anterior left tibial stress fracture with posterior cortical response. *B*, Anterior right mid-third tibial fracture 1 year previously.

nasts as well as coaches about such stress-related injuries so that early recognition and treatment can be established. Rehabilitation of the entire upper extremity was advised prior to return to activity. Read [128] also commented on stress fractures of the distal radius in adolescent girl gymnasts and blamed the rotational vault for producing excessive distal radial physeal stress. Yong-Hing and colleagues [146] reported on a national class 13-year-old gymnast who had ulnar stress fractures of the distal physis, which resolved following immobilization. One year later, after an intense competitive interval, the patient experienced radial distal epiphyseal involvement, and the authors implicated the use of dowel grips to enhance high-bar performance as an etiologic factor in this patient's recurrent injury. They recommended that use of such grips not be allowed by skeletally immature gymnasts because of the enhanced compressive force produced at the distal radial and ulnar physes.

Stress fractures represent bone's response to overuse. The basic principles of diagnosis described in the previous section on overuse injuries apply to stress fractures as well. Stress fractures in certain locations (anterior midtibia, tarsal navicular, femoral neck) require more specific management.

As with any other overuse disorder, identification of the offending factor or factors must be the prelude to any treatment. Education of the athlete, parents, and coaches must be a major part of the treatment program of overuse injuries, focusing on training abuse and improper equipment. Further specific management choices (e.g., orthotics, training modification, surgery) are but one phase of the treatment plan.

References

Musculoskeletal Overuse

1. Adams, J. E. Injuries to the throwing arm: A study of traumatic changes in the elbow joints of boy baseball players. *Calif Med* 102:127–129, 1965.
2. Adams, J. E. Little League shoulder osteochondrosis of the proximal humeral epiphysis in boy baseball pitchers. *Calif Med Assoc J* 105:22, 1966.
3. Albanese, S. L., et al. Wrist pain in gymnasts. *J Pediatr Orthop* 9:23–27, 1989.
4. Albright, J. A., et al. Clinical study of baseball pitchers: Correlation of injury to the throwing arm with method of delivery. *Am J Sports Med* 6:15–20, 1978.
5. Alekseev, B. A. The influence of skiing on the hand and foot skeleton of young sportsmen. *Arkhiv Anatomii, Gistologii Embriologii Lenigrad* 72:35–39, 1977.
6. Andrish, J. G. Overuse syndromes of the lower extremity in youth sports. *In* Boileau R. (Ed.), *Advances in Pediatric Sports Sciences*. Champaign, IL, Human Kinetics, 1984.
7. Blanten, B. Mechanical strength of fetal and adult tissue. *J Anat* 61:223–231, 1981.

8. Burke, B. L., Jr., and McGee, D. P. Sport deficit disorder. *Pediatrics* 85:1118, 1990.

9. Cahill, B. R., Tullos, H. S., and Fain, R. H. Little League shoulder. *Am J Sports Med* 2:150–153, 1974.

10. Caine, D., Roy, S., Singer, K. M., et al. Stress changes of the distal radial growth plate. *Am J Sports Med* 20(3):290–298, 1992.

11. Carter, D. R. et al. Influences of mechanical stress on prenatal and postnatal skeletal development. *Clin Orthop* 219:237–250, 1987.

12. Carter, D. R., et al. Mechanical stresses and endochondral ossification in the chondroepiphysis. *J Orthop Res* 6(1):148–154, 1988.

13. Carter, S. R., et al. Stress changes of the wrist in adolescent gymnasts. *Br J Radiol* 61(722):109–112, 1988.

14. Carter, S. R., et al. Stress injury of the distal radial growth plate. *J Bone Joint Surg* 70B:834–836, 1988.

15. Curwin, S., and Stanish, W. D. *Tendinitis: Its Etiology and Treatment.* Lexington, MA, D. C. Heath, 1984, pp. 25–44.

16. Dalen, N., and Olsson, K. E. Bone mineral content and physical activity. *Acta Orthop Scand* 45:170, 1974.

17. Elkus, R. A. Tarsal coalition in the young athlete. *Am J Sports Med* 14(6):477–480, 1986.

18. Farkas, T., Boyd, R. D., Schaffler, M. B., et al. Early vascular changes in rabbit subchondral bone after repetitive impulsive loading. *Clin Orthop* 219:259–267, 1987.

19. Garrick, J. G., and Requa, R. K. Epidemiology of women's gymnastics injuries. *Am J Sports Med* 8:261–264, 1980.

20. Gelberman, R. H., Goldberg, V. M., An, K., et al. Tendon. *In* Woo, S. L.-Y., and Buckwalter, J. A. (Eds.), *Injury and Repair of the Musculoskeletal Soft Tissues.* Park Ridge, IL, American Academy of Orthopaedic Surgeons, 1988, p. 1.

21. Grana, W. A., and Rashin, A. Pitcher's elbow in adolescents. *Am J Sports Med* 8(5):333–336, 1980.

22. Gugenheim, J. J., Jr., Stanley, R. F., Woods, G. W., et al. Little League survey: The Houston Study. *Am J Sports Med* 4(5):189–200, 1976.

23. Herring, S. A., and Nilson, K. L. Introduction to overuse injuries. *Clin Sports Med* 6(2):225–239, 1987.

24. Jackson, D. W., Silvino, N., and Reiman, P. Osteochondritis in the female gymnast's elbow. *Arthroscopy* 5:129–136, 1989.

25. Kannus, P., et al. Overuse problems in children. *Clin Pediatr* 27(7):333–337, 1988.

26. Kato, S., and Ishiko, T. Obstructed growth of children's bones due to excessive labor in remote corners. *In Proceedings of International Congress of Sports Sciences.* Tokyo, Japanese Union of Sports Sciences, 1976.

27. Konradsen, L., et al. Long distance running and osteoarthrosis. *Adv Orthop Surg* 15(1):35–38, 1991.

28. Kurtz, A. D. Apophysitis of the os calcis. *Am J Orthop Surg* 15:659–563, 1917.

29. Kvist, M., Kujala, U., et al. Osgood-Schlatter's and Sever's disease in young athletes. *Duodecim* 142–150, 1984.

30. Lane, N. E. Does running cause degenerative joint disease? *J Musculoskel Med* 4(7):17–24, 1987.

31. Larson, R. L., Single, K. M., Bergstrom, R., et al. Little League survey: The Eugene Study. *Am J Sports* 4(5):201–209, 1976.

32. Leadbetter, W. B., Buckwalter, J. A., and Gordon, S. L. *Sports-Induced Inflammation.* Park Ridge, IL, American Academy of Orthopaedic Surgeons, 1990.

33. Maffulli, N., Cahn, D., and Aldridge, M. J. Overuse injuries of the olecranon in young gymnasts. *J Bone Joint Surg* 74B:305–308, 1992.

34. Mandelbaum, B. R., Bartolozzi, A. R., et al. Wrist pain syndrome in the gymnast. Pathogenic, diagnostic, and therapeutic considerations. *Am J Sports Med* 17:305–317, 1989.

35. McManama, G. B., Jr., Micheli, L. J., Berry, M. V., et al. The surgical treatment of osteochondritis of the capitellum. *Am J Sports Med* 13(1):11–21, 1985.

36. Micheli, L. J., and Ireland M. L. Prevention and management of calcaneal apophysitis in children: An overuse syndrome. *J Pediatr Orthop* 7(1):34–38, 1987.

37. Micheli, L. J. Overuse injuries in children's sports. *Orthop Clin North Am* 14:337–359, 1983.

38. Morgan, R. C., Jr., et al. Surgical management of tarsal coalition in adolescent athletes. *Foot Ankle* 7(3):183–193, 1986.

39. Nordin, M., and Frankel, V. H. Biomechanics of collagenous tissues. *In Basic Biomechanics of the Skeletal System.* Philadelphia, Lea & Febiger, 1980, pp. 87–110.

40. Ogden, J. A., and Lee, J. Accessory ossification patterns and injuries of the malleoli. *J Pedr Orthop* 10:306, 1990.

41. O'Neill, D. B., et al. Tarsal coalition. A followup of adolescent athletes. *Am J Sports Med* 17(4):544–549, 1989.

42. Panner, H. J. A peculiar affection of the capitellum humeri, resembling Calve-Perthes' disease of the hip. *Acta Radiol* 8:617, 1927.

43. Pettrone, F. A., and Ricciardelli, E. Gymnastic injuries: The Virginia experience, 1982–1983. *Am J Sports Med* 4:145, 1976.

44. Read, M. F. T. Stress fractures of the distal radius in adolescent gymnasts. *Br J Sports Med* 15:272–276, 1981.

45. Roy, S., et al. Stress changes of the distal radial epiphysis in young gymnasts. *Am J Sports Med* 13(5):301–308, 1985.

46. Rowland, T. W. Overtraining hazards in prepubertal athletes. *J Musculoskel Med* 7(2):52–60, 1990.

47. Sever, J. W. Apophysitis of the os calcis. *NY Med J* 95:1025–1029, 1912.

48. Simkin, A., et al. The effect of swimming activity on bone architecture in growing rats. *J Biomech* 22(8–9):845–851, 1989.

49. Singer, K. M., and Roy, S. P. Osteochondrosis of the humeral capitellum. *Am J Sports Med* 12(5):351–360, 1984.

50. Snook, G. A. Injuries in women's gymnastics: A five-year study. *Am J Sports Med* 7:242–244, 1979.

51. Sohn, R. S., and Micheli, L. J. The effect of running on the pathogenesis of osteoarthritis of the hips and knee. *Clin Orthop* 198:106–109, 1985.

52. Stanish, W. D. Overuse injuries in athletes. *Med Sci Sports Exer* 16:1–7, 1984.

53. Stanitski, C. L. Repetitive stress and connective tissue. *In* Sullivan, J. A., and Grana, W. A. (Eds.), *The Pediatric Athlete.* Park Ridge, IL, American Academy of Orthopaedic Surgeons, 1988, pp. 203–209.

54. Stanitski, C. L. Common injuries in preadolescent and adolescent athletes: Recommendations for prevention. *Sports Med* 7(1):32–41, 1989.

55. Stanitski, C. L., and Micheli, L. J. Observations on symptomatic medial malleolar ossification centers. *J Pediatr Orthop* 13:575, 1993.

56. Szot, Z., Boron, Z., and Galaj, Z. Overloading changes in the motor system occurring in elite gymnasts. *Int J Sports Med* 6:36–40, 1985.

57. Tipton, C. M., Matthes, R. D., Maynard, J. A., et al. The influence of physical activity on ligaments and tendons. *Med Sci Sports Exerc* 7:165–175, 1975.

58. Tursz, A., and Crost, M. Sports related injuries in children. *Am J Sports Med* 14(4):294–299, 1986.

59. Videman, T. An experimental study of the effects of growth on the relationship of tendons and ligaments to bone at the site of diaphyseal insertion. *Acta Orthop Scand* 131(Suppl.):1–22, 1970.

60. Wolff, J. Concerning the interrelationship between form and function of the individual parts of the organism. *Clin Orthop* 228:2–11, 1988.

61. Wong, M., et al. Mechanical stress and morphogenetic endochondral ossification of the sternum. *J Bone Joint Surg* 70A:992–1000, 1988.

62. Woo, S. L., and Buckwalter, J. A. (Eds.). *Injury and Repair of the Musculoskeletal Soft Tissues.* Park Ridge, IL, American Academy of Orthopaedic Surgeons, 1988.

63. Yong-Hing, K., Wedge, J. H., and Bowen, C. V. Chronic injury to the distal ulnar and radial growth plates in an adolescent gymnast. *J Bone Joint Surg* 70A:1087–1089, 1988.

64. Zaricznyi, B., et al. Sports related injuries in school aged children. *Am J Sports Med* 8:318–322, 1980.

Stress Fractures

65. Albanese, S. A., Palmer, A. K., Kerr, D. R., et al. Wrist pain and distal growth plate closure of the radius in gymnasts. *J Pediatr Orthop* 9:23–28, 1989.

66. Alfred, R. H., et al. Stress fractures of the tarsal navicular. *Am J Sports Med* 20(6):766–768, 1992.

67. Allen, M. E. Stress fractures of the humerus. *Am J Sports Med* 12:244–245, 1974.

68. Belkin, S. C. Stress fractures in athletes. *Orthop Clin North Am* 11:735–742, 1980.

69. Bellah, R. D., Summerville, D. A., Treves, S. T., et al. Low-back pain in adolescent athletes: Detection of stress injury to the pars interarticularis with SPECT. *Radiology* 180:509–512, 1991.

70. Berkebile, R. D. Stress fracture of the tibia in children. *Am J Roentgenol* 91:588–596, 1964.

71. Blank, S. Transverse tibial stress fractures: A special problem. *Am J Sports Med* 15(6):597–602, 1987.

72. Breithaupt, M. D. Zur Pathologie des Mensch lichen Fussess. *Med Zeit* 24:169–177, 1855.

73. Brill, D. R. Sports nuclear medicine: Bone imaging for lower extremity pain in athletes. *Clin Nucl Med* 8:101–106, 1983.

74. Burks, R. T., and Sutherland, D. H. Stress fracture of the femoral shaft in children: Report of two cases and discussion. *J Pediatr Orthop* 4:614–616, 1984.

75. Cahill, B. R., Tullos, H. S., and Fain, R. H. Little League shoulder. *Am J Sports Med* 2:150–153, 1974.

76. Caine, D. Stress changes of the distal radial growth plate. *Am J Sports Med* 20(3):290–298, 1992.

77. Carter, S. R., Aldridge, M. J., Fitzgerald, R., et al. Stress changes of the wrist in adolescent gymnasts. *Br J Radiol* 61:109–112, 1988.

78. Chamay, A. Mechanical and morphological aspects of experimental overload and fatigue in bone. *Clin Orthop* 127:265–274, 1970.

79. Chamay, A., and Tschantz, P. Mechanical influences in bone remodeling. Experimental research on Wolff's law. *J Biomech* 5:173–180, 1972.

80. Clement, D. B. Tibial stress syndrome in athletes. *Am J Sports Med* 2:81–85, 1974.

81. Dalen, N., and Olsson, K. E. Bone mineral content and physical activity. *Acta Orthop Scand* 45:170, 1974.

82. Darby, R. E. Stress fractures of the os calcis. *JAMA* 200:131–132, 1967.

83. Devas, M. B. Stress fractures in children. *J Bone Joint Surg* 45B:528–541, 1963.

84. Devas, M. B. Compression stress fractures in man and the greyhound. *J Bone Joint Surg* 43B:540–551, 1961.

85. Devas, M. *Stress Fractures.* Edinburgh, Churchill Livingstone, 1975, pp. 130–137.

86. Dickason, J. M, and Fox, J. M. Fracture of the patella due to overuse syndrome in a child: A case report. *Am J Sports Med* 10:248–249, 1982.

87. Dickson T. B., Jr., and Kichline, D. D. Functional management of stress fractures in female athletes using a pneumatic leg brace. *Am J Sports Med* 15(1):86–88, 1987.

88. Donati, R. B., Echo, B. S., and Powell, C. E. Bilateral tibial stress fractures in a six-year-old male. A case report. *Am J Sports Med* 18:323–325, 1990.

89. Drinkwater, B. L., Nilson, K., Chestnut, C. H., III, et al. Bone mineral content of amenorrheic and eumenorrheic athletes. *N Engl J Med* 311:277–281, 1984.

90. Engh, C. H., Robinson, R. A., and Milgram, J. Stress fractures in children. *J Trauma* 10:532–541, 1970.

91. Forwood, M. R., et al. Microdamage in response to repetitive torsional leading in the rat tibia. *Calcif Tissue Int* 45(1):47–53, 1990.

92. Geslien, G. E., et al. Early detection of stress fractures using 99m-Tc-polyphosphate. *Radiology* 121:683–687, 1976.

93. Giladi, M., et al. Stress fractures and identifiable risk factors. *Am J Sports Med* 19:647–652, 1991.

94. Giladi, M., et al. Stress fractures and tibial bone width. *J Bone Joint Surg* 69B:326, 1987.

95. Godshall, R. W., Hansen, C. A., and Rising, D. C. Stress fractures through the distal femoral epiphysis in athletes. *Am J Sports Med* 9: 114–116, 1981.

96. Green, N. E., Rogers, R. A., and Lipscomb, A. B. Nonunions of stress fractures of the tibia. *Am J Sports Med* 13:171–176, 1985.

97. Ha, K., et al. A clinical study of stress fractures in sports activities. *Orthopaedics* 14:1089–1095, 1991.

98. Hille, E., et al. Experimental stress-induced changes in growing long bones. *Int Orthop* 12(4):309–315, 1988.

99. Holder, L., and Michael, R. H. The specific scintigraphic pattern of "shin splints on the lower leg." *J Nucl Med* 25:865–869, 1984.

100. Hullko, A., Orava, S., and Nikula, P. Stress fractures in athletes. *Int J Sports Med* 8:221–226, 1987.

101. Hullko, A., Orava, S., and Nikula, P. Stress fractures of the olecranon in javelin throwers. *Int J Sports Med* 7:210, 1986.

102. Hunter, L. Y. Stress fracture of the tarsal navicular. More frequent than we realize? *Am J Sport Med* 9:217–219, 1983.

103. Keating, T. M. Stress fracture of the sternum in a wrestler. *Am J Sports Med* 15(1)92–93, 1987.

104. Kvidera, D. J., and Pedegana, L. R. Stress fracture of the olecranon. Report of two cases and review of literature. *Orthop Rev* 12(7):113–116, 1983.

105. Leabhart, J. W. Stress fractures of the calcaneus. *J Bone Joint Surg* 41A:1285, 1959.

106. Levin, D. C., et al. Fatigue fractures of the shaft of the femur: Simulation of malignant tumor. *Radiology* 89:883–885, 1967.

107. Li, G., Zhang, S., Chen, G., et al. Radiographs and histologic analyses of stress fractures in rabbit tibias. *Am J Sports Med* 113:285–294, 1985.

108. Mandelbaum, B. R., Bartolozzi, A. R., Davis, C. A., et al. Wrist pain syndrome in the gymnast. Pathogenic, diagnostic, and therapeutic considerations. *Am J Sports Med* 17:305–317, 1989.

109. Matheson, G. O., et al. Stress fractures in athletes. A study of 320 cases. *Am J Sports Med* 15(1):46–68, 1987.

110. Manzione, M., and Pizzutillo, P. D. Stress fracture of the scaphoid: A case report. *Am J Sports Med* 10:365–367, 1981.

111. Michael, R. H., and Holder, L. E. The soleus syndrome: A cause of medial tibial stress (shin splints). *Am J Sports Med* 13(2):87–94, 1985.

112. Miller, J. E. Javelin thrower's elbow. *J Bone Joint Surg* 42B:788, 1960.

113. Moritani, T., and De Vries, H. A. Neural factors versus hypertrophy in the time course of muscles' strength gain. *Am J Phys Med* 58:115–130, 1979.

114. Mubarak, S. J., and Hargens, A. R. Exertional compartment syndromes. *In* Mubarak, S. J., and Hargens, A. R. (Eds). *Compartment Syndromes and Volkmann's Contracture.* Philadelphia, W. B. Saunders Co., 1981.

115. Mubarak, S. J., et al. The medial tibial stress syndrome. A cause of shin splint. *Am J Sports Med* 10:201–205, 1982.

116. Murakami, Y. Stress fractures of the metacarpal in an adolescent tennis player. *Am J Sports Med* 16:419–420, 1988.

117. Mutoh, Y., Mori, T., Suzuki, Y., et al. Stress fractures of the ulna in athletes. *Am J Sports Med* 10:365–367, 1982.

118. Nordin, M., and Frankel, V. H. Biomechanics of whole bones and bone tissue. *In* Frankel, V. J., and Nordin, M. (Eds.), *Basic Biomechanics of the Skeletal System.* Philadelphia, Lea & Febiger, 1980, pp. 15–60.

119. Nuber, G. W., and Diment, M. T. Olecranon stress fractures in throwers. *Clin Orthop* 273:58–61, 1992.

120. Nunamaker, D. M., et al. Fatigue fractures in thoroughbred racehorses: Relationship with age, peak bone strain, and training. *J Orthop Res* 8(4):604–611, 1990.

121. Orloff, A. S., et al. Fatigue fracture of the distal part of the radius in a pool player. *Injury* 17(6):418–419, 1986.

122. Orava, S., and Hulkko, A. Delayed unions and nonunions of stress fractures in athletes. *Am J Sports Med* 16:378–382, 1988.

123. Orava, S., and Hulkko, A. Stress fracture of the mid-tibial shaft. *Acta Orthop Scand* 55:35–37, 1984.

124. Orava, S., et al. Stress fractures in young athletes. *Arch Orthop Trauma Surg* 98:271–274, 1981.

125. Pavlov, H., Torg, J. S., Jacobs, B., et al. Nonunion of olecranon epiphysis: Two cases in adolescent baseball pitchers. *Am J Radiol* 136:819, 1981.

126. Puranen, J. The medial tibial syndrome. *J Bone Joint Surg* 56B:712–715, 1974.

127. Qvarfordt, R., Christenson, J. T., Eklof, B., et al. Intramuscular pressure, muscle blood flow, and skeletal muscle metabolism in chronic anterior tibial compartment syndrome. *Clin Orthop* 179:284–290, 1983.

128. Read, M. T. F. Stress fractures of the distal radius in adolescent gymnasts. *Br J Sports Med* 15:272–276, 1981.

129. Rettig, A. C. Stress fracture of the ulna in an adolescent tournament tennis player. *Am J Sports Med* 13:55–58, 1985.

130. Rettig, A. C., et al. The natural history and treatment of delayed union stress fractures of the anterior cortex of the tibia. *Am J Sports Med* 16(3):250–255, 1988.

131. Rorabeck, C. H., Bourne, R. B., and Fowler, P. F. The surgical treatment of exertional compartment syndrome in athletes. *J Bone Joint Surg* 65A:1245–1251, 1983.

132. Rosen, P. R., et al. Early scintigraphic diagnosis of bone stress and fractures in athletic adolescents. *Pediatrics* 70:11–15, 1982.

133. Roub, L. W., et al. Bone stress: A radionuclide imaging perspective. *Radiology* 132:431, 1979.

134. Roy, S., Caine, D., and Singer, K. M. Stress changes of the distal radial epiphysis in young gymnasts. A report of twenty-one cases and a review of the literature. *Am J Sports Med* 13:301–308, 1985.

135. Rubin, C. T., et al. Osteoregulatory nature of mechanical stimuli: Function as a determinant for adaptive remodeling in bone. Kappa Delta Award paper. *J Orthop Res* 5(2):300–310, 1987.

136. Santi, M., et al. Diagnostic imaging of tarsal and metatarsal stress fractures. Part II. *Orthop Rev* 18(3):305–310, 1989.

137. Scully, T. J., and Besterman, G. Stress fracture. A preventable training injury. *Milit Med* 147:285–287, 1982.

138. Shelbourne, K. D., Fisher, D. A., Rettig, A. C., et al. Stress fractures of the medial malleolus. *Am J Sports Med* 16:60–64, 1988.

139. Spencer, R. P., et al. Diverse bone scan abnormalities in ''shin splints.'' *J Nucl Med* 20:1271–1272, 1979.

140. Stanitski, C. L., McMaster, J. H., and Scranton, P. E. On the nature of stress fractures. *Am J Sports Med* 6:391–396, 1978.

141. Swissa, A., et al. The effect of pretraining sports activity on the incidence of stress fractures among military recruits. A prospective study. *Clin Orthop* 245:256–260, 1989.

142. Torg, J. S., Pavlov, H., Cooley, L. H., et al. Stress fractures of the tarsal navicular. *J Bone Joint Surg* 64A:700–712, 1982.

143. Walter, N. E., and Wolf, M. D. Stress fractures in young athletes. *Am J Sports Med* 5:165–170, 1977.

144. Wolff, J. *Das Gesetz, der Transformation, der Knochen.* Berlin, Hirschwold, 1892.

145. Yngve, D. A. Stress fractures in the pediatric athlete. *In* Sullivan, J. A., and Grana, W. A. (Eds.), *The Pediatric Athlete.* Oklahoma City, American Academy of Orthopaedic Surgeons, 1988.

146. Yong-Hing, K., Wedge, J. H., and Bowen, C. V. Chronic injury to the distal ulnar and radial growth plates in an adolescent gymnast. *J Bone Joint Surg* 70A:1087–1089, 1988.

147. Zlatkin, M. B., et al. Stress fractures of the distal tibia and calcaneus subsequent to acute fractures of the tibia and fibula. *Am J Roentgenol* 149(2):329–332, 1987.

HEAD INJURY

A. Leland Albright, M.D.

Sports-related head injuries are common in children. Each year 50,000 football players and 75,000 bicycle riders sustain a concussion. Approximately 10% of all pediatric brain injuries are attributable to accidents in sports and with bicycles [19]. Each season in organized sports, 39 boys and 21 girls per 100 participants sustain injuries; 1% to 5% of those injuries affect the central nervous system [12]. The majority of such injuries are sustained in contact sports, but most are not serious enough to warrant hospitalization.

Except for bicycle accidents, sports-related head injuries are uncommon in children less than 12 years old. Their immature bodies are less able to generate injuring forces, they do not play with the same win-at-all-costs attitude common in older adolescents (and coaches), and they are less likely to play if they are injured or hurting.

Children participating in sports sustain a range of brain injuries from minimal to catastrophic. The spectrum of those injuries reflects the variety of forces applied to athletes' heads. Small-impact forces momentarily disrupt physiologic function, and the athlete is stunned. Moderate impacts disrupt physiologic function longer and result in serious concussion. Severe impacts cause both physiologic and structural damage, and coma or death may occur.

I will review the spectrum of head injuries that can occur in any sport and then comment on specific sports.

PHYSICAL EXAMINATION

The unconscious athlete should be examined immediately by the nearest trainer or physician, regardless of which team the player is on. Because these examinations often occur under stressful circumstances, it is worthwhile to consider the conduct of such an examination ahead of time. The first priority in examining an unconscious athlete is *not* to roll him or her into a supine position and examine the pupils! The first priority is to determine whether he is breathing and whether the air-

way is adequate. Unconscious athletes usually ventilate adequately, but if the impact has caused a post-traumatic seizure, the airway may be compromised, and a plastic oropharyngeal airway may be needed. Second, examine the pulses. Although they are almost always normal, a severe head injury on rare occasions causes cardiac asystole or severe bradycardia, and cardiopulmonary resuscitation must be given.

If the airway and pulses are adequate, move the unconscious athlete into a supine position as though he had a broken neck: logroll him onto a spine board while immobilizing the neck in a neutral position—not flexed and not extended. The *unconscious athlete must be assumed to have an associated cervical spine injury* unless the cause of the blow, such as a golf ball to the temple, makes that unlikely, and a rigid cervical collar should be applied if one is available. If the athlete is unconscious in a prone or lateral position, it is better to roll him once—onto a spine board—than to roll him into a supine position for an examination and then subsequently onto the spine board. If the unconscious athlete is wearing a helmet, it can be left on; traction can be applied under the helmet edge or in the ear holes while moving him onto the board.

After the athlete is supine, assess the level of consciousness and the presence of associated injuries. Unless consciousness is regained within a few minutes, the athlete should be carried from the area on a stretcher; standing these players up before they are alert may cause systemic and cerebral hypotension. The value of the ammonia capsules that are often placed under the nose of partially conscious players is minimal; ammonia irritates the nasal mucosa and may cause quick neck extension, which theoretically could worsen an unstable cervical spine injury.

CONCUSSION

By definition, a concussion is an immediate, temporary, post-traumatic alteration in consciousness that may last from seconds to 24 hours and may be accompanied by amnesia and confusion. The pathophysiology of concussion is unclear but is more likely related to brief changes in membrane ion potentials than to changes in blood flow or to edema.

Although concussions represent an infinitely graded spectrum of injury, most authors grade concussions in three or four categories. The Congress of Neurological Surgeons classification is as follows:

1. Mild—no loss of consciousness
2. Moderate—loss of consciousness with retrograde amnesia
3. Severe—Unconsciousness greater than 5 minutes

A minimal concussion, however, is the most common sports head injury and has been described as the "threshold" injury. Athletes with minimal concussions are stunned or dazed but do not lose consciousness and have no amnesia or associated symptoms. The impact probably alters their level of consciousness by stunning the cortical projections of the reticular activating system. They should be removed from the contest and examined immediately and every 5 minutes, and can return to the contest if no amnesia or other symptoms develop within 20 minutes [18].

Athletes with mild concussions are also stunned but not unconscious, but they do have amnesia. They describe the injury as being "dinged" or as "having their bell rung." They cannot recall all events or information occurring before and after the impact. They often have the "empty eyes" look and do not focus well. They may have associated symptoms such as headache, ringing in the ears, vertigo, or unsteady gait. They should be removed from the game and not allowed to return to that game, nor to practice until they are asymptomatic for 1 week (in particular, without headache), move with their usual coordination, are perfectly oriented, and answer questions appropriately, criteria that may require more than 2 hours and usually preclude resumption in that particular contest. They may develop the postconcussion syndrome, discussed below.

Amnesia in concussed athletes indicates a physiologic brain injury; the timing and duration of amnesia indicate the severity of the injury. Post-traumatic amnesia prevents memory consolidation, but immediate registration and recall may be preserved. Team physicians should therefore test for post-traumatic amnesia by asking questions such as, "Who helped you get up?" or "How did you get to the sidelines?" rather than questions about digit recall or reverse spelling. Retrograde amnesia can be checked with questions such as, "What is the score?" or "Who are you guarding?"

Athletes with moderate concussions are rendered unconscious but become alert within 5 minutes. They have amnesia for events before and after the impact and may also develop associated symptoms and later the postconcussion syndrome. Athletes with moderate concussions should not return to that contest, nor should they resume contact sports until they are asymptomatic for 2 weeks. There is fairly strong evidence—and it makes sense—that those who return earlier have an increased risk for another, more serious injury [9, 18, 25].

The classic, severe concussion is characterized by flaccid unconsciousness from the moment of impact for 5 minutes or more afterward and is due to an impact that physiologically disconnects the cortex from the brain stem reticular formation. After consciousness returns, headache, nausea, and vertigo are common, and both post-traumatic and retrograde amnesia are present. These athletes should be examined by a physician and should be evaluated and treated like any other child with a serious head injury, usually with observation overnight in a hospital. They obviously must not reenter the contest because of the increased risk of a more serious injury, even if they become alert. Severe head injuries cause unconsciousness for more than 24 hours. The intense acceleration-rotation forces producing such an injury can shear deep white matter tracts [13].

Athletes who sustain head injuries while in motion, especially while falling, may develop symptoms resulting from contrecoup brain injuries. The direct injury at the point of impact is the coup injury. The brain may rebound from the point of impact and strike the opposite side of the skull. The resulting contrecoup injury may cause more symptoms than the direct injury. Ice skaters and horse riders, for example, often fall and strike the occipital area. The direct occipital injury may cause blurred vision or transient cortical blindness, but the contrecoup injury to the frontotemporal lobes causes combativeness and confusion.

A few football players have a history of being knocked unconscious rather easily; these players should be encouraged to pursue another sport. The decision about when to discontinue football after multiple head injuries must be made on an individual basis. Although three severe concussions should probably indicate that continuation in football is inadvisable, in my opinion, a single severe concussion accompanied by either a focal neurologic deficit or an abnormality on computed tomography or magnetic resonance imaging should lead to the same conclusion.

The postconcussion syndrome is a common sequela of severe concussions. Studies by Rimal and colleagues [23] and Gronwall and Wrightson [14] indicate that minor head injuries often produce recurring headaches, minor changes in personality, and difficulty with higher integrative functions. These symptoms may last for 2 to 3 months and are often associated with a temporary decline in school performance.

We must remember that the primary goal of the student athlete is to improve the skull contents. Effects of repeated minor concussions are cumulative [14, 24]. Both coaches and players may ask that the concussed athlete return to the contest as soon as he is awake. But information processing is impaired after a concussion, and the likelihood of an additional concussion is increased if the player returns earlier than the guidelines recommended above. If further brain injury occurs, impairment is greater than if the athlete had not been concussed before.

DIAGNOSTIC STUDIES

Skull radiographs are of little if any help in treating athletes with mild or moderate head injuries. Linear skull fractures are occasionally seen, but, unlike the situation in adults, these are often not visible in children who develop hematomas. Children with serious head injuries should be evaluated with computed tomographic (CT) or magnetic resonance imaging (MRI) scans.

A scan should be obtained in athletes with decreased levels of consciousness, persistent headache, signs or symptoms of increased intracranial pressure, and focal neurologic deficits. Scans are probably indicated for athletes who have had a single post-traumatic seizure because management of these individuals would be altered if cerebral contusion or edema were demonstrated. Athletes should never be discharged from the emergency room after a sports head injury unless they are absolutely alert; listlessness alone may be the first sign of an epidural hematoma.

Athletes who are agitated or combative after head injuries should not be sedated so that they will lie quietly for a CT scan unless careful attention is paid to their airway and ventilation. Sedation depresses respiration, causing hypercarbia, increased intracranial pressure, and possible brain herniation. This problem can be prevented by instituting controlled intubation and ventilation before scanning. The most common abnormality evident on CT scans after athletic head injury is a small amount of blood in the subarachnoid space. Second most common is cerebral hyperemia, followed by contusion or edema, and least common is intracranial hematoma.

STRUCTURAL LESIONS

Acute Epidural Hematoma

A few athletes develop intracranial hematomas after sports head injuries. Acute epidural hematomas are usually of arterial origin and can develop if a hard localized blow to the temple fractures the temporal bone, which is only 2 to 4 mm thick in older children, and tears the underlying middle meningeal artery. The artery is not as embedded in the temporal bone as it is in older adults, and therefore the frequency of such hematomas after temporal bone fractures is lower in children than in adults. Acute epidural hematomas develop more often in golfers or baseball players than in helmeted football players. Although the classic history of a child with an acute epidural hematoma is a lucid interval of minutes to hours after the injury, followed by deterioration, that pattern is not invariable; acute epidural hematomas may occur in athletes who never lost consciousness and in those who never regained it.

If the athlete is conscious, the enlarging hematoma usually causes worsening headache, nausea, and vomiting. Later, the hematoma distorts the ipsilateral corticospinal tract and causes weakness of the contralateral arm; it also compresses the ipsilateral oculomotor nerve, causing first pupillary asymmetry and later pupillary unreactiveness. If the hematoma enlarges further, the uncus of the temporal lobe compresses the midbrain, small hemorrhages develop within the midbrain, and the result is either severe disability or death. The brain underneath the hematoma is usually not bruised or edematous, and removal of the clot relieves the problem if the removal is accomplished before the midbrain is injured.

An epidural hematoma should be suspected in children who have sustained hard blows to the temple, even if the neurologic examination is initially normal and skull radiographs show no fracture. Computed tomography or MRI scans should be obtained if persistent headache, drowsiness, or other neurologic symptoms develop. Scans clearly demonstrate the size of the hematoma and the extent of brain shift (Fig. 9–1). Although many epidural hematomas need to be removed, not all do. Small epidural hematomas can be left in place in children who are asymptomatic except for mild headache if the neurologic examination is normal and they remain under close neurosurgical observation for several days.

Acute Subdural Hematomas

These are the hematomas that occur in football players. Nearly all football players who die because of a head injury have an acute subdural hematoma [13]. The hematoma results from a severe blow to the head that causes angular acceleration of the brain and tears the vessels, usually veins, between the cortex and the dura. In contrast to acute epidural hematomas, acute subdural hematomas are associated with contusion (bruising) and edema of the underlying brain, and the mortality is considerably higher, approximately 60%.

Athletes with acute subdural hematomas may be unconscious from the moment of impact or they may have

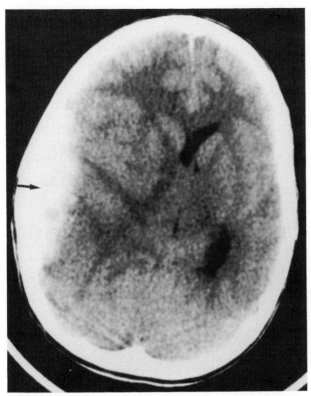

FIGURE 9–1
Axial CT scan, without contrast enhancement, of a 5-year-old boy who was struck in the right temporal area by a thrown baseball. The scan demonstrates a large epidural hematoma (→) and considerable brain displacement.

a lucid interval. They may have a history of a recent concussion. If they are conscious after the injury, they usually complain of headache and nausea, often vomit, and may develop focal or generalized seizures, followed by decreasing levels of consciousness and increasing neurologic deficits. Emergency CT scans are needed to demonstrate the size of the hematoma, the extent of associated contusion and edema, and the extent of brain shift. The mortality of acute subdural hematoma can be reduced if the hematoma is diagnosed and removed within 4 hours [26]. Not all athletes with acute subdural hematoma develop signs within 4 hours, however, a factor that increases the importance of examining the athlete during the night after a severe concussion.

Intracerebral Hematomas

Intracerebral hematomas are the least frequently seen hematomas associated with athletic head injuries and with head injuries due to falls or vehicular accidents. They usually occur in boxers, who often do not recover consciousness after the blow. Intracerebral hematomas result from a blow severe enough to shear intracerebral vessels. They are associated with cerebral contusions

and edema and are diagnosed by CT scans. Small intracerebral hematomas need not be removed; large ones causing a mass effect are removed if intracranial pressure cannot be controlled medically.

Contusions

Contusions—brain bruises—are associated with acute subdural hematomas and intracerebral hematomas but may occur with no hematoma. Contusions result from a severe focal impact and can occur either focally (under the site of impact) or contrecoup. They are associated with typical signs and symptoms of a serious head injury, headache, lethargy, and vomiting, and often cause post-traumatic seizures and neurologic deficits. They require no débridement and may leave an area of permanently damaged brain (encephalomalacia, Fig. 9–2).

PRIMARY AND SECONDARY BRAIN INJURY

Serious head injuries in athletes, as in other children, have two components: the primary injury—whether physiological or structural, caused by the mechanical blow to the brain—and the secondary injury caused by the deleterious effects of hypoxia, hypercarbia, hypotension, increased intracranial pressure, or infection [13]. The primary injury cannot be altered once it occurs, but the secondary injury can be minimized or prevented, initially by paying meticulous attention to the airway and blood pressure, and after hospitalization by controlling intracranial pressure.

A common phenomenon after pediatric head injuries is cerebral hyperemia [5]. This condition is analogous to the blush after a facial slap. After a diffuse head injury, cerebral vessels reflexly and diffusely dilate, intracranial pressure rises, and children develop headache, vomiting, and lethargy [6, 18]. Cerebral hyperemia rather than edema is the usual cause of these symptoms in children. Hyperemia develops minutes to a few hours after injury but usually subsides within 12 hours. The diagnosis of hyperemia is implied by CT scans that demonstrate extreme narrowing of the cerebral ventricles and absence of basal cisterns, changes due to the increase in brain volume owing to increased blood volume. Brain density measurements by CT scan indicate that brain density is increased by 2 to 3 Hounsfield units above normal. If hyperemia persists, it promotes the formation of cerebral edema.

Cerebral edema also develops within hours after athletic head injuries but less commonly than hyperemia. Edema is usually localized to the area of injury. It may

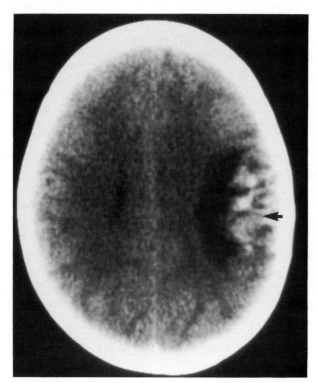 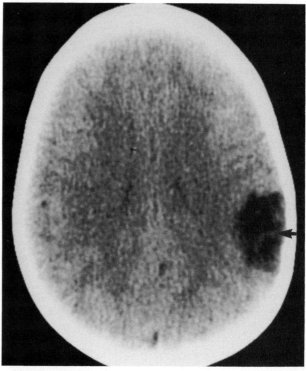

FIGURE 9–2
Axial CT scans, without contrast enhancement, of a 4-year-old boy who was struck in the left parietal region by a line drive foul ball off a professional baseball player's bat. The left scan demonstrates brain contusion (irregular white area, ←) and underlying edema (black). A scan 6 months later (right) demonstrates encephalomalacia (←).

cause post-traumatic seizures, symptoms of increased intracranial pressure, or focal neurologic deficits. Cerebral edema associated with serious head injuries may persist for 1 to 2 weeks. The severity of edema or hyperemia does not correlate well with the severity of head injury; seemingly minor injuries are occasionally followed by malignant cerebral edema [5, 21]. The likelihood of malignant cerebral edema may be increased if the first brain injury is not healed before the second occurs. The exact cause of edema and hyperemia is uncertain; either condition causes neurologic symptoms, and athletes need to be examined by a physician. The use of corticosteroids for post-traumatic cerebral edema is declining. A randomized double-blind study showed no benefit of steroids in head-injured adults [10], although previous less well designed studies had indicated otherwise. Steroids may lessen the meningeal inflammation caused by blood in the subarachnoid space, a common occurrence after athletic head injuries.

POST-TRAUMATIC SEIZURES AND EPILEPSY

Post-traumatic seizures occur in 2.6% of all children after head injuries, in 30% of those with severe head injuries, but in only 1% of those with mild or moderate injuries [1]. Post-traumatic seizures occur more often in athletes who sustain localized brain injuries, whether by pucks, balls, elbows, or falls, especially if a cortical contusion or subdural hematoma is present. The underlying brain is injured at least microscopically and often macroscopically. The initial concern for an athlete who is having a post-traumatic seizure is to maintain the airway, usually by head extension, until the seizure subsides. Efforts to withdraw the tongue result in far more lip lacerations and bitten fingers than in airway improvement. If an athlete has a single post-traumatic seizure and no CT evidence of brain injury, chronic anticonvulsant medications are not indicated. They are indicated, however, if multiple post-traumatic seizures occur or if the athlete has sustained a severe head injury. Epilepsy (i.e., repeated seizures) develops in 7.4% of children with severe head injuries. In those with moderate or minor injuries, epilepsy develops in 1.6% and 0.2%, respectively, a frequency no different from that in nontraumatized children [1].

Some children with epilepsy want to play "contact" sports (A noted collegiate coach used to say that dancing is a contact sport, football is a collision sport). In general, children with epilepsy should be encouraged to play noncontact sports, but each child must be evaluated individually. The frequency, time, and type of seizures and the degree of seizure control should be determined. Children with frequent daytime seizures, petit mal seizures, or psychomotor seizures should not participate in contact sports. Children with generalized seizures may participate if their seizures are well controlled, for example, less than one daytime seizure every 6 months. There is no evidence that repeated head impacts in football worsen the child's seizure disorder [20].

POST-TRAUMATIC MIGRAINE

Athletes with no previous migraine attacks may develop a classic migraine headache after a sports head injury [4, 16]. The headache may begin within a few minutes after the injury or days later, with an initial vasoconstrictive phase causing visual disturbances or focal symptoms such as aphasia, numbness, and confusion, followed by a phase of generalized vasodilation with pounding diffuse headache, nausea, and vomiting. Symptoms persist 15 to 30 minutes and then resolve completely. These symptoms and signs may simulate a structural brain lesion and warrant evaluation by a scan the first time a post-traumatic migraine headache occurs. These headaches may recur for months afterward. The headaches occasionally recur after a subsequent impact but usually do not require (or respond to) prophylactic medication. The symptoms are similar to those of cerebral hyperemia, but a family history of migraine is present in three-fourths of athletes who develop migraine headaches after a sports head injury.

FOOTBALL HEAD INJURIES

Football is a rough, competitive game with a definite but declining risk of head injury. In my experience, football players (perhaps young athletes) are far more likely to injure the cervical spine, particularly with the SCIWORA syndrome (spinal cord injury without radiographic abnormality), than they are to injure the brain. The incidence of death, intracranial hematoma, and concussion has declined in football players during the past 20 years. In 1964, 2.5/100,000 athletes died from football head injuries; in 1980, 0.2/1,000,000 (three players) died (Carl S. Blyth, personal communication). Since 1977 the fatality rate in high school and college football has been 1/10,000,000 athlete exposures. The 1980 incidence of permanent head injury in high school and college football players was 1/1,000,000 [7]. This change has resulted mainly from improved helmet design and rule changes regarding use of the head. A high school or college football player now has no greater statistical risk of death from playing football than the nonplayer; the risk of death for either is 27 times greater while riding in a car than while playing football [8].

The few players (0.75/100,000 per season) who do develop intracranial hematoma after a football head injury do poorly. In Torg's study, 81% of 72 football players with intracranial hematomas during 1971 to 1975 died; the times elapsed between injury and operation were not known [28]. This mortality is far higher than that for children with intracranial hematomas due to other causes [6], perhaps because hematomas are infrequently suspected in healthy athletes or because the hematomas develop insidiously during the night after games. The importance of removing acute subdural hematomas within 4 hours of injury was noted previously.

Most football concussions occur when the player's head is in a flexed position. Players must be taught that leading with the head endangers *both* the brain and the spinal cord. Since 1980 high school football players have been required to wear helmets with the National Operating Committee on Standards for Athletic Equipment seal. All such helmets provide adequate brain protection if they are properly fitted. Large forces (up to 450 Gs for 350 msec) glance off the slick helmets. Nonslick helmets permit the forces to remain in contact with the head for longer periods of time.

Rarely, football players develop neurologic symptoms because of injury to the extracranial vessels. Neck trauma to the carotid arteries can cause carotid thrombosis and secondary cerebral embolization. Compression of the vertebral arteries at the C1 level by hyperextension can cause vasospasm and thrombosis of the vertebral and basilar arteries and can result in transient quadriparesis or death.

HEAD INJURIES IN OTHER SPORTS

In the United States four other sports associated with a significant frequency of head injury are bicycling, baseball, horse riding, and golf. The sporting activity that accounts for the largest number of deaths from head injury is bicycling. Approximately 1000 persons in the United States per year die of head injuries sustained while on bicycles, and thousands more have injuries requiring hospitalization [22]. Approximately 60% of persons with bicycling head injuries are children less than 14 years old, and 68% of persons with serious head injuries are less than 15 years old [27]. Head injuries result mainly from bicycle falls (37%), contact with stationary objects (24%), or contact with moving vehicles (23%). The most common bicycling head injuries (37%) are unconsciousness for less than 15 minutes, skull fracture, and lethargy without unconsciousness; 6% of patients are unconscious for more than 1 hour or have structural brain lesions, and 3% are unconscious for more than 24 hours or have severe structural lesions. Thompson and colleagues have conclusively documented that wearing helmets significantly reduces the risk of bicycling head and brain injuries [27]. In their study, bicyclers who wore helmets had an 85% reduction in risk of head injury and 88% reduction in risk of brain injury. Physicians should strongly advocate the use of bicycle helmets. Hard-shell and rigid helmets with a solid liner provide significantly better protection than helmets consisting of padded strips without a solid liner or helmets that are bendable. Ballantyne's comment is pertinent: "Wear a helmet. It's inconvenient, but so is not being able to think or talk because your head has been pounded into jelly" [2].

Head injuries in golf and baseball are caused more often by backswings or slung bats than by hit balls. Injuries are usually focal, often depressed skull fractures and brain contusions. The most common equestrian injury is a closed head injury, which occurs two to three times more often in girls, who ride more frequently than boys. One study of equestrian injuries found no correlation between injury occurrence and age, sex, or experience of amateur riders; fewer than 20% of riders wore protective helmets [15]. Approximately 18% of equestrian head injuries cause post-traumatic amnesia for more than an hour, and 15% cause a skull fracture [3]. The frequency of equestrian head injuries in school-aged children is unknown but can certainly be decreased by insisting on use of helmets and checking tack. In ice hockey, facial and eye injuries are common, but head injuries are uncommon because high school and junior high school players wear protective helmets.

Boxing head injuries are rare in children less than 17 years old because few children have sufficient strength to knock out their opponent and partly because boxing, the only sport intending harm to the opponent, is relatively unpopular in high school. Boxing head injuries are common, however, in 18- to 22-year-olds and account for 68% of all boxing-related injuries. From 1980 to 1985, there were 67 boxing injury hospitalizations annually in U.S. Army hospitals, with average hospitalization stays of 5.1 days. One soldier died and one became unilaterally blind [11]. MRI scans in amateur boxers have been reported. The scans were performed an average of 1.9 months after a knockout or excessive head blow, however, and were all normal, probably due to the length of time that elapsed before the scan [17]. CT scans performed in 38 retired professional boxers demonstrated a significant relationship between the number of bouts and CT changes indicating cerebral atrophy [24]. Physicians should discourage teenagers from participating in boxing, in which intentional brain injury is the primary objective.

References

1. Annegers, J.F., Grabow, J.D., Groover, R.J., et al. Seizures after head trauma: A population study. *Neurology* 30:683–689, 1980.
2. Ballantyne, R. *Richard's Bicycle Book.* London, Pan, 1975.
3. Barber, H.M. Horse play: Survey of accidents with horses. *Br Med J* 3:532–534, 1973.
4. Bennett, D.R., Fuenning, S.I., Sullivan, G.S., et al. Migraine precipitated by head trauma in athletes. *Am J Sports Med* 8:202–205, 1980.
5. Bruce, D.A., Alvani, A., Bilaniuk, L., et al. Diffuse cerebral swelling following head injuries in children: The syndrome of "malignant brain edema." *J Neurosurg* 54:170–178, 1981.
6. Bruce, D.A., Gennarelli, T.A., and Langfitt, T.W. Resuscitation from coma due to head injury. *Crit Care Med* 6:254–268, 1978.
7. Clarke, K.S. An epidemiologic view.
8. Clarke, K.S., and Braslow, A. Football fatalities in actuarial perspective. *Med Sci Sports* 10:94–96, 1978.
9. Cooper, D.L. This sporting life. *Emerg Med* 11:287–314, 1979.
10. Cooper, P.R., Moody, S., Clark, W.K., et al. Dexamethasone and severe head injury: A prospective double-blind study. *J Neurosurg* 51:307–316, 1979.
11. Enzenauer, R.W., Montrey, J.S., Enzenauer, R.J., et al. Boxing-related injuries in the U.S. Army, 1980 through 1985. *JAMA* 261:1463–1466, 1989.
12. Garrick, J.G., and Regua, R.K. Injuries in high school sports. *Pediatrics* 61:465–469, 1978.
13. Gennarelli, T.A. Cerebral concussion and diffuse brain injuries. *In* Torg, J.S. (Ed.), *Athletic Injuries to the Head, Neck and Face.* Philadelphia, Lea & Febiger, 1982, pp. 83–104.
14. Gronwall, D., and Wrightson, P. Delayed recovery of intellectual function after minor head injury. *Lancet* 2:605–609, 1974.
15. Grossman, J.A.I., Kulund, D.N., Miller, C.W., et al. Equestrian injuries. Results of a prospective study. *JAMA* 240:1881–1882, 1978.
16. Guthkelch, A.N. Benign post-traumatic encephalopathy in young people and its relation to migraine. *Neurosurgery* 1:101–106, 1977.
17. Jordan, B.D., and Zimmerman, R.D. Magnetic resonance imaging in amateur boxers. *Arch Neurol* 45:1207–1208, 1988.
18. Kelly, J.P., Nichols, J.S., Filley, C.M., et al. Concussion in sports. Guidelines for the prevention of catastrophic outcome. JAMA 266:2867–2869, 1991.
19. Kraus, J.F., Fife, D., Cox, P., et al. Incidence, severity and external causes of pediatric head injury. *Am J Dis Child* 140:687–693, 1986.
20. Livingston, S., and Berman, W. Participation of the epileptic child in contact sports. *J Sports Med* 2:170–174, 1974.
21. McQuillen, J.B., McQuillen, E.N., and Morrow, P. Trauma, sport, and malignant cerebral edema. *Am J Forensic Med Pathol* 9:12–15, 1988.
22. National Safety Council. *Accident Facts.* Chicago, National Safety Council, 1982, pp. 45–91.
23. Rimel, R.W., Giordani, B., Barth, J.T., et al. Disability caused by minor head injury. *Neurosurgery* 9:221–228, 1981.
24. Ross, R.J., Cole, M., Thompson, J.S., et al. Boxers—computed tomography, EEG, and neurological evaluation. *JAMA* 249:211–213, 1983.
25. Saunders, R.L., and Harbaugh, R.E. The second impact in catastrophic contact-sport head trauma. *JAMA* 252:538–539, 1984.
26. Seelig, J.M., Becker, D.P., Miller, J.D., et al. Traumatic acute subdural hematoma. Major mortality reduction in comatose patients treated within four hours. *N Engl J Med* 304:1511–1518, 1981.
27. Thompson, R.S., Rivara, R.P., and Thompson, D.C. A case-control study of the effectiveness of bicycle safety helmets. *N Engl J Med* 320:1361–1367, 1989.
28. Torg, J.S., Truex, R., Quedenfeld, T.C., et al. The national football head and neck injury registry. Report and conclusions 1978. *JAMA* 241:1477–1479, 1979.

THE CERVICAL SPINE

Peter D. Pizzutillo, M.D.

The pursuit of excellence in athletic endeavors has resulted in the development of highly effective training programs for adolescent athletes that have made them bigger, stronger, and faster than young athletes of a generation ago. The emphasis on winning is generated by pressures within the athlete and is enhanced by peers, parents, coaches, and society in general. Society likes "a winner." Tremendous pressures are placed on young athletes to perform well not only for the satisfaction enjoyed in sports but also as a passport to a lifetime of success. This milieu has led to significant medical problems in athletes with the popularization of steroids, psychological turmoil due to unrealistic expectations, and the "burnout" phenomenon.

Competitive behavior has become more aggressive and physical. Even a highly skilled finesse sport such as basketball is now played as a contact sport. Football and ice hockey have evolved from contact sports to the level of collision sports. The result is an increased incidence of injury in young athletes. Forty-four percent of injuries sustained in students 14 years of age and older are due to sports activity [41]. In a high school survey conducted by Paulson [41], 80 of 100 participants in football sustained an injury during the playing season. This compares to 75 of 100 participants in wrestling, 44 of 100 participants in softball, 40 of 100 female participants in gymnastics, 28 of 100 male participants in gymnastics, 35 females and 29 males of 100 participants in track and cross-country, 31 of 100 male participants in basketball, 30 of 100 participants in soccer, and 18 of 100 male participants in baseball. This survey reflects all levels of severity; however, it is significant that 7% of high school teenagers were hospitalized as the result of sports injuries. Football injuries accounted for 20% of these cases, and basketball injuries accounted for 17.4%.

A review of patients with spinal cord injury at several regional rehabilitation centers revealed that 10% to 20% of spinal cord injuries were due to sports-related accidents [7, 49]. From 1950 to 1989, 90% of fatal football injuries involved head or neck injuries [8]. The modern helmet and face mask were developed in the 1950s and 1960s, and these devices led to increased use of the head in blocking and tackling techniques, resulting in an increase in deaths from head injury [51]. In the 1970s helmets were improved to protect the brain. A subsequent decrease in fatalities due to head injury followed, but the level of cervical spine injuries was sustained, primarily due to "spearing" techniques in tackling [60]. In January 1976 the National Collegiate Athletic Association (NCAA) and the National Federation of State High School Associations (NFSHSA) formally adopted high school, college, and coaching rules that prohibited tackling or blocking with a helmeted head because of the vulnerability of the cervical spine to injury in this position. This single step has resulted in a significant decrease in serious cervical spine injury [64]. Since 1977 there has been one fatality for every 10 million athlete exposures in football at the high school, college, and professional levels.

The incidence of nonfatal but catastrophic injuries is difficult to report reliably because of incomplete recording of injuries [37, 47]. The National Football Head and Neck Injury Registry has been functional since 1955 and has provided much of the information that is used today for analysis. The decreasing rate of cervical spine injury in football is attributed to improvements in equipment, changes in game rules that better protect the athlete, more effective conditioning of the athlete, and better coaching of basic playing techniques, especially blocking and tackling. Similar developments are necessary to reverse the increasing incidence of cervical spine injury in other sports.

From 1978 to 1982, the National Registry of Gymnastic Catastrophic Injuries documented 20 incidents of injury including 17 patients with permanent quadriplegia and three deaths [9]. These injuries occurred in skilled performers during practice settings. Analysis of this group revealed that permanent spinal cord injury was closely associated with use of the trampoline [53], especially when attempting to perform a somersault. In many states the trampoline has now been banned from physical education classes and is only used with spotters and physical restraints in teaching new skills in gymnastics.

Catastrophic neurotrauma involving the cervical spinal cord has also occurred in diving [6, 31, 38], rugby [9, 25, 35], ice hockey [15, 16], and wrestling [30]. Diving injuries account for 4% to 14% of spinal cord injuries in young patients [17]; the majority of these occur outside of organized programs [6]. Downhill skiing has a reported mortality of 1.7% in 430 patients reported from Lake Tahoe in a 14-year study [20]. Thirteen patients in this group had permanent radiculopathy, and four had permanent myelopathy. Cervical spine injury in skiers is frequently associated with concurrent head injury. The martial arts have contributed to cervical spine fractures and dislocations, usually as the result of a forceful foot strike to the head or a fall onto the head and neck area. At least 17 deaths have been reported in judo and karate as a result of this mechanism [5]. Interestingly, soccer [5] and boxing [29] have not been associated with a high incidence of cervical spine injury.

ANATOMY OF THE CERVICAL SPINE

Cervical spine injury in children younger than 8 years of age is uncommon and differs from injury in older adolescents and adults by virtue of site and mechanism of injury [24, 26]. The problem of evaluation of the cervical spine in childhood is complicated by the fact that much of the cervical spine is unossified and is undergoing progressive radiographic changes as ossification and growth proceed. By 8 years of age, the cervical spine has developed the adult configuration. Under the age of 1 year, the anterior ring of C1 is unossified, and it may be difficult to determine whether the upper cervical spine is unstable (Fig. 10–1). At between 3 and 6 years of age, the basilar synchondrosis becomes visible and may be mistaken for fracture at the base of the odontoid. By 6 years of age, the inner diameter of the spinal canal of the entire cervical spine has reached the adult level. In the child under 8 years of age, extension of the spine causes a spurious impression of subluxation of the anterior arch of the atlas over the superior aspect of the dens, which is not yet ossified. From infancy to 8 years of age, lateral neutral radiographs of the cervical spine reveal an increase in the angulation of the facet joint from 30 degrees to 60 degrees. In the younger child with a facet joint angle of 30 degrees, a greater degree of freedom in flexion and extension exists that may contribute to the appearance of ''pseudosubluxation'' commonly seen at the C2–C3 and C3–C4 levels. In the first decade of life, flexion-extension lateral radiographs of the cervical spine may reveal an atlantodens interval up to 5 mm, whereas the adult interval should not exceed 3.5 mm. Incomplete ossification of the cervical spine

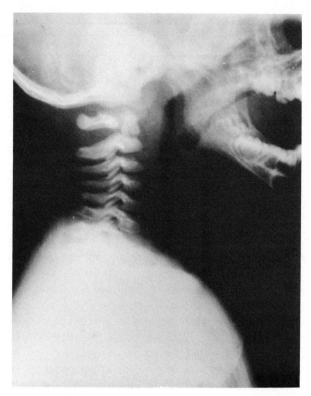

FIGURE 10–1
Lateral radiograph of the immature cervical spine reveals absence of the anterior arch of C1, presence of the basilar synchondrosis, and apparent wedging due to unossified vertebral bodies.

creates the appearance both of a truncated odontoid, until its tip ossifies at 10 to 12 years of age, and of apparent wedging of the vertebral bodies on lateral radiographs until ossification is more complete at 10 years of age.

Whereas the majority of fractures in adults occur in the lower cervical spine, the upper cervical spine is involved in up to 70% of cervical spine fractures in children. The relatively large size of the child's skull may be a significant factor in injury of the upper cervical spine in this age group.

A marked differential in elasticity between the spinal column and the spinal cord has been identified in the young child. The clinical expression of this differential in elasticity has been popularized by Pang and Wilberger [39] in their report of spinal cord injury without radiographic abnormality (SCIWORA) in children. Pang and Wilberger's study documents the presence of serious neurologic damage of the upper cervical cord in the absence of cervical spine osseous damage on initial radiographic evaluation in children less than 8 years of age.

RECOGNITION AND PRIMARY TREATMENT

The lifelong consequences of catastrophic spinal cord injury are of such magnitude that it is imperative that personnel dealing with athletes on a regular basis be well educated about the possibility of injury during practice and game conditions. Education alone can increase awareness of this problem and may indeed spare the injured athlete from further neural damage caused by mismanagement on the field. There is considerable difficulty in maintaining a high index of suspicion for spinal injury because severe neck injury does not frequently occur. The very mention of spinal cord injury creates an immediate emotional response among athletes, coaching staff, and the athletes' families. In competitive conditions, whether in practice or in actual game situations, it can be quite difficult to evaluate the injured athlete adequately and manage problems on the field. Preparation and education of everyone involved in the athlete's care in the event of nonfatal catastrophic spinal cord injury is of the utmost importance. A properly equipped ambulance with attendants trained in safe transport of individuals with neurologic damage as well as identification of hospital facilities that have the capability of dealing with catastrophic neurologic injury must exist well in advance of injury in order to provide the optimum environment for the athlete's treatment. The development of regional spinal cord injury centers has provided a network of experienced staff throughout the country that can provide the very best of care for the spinal cord-injured athlete. Education of emergency medical technicians has significantly decreased the incidence of secondary neural injury that was formerly caused by improper immobilization during transport. Ongoing educational efforts are needed to maintain current proficiency and to improve our existing level of care.

The management of the athlete with a severe spinal injury requires rapid assessment with protection of vital structures [4]. If the athlete is unconscious, quadriparetic, quadriplegic, or has significant paresthesias or dysesthesias involving the upper and lower extremities, the cervical spine must be considered unstable and must be protected [33]. The head and neck should immediately be immobilized in a neutral position. If the patient is in the prone position, an organized logroll maneuver may be performed in which the head and neck are turned as one unit with the patient's trunk. This can be managed by having one member of the emergency team control the head and neck while grasping the shoulder area in order to prevent changes in flexion or extension. In addition to level of consciousness, it is important to determine the patient's respiratory and circulatory status. If the athlete uses a mouthpiece during sports activity, the mouthpiece should be removed. Football players should have their face masks removed, but the helmet and chin strap should be left in place until the athlete is evaluated neurologically. If the patient is not breathing, it is important to position the jaw in an appropriate forward attitude to open the airway without overextending the neck. If the jaw-thrust maneuver is not successful in restoring breathing, rescue breathing must be initiated. The athlete must be transported in an expedient manner but under safe conditions to an appropriately identified medical facility capable of dealing with these problems. In athletes younger than 8 years of age, care must be taken to avoid the forced flexion of the cervical spine that occurs on a flat spine board because of the relative increased size of the head in relation to the size of the chest [23]. A standard flat board can be used with a towel roll beneath the shoulders to create a more neutral position of the cervical spine. The minimum components provided by the evaluating facility should include a neurosurgeon, an orthopedic surgeon, and adequate radiographic capability.

ACUTE SOFT TISSUE INJURY

Acute soft tissue injury of the cervical spine may involve the disc, ligaments, muscle, and fascia. Typically, these injuries are the result of a collision or fall onto the head and neck complex. The athlete usually complains of neck pain or neck and shoulder pain without distal radiation of pain or paresthesias. Physical examination reveals a limited range of motion of the cervical spine, usually in the presence of mild to moderate paraspinal muscle spasms, with no evidence of motor, sensory, or reflex changes in the upper or lower extremities. Radiographs of the cervical spine are normal and show no evidence of subluxation or dislocation but may reveal straightening of the cervical lordosis.

Acute injury involving the fascia, muscle, or ligaments of the neck without disruption and instability should be treated symptomatically. A rehabilitation program comprising range of motion exercises and restitution of strength of the neck and shoulder girdle is important prior to gradual resumption of sports activity. The painful phase of soft tissue injury usually does not last more than 5 to 10 days and will allow the athlete to resume sports activity. If rehabilitation is not included as an integral part of the return-to-play program, the athlete will demonstrate a chronic decrease in range of motion of the cervical spine and diminished strength of the neck, especially in the flexor muscle group. Limitation of motion and weakness of the neck may lead to secondary injury with low-grade fascial, muscular, or ligamentous injury that perpetuates a vicious cycle of disability. Effective treatment of chronic cervical sprains and strains, therefore, includes a rehabilitation program designed to stretch out contracture of the cervical soft tissues and reconstitute the strength of the surrounding cervical and shoulder musculature.

It is extremely important that children and adolescents

who have sustained apparent innocuous injury to the cervical spine be reevaluated on a serial basis. Herkowitz and Rothman [21] reported development of instability of the cervical spine in individuals who initially demonstrated no radiographic evidence of bony or soft tissue abnormality. Subacute instability of the cervical spine is due to elastic and plastic deformation of the ligamentous and disc structures and may result in neurologic deficits in individuals who were initially neurologically normal. Children in the first decade of life who sustain neck injuries but appear to be normal by radiographic and neurologic testing need careful follow-up. Pang and Wilberger's report [39] primarily involved victims of vehicular injury and included only four sports injuries, but it demonstrated that 52% of patients with spinal cord injury without radiographic abnormality experienced the onset of serious neurologic problems an average of 4 days after their initial injury. Pollack and colleagues [45] reviewed 42 children with spinal cord injury and found that within 10 weeks of the first injury eight children had a second spinal cord injury with more serious neurologic consequences; central or partial cord injury occurred in all eight, and three patients had severe quadriparesis or paraparesis [45]. Pollack and colleagues proposed an arbitrary protocol that includes immobilization of the cervical spine in a brace for 3 months with no sports activity, close clinical follow-up, and repeat somatosensory evoked potentials (SSEPs) at 6 weeks. If dynamic radiographic studies and physical examination of the cervical spine are normal at the 3 months follow-up examination, the individual is ready to begin the return to sports. Full range of motion of the neck with demonstrated stability of the cervical spine on flexion-extension lateral radiographs and the absence of sensory or motor loss are required before the athlete is allowed to return to competitive sports activity.

Acute herniation of the cervical nucleus pulposus has been reported in adult sports activity [28] but is rare in the child or adolescent athlete. Its presence can result in catastrophic neurologic injury with compromise of the anterior spinal cord [36]. These patients experience a sudden onset of neck pain with radiation to both shoulders, arms, and hands, and tend to hold the head tilted to the side of the disc lesion. Interscapular pain is commonly reported. When the head is tilted to the side of the lesion and then extended, there is an increase in pain. Herniation of the cervical disc most commonly occurs at the C5–C6 and C6–C7 levels. The immediate concern is to differentiate the acute herniated disc from the "burner lesion" that results in searing pain in a radicular distribution. A detailed neurologic assessment as well as an appropriate radiographic evaluation including CT scan and magnetic resonance imaging (MRI) are usually required. Treatment of acute disc herniation in adolescent athletes requires decompression of the spinal canal. Re-

petitive axial compression of the cervical spine may result in chronic changes involving the disc. Albright and colleagues [2, 3] reported radiographic evidence of neck injury in 32% of freshman college football players in their preseason evaluations. Half of this study group had a past medical history of neck pain and showed abnormal radiographic findings involving the cervical spine. Linebackers and defensive halfbacks were most commonly involved; running backs and wide receivers were at greater risk than linemen. Among athletes in whom the preseason physical examination or past medical history suggested a cervical spine problem, half demonstrated radiographic abnormalities of the cervical spine involving disc degeneration. Most of the athletes were unaware of any significant neck problems and had not sought prior medical evaluation.

Axial loading appears to be the most important injury of the cervical spine. Torg and colleagues [57] demonstrated that axial forces transmitted to the cervical spine in slight extension are dissipated primarily by the cervical muscles. When the neck is flexed 30 degrees, it becomes a straight segmented column. Axial forces applied under these conditions are transmitted directly to the vertebrae, ligaments, and disc rather than being dissipated by muscle. These observations have led to improvements in tackling and blocking techniques to reduce the frequency of cervical spine injury.

FRACTURES AND DISLOCATIONS
Atlanto-Occipital Instability

Atlanto-occipital instability is usually the result of violent forces and is frequently fatal [10, 14, 32]. Although atlanto-occipital instability has not been reported in sports injuries, it is conceivable that its incidence may be higher than suspected because appropriate diagnostic tests for spinal stability are not always conducted in acute fatalities, and there has not been very much attention directed at the atlanto-occipital junction in the past.

Athletes with Down's syndrome are of special concern. The recent observation that individuals with Down's syndrome may have atlanto-occipital hypermobility that excludes them from contact sports and from axial loading sports is important. In addition to the more commonly reported atlantoaxial instability, atlanto-occipital instability must be ruled out before athletes with Down's syndrome can be medically cleared for sports activities (Fig. 10–2).

Injury to the Atlas and Axis
Jefferson Fracture [27]

When a high axial load is delivered from the apex of the skull to the cervical spine, tremendous forces are

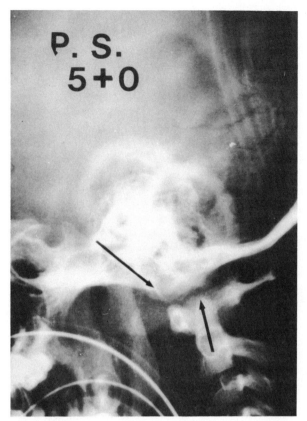

FIGURE 10–2
Lateral radiograph of the upper cervical spine reveals significant anterior translation (arrows) of the occiput on the cervical axis.

generated at the junction of the occipital condyle and the ring of the atlas. Low level forces result in fractures of the posterior atlantal arch that are stable and can be successfully treated with immobilization by orthotics. When severe force is applied, a burst fracture of the atlas involving disruption of both anterior and posterior arches allows progressive displacement of the lateral masses of the atlas, producing consequent vascular and neurologic compromise. The great majority of patients who have sustained injuries to the ring of the atlas are neurologically intact and must be evaluated in an expedient manner to avoid delay in diagnosis and secondary neurologic compromise.

Patients with an injury of the ring of the atlas complain of neck pain and have severely restricted motion of the cervical spine in flexion, extension, lateral side bending, and lateral rotation. In the presence of a normal neurologic examination, a high index of suspicion of fracture of the atlas is required when evaluating patients with a skull fracture or severe laceration of the scalp that suggests axial loading.

Routine radiographs of the upper cervical spine are difficult to interpret, especially when the head is tilted in response to paravertebral muscle spasm. Detailed inspec-

tion of the ring of the atlas on both lateral and open mouth anteroposterior (AP) radiographs is required to determine the relationship between the lateral masses of the atlas and the axis. When the open mouth AP radiograph reveals combined overhang of the lateral masses of the atlas on the axis of more than 7 mm, instability and disruption of the transverse ligament must be assumed. If there is difficulty in obtaining adequate information from routine radiographs, CT scans provide excellent detail in evaluation of an injury of the atlas (Fig. 10–3). Fractures of the anterior and posterior arches of the atlas as well as the relationship of the odontoid to the anterior arch of the atlas can be precisely evaluated on CT scans. Although the majority of fractures of the atlas heal by nonoperative immobilization techniques, such as a halo brace, there is an occasional need for surgical fusion [18].

Acute Atlantoaxial Instability

Acute atlantoaxial instability is usually the result of severe flexion forces imposed on the cervical spine. If the atlanto-dens interval is greater than 5 mm in children, the transverse ligament is compromised, and instability is present (Fig. 10–4). Posterior fusion of the atlas and axis is required to avoid spinal cord compression.

Special concern exists about individuals with Down's syndrome who are athletically active. The standard radiographic parameters of stability of the cervical spine in individuals without Down's syndrome are not appropriate for judging stability in individuals with Down's syndrome. Natural history studies indicate that one-third of adults with Down's syndrome demonstrate a radiographic appearance of instability at all levels of the cervical spine, but only 3% of these individuals experience neurologic problems. Caution must be exercised in evaluating individuals with Down's syndrome to avoid undertreatment or overtreatment. Many children and adolescents with Down's syndrome are actively involved in sports activities such as basketball, swimming, and horseback riding. Like other athletes, these individuals and their families derive a great deal of satisfaction, pride, and joy in their athletic accomplishments. A blanket prescription against sports involvement needlessly deprives these athletes of the sense of accomplishment that accompanies athletic endeavor and diminishes their self-esteem. On the other hand, children and adolescents with Down's syndrome who demonstrate radiographic evidence of cervical instability should be advised against participation in sports activities that potentially endanger neural function, such as diving and gymnastics. In the presence of neurologic dysfunction and radiographic cervical instability, surgical stabilization of the cervical

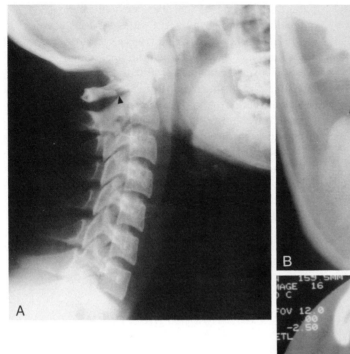

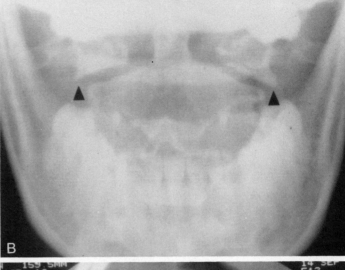

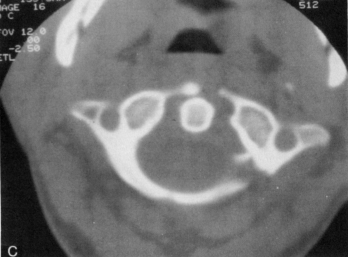

FIGURE 10–3
A, Lateral radiograph reveals a break in the cortex of the posterior arch of C1. *B,* Open-mouth view reveals bilateral symmetrical overhang of the lateral masses of C1 on C2. *C,* CT scan reveals a disruption in the ring of C1 in both the anterior and posterior arches.

spine is necessary to preserve existing neural function and to prevent progressive loss.

Rotary Atlantoaxial Subluxation

Children may demonstrate the insidious onset of wry neck deformity in association with posterior pharyngeal inflammation. Clinical examination of the involved child reveals a "cock-robin" attitude of the head with tilt of the head toward one shoulder and rotation of the chin toward the opposite shoulder. The patient demonstrates mild to moderate limitation of flexion and extension and nearly full lateral rotation to the side opposite the head tilt. In contrast, there is minimal lateral rotation toward the side of the head tilt. Cervical muscle spasm or localized soft tissue tenderness is usually absent. In addition, there is no prominence of the sternocleidomastoid muscle on the side of the head tilt as is seen in congenital

muscular torticollis. The great majority of involved children are neurologically intact.

Routine radiographs of the cervical spine should be supplemented by open mouth as well as lateral flexion-extension views of the upper cervical spine. Adequate lateral evaluation may be quite difficult to obtain if the radiology technician aligns the patient in the standard fashion for a lateral view of the cervical spine because of the rotation and tilt of the skull and atlas. To avoid the confusing features caused by rotation and lateral tilt, the technician should be instructed to obtain a lateral radiograph of the skull to include the upper cervical spine. A lateral view of the skull using this technique will reveal a true lateral view of the atlas and permit more reliable interpretation of the relationship between the atlas and the axis. In the presence of malrotation, the lateral radiograph may spuriously suggest instability at the atlanto-occipital junction as well as at the atlantoaxial junction. In addition, the lateral mass of the atlas may

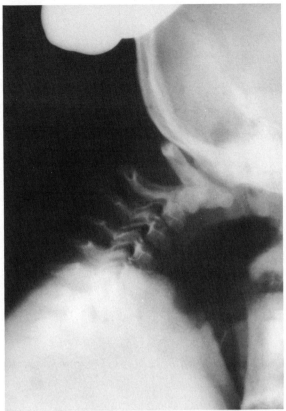

FIGURE 10–4
Lateral flexion radiograph of the cervical spine reveals significant anterior displacement of the ring of C1 from the odontoid in a patient with Down's syndrome with hypoplastic odontoid.

appear anteriorly as a triangular wedge, the so-called sail sign (Fig. 10–5A). Lateral flexion-extension radiographs in neutral rotation are needed to reliably evaluate the degree of stability of the upper cervical spine as well as the existence of fixed rotary displacement between the atlas and axis. CT scans have been extremely helpful in documenting the degree of displacement of the lateral mass of the atlas in relationship to the axis, the spatial relationship of the odontoid to the anterior arch of the atlas, and the space available for the cord dorsal to the odontoid (Fig. 10–5B).

Parke and colleagues [40] demonstrated a rich network of sinusoidal vessels draining directly from the posterior pharynx to the soft tissues about the atlas and axis. During inflammatory states, such as those occurring with upper respiratory tract infection, hyperemia results in dissolution of the attachment of the transverse ligament to the anterior arch of the atlas. With progressive dissolution, gross instability occurs with loss of orientation of the lateral masses of the atlas and axis. Treatment initiated before 4 weeks of clinical expression is successful in resolving rotary subluxation of the atlas and axis by nonsurgical methods. After 4 weeks, surgical stabilization is frequently required to maintain stability

even when anatomic alignment can be regained by traction techniques (Fig. 10–5C) [42].

Children and adolescents who present with a mild degree of rotary subluxation of the atlas and axis should be placed in a cervical collar and prohibited from recreational and sports activity. With more severe degrees of subluxation or fixed rotary subluxation, the patient should be protected and treated as an inpatient. Patients are initially treated by halter cervical spine traction or by halo traction in mild hyperextension and longitudinal traction. Once anatomic reduction has been obtained, the patient is immobilized either in a halo vest or a Minerva cast. After a 6- to 8-week period of immobilization, lateral flexion-extension radiographs of the cervical spine out of the cast or brace are needed to document stability. If stability is proved, the patient may be weaned to a soft cervical collar and begun on gentle range of motion exercises as well as isometric strengthening exercises. Repeat lateral flexion-extension radiographs of the cervical spine should be performed 6 weeks later to rule out recurrent instability. If instability persists following immobilization or if recurrent instability develops, posterior atlantoaxial surgical fusion is indicated.

Fracture of the Odontoid

Fractures of the odontoid in children may be difficult to assess, especially in the presence of an unossified basilar synchondrosis. Acute separation of the odontoid through the basilar synchondrosis can occur in children younger than 7 years of age. Spontaneous reduction may occur, but marked widening of the retropharyngeal space is usually observed on radiographic evaluation of these patients [10]. MRI evaluation may also reveal occult injury. With ossification of the ossiculum terminale, avulsion of the tip of the odontoid may be inadvertently suspected on radiographs. Lateral flexion extension radiographs document the presence or absence of stability. In children older than 7 years, a type II odontoid fracture is more common and may be associated with nonunion as it is in adults. The majority of type II odontoid fractures heal through the use of nonsurgical techniques of immobilization such as halo vest stabilization but may require surgical fusion [19].

Hangman's Fracture

The term hangman's fracture refers to fractures involving the pedicle of the second cervical vertebra. These fractures are frequently the result of motor vehicle accidents or falls and do occur in children and adolescents [43]. The most common mechanism of injury is

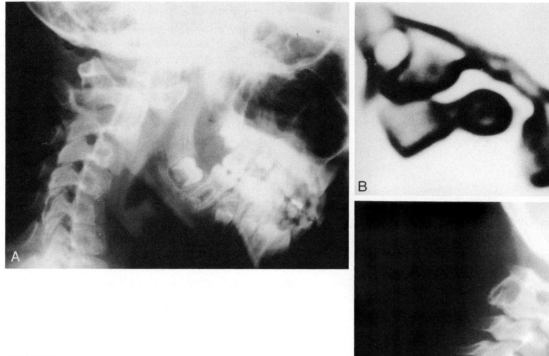

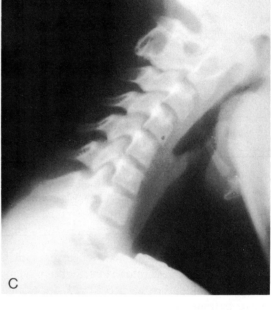

FIGURE 10–5
A, Lateral radiograph of the cervical spine in a patient with rotary subluxation of C1–C2 presents a triangular wedged appearance of the anterior arch of C1. *B,* CT scan of C1–C2 reveals malalignment of the axis of the vertebrae with anterior translation of the lateral mass of C1 on C2. *C,* Lateral flexion radiograph reveals solid fusion between C1 and C2 without evidence of displacement.

that of extension and distraction, although other mechanisms have been suggested, including axial loading in extension and flexion. With bilateral disruption of the axial pedicles, the atlas and the anterior elements of the axis move as a single unit in flexion and extension. Schneider and associates described anterior displacement of the ''cervicocranium'' with enlargement of the upper cervical spinal canal in flexion that spares the spinal cord from injury [50].

The patient with hangman's fracture may present with neck pain and cradling of the head in the absence of objective neurologic abnormalities. With persistent anterior displacement of the ''cervicocranium,'' neurologic deficits will eventually develop. Early identification is of paramount importance. In addition to routine radiographs, CT scans of the cervical spine have allowed precise delineation of fracture patterns. The majority of patients with hangman's fracture may be treated with gentle traction followed by halo vest or cast for 3

months. Lateral flexion and extension radiographs are necessary to demonstrate osseous healing and intersegmental stability. In the presence of nonunion or disruption of the C2–C3 disc, surgical fusion is indicated either by anterior fusion of C2 to C3 or posterior cervical fusion involving C1, C2, and C3.

The Subaxial Cervical Spine

Injury to the lower cervical spine from C3 to C7 may involve injury to the anterior elements of the spinal column, to the posterior elements, to the lateral elements, or to a combination of sites. Clinical problems include facet dislocation with or without fracture, laminar fractures, and avulsion fractures of the spinous processes. Lateral mass fractures and pedicle fractures are uncommon in the subaxial spine compared to the incidence of injury in the upper cervical spine. The anterior elements of the spinal column are usually injured in flexion with resultant compression fractures of the vertebral body and injury to the disc. Although disruption of the posterior longitudinal ligament is not common in athletic injuries, disruption may occur, especially with a flexion-distraction mechanism associated with significant intersegmental instability and the potential for neurologic catastrophe. As with injury at other levels, immediate immobilization of the spine is of extreme importance to prevent additional loss of neurologic function.

Fracture at the C3–C4 vertebral level is rare [32]. Athletic injuries most commonly result in injury at vertebral levels ranging from C4 to C7 [1, 11–13, 30, 45, 46, 56, 59]. Facet dislocation may be unilateral or bilateral and may occur with or without associated fracture. Unilateral facet dislocation is usually the result of axial loading in combination with flexion and rotation and does not usually result in neurologic damage. In the absence of facet fracture, the injury is primarily ligamentous and capsular, and the spine maintains its stability. Lateral radiographs of the cervical spine with unilateral facet dislocation reveal anterior translation of one vertebra on another of approximately 25%. Reduction of facet dislocation is obtained by closed traction techniques; occasionally, inability to reduce facet dislocation caused by closed methods necessitates open reduction with posterior fusion of the involved levels.

Bilateral facet dislocation is a much more serious injury and occurs primarily through a mechanism of flexion. The spine is unstable in this situation and is associated with severe neurologic deficit including quadriplegia. Lateral radiographs of the cervical spine with bilateral facet dislocation reveal translation of more than 50% of one vertebra on another. These dislocations can usually be reduced by traction, immobilized in a halo cast, and stabilized by posterior fusion of the involved cervical vertebrae.

Laminar fractures are difficult to diagnose on routine radiographs owing to the obliquity of the lamina in relation to the axis of the x-ray. CT scan is more reliable in identification of laminar fractures. Fractures of the lamina do not usually participate in compression of neural tissue and heal with immobilization. Avulsion fractures of the spinous process are the result of vigorous exertion and are termed the ''clay shoveler's fracture.'' The spinous process of the seventh cervical vertebra is most frequently involved. Treatment of the clay shoveler's fracture is symptomatic because no subsequent instability results from this avulsion fracture.

Injury of the anterior elements of the spinal column primarily involves axial loading resulting in compression fracture of the vertebral body. The extent of injury varies from a wedge fracture, which is stable, to the severely comminuted burst fracture, which is unstable and involves intrusion of bony elements into the spinal canal.

The wedge fracture is common and is not associated with neurologic compromise. The posterior elements, including the ligamentous structures, are intact, and the spinal column remains stable. If disruption of the posterior elements is associated with anterior compression fracture of the vertebral body, stability is most likely compromised, and surgical stabilization is necessary. When progressive escalation of forces is experienced by the neck with axial loading, more severe injury of the vertebral body occurs ranging from nondisplaced fracture fragments to wide displacement of bone and compromise of the spinal canal. Disruption of the posterior elements is more frequent with severe flexion and distraction forces and creates an extremely unstable clinical situation with severe neurologic compromise including quadriplegia. Anterior decompression of the spinal canal with fusion is required followed by posterior spinal fusion.

Patients with facet dislocation or moderate to severe degrees of compression fracture require evaluation of the spinal canal to eliminate the possibility of concomitant extruded disc material (Fig. 10–6). Neurologically intact individuals with facet dislocation have been rendered quadriplegic following closed reduction owing to com-

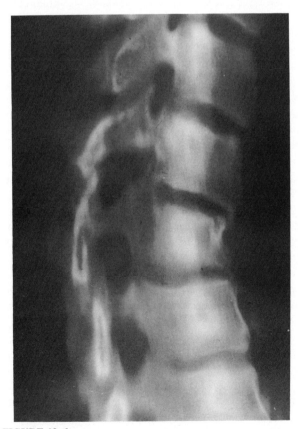

FIGURE 10–6
Patients with a severe compression fracture and disruption of the posterior soft tissues require further evaluation to rule out disc extrusion into the spinal canal.

promise of the anterior spinal cord by extruded disc material. If a disc is extruded, anterior surgical decompression of the disc should be performed, followed by reduction of facets with anterior and posterior spinal stabilization.

Subacute or late instability of the cervical spine should be suspected in the presence of facet dislocation. Herkowitz and Rothman [21] reported on six neurologically intact patients with no bone or soft tissue abnormalities on initial radiographs. Four patients had unilateral facet dislocations; one had a perched facet at C5–C6; and one had subluxation at C4–C5. Each patient subsequently developed radiographic changes indicating intersegmental instability with attendant neurologic compromise. It is important to perform repeat physical examinations and radiographic studies within 3 weeks of injury to rule out the existence of subacute instability. Once instability has been identified, surgical stabilization is required.

SPINAL CORD INJURY

Spinal cord injury results from violent forces imposed on the spinal column. Injury may be direct, as in complete transection or bony compression of the spinal cord, or indirect as a result of hemorrhage, swelling, or secondary ischemia. With the clinical presentation of complete motor and sensory loss, transection of the spinal cord is likely and is irreversible. Incomplete lesions of the spinal cord usually present as mixtures of described syndromes. When severe forces are imposed by axial load on the cervical spine, a burst fracture of the vertebral body may result, producing bony impingement on the anterior spinal artery with motor loss below the injury level and loss of sensations of pain and temperature. These deficits are usually permanent, and the degree of loss is equal in both upper and lower extremities.

Severe flexion-extension moments applied to the cervical spine in the presence of spinal stenosis or secondary degenerative changes, which may occur in high school athletes, result in central cord hemorrhage and ischemia with primary involvement of the corticospinal tracts. Nonspecific sensory loss may be observed in the presence of incomplete motor loss involving all extremities. The upper extremities are usually significantly weaker than the lower extremities. Central cord involvement has a relatively favorable prognosis with varying degrees of recovery.

Hemisection of the spinal cord results in loss of ipsilateral motor function and contralateral pain and temperature and is designated the Brown-Sequard syndrome. Posterior spinal cord syndrome is a rare lesion in sports with ischemia of the posterior spinal artery resulting in loss of dorsal column function and preservation of ante-

rior cord function. These clinical syndromes do not usually appear in pure form but rather as parts of more complex lesions, most commonly involving a combination of central cord injury and the Brown-Sequard syndrome.

The "burning hands syndrome" was first described by Maroon in 1977 as severe burning dysesthesias and paresthesias of both hands due to injury to the central fibers of the spinal tract [34]. The injury is usually the result of ischemia. Wilburger and colleagues [63] used MRI and SSEP to demonstrate that the burning hands syndrome was a reversible insult to the sensory pathways of the spinal cord.

Vascular insults may result in thrombosis or embolization. In 1970 Schneider and associates [52] reported seven cases of cervicomedullary injury in football players that resulted from "spearing." Five of the athletes had no radiographic evidence of fracture or dislocation, although two showed evidence of atlantoaxial instability. Schneider and co-workers postulated that vertebrobasilar insufficiency with hypoperfusion of either the vertebral or basilar arteries could result in intramedullary cavitation and hemorrhage. A second possible mechanism of injury suggested by these authors involved acute arterial or venous obstruction from the brain due to uncal herniation through the tentorial notch. The final mechanism postulated by Schneider and colleagues involved high-velocity impact to the top of the head such that the brain interacts with the cervicomedullary junction, which is tethered by the dentate ligaments, resulting in secondary hemorrhages of the cervicomedullary junction. Fortunately, vascular injury of this sort in athletic events is uncommon.

Of great concern is the problem of transient quadriplegia. Torg and his colleagues [58, 59] described this problem as acute but transient episodes of sensory changes that may be associated with motor paresis in either both arms, both legs, or all four limbs following a forced hyperextension, hyperflexion, or axial load to the cervical spine. Complete recovery usually occurs in less than 15 minutes. Of interest is Torg's report of 32 athletes with transient quadriparesis and associated developmental cervical spine stenosis [58]. The degree of canal stenosis may be enhanced in flexion and extension by the "pincer mechanism" described by Penning [41A] or by infolding of the laminar ligaments, which are capable of narrowing the spinal canal by 30% in hyperextension. Torg notes that 17 of the reported 32 athletes demonstrated developmental spinal stenosis. Only 4 of the 17 were able to return to play without permanent problems. Of the remaining 15 athletes without stenosis, five had congenital cervical fusions, and only one of these returned to play; four athletes had evidence of cervical instability, and one of these returned to competition; and of six athletes with degenerative disc changes, none returned to sports without problems. Therefore, of the group of 32 patients reported by Torg and associates, only six were able to return to play without problems. Although Torg and his group imply that athletes who have sustained transient quadriplegia with coincident developmental spinal stenosis should be discouraged from returning to competition, they conclude that athletes with transient quadriplegia and no demonstrated stenosis should be able to return to sports activity without a predisposition to permanent neurologic injury. The subset sample size is small in this study and does not allow formulation of a firm conclusion about the safety of return to competition. Transient quadriplegia in young athletes demands a detailed orthopedic, neurologic, and imaging evaluation to rule out factors that may prohibit continued sports participation [54, 68]. Evaluation of larger study groups of involved athletes is required before strong recommendations can be formulated about return to competition. The human cost of premature conclusions is too great.

''Burners'' are described as episodes of searing pain in the upper extremities that follow the radicular distribution [8, 22, 44, 48, 57, 62]. Burners tend to occur after acute extension of the neck or a lateral stretch of the neck to the side opposite the painful arm with depression of the shoulder, as in a tackling maneuver. The symptoms usually last a few seconds in the initial episodes. The involved athlete allows his arm to hang limply at the side and then shakes or rubs the hand or arm vigorously to diminish the unpleasant searing pain. Numbness tends to last longer than the weakness; however, with repeated episodes, progressive residual weakness is observed. College football players have reported that burners last longer with increased frequency of the episodes, and occasionally persistent weakness, sensory loss, and pain are experienced whenever the arm is used. Rockett's observations [48] during surgical exploration of patients with burners document scarring at the C5–C6 nerve roots as they emerge between the anterior and posterior lamellae of the transverse processes. He subsequently recommended decompression of the nerve roots with lysis of nerve adhesions. Poindexter and Johnson [44] performed electromyographic (EMG) evaluation of burners and suggested that they are the result of C6 radiculopathy rather than stretch of the brachial plexus.

The initial complaints of athletes with burners suggest the diagnosis of acute herniated nucleus pulposus; however, with burners the range of motion of the cervical spine remains normal, and symptoms are short lived. Burners, or stingers as they are also known, have been reported at least once in the careers of more than 50% of football players [22]. During on-field evaluation the affected player holds his head in a forward, stiff position to avoid extension and rotation of the neck. The presence of motor or sensory loss or arm or neck pain precludes return to play during that game until further evaluation is performed.

In players who have sustained repeated injuries, full range of motion of the cervical spine as well as normal strength of the neck and shoulder girdle should be present before the athlete is permitted to return to competition [61]. If weakness persists despite rest and rehabilitation, radiographic evaluation, EMG analysis, and MRI are needed to rule out less common lesions such as a herniated nucleus pulposus. EMG changes may persist in the absence of objective neurologic deficits for several years and cannot be used as a parameter for determining return to competition. Preventive measures that have been recommended to decrease the frequency of burners include neck and shoulder strengthening exercises, increasing the thickness of shoulder pads, and using neck rolls.

CONGENITAL ANOMALIES

Congenital anomalies of the cervical spine primarily involve failure of formation or failure of segmentation of the vertebrae. Occipitalization of the atlas has been associated in neurosurgical literature with neurologic compromise; however, occipitalization is not usually associated with stenosis at the foramen magnum or with instability. The exception is the patient with occipitalization of the atlas and congenital fusion of C2–C3 in whom secondary hypermobility and instability frequently develop at the atlantoaxial junction. Instability has also been reported in individuals with hypoplasia of the odontoid in the presence of occipitalization of the atlas. Instability at this level requires posterior fusion of the occiput to the axis.

Congenital absence of the posterior arch of the atlas is a rare congenital anomaly that is not usually associated with instability (Fig. 10–7). Lateral flexion-extension radiographs of the cervical spine as well as MRI evaluation are helpful to rule out cervical spine instability and chronic spinal cord impingement. In the absence of the posterior arch of the atlas, it is the author's recommendation that athletes refrain from high-impact loading activities such as contact or collision sports and diving.

Os odontoideum may be the result of nonunion or fracture through the body of the odontoid or congenital deformity. Lateral flexion-extension radiographs are required to document stability. Athletes with a stable os odontoideum should avoid impact-loading sports including contact and collision sports. Individuals with an unstable os odontoideum require posterior surgical stabilization of the atlas and axis. The normal spine that has undergone single level spinal fusion should not be con-

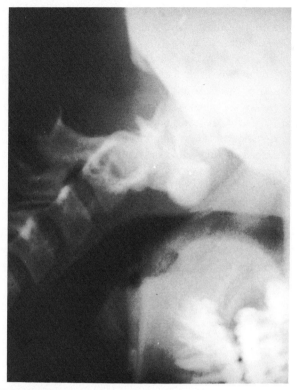

FIGURE 10–7
Lateral radiograph of the cervical spine reveals a complete absence of the posterior arch of C1 with no instability at C1–C2.

sidered normal, and such an individual should not be allowed to return to full sports activity. There are no scientific data on the response of the surgically fused spine to forces imposed by sudden motion and the forces experienced in athletic activity. High-impact loading in the form of contact and collision sports and high diving should be avoided by this patient population.

Congenital absence of the pedicles is a rare congenital anomaly that is usually alarming when viewed radiographically. If lateral flexion-extension radiographs demonstrate stability, however, there is no known reason to restrict the athlete's activity.

Congenital scoliosis of the cervical spine is not associated with instability. Mixed bony lesions may be noted with widening of the interpedicular distances suggestive of intraspinal lesions such as diastematomyelia. If appropriate radiographic studies and MRI eliminate the existence of intraspinal lesions and instability, involved athletes should be permitted to participate in all sports activities.

Congenital fusion of the cervical spine, referred to as the Klippel-Feil syndrome, presents with a host of patterns that span the spectrum from one-level fusion to multiple levels of fusion to complete fusion from C2 to C7 (Fig. 10–8). It is extremely important to document the integrity of the occipitocervical junction in patients with Klippel-Feil syndrome to rule out instability. In the

subaxial cervical spine, lateral flexion-extension radiographs may demonstrate anteroposterior translation of vertebrae as well as anterior gaping of open disc spaces. In the absence of progressive radiographic changes in stability and of neurologic deficits, individuals with Klippel-Feil syndrome should be observed; however, progressive translation or angular deformation at an open disc space should lead to exclusion of these patients from contact and collision sports and possibly to surgical stabilization of the unstable segment. The high association of renal anomalies in those with congenital scoliosis or congenital fusion of the cervical spine demands evaluation of the renal system by ultrasound to rule out clinically important anomalies. Unilateral absence of a renal system is the most common anomaly and is a significant factor in restricting involved individuals from contact sports (Fig. 10–9).

CONCLUSION

Neglect of injury to the cervical spine can result in catastrophic neurologic damage as well as death. During the past decade, the study of mechanisms of sports injuries involving the neck has resulted in a significant de-

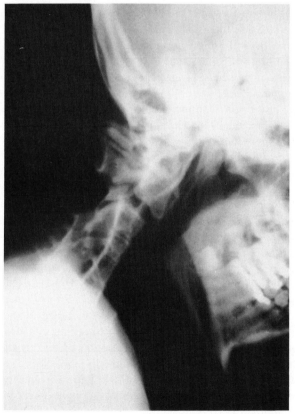

FIGURE 10–8
Lateral radiograph of the cervical spine reveals congenital fusion of C1 and C2 and also of C3, C4, C5, and C6.

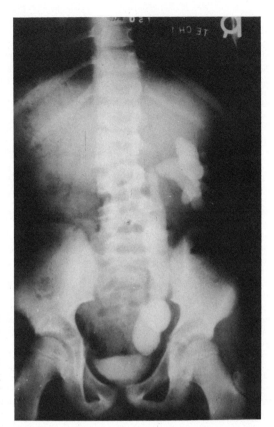

FIGURE 10–9
Intravenous pyelogram demonstrates complete absence of one renal system with hydronephrosis of the remaining system.

crease in the incidence of catastrophic and fatal injuries involving the cervical spine by means of alterations in competitive rules and the education of athletes and coaches in safe techniques of play. Comprehensive conditioning programs tailored to the neck and shoulder girdle improve the athlete's ability to resist damaging forces. Equipment deficits have been responsibly addressed by manufacturers with design improvement in such items as football pads, cervical rolls, and helmets.

The "unexpected" contributes to the excitement experienced in sports. Unfortunately, it is a limiting factor that precludes the reduction of serious or fatal injury to zero. The majority of serious cervical spine injuries can be eliminated by strict adherence of coaches and officials to the rules of competition, use of effective equipment, instruction of athletes in safe techniques, and identification of high-risk athletes combined with subsequent conditioning prior to competition [4]. Team orthopedic surgeons should educate the coaching staff about the serious nature of injury to the cervical spine. Injury to the soft or hard tissues of the neck requires attention to treatment guidelines and a comprehensive rehabilitation program that fosters full range of motion of the neck as well as normal strength. There have been no rigorous studies designed to prove that proper conditioning and

preparation for competition decreases the incidence of injury of the cervical spine; however, the uncertainty of sports demands that the competitive athlete be in optimum physical condition during competition. Safe and effective competition requires appropriate mental and psychological preparation as well as physical conditioning to complement the state-of-the-art equipment available. It is only by adherence to a disciplined program that the incidence of serious and catastrophic cervical spine injuries can be lowered.

References

1. Albrand, O.W., and Corkill, G. Broken necks from diving accidents: A summer epidemic in young men. *Am J Sports Med* 4(3):107–110, 1976.
2. Albright, J.P., et al. Nonfatal cervical spine injuries in interscholastic football. *JAMA* 236(11):1243–1245, 1976.
3. Albright, J.P., et al. Head and neck injuries in college football: An eight-year analysis. *Am J Sports Med* 13(3):147–152, 1985.
4. Bailes, J.E., and Maroon, J.C. Management of cervical spine injuries in athletes. *Clin Sports Med* 8(1):43–58, 1989.
5. Birrer, R.B. Neurologic injury in the martial arts. *In* Jordan, B.D., Tsairis, P., and Warren, R.F. (Eds.), *Sports Neurology.* Rockville, MD, Aspen, 1989.
6. Bruce, D.A., Schut, L., and Sutton, L.N. Brain and cervical spine injuries occurring during organized sports activities in children and adolescents. *Clin Sports Med* 1(3):495–514, 1982.
7. Carter, R.E. Etiology of traumatic spinal cord injury: Statistics of more than 1,100 cases. *Texas Med* 73:61–65, 1977.
8. Clark, K.S. Epidemiology of neurologic injuries in sports. *In* Jordan, B.D., Tsairis, P., and Warren, R.F. (Eds.), *Sports Neurology.* Rockville, MD, Aspen, 1989.
9. Davies, J.E., and Gibson, T. Injuries in Rugby Union Football. *Br Med J* 2:1759–1761, 1978.
10. Fielding, J.W., Fietti, V.G., and Mardam-Bey, T.H. Athletic injuries to the atlantoaxial articulation. *Am J Sports Med* 6(5):226–231, 1978.
11. Fife, D., and Kraus, J. Anatomic location of spinal cord injury. *Spine* 11(1):2–5, 1986.
12. Frankel, H.L., Montero, F.A., and Penny, P.T. Spinal cord injuries due to diving. *Paraplegia* 18:118–122, 1980.
13. Funk, F.J., and Wells, R.E. Injuries of the cervical spine in football. *Clin Orthop* 109:50–58, 1975.
14. Georgopoulos, G., Pizzutillo, P.D., and Lee, M.S. Occipito-atlantal instability in children. *J Bone Joint Surg* 69A:429–436, 1987.
15. Gerberich, S.G., et al. Neurologic injury in ice hockey. *In* Jordan, B.D., Tsairis, P., and Warren, R.F. (Eds.), *Sports Neurology.* Rockville, MD, Aspen, 1989.
16. Gerberich, S.G., et al. An epidemiological study of high school ice hockey injuries. *Child's Nerv System* 3:59–64, 1987.
17. Good, R.P., and Nickel, V.L. Cervical spine injuries resulting from water sports. *Spine* 5(6):502–506, 1980.
18. Hadley, M.N., et al. Acute traumatic atlas fractures: Management and long term outcome. *Neurosurgery* 23(1):31–35, 1988.
19. Hadley, M.N., et al. Acute axis fractures: A review of 229 cases. *J Neurosurg* 71:642–647, 1989.
20. Harris, J.B. Neurologic injury in skiing and winter sports in America. *In* Jordan, B.D., Tsairis, P., and Warren, R.F. (Eds.), *Sports Neurology,* Rockville, MD, Aspen, 1989.
21. Herkowitz, H.N., and Rothman, R.H. Subacute instability of the cervical spine. *Spine* 9(4):348–357, 1984.
22. Hershman, E.B. Brachial plexus injuries. *Clin Sports Med* 9(2):311–329, 1990.
23. Herzenberg, J.E., Hensinger, R.N., Dedrick, D.K., et al. Emergency transport and positioning of young children who have an injury of the cervical spine. *J Bone Joint Surg* 71A:15–22, 1989.

24. Hill, S.A., et al. Pediatric neck injuries. *J Neurosurg* 60:700–706, 1984.

25. Hoskins, T.W. Prevention of neck injuries playing rugby. *Public Health* 101:351–356, 1987.

26. Hubbard, D.D. Injuries of the spine in children and adolescents. *Clin Orthop* 100:56–65, 1974.

27. Jefferson, G. Fracture of the atlas vertebra. *Br J Surg* 7:407–422, 1920.

28. Jordan, B.D., et al. Acute cervical radiculopathy in weight lifters. *Physician Sportsmed* 18(1):73–76, 1990.

29. Jordan, B.D. Neurologic injuries in boxing. *In Sports Neurology.* Rockville, MD, Aspen, 1989.

30. Kewalramani, L.S., and Krauss, J.F. Cervical spine injuries resulting from collision sports. *Paraplegia* 19:303–312, 1981.

31. Kiwerski, J. Cervical spine injuries caused by diving into water. *Paraplegia* 18:101–105, 1980.

32. Marks, M.R., Bell, G.R., and Bumphrey, F.R.S. Cervical spine fractures in athletes. *Clin Sports Med* 9(1):13–29, 1990.

33. Marks, M.R., Bell, G.R., and Bumphrey, F.R.S. Cervical spine injuries and their neurologic implications. *Clin Sports Med* 9(2):263–278, 1990.

34. Maroon, J.C. Burning hands in football spinal cord injury. *JAMA* 238:2049–2051, 1977.

35. McCoy, G.F., et al. Injuries of the cervical spine in schoolboy rugby football. *J Bone Joint Surg* 66B(4):500–503, 1984.

36. McKeag, D.B., and Cantu, R.C. Neck pain in a football player. *Physician Sportsmed* 18(3):115–120, 1990.

37. Mueller, F., and Blyth, C. Epidemiology of sports injuries in children. *Clin Sports Med* 1(3):343–352, 1982.

38. Ohry, A., and Rozin, R. Spinal cord injuries resulting from sport. The Israeli experience. *Paraplegia* 20:334–338, 1982.

39. Pang, D., and Wilberger, J.E. Spinal cord injury without radiographic abnormalities in children. *J Neurosurg* 57:114–129, 1982.

40. Parke, W., Rothman, R.H., and Brown, M.D. The pharyngovertebral veins: An anatomical rationale for Grisel's syndrome. *J Bone Joint Surg* 66A:568, 1984.

41. Paulson, J.A. The epidemiology of injuries in adolescents. *Pediatr Ann* 17:84–96, 1988.

41A. Penning, L. Some aspects of plain radiographs of the cervical spine in chronic myelopathy. *Neurology,* 12:513–519, 1962.

42. Phillips, W.A., and Hensinger, R.N. The management of rotatory atlantoaxial subluxation in children. *J Bone Joint Surg* 71A:664–668, 1989.

43. Pizzutillo, P.D., et al. Bilateral fracture of the pedicle of the second cervical vertebra in the young child. *J Bone Joint Surg* 68A:892–896, 1986.

44. Poindexter, D.P., and Johnson, E.W. Football shoulder and neck injury: A study of the "stinger." *Arch Phys Med Rehabil* 65:601–602, 1984.

45. Pollack, I.F., Pang, D., and Sclabassi, R. Recurrent spinal cord injury without radiographic abnormalities in children. *J Neurosurg* 69:177–182, 1988.

46. Rapp, G.F., and Nicely, P.G. Trampoline injuries. *Am J Sports Med* 6(5):269–271, 1978.

47. Reid, S.E., and Reid, S.E., Jr. Advances in sports medicine: Prevention of head and neck injuries in football. *Surg Annu* 13:251–270, 1981.

48. Rockett, F.X. Observations on the "burner:" traumatic cervical radiculopathy. *Clin Orthop* 164:18–19, 1982.

49. Shields, C.L., Fox, J.M., and Stauffer, E.S. Cervical cord injuries in sports. *Physician Sportsmed* 6:71–76, 1978.

50. Schneider, R.C., et al. Hangman's fracture of the cervical spine. *J Neurosurg* 22:141, 1965.

51. Schneider, R.C. Serious and fatal neurosurgical football injuries. *Clin Neurosurg* 12:226–236, 1966.

52. Schneider, R.C., et al. Vascular insufficiency and differential distortion of brain and cord caused by cervicomedullary football injuries. *J Neurosurg* 33:363–375, 1970.

53. Silver, J.R. Spinal injuries as a result of sporting accidents. *Paraplegia* 25:16–17, 1987.

54. Starshak, R.J., Kass, G.A., and Samaraweera, R.N. Developmental stenosis of the cervical spine in children. *Pediatr Radiol* 17:291–295, 1987.

55. Steinbruck, D., and Paeslack, V. Analysis of 139 spinal cord injuries due to accidents in water sports. *Paraplegia* 18:86–93, 1980.

56. Thompson, R.C., Morris, J.N., and Jane, J.A. Current concepts in management of cervical spine fractures and dislocations. *J Sports Med* 3(4):159–167, 1975.

57. Torg, J.S. Severe and catastrophic neck injuries resulting from tackle football. *Del Med J* 49(5):267–275, 1977.

58. Torg, J.S., et al. Neurapraxia of the cervical spinal cord with transient quadriplegia. *J Bone Joint Surg* 68A(9):1354–1370, 1986.

59. Torg, J.S. Cervical spinal stenosis with cord neurapraxia and transient quadriplegia. *Clin Sports Med* 9(2):279–296, 1990.

60. Virgin, H. Cineradiographic study of football helmets and the cervical spine. *Am J Sports Med* 8(5):310–317, 1980.

61. Warren, R.F. Neurologic injuries in football. *In Sports Neurology.* Rockville, MD, Aspen, 1989.

62. Watkins, R.G. Neck injuries in football players. *Clin Sports Med* 5(2):215–246, 1986.

63. Wilberger, J.E., Adnan, A., and Maroon, J.C. Burning hands syndrome revisited. *Neurosurgery* 19(6):1038–1040, 1986.

64. Wilberger, J.E., and Maroon, J.C. Cervical spine injuries in athletes. *Physician Sportsmed* 18(3):57–70, 1990.

65. Williams, P., and McKibbin, B. Unstable cervical spine injuries in rugby—a 20-year review. *Injury* 18:329–332, 1987.

66. Wroble, R.R., and Albright, J.P. Neck and low back injuries in wrestling. *Clin Sports Med* 5(2):295–325, 1986.

67. Wu, W.Q., and Lewis, R.C. Injuries of the cervical spine in high school wrestling. *Surg Neurol* 23:143–147, 1985.

68. Zwimpfer, T.J., and Bernstein, M.B. Spinal cord concussion. *J Neurosurg* 72:894–900, 1990.

ACUTE MUSCULOTENDINOUS INJURIES

Richard H. Gross, M.D.

Until quite recently, the musculotendinous unit was unquestionably the least studied and least understood component of the musculoskeletal system. Considering the size and importance of skeletal muscle, this is modestly surprising; however, debilitating injuries were not as common as ligamentous injuries and not as dramatic as fractures, so those interested in problems related to sports medicine directed their attention toward more high-profile injuries. Hamstring tears and ''pulled muscles'' were always there, but not often in the pediatric athlete, who was regarded as having the resiliency of a rubber band. More recently, the musculotendinous unit has been intensively studied, although our knowledge of this structure in the pediatric athlete is still far from complete.

There are approximately 450 skeletal muscles, and they comprise 40% to 45% of total body weight in the adult. As is the case for any structure prone to injury, an understanding of normal muscle anatomy and physiology is essential before rational treatment plans can be formulated.

ANATOMY

A muscle is composed of many multinucleated cells called *muscle fibers* [4, 8, 12, 15]. Fibers are multinucleated because they are formed by the fusion of hundreds of myoblasts (see next section, Muscle Growth and Development). The length of fibers varies greatly, from a few millimeters to as much as 30 cm in long adult muscles such as the sartorius. Groups of muscle fibers are characteristically grouped into bundles, or *fasciculi*. The arrangement of fasciculi determines whether a muscle is pennate, bipennate, fusiform, or other form. In general, velocity is related to length (number of sarcomeres acting in series) and force is related to bulk (number of sarcomeres acting in parallel). Thus, long muscles (sartorius, brachialis) have greater velocity, and short muscles (deltoid, soleus) have greater power. In some muscles, such as the rectus abdominis, the fasciculi insert into transverse tendinous bands. *Endomysium* is the connective tissue that fills the space between fibers. *Perimysium* surrounds fascicles and is thus the material found between fascicles. The entire muscle, composed of many fasciculi, is enveloped by *epimysium*. The epimysium changes its name to epitenon, or tendon sheath, when it overlies that part of the muscle-tendon unit. The epimysium is continous at times with the deep fascia. Epimysium and perimysium also are continuous with tendon, the largely collagenous structure that connects muscle to bone. Skeletal muscles have a proximally fixed bony attachment, called the origin, and a distal and more mobile fixation site, the insertion.

The neurovascular supply usually enters at a site near the origin, the neurovascular hiatus. Vessels branch in the perimysium, and capillaries course in the endomysium, between fibers. Blood flow is increased during moderate exercise; strong contractions have been shown to be associated with an obstruction of capillary flow [12]. The nerve supply contains both motor and sensory fibers. Motor fibers include alpha efferents, which branch to supply the *neuromuscular junction* (motor end plate), and gamma efferents supply the muscle spindle.

The *muscle spindle* is a specialized structure within the muscle that controls tension. Motor centers in the brain control the rate of firing of gamma efferents to the muscle spindle. The gamma efferents cause contraction of the intrafusal fibers, increasing their sensitivity to stretch, and thus, by way of messages traveling through the alpha afferent neuron to the anterior horn cells, they increase the reflex tone of the muscle. When central control of the gamma efferents is lost or impaired (e.g., by head or high spinal cord injury), the output of the gamma efferents is uncontrolled, and spastic paralysis results. The spindle itself consists of about 6 to 14 specialized intrafusal fibers, encased in a connective tissue shell. The bulk of muscle fibers outside the muscle spindle are extrafusal. Extrafusal fibers do the work of muscular contraction. Due to its specialized task of holding up the head, the neck has more muscle spindles per unit of muscle than any other site in the body.

Muscle is 75% water, and 20% to 25% protein. The remaining portion includes phosphates, lactates, carbohydrates, and inorganic salts. Of the 25% of muscle that is protein, about three-fourths is in the form of actin or myosin. These specialized proteins provide the configuration that allows for contraction of muscle fibers.

Ultrastructure

A muscle fiber may be defined as a multinucleated cell that contains a larger number of *myofibrils* embedded in a matrix of specialized cytoplasm, all enclosed within a fine sheath, the *sarcolemma* (Fig. 11–1). Outside the sarcolemma is the *basement membrane*. Between the sarcolemma and the basement membrane is the *satellite cell,* which is believed to activate the repair process at the time of injury in addition to providing the extra nuclei necessary for muscle growth during childhood. The myofibrils are about 1 μm (1/1000 mm) in diameter and extend the entire length of the fiber. Under light microscopy, myofibrils have a striated appearance, with alternating light and dark bands; these bands have been named according to their influence on polarized light. The *A (anisotropic) bands* are dark and rotate the plane of polarized light away from the eye. The *I (isotropic) bands* are light and do not deflect polarized light. The I bands are bisected by the *Z lines* (Zwischenscheibe), and the A bands are bisected by the *H zones* or Hensen's zones. The distance between two Z lines represents the basic repeating unit of the muscle fiber, the *sarcomere.* Growth in length of muscle fibers occurs as a result of adding sarcomeres.

In each sarcomere are specially arranged sets of parallel, partially overlapping protein filaments. The thick filaments comprise the A bands (which are thick enough to deflect polarized light) and consist primarily of myosin. The thin filaments are predominantly actin, contain smaller amounts of tropomyosin and troponin, do not deflect polarized light, and thus comprise the I bands.

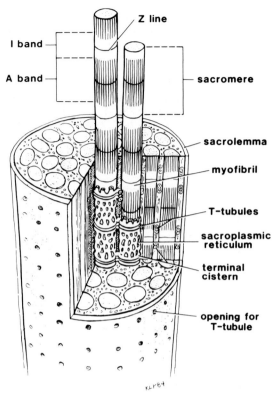

FIGURE 11–1
The ultrastructure of muscle. The Z lines define the limit of the sarcomere, the basic repeating unit of muscle. Many myofibrils constitute a muscle fiber. Not illustrated are the satellite cells that would lie between the sarcolemma and the overlying basement membrane. (From Siegel, I.M. *Muscle and Its Diseases.* Chicago, Year Book, 1986.)

At the region of the Z band, *transverse or T tubules* form an inner extension of the sarcolemma, penetrating between the myofibrils. The *sarcoplasmic reticulum* extends longitudinally. These structures are believed to provide a mechanism for transmitting the excitatory impulse from the sarcolemma to the myofibrils.

At the *neuromuscular junction* the sarcolemma is folded into troughs that contain acetylcholine receptor sites. Stimulation of these receptor sites by neural impulses depolarizes the sarcolemma and T tube system, initiating muscle contraction.

At the *musculotendinous junction* the terminal fibers are stiffer, and the sarcomeres are shorter. Each muscle cell appears to have terminal connections directly to the tendon on which it acts. The cell membrane (sarcolemma) is continuous between intracellular (muscle) and extracellular (tendon) components. The membrane is extensively folded at this site (allowing more contact between muscle and tendon), and the cellular and extracellular connective tissues appear to interdigitate. There are increased numbers of mitochondria, nuclei, and Golgi complexes, and a greater density of sarcoplasmic reticulum at the musculotendinous junction, all of which are felt to indicate greater synthetic activity at this site. This area is currently being actively investigated because it is the site of nearly all muscle strains. This is not surprising when one considers the function of the musculotendinous junction—to transfer force from a contracting muscle cell to an extracellular tendon.

Contraction

The model proposed by A. Huxley and H.E. Huxley and their co-workers has stood the test of time and is presently accepted as an accurate depiction of the process of contraction [8]. During contraction, the I band decreases in length, as does the sarcomere. The myosin molecules have globular heads, and ''walk'' along the actin filaments by successive bonding and rebonding of these globular heads to the thinner actin filaments (Fig. 11–2). Energy is provided by hydrolysis of adenosine triphosphate (ATP) to adenosine diphosphate (ADP).

Muscle Fiber Type

Based on contraction velocity and metabolic characteristics, muscle fibers are classified as either *type I*

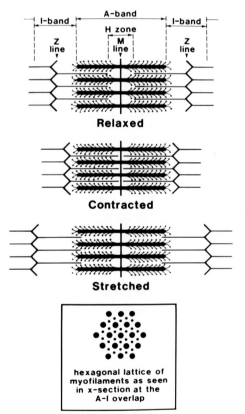

FIGURE 11–2
The configuration of the A bands and I bands. During contraction, the bands overlap, and the I band appears to shorten. Filaments in the A band are thick and are composed of myosin. The globular myosin heads ''walk'' along the actin filaments in the I band by successive bonding and rebonding. (From Siegel, I.M. *Muscle and Its Diseases.* Chicago, Year Book, 1986.)

(slow-twitch) or *type II (fast-twitch)* [11]. The particular fate of a muscle is dependent on its nerve supply, because every motor unit (efferent neuron, axon, plus all the muscle fibers supplied) has identical metabolic and contractile properties. In most muscles, there is a mixture of both types; although one often predominates. Type I fibers have a relatively slow contraction time and are not easily fatigued. Type II fibers are fast-twitch and are capable of intense activity of short duration. Type II fibers are now often further subdivided into type IIa (high levels of glycotytic and oxidative enzymes), type IIb (high levels of glycolytic enzymes), and type IIc (mixed). The fiber type is dependent on the composition of the myosin heavy chains. Coding of the myosin heavy chains is genetically determined and in the human is clustered on chromosome 17 [4]. However, reports of fiber type in twins are confusing, and the genetic influence, albeit very strong, does not appear to be the only factor affecting fiber type [3, 13]. There is much current interest in fiber typing, and it is likely that more sophisticated typing will become available in the future. Fiber type is also neurally controlled because cross-innervation experiments have been shown to partly reverse the muscle's fiber type. Training does not alter fiber type, but of course it can increase the size of a particular type of fiber.

MUSCLE GROWTH AND DEVELOPMENT

Skeletal muscle derives from the mesodermal somites, formed when the embryo is 2 to 3 weeks old. Myoblasts, initially with single nuclei, are produced by the middle germ layer of mesoderm. By the seventh to ninth week, the myoblasts are elongating and fusing to form primitive myotubes. Actin and myosin filaments are synthesized at this time. Individual skeletal muscles are well constructed by the tenth week, but new myotubes are also still being formed, giving a somewhat random appearance to muscle fibers at this age. From the sixteenth week until term, the muscle fibers enlarge, and the striations become better developed (Fig. 11–3). No other histologic changes occur [12]. During childhood, muscle growth appears to be the result of adding sarcomeres at the myotendinous junction [10]; Ziv and colleagues designated this area as a ''muscle growth plate'' [17]. Muscle growth is impaired in the presence of spasticity. The mode of formation of tendon has not been settled, although Crawford believed that the greatest amount of tendon formation also occurred at the myotendinous junction [7]. The process of muscle repair and regeneration after injury is very similar to the process of the original formation of skeletal muscle (Fig. 11–4).

The size of muscle fibers varies with age. In general,

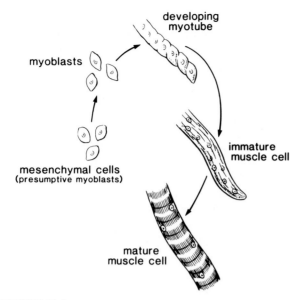

FIGURE 11–3
Skeletal muscle fiber development. Mesenchymal cells fuse to form a myotube, the precursor of the mature muscle fiber. (From Siegel, I.M. *Muscle and Its Diseases.* Chicago, Year Book, 1986.)

fiber size increases with age during childhood, reaching a peak in early adult life (Fig. 11–5). Fiber size then slowly declines, and in old age there is an additional loss in number of fibers (Fig. 11–6). At 1 year of age, fiber diameter is roughly 30% of adult size; at 5 years, it is 50% [2]. Boys have approximately 5% greater muscle size than girls [2]. In the first year of life there is a gradual increase in numbers of type I and type II fibers (as the number of undifferentiated fibers decreases) [6]. Composition and distribution of fiber type in the child over age 1 does not appear to differ significantly from that in the adult [14] (Fig. 11–1). A study of muscle composition in 6-year-olds showed no difference from the adult pattern [1].

INJURY TO MUSCLE

The vast majority of sports injuries involving muscle are either strains or contusions. Both injuries are unusual in early and midchildhood but become quite common after the growth spurt. The repair processes for these two injuries are somewhat similar because they both involve the same tissue, muscle. However, strains, which have only recently been intensively investigated, occur at the musculotendinous junction, whereas contusions, which occur in the muscle belly, are more problematic. Because the underlying pathology is different in these two entities, they are discussed separately. The term Charley horse is said to be a synonym for quadriceps contusion resulting from jumping on the padded wooden horse used in gymnastics; it has also been attributed to a lame

horse named Charley [8, 40]. "Charley horse," although colorful and long included in standard nomenclature of athletic injuries, is presently thought to be a confusing term, and its usage is discouraged [20].

MUSCLE CONTUSIONS

Soft tissue contusions are probably the most common injury in the pediatric athlete, but this is largely dependent on the definition of injury. Watson [27] reported 116 sports injuries (defined as an incident resulting in at least 1 day of incapacity or necessitating medical treatment) in 6799 Irish schoolchildren aged 10 to 18 in one academic year. Of the 116 injuries, 18 were strains, and 14 were contusions (12%). Backous and colleagues [19], in a study of youth soccer injuries sustained at a summer training camp, found contusions to be the most common injury (35.2%). Injury was defined as any soccer-related medical problem that caused the player to miss at least one of the three 2-hour sessions in a day, a less stringent definition than Watson's. Eighty-one percent of the injuries reported caused the player to miss only one session; only 3% of injuries resulted in more than one day's

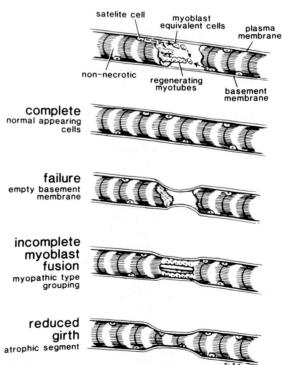

FIGURE 11–4
Response of muscle to injury. The peripherally placed satellite cells retain some stem cell potential and are mobilized at the time of injury. The regenerating myotubes are very similar to embryonic myotubes. In the child with an intact basement membrane, complete healing can be expected. With more severe injury or advanced age, less complete forms of repair are noted. (From Siegel, I.M. *Muscle and Its Diseases.* Chicago, Year Book, 1986.)

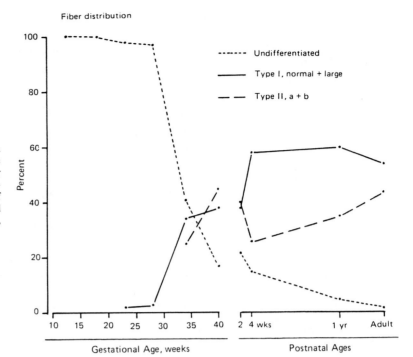

FIGURE 11–5

Distribution of fiber size related to age, from the data of Colling-Saltin, 1978. At birth, the number of type I and type II fibers are essentially equal, but a greater increase occurs postnatally in type I fibers at the expense of the undifferentiated fibers in the first year of life. (From Malina, R.M. Growth of muscle tissue and muscle mass. *In* Falkner, F., and Tanner, J.M. (Eds.), *Human Growth,* 2nd ed. New York, Plenum, 1986.)

loss of participation. Obviously, most contusions in this population were very minor. Contusion was also (barely) the most common injury reported by Sullivan and colleagues [26] in youth soccer players, and both studies reported higher injury rates in older children. Jackson and Feagin [20] reported 65 quadriceps contusions in 4000 young male cadets at the U.S. Military Academy in one year. The incidence of quadriceps contusion in this population of athletically active young men is 1.4/100/year, which is remarkably high compared with other reports on the subject. There is no question that the rate of injury in the pediatric athlete increases with

age, and that the male has a higher risk of injury, so the population studied by Jackson and Feagin is representative of the population at greatest risk for injury. Their numbers emphasize the frequency of this injury near the time of skeletal maturation in males [36].

Despite the frequency of minor contusions, this subject has received scanty attention in the literature. For instance, in the current edition of Kakulas and Adams' *Diseases of Muscle,* the term contusion is not even listed in the index [12]. Hemorrhage, myositis ossificans, crush syndrome, and compartment syndromes all earned attention, but not contusion. Most published work on muscle

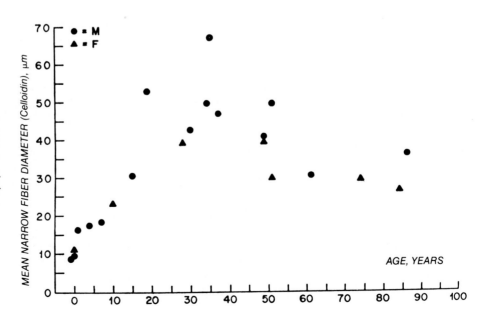

FIGURE 11–6

Diameters of biceps muscle fibers for birth to old age. The fiber size for males is greatest in adolescence and young adult life, with fiber size diminishing in old age. (From Kakulas, B.A., and Adams, R.D. *Diseases of Muscle. Pathologic Foundations of Clinical Myology,* 4th ed. Philadelphia, Harper & Row, 1985.)

contusion has concerned the relationship of contusion to myositis ossificans, but Jarvinen and co-workers have extensively studied muscle contusions experimentally in the rat [21–24]. The initial response is hematoma and inflammation; regeneration of muscle and connective scar tissue formation followed. The rate of healing depended on the formation of connective tissue scar, which in turn depended on vascular ingrowth. This process was delayed in old rats compared to young ones [25]. Although blood flow was not measured in the study comparing age and repair, the histologic patterns noted in aged rats were similiar to those of attempted repair in immobilized limbs with muscle contusions. Animals allowed to mobilize their contused limbs demonstrated increased capillary production and faster healing times [23]. Subsequent studies by the same authors noted the deleterious effects of immobilization of contused muscle, with the force necessary to rupture the muscle lessened 20% to 30% after 2 weeks of immobilization [24]. Importantly, immobilized muscle tendon units strained to rupture failed in the muscle belly instead of in the usual site, the musculotendinous junction.

Thus, the age of the pediatric athlete is undoubtedly important in the response to contusion [5]. Development, maturation, and aging form a continuum wherein cells and tissues are regularly replaced by structures of greater specialization and reduced developmental potential [4]. Muscle formation is dependent on a cooperative interplay between cells of two separated lineages, one involved with formation of the muscle cells themselves and the other with mesenchymal cells—the connective tissue that provides the bed for the muscle fiber. An intact blood supply is obviously necessary for both pathways, and therefore the response to injury will be temporally dependent on the degree of ischemia and vascular impairment accompanying the contusion. The amount of muscle mass that can spontaneously revascularize is reported to be 3 gm [4]. Macrophage invasion is the initiating step in repair. If muscle injury occurs without vascular injury, macrophages can be seen in the muscle fibers 12 hours after injury. Obviously, with more extensive hematoma formation or necrosis, the repair process is delayed until vascular invasion occurs.

Allbrook and associates corroborated this sequence of repair and also noted the deleterious effects of immobilization in a study of muscle regeneration in a monkey model and in human patients with a fracture of the tibia and fibula [18]. Although contusion was not an isolated injury in their study, the process of muscle repair was well documented, and muscle regeneration was found to be complete in about 3 weeks.

The satellite cell between the basement membrane and the sarcolemma has been conclusively shown to be the origin of the myoblasts that fuse to form new myotubes with centrally placed nuclei (similar to embryonic my-

ogenesis) [4]. The myotubes possess the cellular components necessary for formation of contractile proteins. Thus, most contusions seen in clinical practice, which are not accompanied by extensive neurovascular injury, heal uneventfully with normal function. The factors influencing regeneration of contused muscle fibers have not been extensively studied; these include the effects of anti-inflammatory agents, rehabilitation programs, steroids, and other muscle growth factors [4].

Treatment

Treatment of contusions is straightforward. The time-honored principles of rest, ice, compression (but not too tight), and elevation (RICE) are ingrained as initial measures to the point where little further emphasis is necessary. This phase of treatment in West Point cadets generally lasted for less than 24 hours with mild contusions and for about 48 hours with more severe contusions [20]. Isometric quadriceps exercises were started at soon as the patient was capable. After quadriceps control was regained, active range of motion was begun. Physical modalities such as ultrasound, heat, and whirlpool treatments were described as pleasing to the patient but did not influence the rate of recovery. Recovery of extension was emphasized. Touch-down weight bearing with crutches was allowed. Once the patient had recovered 90 degrees of knee flexion, progressive resistance exercises were begun along with participation in noncontact sports to regain agility.

This study provides a good model for the treatment of contusions, allowing for individualization of recovery time consonant with the severity of injury and the patient's rehabilitative effort. The initial inflammatory reaction is controlled with rest, ice, elevation, and gentle compression. Active range of motion exercises follow, with restriction from vigorous activity until a painless functional range of motion is regained. At that point, resistive exercises are begun, accompanied by agility training. Return to sport follows recovery of functional use and requires functional motion, good strength, and the ability to use that motion and strength (for example, in performing cutting maneuvers without favoring the injured limb). There does not seem to be any demonstrable advantage to using other modalities, such as anti-inflammatory agents, especially in children. The connective and vascular tissue of children favors the healing of muscle injuries. Experimentally grafted muscle from young to old animals heals slowly; muscles grafted from old to young heal rapidly.

Reinjury of an injured muscle seems to be a major factor in developing myositis ossificans as a complication of muscular hematoma. In the series of Jackson and Feagin [20] not only did reinjury occur in the form of a repeat blow due to premature return to sports, it also resulted from falls, trips, or uncontrolled forced flexion. Passive stretching of a previously immobilized limb is a reliable method of producing myositis ossificans in rabbits (the animal that did not develop myositis ossificans from external blows to the muscle) [29, 40, 48]. Thus, there is both clinical and basic science evidence for *avoiding passive stretching in any form* in an injured muscle. Tearing a healing muscle unit appears to be a critical factor in producing myositis ossificans.

For the pediatric athlete with a muscle contusion, the best initial management appears to be a loosely appled compression bandage with ice. The method of application described by Dyment is useful [50]. Crushed ice is placed in a sandwich bag. A single layer of wet elastic bandage is applied between the ice bag and the skin; the remainder of the elastic bandage holds the ice in place. The patient undergoing cryotherapy for acute injury experiences several stages of sensation [61]. For the first minute or two, a cold feeling is noted. The second stage of an aching or burning sensation lasts until about 7 minutes after application. The third stage is numbness or anesthesia, with inhibition of reflexes and spasm. Reflex deep tissue dilation with no increase in metabolic activity comprises the fourth stage, reached about 12 to 15 minutes after application of ice. Although I could find no experimental evidence of a salubrious effect of cryotherapy in muscle contusions, its value in the treatment of sprains is well established. However, given the minor nature of the great majority of contusions in the pediatric athlete, it may be difficult to convince the child that the discomfort associated with the second stage of cryotherapy is worthwhile. For severe contusions, the principles of treatment outlined by Jackson and Feagin [20] are recommended. Active use of the limb is encouraged, functional strengthening is commenced when a functional range of motion (90 degrees in the knee) has been achieved. Return to play is dependent on the demonstration of full strength and full range of motion of the injured limb. The importance of avoiding reinjury before healing is complete was emphasized in Jackson and Feagin's study.

MYOSITIS OSSIFICANS

Myositis ossificans (traumatica) is an unfortunate sequela of some severe muscle contusions [28, 34, 35, 37, 45, 46]. Nomenclature in this area can sometimes be a problem because similiar terms are employed to describe very different pathologic conditions. For this chapter, the term myositis ossificans refers to the phenomenon of new bone formation in muscle following injury. This condition is sometimes described as myositis ossificans traumatica to differentiate it from myositis ossificans progressiva (now known as fibrodysplasia ossficans progressive, or FOP), a rare heritable condition characterized by progressive extraskeletal ossification with no established effective treatment. Heterotopic ossification and ectopic ossification are other terms often encountered, especially when describing unwanted soft tissue ossification following surgery (especially on the hip or elbow) or trauma in the presence of head or spinal cord injury. The latter conditions may have some similarity to myositis ossificans traumatica, but the predisposing soft tissue equilibrium is quite different from that in the athlete, and treatment recommendations based on experience with heterotopic ossification may not necessarily transfer to the patient with myositis ossificans. Finally, the term pseudomalignant myositis ossificans has been used to describe nontraumatic localized myositis ossificans [42].

Myositis ossificans has been noted since the eighteenth century and was very well described in the early twentieth century, with emphasis placed on a noninterventive approach [12]. The quadriceps and brachialis have long been documented as favorable sites of involvement. Myositis ossificans appears most often in the second and third decades, but a typical lesion has been reported in a 5-year-old following a motor vehicle accident [32].

The lesion has also been studied experimentally in a variety of animal models. There appears to be some degree of difference among species in susceptibility to traumatic myositis ossificans because Zaccalini and Urist [48] could not produce the lesion in rabbits, who developed only periosteal new bone regardless of the site of the offending blow. Walton and Rothwell [47] produced the lesion in anesthetized sheep, noting the anatomic similiarity of the sheep midthigh to that of the human. However, multiple blows were necessary to produce the lesion in the sheep, whereas a single blow appears adequate in the human. Swelling was not prominent in the sheep. However, the incidence of ossification following trauma in sheep (16.6%) was remarkably similar to a controlled study of quadriceps hematomas by Rothwell (also 16.6%) [45] and to that reported by Jackson and Feagin (20%) [20]. The major damage in the sheep occurred in the vastus intermedius, close to the bone. The pathologic findings were those of a severe contusion, with necrosis of the muscle and replacement by scar tissue. Subperiosteal hemorrhage was never observed. However, appositional periosteal new bone was regularly noted, and in one case the heterotopic bone was connected to the periosteum by a bony stalk. Walton and Rothwell [47] felt that the predilection of the vastus intermedius for this lesion was a result of the shock wave from the injuring blow passing unimpeded through the soft tissue of the thigh until it reached the incompressible bone. As the structure adjacent to bone, the vastus intermedius absorbed the shock and injury. Creatine kinase determinations did not correlate with the extent of damage, and no reliable laboratory findings for diagnosing myositis ossificans have been reported.

In the human, the classic description of the process was by Ackerman in 1959, who credited Johnson with the concept described [28, 38] (Fig. 11–7). Histologic study revealed a zonal type of maturation, with a relatively mature outer zone clearly demarcated from the surrounding muscle. The middle zone was more cellular, with immature osteoblasts, and the inner zone was composed of immature fibroblasts along with hemorrhage and necrosis. With improved imaging techniques and awareness of the characteristic zonal nature of myositis ossificans, the confusion with malignancy that dogged the surgeon of a generation ago is less likely. Of course, the changes just described are not present until ossification has begun, and the early changes are those of a soft tissue mass. Ultrasound and computed tomography have been reported to be helpful in the early diagnosis [30, 33, 39, 43]. Technetium scanning has also been found to herald the appearance of extraskeletal ossification in myositis ossificans [45], but is more nonspecific than other types of imaging. The major masqueraders of myositis ossificans that behave poorly are parosteal and periosteal osteosarcoma [41]. Inasmuch as both varieties of osteosarcoma are attached to bone, the appearance of a radiolucent line between an ossifying soft tissue mass is an extremely helpful diagnostic finding (Fig. 11–8). The

absence of such a finding, however, does not establish the presence of a neoplasm, because the periosteum may also be intimately involved in myositis ossificans [20, 44].

Most cases of myositis ossificans traumatica should present little difficulty in diagnosis. A clear history of injury in a patient with no previous symptoms referable to the injured limb and accompanied by soft tissue swelling should leave little doubt about the etiology. Specialized imaging studies can be done if the history or findings on routine radiography are obfuscatory [44], but I see no reason for their routine use.

Treatment

The management of established myositis ossificans is expectant because resection of an immature lesion can magnify morbidity. Protection from reinjury is the key with resumption of activities as the lesion matures. Despite the benign nature of the condition, restriction of activity for this period can be trying for the young athlete. The average period of disability in patients with myositis ossificans reported by Jackson and Feagin was 73 days [20]. In the more usual situation, in which the physician has less control over the patient's activity than a military academy, the physician's persuasive powers may be taxed to their utmost. Obviously, the avoidance of reinjury includes that from the surgeon, and the "hands off" approach to a maturing myositis ossificans ideally needs little further emphasis. When a mature lesion restricts function, excision can be helpful, but the maturation process is incomplete for about a year after the initial appearance of ectopic ossification. Symptoms warranting excision persist in less than 10% of individuals with myositis ossificans [20, 31].

MUSCLE STRAIN

Muscle strain is such an unglamorous injury that many practitioners have difficulty remembering which tissue is injured in a strain versus a sprain. A *strain* is an injury incurred in the muscle-tendon unit as a result of contraction of the muscle. (Strain is also an engineering term describing deformation of a material body resulting from applied forces. Although this is an appropriate depiction of muscle injury resulting from applied stresses, the opportunity for confusion in terms is unfortunately obvious.) Webber lists three degrees of severity of muscle strain [75]. A first-degree strain involves only mild tenderness, pain with stretch of the muscle, and no palpable defect. A second-degree strain involves spasm of the limb, holding the knee (in the case of a hamstring strain) in 20 to 45 degrees of flexion. Third-degree

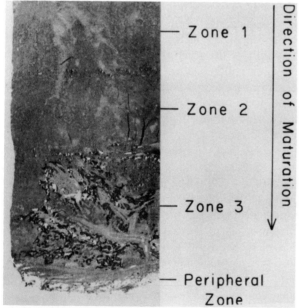

FIGURE 11–7
The zonal nature of maturation in myositis ossificans, described by Ackerman and Johnson. The more mature periphery and cellular central zone are easily evident. (From Ackerman, L.V. Extraosseous localized nonneoplastic bone and cartilage formation [so-called myositis ossificans]. *J Bone Joint Surg [Am]* 40:279, 1958.)

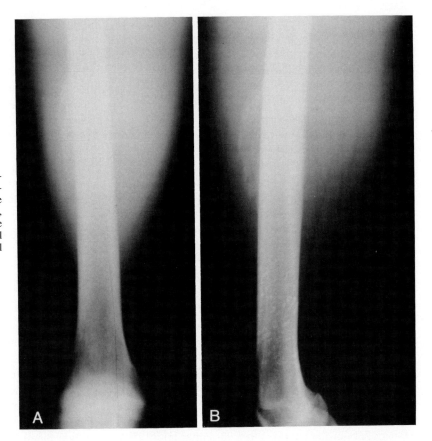

FIGURE 11–8
The radiographic appearance of myositis ossificans in a male nearing skeletal maturity, a characteristic time of appearance of this lesion. The lesion is confined to the vastus intermedius. *A,* The anteroposterior view shows a radiolucent line in the distal part of the lesion, but the proximal portion appears connected by a stalk. *B,* Lateral view. (Courtesy of John Eady, M.D.)

strains imply complete tearing of the musculotendinous junction. A palpable defect can be found if examination permits. Pain and spasm are marked.

Micheli and Smith report that the rapidly growing child is more susceptible to avulsion of the apophysis than strain [68]. They believe that bony growth outpaces muscle tendon growth, leading to a marked degree of inflexibility at this stage of growth. Although avulsion fractures are certainly characteristic of rapidly growing athletes, inflexibility has not been documented, and the relationship of growth to muscle strain rate is unclear at present. In fact, despite a recent explosion of literature investigating muscle strain, there is still much we do not know, especially in the pediatric athlete.

Muscle contraction can be concentric, eccentric, or isometric [8]. Concentric contraction moves an object in accordance with the contracting muscle, such as curling a weight held in the hand results from concentric contraction of the biceps. Concentric contraction at a controlled angular velocity is isokinetic and is a commonly used exercise and testing mode at present. Isometric contraction implies contraction without motion—the resisting forces are such that the contracting force is met by an equal opposing force, and no motion occurs. Attempting to push a heavy boulder usually results only in isometric contraction.

Eccentric contraction allows smooth deceleration of a force tending to pull away from the direction of the contracting muscle. Eccentric contraction, though not measured as often as concentric contraction, occurs regularly in each gait cycle (the hamstrings slowing the acceleration of the leg in swing phase). Eccentric contraction also provides shock absorption, as in landing from a jump off a step. The quadriceps contract eccentrically to dampen the impact, lessening the likelihood of injury. More energy and tension are generated in a muscle as a result of eccentric contraction than of other types of contraction because the preexisting tension from the passive stretch is combined with the tension generated by contraction [71]. Eccentric contraction has been demonstrated to play a key role in the production of muscle strain. Muscles with a high content of type II fibers are more susceptible to strain, as are muscles that cross two joints. Thus, the hamstrings, which often contract eccentrically in running and deceleration maneuvers and have a high content of type II fibers, are a frequent site of muscle strain [54].

The classic study on muscle strain was done by McMaster in 1933 [66]. He found that muscle-tendon units, when strained to failure, sustained injury at the tendon-bone or muscle-tendon interface but not in the muscle belly or in normal tendon. The subject lay fallow for decades, but in recent years Garrett and his associates have recently studied this subject extensively [54, 55, 56, 57, 70]. They have confirmed the propensity of the muscle-tendon unit to fail under a variety of experimental conditions. An exception appears to occur in previously injured muscle, in which failure can occur in the fiber itself rather than in the muscle-tendon junction [24, 73]. As discussed previously in relation to myositis ossificans, these findings obviously underscore the importance of protecting the injured muscle from further injury before healing has occurred.

Although original studies used passive stretching to study muscle strain, more recent studies have used an active experimental model, in which muscle activation is accomplished with electrical stimulation before stretching to failure [55]. This is more relevant to the usual mode of injury, eccentric contraction. Eccentric exercise also leads to more postexercise stiffness and soreness. McCully and Faulkner noted injury to muscle fibers after as few as 15 eccentric contractions [65]. A loss of range of motion can be noted after exhausting eccentric muscle action. Despite earlier reports that spasm was responsible for the decreased motion, recent reports have not found any increased electrical activity in the exercised muscle at rest [16]. The relationship of previous exercise and myofiber damage to risk of subsequent strain appears likely but is not documented. A study of acute strains by MRI concluded that the earliest changes were centrally located in the muscle; these were followed by a "rim" of altered signal density around the periphery of the muscle 2 to 5 days after injury [53]. The pathologic changes responsible for the altered imaging patterns have not been established, but Howell and colleagues [62] suggested that the muscle may be swollen, thus accounting for restricted motion analogous to a rubber balloon in a nylon stocking, which would shorten the length of the stocking [62]. An analysis of CT scans of hamstring muscle strains also concluded that the muscle was edematous but that the edema was secondary to tearing at the musculotendinous junction [57]. The authors emphasized the length of the musculotendinous junction in the hamstrings, noting that the proximal tendon and musculotendinous junction of the biceps femoris extended for approximately 60% of the length of the muscle. The distal tendon also extended about 60% of the length of the muscle, so there is a musculotendinous junction somewhere along the entire biceps. Most of the injuries studied by CT scan in young adult athletes involved the biceps. Another factor that may predispose the hamstrings to strain is the finding that type II fibers appear to be more susceptible to fiber damage induced by eccentric exercise [64].

The preponderance of opinion at present implicates the myotendinous junction as the site of most if not all muscle strains. However, Tidball and Chan [73] found that previously injured muscle failed within the muscle fiber rather than the myotendinous junction, and it is conceivable that damaged fibers secondary to eccentric exercise could fail in the fiber itself. Despite mounds of

evidence, the early pathologic changes in muscle strain are still poorly defined. Furthermore, pathologic events leading to a specific histologic picture are still conjectural, and differing interpretations of the same histologic specimen are likely [72].

Nonetheless, some clinically useful current concepts have evolved. Eccentric contraction, which stretches a preloaded muscle, is almost always responsible for muscle strain. The hamstrings have a high percentage of type II fibers, cross two joints, are commonly loaded eccentrically, and are commonly strained. There is no evidence that a hematoma accompanies strain; soft tissue swelling within the muscle (and surrounding soft tissue) is apparently edematous and is a reaction to injury.

Treatment

The tried and true principles of RICE (rest, ice, compression, and elevation), but not too much compression, are effective initial measures. Regeneration of vascularized muscle occurs quickly, so rapid recovery can be expected in most patients with strains. In fact, reported morbidity from strains incurred during youth sports appears to be minimal [19, 26]. The same general rehabilitation measures recommended for a contusion are also applicable to strain. Active range of motion within pain tolerance is encouraged. When a functional range of painless motion has been achieved, muscle strengthening is begun. Return to sport is allowed when the athlete can demonstrate full motion, strength, and agility. Isokinetic testing is helpful when it is available because the graphs produced give the athlete an easily understandable interpretation of his performance. When such means are not feasible, a useful method of assessing functional recovery is the "figure-of-8 test," in which the athlete is asked to run a figure-of-8 pattern in a constrained space (perhaps 5 yards). Loss of strength or agility are easily noted by the asymmetry of gait in the incompletely rehabilitated athlete. Informing the athlete and coach (and, on many occasions, the parents) of the details of the rehabilitation program at the time of initial assessment, including the physical requirements, before allowing a return to competition is highly recommended. Athletes with even severe muscle strains often recover symptomatically for nonathletic activity in a few days, and the affected athletes consider themselves ready for action at that time unless they are properly counseled. Waiting until the injury is asymptomatic before telling the athlete to start a rehabilitation program and advising him that competition is not yet permissible is an invitation to frustration and resentment. Allowing return to play before rehabilitation is complete is not in the young athlete's best interest. Explaining the nature of the injury, the healing process, and the requirements for return to play at the outset is preferred.

An experimental study of anti-inflammatory medication for treatment of muscle strains (in rats) showed that strained muscles continued to weaken in the early postinjury period regardless of management [49]. Anti-inflammatory medication did reduce the inflammatory reaction and delayed the time of greatest weakness of the muscle postinjury by a day or two. By the eleventh day, the strength of the treated and nontreated muscles was essentially the same. With such inconclusive results, usage of anti-inflammatory medications for treatment of muscle strains in children hardly seems worth the cost or risk of side effects other than for the pain relief that they provide.

Prevention

The role of stretching, although intuitively beneficial, has still not been documented to reduce the rate of strain consistently. In a study of adult male soccer players, players with decreased flexibility showed a higher, though not significantly higher, incidence of strain. The kicking, or dominant, leg suffered a significantly increased number of strains compared with the nondominant leg [51]. A recent article entitled, "Can stretching prevent athletic injuries?", which emphatically advocated regular stretching for athletes, could only conclude, "Although it has not yet been conclusively proved that stretching can reduce the risk of athletic injury, physiologic studies do indicate that stretching can effectively increase a muscle's compliance and extend a joint's range of motion" [63]. Although initially this statement may seem at odds with the dictum of insisting on a full, functional, painless range of motion after injury before permitting return to sport, there is ample evidence that stretching stiff or injured muscles is deleterious [29, 40, 73]. The question of whether individual variations in range of motion in the uninjured state determine susceptibility to strain appears much more difficult to determine. Nicholas linked flexibility to injury pattern in professional football players [69], but others were unable to reproduce his findings in secondary school athletes [59]. High school athletes tested longitudinally became less flexible with maturity [58].

In a study of collegiate football players at the University of Nebraska, a program of isokinetic strengthening and flexibility training was found to be effective in reducing the rate of morbidity from hamstring strains [60]. These measures have become widely used and are very probably effective, but further corroboration is still needed. Stretching exercises do increase flexibility [74]. However, the benefits of increased flexibility per se in terms of decreased injury rates are still unsubstantiated.

Safran and colleagues [70] found that, in rabbits, a preconditioned muscle (stimulated to maximal force generated by the muscle, an average of 15 seconds of contraction) absorbed more force before failing in tension than the unstimulated similar muscle on the other leg [70]. The intramuscular temperature rose an average of 1°C during contraction. They concluded that warming up is of benefit in preventing injury to the muscle-tendon unit. Stretching programs generally are designed to follow a few minutes of activity to allow increased intramuscular temperature before stretching is initiated on the premise that it is safer and more effective to stretch a warm muscle than a cold one. Although this seems to be a very logical sequence, Williford and associates [76] were unable to demonstrate any superiority of a jog-stretch routine over simply stretching cold muscles.

Undoubtedly, we will learn more about the role of stretching and flexibility in sports performance and injury prevention in the future because there is currently considerable interest in this field. At present, however, there is no firm evidence of the effect of stretching in either sphere, especially in children. Despite this, I advocate a routine stretching program for youth sports programs. There is no risk, and there may be some benefit. The only well-established caution is the avoidance of passive stretching of an injured muscle, which, as noted previously, contributes to the formation of myositis ossificans or extensive scar formation.

Much less protective equipment is worn for the purpose of protecting the muscle-tendon complex than for protecting joints or other vital organs. Thigh pads are certainly vital for football but are awkward for other sports with some risk such as basketball and soccer. Contusions and strains are inevitable byproducts of any contact sport, and it is unlikely that risk can be eliminated without altering the essence of the game. However, *reinjury* is preventable with the common sense approach to muscle injuries already described—the use of RICE, early mobilization, functional strengthening, and restriction of return to sport until the limb has been rehabilitated [52].

Acute Tendinous Injuries

Except for overuse syndromes, described in Chapter 8, I have been unable to find any reports of acute tendinous injuries in children.

SUMMARY

Muscle contusions and strains are common in youth sports. The benign natural history of most of these injuries has deflected serious study of these problems in the pediatric athlete until the very recent past. There is no question that the contused or strained muscle is vulnerable to reinjury, and the mainstay of an effective treatment plan is the avoidance of reinjury before functional recovery has occurred. Sequelae of reinjury include myositis ossificans and more incapacitating strains. Muscle heals promptly in children compared to adults, but full motion and full strength are still prerequisites for return to sport. Acute tendinous injuries are essentially nonexistent in children.

References

Anatomy, Physiology and Growth

1. Bell, R.D., Macdougall, J.D., Billeter, R., et al. Muscle fiber types and morphometric analysis of skeletal muscle in six-year-old children. *Med Sci Sports Exerc* 12:28, 1980.
2. Blimkie, C.J.R. Age and sex-associated variation in strength during childhood: Anthropometric, morphologic, neurologic, biomechanical, endocrinologic, genetic, and physical activity correlates. *In* Gisolfi, C.Y., and Lamb, D.R. (Eds.), *Perspectives in Exercise Science and Sports Medicine,* Vol. 2. *Youth, Exercise, and Sport.* Indianapolis, Benchmark Press, 1989.
3. Bouchard, C., Simoneau, J.A., Lortie, O., et al. Genetic effects in human skeletal muscle fiber type distribution and enzyme activities, *Can J Physiol Pharmacol* 64:1245, 1986.
4. Caplan, A., Carlson, B., Faulkner, J., et al. Skeletal muscle. *In* Woo, S.L.-Y., and Buckwalter, J.A. (Eds.), *Injury and Repair of the Musculoskeletal Soft Tissues.* Park Ridge, Il, American Academy of Orthopaedic Surgeons, 1987.
5. Carlson, B.M., and Faulkner, J.A. Muscle transplantation between young and old rats: Age of host determines recovery. *Am J Physiol* 256:C1262, 1989.
6. Colling-Saltin, A.S. Enzyme histochemistry in skeletal muscle of human foetus. *J Neurol Sce* 39:169, 1978.
7. Crawford, G.N.C. An experimental study of tendon growth in the rabbit. *J Bone Joint Surg* 32B:234, 1950.
8. Gamble, J.G. *The musculoskeletal system: Physiological Basis.* New York, Raven Press, 1988.
9. Garrett, W., and Tidball, J. Myotendinous junction: Structure, function, and failure. *In* Woo, S.L.-Y., and Buckwalter, J.A. (Eds.), *Injury and Repair of the Musculoskeletal Soft Tissues.* Park Ridge, Il, American Academy of Orthopaedic Surgeons, 1987.
10. Goldspink, G. Postembryonic growth and differentiation of striated muscle, *In* Bourne, G.H. (Ed.), *The Structure and Function of Muscle.* New York, Academic Press, 1972, pp. 179–236.
11. Gollnick, P.D., and Matoba, H. The muscle fiber composition of skeletal muscle as a predictor of athletic success. An overview. *Am J Sports Med* 12:212, 1984.
12. Kakulas, B.A., and Adams, R.D. *Diseases of Muscle. Pathological Foundations of Clinical Myology* (4th ed.). Philadelphia, Harper & Row, 1985.
13. Komi, P.V., and Karlsson, J. Physical performance, skeletal muscle enzyme activities, and fiber types in monozygous twins of both sexes. *Acta Physiol Scand* Suppl. 462:1, 1979.
14. Malina, R.M. Growth of muscle tissue and muscle mass. *In* Falkner, F., and Tanner, J.M. (Eds.), *Human Growth* (2nd ed.). New York, Plenum Press, 1986, pp. 77–99.
15. Siegel, I.M. *Muscle and Its Diseases. An Outline Primer of Basic Science and Clinical Material.* Chicago, Year Book, 1986.
16. Stauber, W.T. Eccentric action of muscle. Physiology, injury, and adaptation. *Exerc Sports Sci Rev* 17:157, 1989.
17. Ziv, I., Blackburn, H., Rang, M., et al. Muscle growth in normal and spastic mice. *Dev Med Child Neurol* 26:94, 1984.

Contusion

18. Allbrook, D., Baker W.C., and Kirkaldy-Willis, W.H. Muscle regeneration in experimental animals and man. The cycle of tissue change that follows trauma in the injured limb syndrome. *J Bone Joint Surg* 48B:153, 1966.
19. Backous, D.D., Friedl, K.E., Smith, N.J., et al. Soccer injuries and their relation to physical maturity. *Am J Dis Child* 142:839, 1988.
20. Jackson, D.W., and Feagin, J.A. Quadriceps contusions in young athletes. Relation of severity of injury to treatment and prognosis. *J Bone Joint Surg* 55A:95, 1973.
21. Jarvinen, M., and Sovari, T. Healing of a crush injury in rat striated muscle: 1. Description and testing of a new method of inducing a standard injury to the calf muscles. *Acta Pathol Microbiol Scand* 83:259, 1975.
22. Jarvinen, M. Healing of a crush injury in rat striated muscle: 2. A histological study of the effect of early mobilization and immobilization on the repair processes. *Acta Pathol Microbiol Scand* 83:269, 1975.
23. Jarvinen, M. Healing of a crush injury in rat striated muscle: 3. A microangiographical study of the effect of early mobilization and immobilization on capillary ingrowth. *Acta Pathol Microbiol Scand* 84:85, 1976.
24. Jarvinen, M. Healing of a crush injury in rat striated muscle: 4. Effect of early mobilization and immobilization on the tensile properties of gastrocnemius muscle. *Acta Chir Scand* 142:47, 1976.
25. Jarvinen, M., Aho, A.J., Lehto, M., et al. Age-dependent repair of muscle rupture. A histological and microangiographical study in rats. *Acta Orthop Scand* 54:64, 1983.
26. Sullivan, J.A., Gross, R.H., Grana, W.A., et al. Evaluation of injuries in youth soccer. *Am J Sports Med* 8:325, 1980.
27. Watson, A.W.S. Sports injuries during one academic year in 6799 Irish school children. *Am J Sports Med* 12:65, 1984.

Myositis Ossificans

28. Ackerman, L.V. Extraosseous localized nonneoplastic bone and cartilage formation (so called myositis ossificans). *J Bone Joint Surg* 40A:279–298, 1958.
29. Aho, H.J., Aro, H., Juntunin, S., et al. Bone formation in experimental myositis ossificans. Light and electron microscopic study. *Acta Pathol Microbiol Scand* 96:933, 1988.
30. Amendola, M.A., Glazer, G.M., Agha, F.P., et al. Myositis ossificans circumscripta: Computed tomographic diagnosis. *Radiology* 49:775–779, 1983.
31. Carlson, W.O., and Klassen, R.A. Myositis ossificans of the upper extremity. A long-term followup. *J Pediatr Orthop* 4:693–696, 1984.
32. Dickerson, R.C. Myositis ossificans in early childhood. Report of an unusual case. *Clin Orthop* 79:42, 1971.
33. Fornage, B.D., and Eftekhari, F. Sonographic diagnosis of myositis ossificans. *J Ultrasound Med* 8:463–466, 1989.
34. Geschickter, C.F., and Maseritz, I.H. Myositis ossificans. *J Bone Joint Surg* 20:661–674, 1938.
35. Gilmer, W.S., and Nanderson, L.D. Reactions of soft somatic tissue which may progress to bone formation. *South Med J* 52:1432–1448, 1959.
36. Hughston, J.C., Whatley, G.S., and Stone, M.M. Myositis ossificans traumatica (myo-osteosis) *South Med J* 55:1167–1170, 1962.
37. Huss, C.D., and Puhl, J.J. Myositis ossificans of the upper arm. *Am J Sports Med* 8:119–124, 1980.
38. Johnson, L.C. Histogenesis of myositis ossificans. *Am J Pathol* 254:681, 1948.
39. Kirkpatrick, J.S., Koman, L.A., and Rovere, G.D. The role of ultrasound in the early diagnosis of myositis ossificans. A case report. *Am J Sports Med* 15:179–181, 1987.
40. Michelsson, J.-E., and Rauschning, W. Pathogenesis of experimental heterotopic bone formation following temporary forcible exercising of immobilized limbs. *Clin Orthop* 176:265, 1983.
41. Norman, A., and Dorfman, H.D. Juxtacortical circumscribed myositis ossificans: Evolution and radiographic features. *Radiology* 96:301–306, 1970.
42. Ogilvie-Harris, D.J., and Fornasier, V.L. Pseudomalignant myositis ossificans: Heterotopic new-bone formation without a history of trauma. *J Bone Joint Surg* 62A:1274–1283, 1980.
43. Peck, R.J., and Metreweli, C. Early myositis ossificans: A new echographic sign. *Clin Radiol* 39:586, 1988.

44. Resnick, D., and Niwayama, G. Soft tissue. *In* Resnick, D., and Niwayama, G. (eds.), *Diagnosis of Bone and Joint Disorders.* Philadelphia, W.B. Saunders Co., 1988, p. 4253.

45. Rothwell, A. Quadriceps hematoma. A prospective clinical study. *Clin Orthop* 171:97–103, 1982.

46. Thorndike, A. Myositis ossificans traumatica. *J Bone Joint Surg* 22:315–323, 1940.

47. Walton, M., and Rothwell, A. Reactions of thigh tissues of sheep to blunt trauma. *Clin Orthop* 176:273–281, 1983.

48. Zaccalini, P.S., and Urist, M.R. Traumatic periosteal proliferations in rabbits. The enigma of experimental myositis ossificans traumatica. *Trauma* 4:344–357, 1964.

Strain

49. Almekinders, L.C., and Gilbert, J.A. Healing of experimental muscle strains and the effects of nonsteroidal antiinflammatory medication. *Am J Sports Med* 14:303, 1986.

50. Dyment, P.G. Initial management of minor acute soft-tissue injuries. *Pediatr Ann* 17:99, 1988.

51. Ekstrand, J., and Gillquist, J. The frequency of muscle tightness and injuries in soccer players. *Am J Sports Med* 10:75, 1982.

52. Ekstrand, J., and Gillquist, J. Soccer injuries and their mechanisms: A prospective study. *Med Sci Sports Exerc* 15:267, 1983.

53. Fleckenstein, J.L., Weatherall, P.T., Parkey, R.W., et al. Sports-related muscle injuries. Evaluation with MR Imaging. *Radiology* 172:793, 1989.

54. Garrett, W.E., Califf, J.C., and Bassett, F.H. Histochemical correlates of hamstring injuries. *Am J Sports Med* 12:98, 1984.

55. Garrett, W.E., Safran, M.R., Seaber, A., et al. Biomechanical comparison of stimulated and nonstimulated skeletal muscle pulled to failure. *Am J Sports Med* 15:448, 1987.

56. Garrett, W.E., Nikolaou, P.K., Ribbeck, B.M., et al. The effect of muscle architecture on the biomechanical failure of properties of skeletal muscle under passive extension. *Am J Sports Med* 16:7, 1988.

57. Garrett, W.E., Rich, F.R., Nikolaou, P.K., et al. Computed tomography of hamstring muscle strains. *Med Sci Sports Exerc* 21:506, 1989.

58. Godshall, R.W. The predictability of athletic injuries: An eight year study. *J Sports Med* 3:50, 1975.

59. Grana, W.A., and Moretz, J.A. Ligamentous laxity in secondary school athletes. *JAMA* 240:1975, 1978.

60. Heiser, T.M., Weber, J., Sullivan, G., et al. Prophylaxis and management of muscle injuries in intercollegiate football players. *Am J Sports Med* 12:368, 1984.

61. Hocutt, J.E., Jaffe, R., Rylander, C.R., et al. Cryotherapy in ankle sprains. *Am J Sports Med* 10:316, 1982.

62. Howell, J.N., Chila, A.G., Ford, G., et al. An electromyographic study of elbow motion during postexercise muscle soreness. *J Appl Physiol* 58:1713, 1985.

63. Hubley-Kozey, C.L., and Stanish, W.D. Can stretching prevent athletic injuries? *J Musculoskel Med* (March): 21, 1990.

64. Jones, D.A., Newham, D.J., Round, J.M., et al. Experimental human muscle damage: morphological changes in relation to other indices of damage. *J Physiol* 375:435, 1986.

65. McCully, K.K., and Faulkner, J.A. Characteristics of lengthening contractions associated with injury to skeletal muscle fibers. *J Appl Physiol* 61:293, 1986.

66. McMaster, P.E. Tendon and muscle ruptures: Clinical and experimental studies on the causes and location of subcutaneous ruptures. *J Bone Joint Surg* 15:705, 1933.

67. McMaster, W.C., Liddle, S., and Waugh, T.R. Laboratory evaluation of various cold therapy modalities. *Am J Sports Med* 6:291, 1978.

68. Micheli, L.J., and Smith, A.D. Sports injuries in children. *Curr Probl Pediatr* 12(9), 1982.

69. Nicholas, J.A. Injuries to knee ligaments. Relationship to looseness and tightness in football players. *JAMA* 212:2236, 1970.

70. Safran, M.R., Garrett, W.E., Seaber, A.V., et al. The role of warmup in injury prevention. *Am J Sports Med* 16:123, 1988.

71. Singh, M., and Karpovich, P.V. Isotonic and isometric forces of forearm flexors and extensors. *J Appl Physiol* 21:1435, 1966.

72. Stauber, W.T., Fritz, V.K., Vogelbach, D.W., et al. Characterization of muscles injured by forced lengthening I. Cellular infiltrates. *Med Sci Sports Exerc* 20:345, 1988.

73. Tidball, J.G., and Chan, M. Adhesive strength of single muscle cells to basement membrane at myotendinous junction. *J Appl Physiol* 67:1063, 1989.

74. Toft, E., Espersin, G.T., Kalund, S., et al. Passive tension of the ankle before and after stretching. *Am J Sports Med* 17:489, 1989.

75. Webber, A. Acute soft-tissue injuries in the young athlete. *Clin Sports Med* 7:661, 1988.

76. Williford, H.N., East, J.B., Smith, F.H., et al. Evaluation of warmup for improvement in flexibility. *Am J Sports Med* 14:316, 1986.

PHYSEAL INJURIES IN YOUNG ATHLETES

Daniel C. Wascher, M.D.
Gerald A. M. Finerman, M.D.

The past 20 years have seen a large increase in organized athletic participation by children. Although these programs promote fitness and health consciousness among youth, sporting activities also carry inherent risks of injury. In the growing child, excessive force applied to the appendicular skeleton often results in growth plate injuries. Sports trauma remains an important cause of physeal injuries, particularly physeal damage about the knee [52]. Fortunately, the majority of these injuries heal without permanent sequelae; however, accurate recognition and prompt appropriate treatment are required to minimize complications.

The first description of physeal injuries may well date back to Hippocrates. Poland [44] published an extensive review of growth plate injuries in 1898 that included an early classification system. With the advent of roentgenograms in the late nineteenth century, physicians were able to diagnose physeal injuries more easily. The past 25 years have seen an increased understanding of physeal anatomy and biomechanics as well as a variety of newer classification systems. This information has led to improved recognition and treatment of these injuries. When growth arrest follows trauma to the physis, the surgeon can now employ a variety of techniques to correct the deformity.

In addition to acute traumatic damage to the physis, the physician caring for young athletes must also be aware of chronic injuries to the growth plate. The increased organized sports participation by youth has led to a rise in the number of overuse injuries seen. These injuries are caused by excessive training demands placed on the immature musculoskeletal system. The physis is not immune from chronic repetitive damage, and many examples of physeal stress injuries have been reported in the past few years.

ANATOMY OF THE PHYSIS

In the embryo the limb buds appear at about the fifth week. A condensation of mesenchymal cells in the buds differentiates into a cartilaginous precursor of the long bones. Vascular invasion of this cartilage anlage causes ossification in the central portion, producing the primary ossification center. Depending on the exact bone, at various times the cartilage caps at the ends of the bone are invaded by blood vessels, causing formation of secondary ossification centers. A well-organized layer of cartilage separates the primary and secondary ossification centers until late adolescence. This cartilage layer is the physis. The physis is where the axial and circumferential growth of the bone occurs. Eventually, the physis is penetrated by metaphyseal vascular channels, resulting in ossification of the growth plate and bony fusion of the ossification centers. Various physis close at various ages, but the progression of closure follows an organized, predictable sequence.

The growth plate can be divided into several anatomic layers (Fig. 12–1). Beginning at the top, the epiphysis with its layer of articular hyaline cartilage is the first layer. Beneath this lies the true cartilaginous physis, and below this lies the metaphyseal bone. The physis is not a flat plane of cartilage. Viewed macroscopically, the physis is a wavelike layer that separates the ossification centers. The nature and complexity of these convolutions vary with the different physes. On a microscopic level there are small surface irregularities along the physeal-metaphyseal junction known as mammillary processes. It is theorized that these major and minor interdigitations help to increase the strength of the physis to shear forces [8]. These interdigitations appear to play a greater role in physeal strength during puberty [15].

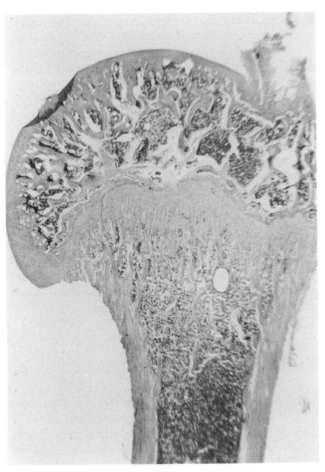

FIGURE 12–1
Histologic section of a proximal femur at low power. The physis is a cartilaginous layer lying between the metaphysis and epiphysis. The wavelike structure of the physis helps to increase its strength against shear stresses.

Histologically, the growth plate can be divided into several discrete layers [11, 48] (Fig. 12–2). On the epiphyseal end of the physis is a zone of small isolated chondrocytes. This layer is referred to as the reserve

zone. It was previously called the resting zone or the germinal zone; however, these cells are metabolically quite active but proliferate only sporadically. They do not give rise to the columns of cells seen in the deeper zones of the physis. The cells in the reserve zone are spherical, exist singly with occasional couplets, and are surrounded by an abundant extracellular matrix. The exact function of these cells is unclear; a high lipid body and vacuole content suggest that this layer provides storage for later nutritional requirements.

Below the reserve zone lies the proliferative zone. This layer contains the true "mother" cells that divide, forming palisading columns of chondrocytes. The growth of the physis is equal to the rate of production of new chondrocytes multiplied by the maximum size of the chondrocytes at the bottom of the hypertrophic zone. In addition to cell division, these cells also play a role in matrix production.

The bottom layer of the physis is the hypertrophic zone. In this zone the proliferating chondrocytes become spherical and undergo a fivefold enlargement. The cells in the upper portion of the hypertrophic zone remain metabolically active, but as the cells are pushed further away from the physeal blood supply, they eventually undergo a process of vacuolization and ultimately cell death. At the bottom of each column of chondrocytes lie empty lacunae. Cell death leads to calcium release from the mitochondria, which probably plays a role in initiation of calcification of the matrix. Some authors refer to the bottom area of this layer as the zone of provisional calcification [47].

Beneath the physis lies the metaphyseal bone. There is a transverse septum of bone adjacent to the physis, and then the normal pattern of trabecular metaphyseal bone is encountered. Vascular invasion of the physeal extracellular matrix occurs from the metaphyseal capillary loops, which deliver osteoprogenitor cells. The vascularized calcified cartilage layer is referred to as the

FIGURE 12–2
Schematic drawing illustrating the layers of the physeal plate. The epiphyseal side of the growth plate is at the top of the drawing. (From Brighton, C. T., Structure and function of the growth plate. *Clin Orthop* 136:24, 1978.)

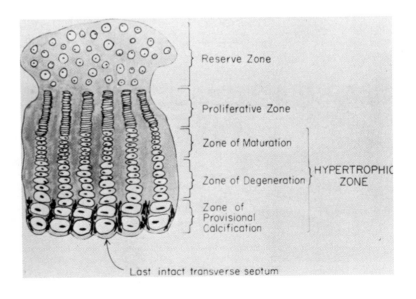

Reserve Zone

Proliferative Zone

Zone of Maturation

Zone of Degeneration

Zone of Provisional Calcification

HYPERTROPHIC ZONE

Last intact transverse septum

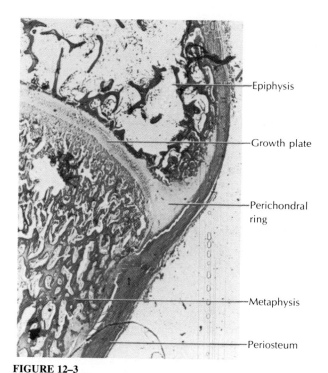

Epiphysis

Growth plate

Perichondral ring

Metaphysis

Periosteum

FIGURE 12–3
Histologic section through the peripheral portion of a rodent's growth plate. The ossification groove of Ranvier, the wedge of fibrous tissue at the rim of the physis, is clearly visible. The perichondral ring of Lacroix lies peripheral to the ossification groove and provides mechanical support to the growth plate. (From Rockwood, C. A., and Green, D. P. [Eds.]. *Children's Fractures*, 3rd ed. Philadelphia, J. B. Lippincott, 1991.)

primary spongiosum. Just below this layer, osteoblasts cause enchondral ossification on the calcified cartilage bars; this is the secondary spongiosum. Below this layer, the calcified cartilage and the woven bone initially produced are replaced with lamellar bone. Osteoclasts are seen in this region of remodeling. This region takes on the characteristics of trabecular bone.

Surrounding the physeal cartilage is a wedge of fibrous cells termed the ossification groove of Ranvier

[55] (Fig. 12–3). This groove has been shown to contain undifferentiated cells that contribute chondrocytes to the physis, thus allowing circumferential growth of the physis to occur. Fibroblasts in the groove of Ranvier also help to anchor the growth plate to the perichondrium of the hyaline cartilage above the growth plate. In addition to the groove of Ranvier, a dense fibrous band encircles the growth plate at the physeal-metaphyseal junction. This band has been labeled the perichondral ring of Lacroix. This ring is contiguous with the periosteum of the metaphysis and the fibroblasts in the groove of Ranvier [48]. The ring of Lacroix provides mechanical support, acting as a limiting membrane to the physis. Chung and colleagues [15] showed that the perichondral ring provides much of the resistance to shear forces seen in younger children. As the child matures, the perichondral ring thins out and plays a smaller role in the strength of the physis. Injury to these peripheral structures can cause formation of peripheral physeal bars [47].

VASCULARITY

Each portion of the growth plate has a unique blood supply (Fig. 12–4) [63]. The metaphyseal circulation is derived primarily from branches of the nutrient artery. Additional blood supply occurs from perforating vessels from the periosteal arteries. These metaphyseal vessels end in vascular capillary loops just below the base of the cartilaginous zones. No vascular channels cross the bone-cartilage junction; hence, the metaphyseal vessels do not contribute at all to the nutrition of the physeal cartilage cells.

The epiphysis is supplied by epiphyseal arteries. The majority of physes are located extracapsular [6]; in these physes, arteries penetrate the epiphysis through soft tissue attachments. However, the proximal radial and the proximal femoral physes are unique. These physes are located completely intracapsularly, and there

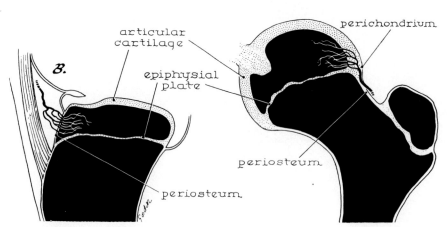

articular cartilage

B.

epiphysial plate

periosteum

perichondrium

periosteum

FIGURE 12–4
The blood supply to the growth plate can arrive by one of two paths. Most commonly, the vessels enter from soft tissues surrounding the epiphysis (left). When the entire physis is located intracapsularly (right), the vasculature arises from soft tissues overlying the metaphysis; the blood vessel must then travel along the articular surface before penetrating the epiphysis. (From Dale, G. G., and Harris, W. R. Prognosis of epiphyseal separation. An experimental study. *J Bone Joint Surg* 40B:117, 1958.)

are no soft tissue attachments to the epiphysis. Their epiphyseal vessels arise from soft tissue overlying the metaphysis, and these vessels then crawl along the surface of the epiphysis to penetrate it intracapsularly. The proximal femoral and proximal radial epiphyseal vessels are thus at great risk for injury with physeal disruption. Branches of the epiphyseal vessels supply the reserve and the proliferating zones of the physis; no vessels pass through the proliferative zone to supply the hypertrophic zone. Hence, the hypertrophic zone is avascular and relies on diffusion for its nutrition; cell death eventually occurs when the hypertrophic cells become too remote from the physeal vessels. This avascularity also plays an important role in matrix calcification, which results in part from decreased oxygen tension in the lower portion of the hypertrophic zone [11]. The peripheral fibrous structures receive a rich blood supply from perichondral arteries [55].

The vascular supply of the growth plate has important implications for physeal injuries. Even minor physeal injuries of the proximal femur and the proximal radius can completely disrupt the physeal blood supply, leading to premature closure of the physis and avascular necrosis of the epiphysis. In addition, disruption of the physis that allows communication between the metaphyseal and epiphyseal circulations allows osteoprogenitor cells to enter the physis, resulting in localized or complete growth plate arrest. As discussed later in this chapter, the vascular damage that occurs at the time of physeal injury is an important predictor of complications.

INCIDENCE

A number of authors have analyzed the incidence of growth plate injuries [23, 36, 38, 43, 50]; although the exact numbers vary from study to study, remarkably constant findings are seen. Some general conclusions are readily drawn. Approximately 15% to 20% of injuries to the long bones of children involve the growth plate. The upper extremities are involved more frequently than the lower extremities by a ratio of 2:1. The distal radial physis is the most commonly injured, accounting for approximately one-third of all growth plate injuries. Although not included in early reports, it is now recognized that collectively the phalangeal physes constitute the second most common site of growth plate injury [23, 30, 62], followed closely by the distal tibial physis. Physeal disruptions about the knee are rare, constituting only about 2% of all growth plate injuries; however, they represent half of all growth arrests requiring surgical correction.

Most studies have found that the incidence of physeal injuries in boys is twice that in girls. This is thought to be secondary to an increased exposure to trauma in

young males as well as to a longer period of exposure because physeal closure occurs at a later date in males. Hormonal differences may also cause a qualitatively weaker growth plate in males during puberty [37].

The peak incidence of injury occurs during the period of rapid growth in early adolescence (Fig. 12–5). This occurs at about age 11 in girls and at age 12 to 13 in boys. Again, these peaks result from increased exposure to trauma at this age combined with a weakening of the growth plate during puberty. Peterson and Peterson [43] and Rogers [50] noted in their studies that the distal humeral physis was an exception in that it was associated with an early peak incidence of injury (occurring at age 4 to 5 in girls and 5 to 8 in boys) as well as the peak

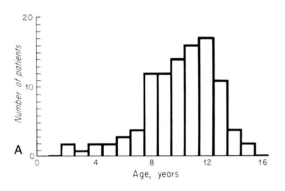

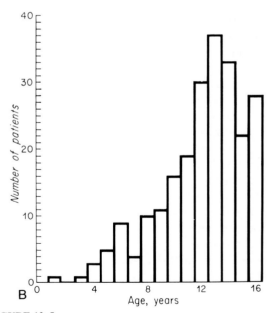

FIGURE 12–5
Incidence ratio of acute physeal injuries in females *(A)* and males *(B)*. Note that boys have an incidence of growth plate fractures twice that of girls; the peak incidence for males (ages 12 to 16) also occurs later than that for females (ages 8 to 13). (From Peterson, C. H., and Peterson, H. A. Analysis of the incidence of injuries to the epiphyseal growth plate. *J Trauma* 12:279. Copyright Williams & Wilkins, 1972.)

seen in adolescence. These authors suggested that the early peak represented complete epiphyseal separation, whereas the adolescent injuries involved predominantly only the medial or lateral epicondyle. It should also be noted that most epidemiologic studies excluded slipped capital femoral epiphyses and vertebral physeal injuries. The physician frequently has difficulty in differentiating traumatic and chronic injuries of the proximal femoral physis. Physeal injuries have been reported in the cervical, thoracic, and lumbar spine, but they appear to be unusual [29].

The exact role of athletics in causing physeal injuries is unknown, but several studies suggest that sports cause a large proportion of physeal injuries about the knee and ankle; these locations are common sites of growth arrest requiring treatment [17, 31, 61]. In one study 15 of 23 triplane fractures of the distal tibia occurred during sporting activities [17]. Twenty percent of all distal femoral epiphyseal injuries in one series were related to athletic pursuits [31]. Over half of Salter-Harris III injuries of the medial femoral condyle are reported to be secondary to clipping injuries in football or soccer [49, 61]. Certainly sports trauma represents a significant source of physeal injury, particularly about the knee, a location prone to physeal bar formation and subsequent growth deformity.

MECHANISMS OF INJURY

A variety of forces, both acute and chronic, can result in physeal injury. The most common form of injury results from acute mechanical overload. The cartilaginous physis represents the weakest biomechanical link in the growth plate [53]. The physis is most susceptible to shear forces. Bright and colleagues [10] showed that the physis exhibits viscoelastic properties, requiring higher loads to failure with increasing rates of load. Bright and associates [10] and others [15, 37] also observed that female physes are stronger than their male counterparts. A decrease in physeal strength has been noted at puberty [37] Chung and colleagues [15] noted the importance of the ring of Ranvier in resisting shear stress in younger children; this role decreased concomitant with the thinning of the ring seen during puberty. These observations may explain some of the increased incidence of physeal injury seen in pubescent males.

Salter and Harris [53] noted that the plane of cleavage in physeal separations almost always occurs between the hypertrophic zone and the metaphyseal bone. The strength of the physis is derived from the extracellular matrix. At the bottom of the hypertrophic zone there is a paucity of matrix, and intuitively one would expect physeal failure at this level. Bright and associates [10] noted cleavage of the physis through this plane, but they also observed short linear cracks deep within the physis.

Subfailure loads of 50% also initiated these cracks (Fig. 12–6). They suggested that the primary failure occurred through these short linear breaks in the deeper layers of the physis along the planes of highest shear stress. With continuing load, a tensile failure occurred, causing a secondary crack along the cleavage plane between the zone of hypertrophy and the metaphysis. The secondary cracks often coalesced with the primary cracks, especially in older animals. With additional load application, rupture of the periosteal sleeve occurred, allowing epiphyseal displacement. Using torsional forces, Peltonen and associates [40] observed a pure cleavage plane through the physeal-metaphyseal junction in younger animals. In older animals, however, a more sinuous separation pattern appeared, with the fracture also occurring through metaphyseal bone. In summary, the major cleavage plane in physeal injuries occurs through the zone of hypertrophy. Both clinical experience and animal studies suggest that younger children sustain more pure physeal separations without bone fractures. Other areas fail also, more frequently in older children, giving rise to the varied physeal fracture patterns seen.

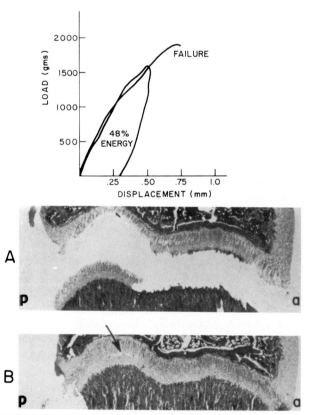

FIGURE 12–6
Histologic sections through proximal tibial physes of rats subjected to shear loads. *A,* The typical failure path when the physis is loaded to failure. The majority of the separation occurs between the hypertrophic zone and the metaphyseal bone. *B,* A physis loaded to 48% of failure energy. A short linear crack (arrow) is seen deep within the physis where primary failure to shear stress occurs. (From Bright, R. W., et al. Epiphyseal-plate cartilage. A biomechanical and histological analysis of failure modes. *J Bone Joint Surg* 56A:699, 1974.)

Pressure applied perpendicular to the growth plate can have profound effects on physeal function. Arkin and Katz [4] used serial casts to apply pressure to rabbit tibial physes and demonstrated marked angular deformities with relative growth arrest on the side of the physis exposed to increased pressure from the casts. They also observed increased physeal longitudinal growth in rabbit limbs that were kept nonweight-bearing. Slight and even intermittent pressures were shown to slow or hinder physeal growth. Simon [59] found that excessive dynamic loading could decrease physeal growth, but he noted that slight increases in dynamic loading could cause increased growth. Short-acting high-energy forces cause metabolic changes in the physeal layers indicative of permanent growth plate injury [20]. Distal radius growth arrest has been seen in young gymnasts who train excessively. Markolf and colleagues [34] studied the forces generated in gymnasts' wrists and showed that forces almost three times body weight (BW) are applied to the distal radius during pommel horse routines. Loading rates reached 28 BW/second. This repetitive, rapid, high loading probably produces the physeal changes in the distal radius seen in young gymnasts.

Physeal damage also results from nonmechanical causes. Children with frostbite have been noted to have premature physeal closure [54]; this effect results from both ischemia and thermal damage. Stark and associates [60] showed that 7 hours of warm ischemia cause severe damage to the central region of the physis; 12 hours of warm ischemia lead to infarction. Infection due to metaphyseal hematogenous osteomyelitis or open physeal injuries often causes growth arrest [41]. A stable environment must be maintained to ensure continued physeal growth.

Iatrogenic physeal arrest has also been demonstrated. Epiphysiodesis has been used as a surgical procedure to correct limb length discrepancies. Siffert [58] showed that staples bridging the physis caused permanent growth arrest of the physis. Large or threaded wires crossing the physis have been reported to cause growth arrest. Makela and colleagues [32] demonstrated that destruction of only 7% of the cross-sectional area of the growth plate caused permanent growth disturbances. When internal fixation is required for physeal injuries, the surgeon should use thin smooth wires and avoid fixation that crosses the physeal cartilage if possible [8, 53].

CLASSIFICATION OF PHYSEAL INJURIES

Many classification schemes for physeal injuries have been proposed [1, 14, 18, 44, 45, 53]. Foucher [18] in 1860 was the first to propose a system for classifying physeal injuries. Poland [44] in 1898 proposed four types of epiphyseal injuries. His types I to III are identical to the types I to III used in the Salter-Harris system of today. Poland's type IV was an intercondylar T-type fracture. Aitken [1] and later Weber [65] categorized physeal injuries based on the presence or absence of intra-articular extension. Pollen [45] describes three groups: fracture separation of the epiphysis, transepiphyseal fractures, and crushing injuries of the growth plate. Today in North America, the most commonly used classification system is the Salter-Harris system [53] (Fig. 12–7). Types I to IV of this system are similar to the types listed in the previous classification systems. The Salter-Harris classification is based on the pathoanatomy of the fractures, which is readily apparent from radiographic studies. This feature facilitates communication between physicians when discussing physeal injuries.

Salter-Harris type I injuries involve a purely transphyseal separation with no osseous fracture lines visible. If the periosteal sleeve remains intact, there may be very little displacement. These injuries are more commonly seen in younger children and in rachitic patients.

Type II fractures comprise a transphyseal separation with an extension through the metaphysis on the compression side of the bone. This metaphyseal fragment, which remains attached to the epiphysis, is referred to as the Thurston Holland sign. The size of the metaphyseal piece can be quite variable. The intact periosteal sleeve on the compression side usually facilitates closed reduction. Type II injuries are by far the most common type of physeal injury seen [43, 50].

Salter-Harris type III injuries involve a partial separation through the physis with extension of the fracture line through the epiphysis and exiting out of the joint surface. This injury is uncommon and is usually found around the knee joint or at the distal tibial physis. Anatomic reduction of the fracture fragment is necessary to restore a smooth articular surface.

A type IV Salter-Harris injury is a fracture that extends from the joint surface through the epiphysis and physis, exiting through metaphyseal bone. This injury is most commonly seen about the lateral humeral condyle and the medial malleolus. Anatomic reduction is necessary to restore joint congruity and to prevent metaphyseal-epiphyseal bony bridging.

Salter-Harris type V injuries involve a crush injury of the epiphyseal plate. Radiographs at the time of injury often appear normal. This diagnosis is usually made retrospectively after growth arrest has occurred following a compression injury to a physis. Some authors doubt the existence of this injury [42]; most agree that it occurs but is rare. Distal radial physeal growth disturbances from chronic stresses seen in young gymnasts probably represent a variant of the type V injury [51].

Rang [47] later added a type VI to the Salter-Harris classification. This injury involves damage to a portion of the perichondral ring. There is minimal damage to the

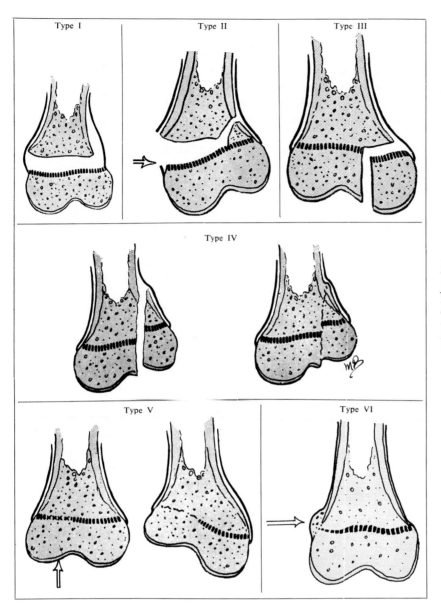

FIGURE 12–7
The Salter-Harris classification of physeal injuries is the most commonly used system in North America. Rang added type VI (perichondral ring injuries) to the initial scheme. (From Rang, M. *The Growth Plate and Its Disorders.* Edinburgh, E & Livingstone, S, 1969.)

true physis, but a bony bridge can develop across the peripheral site of injury, resulting in angular deformity of the physis. Ogden [39] proposed a classification system that subdivides the Salter-Harris groups and adds three additional paraphyseal injury types. With 20 different categories, this system appears overly complex for routine use in practice.

The Salter-Harris classification system was originally intended to serve as a prognostic indicator for the chances of subsequent growth arrest. The authors stated that types I, II, and III had an excellent prognosis for continued physeal function because the blood supply to the injured physis remained intact. Type IV injuries were thought to have a poor prognosis if they were not anatomically reduced because of the communication of the metaphyseal and epiphyseal circulations and subsequent bony bridge formation. Type V injuries were considered to have the worst prognosis because microscopic bony

bridges formed through the crushed physis, causing growth disturbance. Many studies have subsequently found a poor correlation between Salter-Harris type and subsequent development of physeal bars [8, 14, 31, 41]. This discrepancy arises from the failure of the Salter-Harris classification to take into account macroscopic or microscopic physeal vascular damage at the time of injury. For example, even type II radial head fractures cause a high incidence of growth arrest and avascular necrosis because of the precarious epiphyseal blood supply. Additionally, as shown in the experimental work of Bright and colleagues [10], physeal separation is usually not a pure cleavage through the hypertrophic zone. Other cracks and fissuring occur in the physis that can potentially lead to the formation of bony bridges even in type I and II injuries.

Shapiro [57] has proposed a pathophysiologic classification scheme to be superimposed on the Salter-Harris

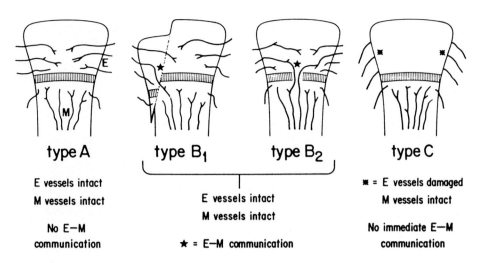

FIGURE 12–8
Shapiro's pathophysiologic classification of growth plate injuries. Type B injuries, which result in communication between the epiphyseal and metaphyseal circulations, have the potential to produce physeal bars and subsequent growth disturbances. (From Shapiro, F. Epiphyseal growth plate fracture-separations. A pathophysiologic approach. *Orthopedics* 5:721, 1982.)

system (Fig. 12–8). In Shapiro's approach, type A injuries have an intact epiphyseal vascularity with no communication between the epiphyseal and metaphyseal circulations. Type B injuries have intact epiphyseal vessels, but communication exists between the epiphyseal and metaphyseal systems. Type B_1 injuries result from gross displacement (i.e., Salter-Harris type IV); type B_2 injuries result from microscopic or macroscopic crushing or fissuring of the physis. Type C injuries have disrupted epiphyseal circulation with subsequent death of the growth plate cartilage. This system helps to explain the poor correlation of Salter-Harris type with eventual outcome, but it remains difficult to identify type B_2 injuries prospectively.

Currently, we continue to use the Salter-Harris classification. It is an anatomic classification, and identification can easily be made from roentgenograms. Although it does not accurately predict the incidence of subsequent growth plate arrest, the Salter-Harris system does help in planning treatment. The pathophysiologic approach of Shapiro accurately emphasizes that vascular injury is the best predictor of potential growth plate damage; however, until better diagnostic techniques for studying the microcirculation in physeal injuries become available, it will have only limited value.

HISTORY AND EXAMINATION

An injury in any child at the end of a long bone should be suspected of being a physeal injury. Likewise, a joint dislocation or ligament injury in any young athlete should be considered to be a physeal injury unless proven otherwise. The physeal plate is by far the weakest structure around the joint in growing children; physeal injuries are far more common than dislocations and ligament tears in this age group. A history should be obtained in an attempt to elicit the mechanism of the injury. For example, distal femoral physeal injuries are commonly caused by clipping injuries in football [49].

The possibility of child abuse should always be kept in mind.

Physical examination should include a careful examination of the entire injured extremity; patients with injuries resulting from high-energy trauma should have a complete examination to rule out visceral injury. Bilateral physeal injuries have been reported [35]. In children with physeal trauma, pain and swelling are almost invariably present. Deformity is often present but may be slight if the fracture is minimally displaced. Crepitus may be absent in patients with pure physeal separations. A careful distal neurovascular examination should be performed before any reduction or casting is undertaken.

Although physeal injuries about the knee are more common in children than ligament disruptions, the presence of a physeal separation does not rule out concomitant ligament injury. Bertin and Goble [5] reported a series of 29 patients with physeal injuries about the knee. At follow-up examination, 14 (48%) had evidence of ligament instability about the knee. Eleven of the fourteen had anterior cruciate ligament (ACL) laxity and 5 of 14 had medial collateral ligament (MCL) laxity of 2 + or greater; two of the patients had combined ACL/MCL instability patterns. Of note, 11 patients in their series were injured during athletic activities, and six of these showed demonstrable ligamentous instability. In physeal injuries about the knee, the physician must maintain a high index of suspicion for coexisting ligamentous injury; reexamination after fracture treatment is mandatory, and treatment is dictated by the patient's age, physical demands, and desires.

DIAGNOSTIC STUDIES

Radiographic examination is required in every child in whom a growth plate injury is suspected. Plain x-rays in two views are requisite; often oblique views are necessary to demonstrate small metaphyseal fragments in Salter-Harris II injuries [50] (Fig. 12–9). The presence of normal physeal lines is often confusing. Fractures can mimic physiologic physeal lines and vice versa [28]. The physician should not hesitate to obtain comparison views of the contralateral extremity to settle any doubts. If no obvious physeal disruption is seen on initial radiographs and physical examination suggests ligamentous laxity, stress radiographs should be taken to look for occult physeal fractures [49] (Fig. 12–10).

CT scanning has been reported to be helpful in evaluating triplane fractures of the distal tibia [17], but it is not required in the evaluation of most physeal injuries. We are not aware of any reports of magnetic resonance imaging (MRI) for physeal injuries, but MRI may have the potential to provide more detailed information about injury to the growth plate. Likewise, bone scanning is being investigated in children with growth plate trauma [56, 67], but its usefulness in predicting subsequent physeal arrest remains to be proved. Plain radiographs remain the workhorse for evaluating physeal injuries.

TREATMENT

The great majority of physeal injuries in children heal without any significant or clinically important growth disturbance. The treating physician should warn the parents of the possibility of physeal arrest at the time of injury. Follow-up examinations after fracture healing are required to search for any signs of altered physeal growth. Some authors recommend clinical and radiographic follow-up until the child attains skeletal maturity, but this seems excessive. A careful clinical examination combined with attention to radiographic detail will allow detection of almost all cases of growth arrest within 1 year of injury. Hynes and O'Brien [24] pointed out that observation of the Harris growth lines after physeal trauma can provide early evidence of partial physeal arrest. If these growth disturbance lines remain parallel to the physis with longitudinal bone growth, then physeal growth is occurring normally.

Almost all Salter-Harris I and II fractures can be treated with closed reduction and immobilization. The intact periosteal hinge on the compression side of the injury prevents overreduction. The manipulation must be done gently. Adequate anesthesia is mandatory; the physician should not hesitate to use general anesthesia if necessary. An imperfect reduction has a great capacity for remodeling in children if the angle of deformity is in the same plane as the angle of joint motion [8, 53]. The younger the child and the greater the contribution of the physis to the overall length of the bone, the greater the capacity for remodeling. For example, in proximal humeral fractures remodeling of almost any residual angulation occurs with excellent final functional results.

Occasionally, a flap of periosteum is interposed at the

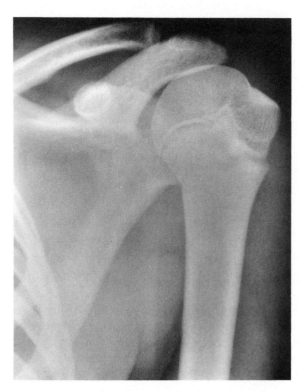

FIGURE 12–9
Radiograph of a 14-year-old boy who sustained a Salter-Harris type II injury to the proximal humeral physis. The fracture line was not readily visible on other views of the shoulder.

fracture site and blocks reduction. If success is not obtained after several attempts at closed reduction, the physician should not be reluctant to proceed with an open reduction. Excessive closed manipulation can lead to further physeal damage and increase the potential for growth plate arrest [52]. After open reduction, many Salter-Harris I and II injuries do not require internal fixation.

Salter-Harris III and IV physeal injuries require anatomic reduction [53, 61]. Because these are intra-articular fractures, articular congruity is requisite for accurate restoration and fixation of the fracture fragments. In addition, type IV injuries require accurate alignment to prevent the formation of bony bridges between metaphyseal and epiphyseal bone. If these injuries are nondisplaced on all radiographic views, they can be treated with immobilization alone. Some authors believe that all of these injuries should have internal fixation [8]; however, with close follow-up, any displacement should be readily detected. If any displacement of the fragments is suggested on the initial or subsequent radiographs, immediate open reduction and internal fixation should be performed (Fig. 12–11). The surgeon should use only small diameter smooth pins for fixing the fracture fragments and should avoid crossing the physis with the pins if possible [58]. These injuries heal rapidly, and fixation

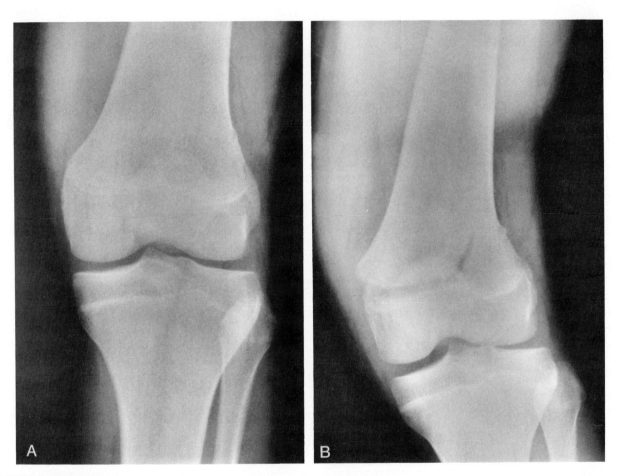

FIGURE 12–10
This 14-year-old boy sustained a valgus injury to his knee in a football game. Examination revealed marked valgus laxity. The initial radiograph (*A*) shows only subtle evidence of a growth plate injury. A stress radiograph (*B*) clearly demonstrates a Salter-Harris type II injury of the distal femur.

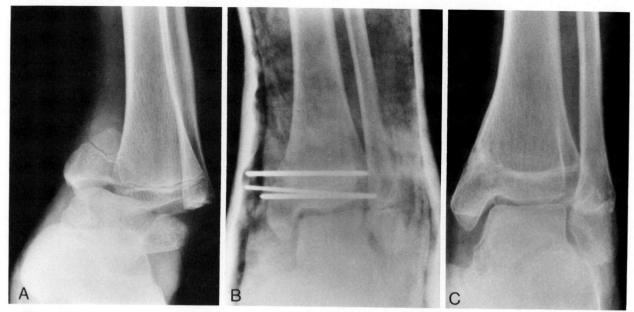

FIGURE 12–11
This 14-year-old boy injured his left ankle during a baseball game. The initial radiograph reveals a Salter-Harris type IV injury to the distal tibial physis (*A*). An anatomic closed reduction could not be obtained and the patient was treated with open reduction (*B*). The reduction is internally fixed with smooth pins that do not cross the physis. Despite anatomic reduction, 6 months later there is evidence of a physeal bar, but minimal growth deformity is present (*C*).

does not need to be rigid, but only secure enough to prevent loss of reduction.

Type V and VI injuries are usually impossible to detect on initial presentation. The physician must maintain a high index of suspicion for significant physeal trauma from a compression injury or direct blow. If the physician is concerned about an occult physeal injury, he should immobilize the patient and keep him or her nonweight-bearing on the affected extremity. Serial radiographs can be taken to detect the occurrence of any physeal bars.

As a rule of thumb, physeal injuries can be expected to heal in half the time of a purely bony injury at the same location [8]. This applies to type I injuries and, if the metaphyseal fragment is small, to type II separations. Thus, if a metaphyseal fracture of the distal radius requires 6 weeks of immobilization, a Salter-Harris type II injury of the distal radial physis will require only 3 weeks of immobilization. Type III and IV injuries will require the same period of immobilization for healing as that needed for nonphyseal injuries in the same location.

The decision about when a patient can return to sports is a difficult one. No good guidelines exist, but the patient should have full use of the injured joint and normal strength for several weeks before returning to contact sports. The physician must use discretion and decide each case on an individual basis, using clinical and radiographic information as well as the social factors involved in the child's need to return to athletics.

GROWTH ARREST

Bony bars have been seen following all Salter-Harris types of physeal injuries [41]. As previously stated, the Salter-Harris classification is not a good predictor of subsequent growth arrest; however, the majority of bony bridges that require treatment occur following Salter-Harris IV injuries [41]. Growth disturbance is also much more common following open fractures involving the physis. Various authors have reported an incidence of growth disturbance following physeal injuries ranging from 1% [36] to 30% [25]. This discrepancy results from the authors' criteria for growth disturbances. If one uses strict radiographic measurements of limb shortening or angulation, a high incidence of growth arrest is found. Fortunately, the majority of these cases do not require treatment for two reasons. First, the incidence of physeal injury is much higher in adolescents near the end of their skeletal growth period. There is not enough longitudinal growth left in this age group for clinically significant deformities to occur. Second, physeal injuries are much more common in the upper extremity, where small angular deformities or limb length discrepancies are not functional liabilities.

Complete growth arrest is unusual following trauma to the growth plate. This usually occurs only in type V compression injuries or in cases of ischemic damage to the physis. Ischemic damage can result from frostbite, from amputation, or from trauma to the vulnerable epiphyseal vessels in the proximal radial or proximal femoral physes. Complete growth arrest is readily detected on plain radiographs. Clinically, these children present with a limb length discrepancy. The long-term functional deficit is dependent on the patient's age and the specific physis involved. Older patients near skeletal maturity have only minor shortening; younger children have a much more noticeable limb length discrepancy. The amount of growth contributed by a particular physis to a bone also plays a role. Complete arrest of the proximal humerus or distal femur results in marked shortening. Likewise, complete physeal arrest in a two-bone unit such as the forearm or calf may cause joint deformities if untreated. There is some evidence that growth is accelerated at the other end of a bone with a complete growth arrest [41]. It is difficult to quantitate the growth potential of this remaining physis, but this phenomenon must be considered before treatment is undertaken.

Patients with partial physeal arrest present clinically with angular deformities or limb shortening (Fig. 12–12). Again, the age of the patient and the location of the physis play a major role in predicting the long-term effects of the growth arrest. Bright [8] classified partial growth arrest into three types (Fig. 12–13). Type I is a peripheral bony bar. These injuries can cause rapid angular deformity of the involved physis. Type II partial growth arrest is a central bony bridge with a perichondral ring that is completely intact. Growth of the peripheral plate continues, and a tenting phenomenon occurs with the apex pointing toward the metaphysis. Type III

lesions are combination injuries that are usually associated with Salter-Harris type III or IV fractures. A linear bone bridge occurs along the fracture plane involving portions of the periphery as well as the central areas. In his series of patients requiring surgery for partial growth arrest, Bright reported that 60% of injuries were type I, 21% were type II, and 19% were type III.

The majority of bony bars requiring treatment occur after physeal injuries about the knee [8, 41]. These physes account for most of the growth occurring in their respective bones. Angular deformity about the knee causes marked cosmetic deformity and functional disability. Therefore, although physeal injuries about the knee account for only 3% of physeal injuries, they comprise more than 50% of patients requiring operative correction for partial growth arrest.

An attempt should be made in all patients with bony bars to assess the complete extent of involvement. Tomograms using thin cuts (1 mm) taken every 3 mm in both the anterior-posterior and lateral planes should be obtained [41]. Careful evaluation of the tomograms allows the surgeon to construct a map of the physeal bar on graph paper, from which he can then estimate the percentage of physeal involvement. CT scanning has not been useful because the irregularity of the physis can cause undulations of the physis to be misinterpreted as bony bars. More sophisticated computer-assisted imaging may improve the value of CT or MRI, but currently tomograms remain the standard means of assessing the extent of the bony bridge. Scanograms should also be

FIGURE 12–12
This 10-year-old girl sustained a Salter-Harris type IV injury to her left distal tibial physis (*A*). Despite an anatomic reduction, 1 year later she had developed a peripheral physeal bar and an angular deformity of her left ankle (*B*).

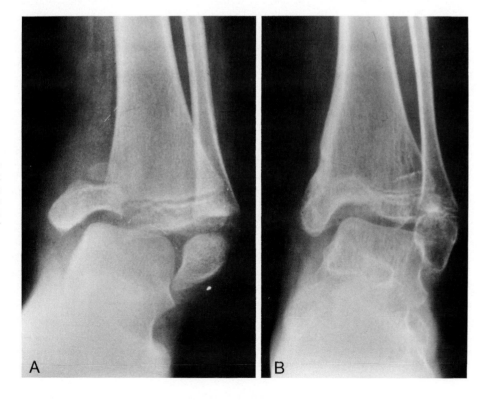

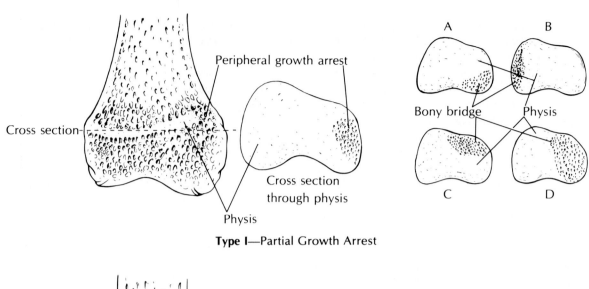

Type I—Partial Growth Arrest

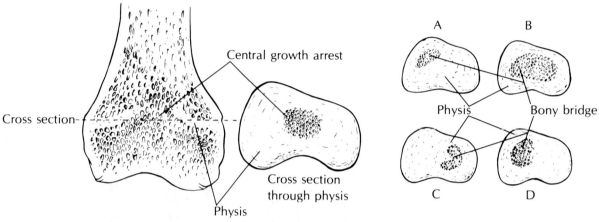

Type II—Partial Growth Arrest

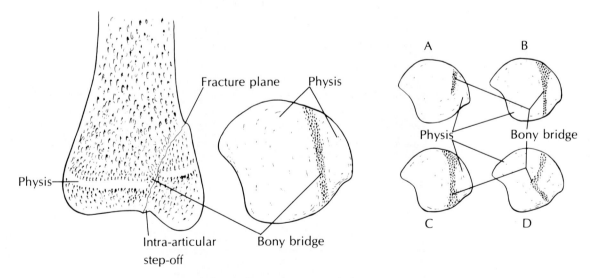

Type III—Partial Growth Arrest

FIGURE 12–13
Bright's classification of partial growth arrest. Type I results from a peripheral bony bar and causes rapid angular deformity. Type II is a central growth arrest that results in limb shortening. Type III partial growth arrests are linear bony bridges that occur after Salter-Harris type III or IV fractures. (From Rockwood, C. A., and Green, D. P. [Eds.]. *Children's Fractures*, 3rd ed. Philadelphia, J. B. Lippincott, 1991.)

obtained to assess the shortening of the involved bone and to obtain a baseline measurement. Bone age determination is required to evaluate the remaining growth potential. Accurate determination of the extent of the physeal bar and assessment of future growth of the physis is mandatory before treatment is pursued for partial physeal arrest.

Treatment of Growth Arrest

The orthopedic surgeon evaluating a child with growth arrest has a variety of treatment options at his disposal. First, it must be remembered that many physeal arrests cause no significant disability. Central physeal bars in adolescents with little growth remaining often do not require treatment. Anticipated arm length discrepancies of 9 cm or less are best left untreated [41]. Leg length discrepancies under 2 cm cause only a mild functional scoliosis and can be readily treated with a shoe lift [41].

Early angular deformities in adolescents should be treated by arresting the remaining physis if the projected limb length discrepancy is minor. In two-bone units such as the forearm, arrest of the physis of the adjacent bone is also required. Contralateral epiphysiodesis can be performed to prevent any worsening of the limb length discrepancy. The above techniques can be combined with angular osteotomies to correct any existing angular deformity. Osteotomy without epiphysiodesis will lead to recurrent angular deformity and the need for future correction.

Surgeons prefer to avoid using physeal arrest to prevent limb length discrepancy or angular deformity in the younger child. The overall loss of height and the malproportion of the extremities that results from the previous options make these choices unattractive in preadolescents. In this situation the surgeon can attempt a bone lengthening procedure. Osteotomy can correct angular deformities; however, if the physeal bar remains in a younger child, the deformity will recur. More recently, epiphyseal distraction has been utilized to correct angu-

lar deformities, and the correction has been maintained in 77% of patients [3]. The physeal bar should not occupy more than 20% to 30% of the growth plate area, and this procedure is more successful in children who are near the end of skeletal growth.

During the past 20 years, much progress has been made in surgical resection of physeal bars. Bony bridges should involve less than 50% of the physeal area to be suitable for resection [27, 41]. Type I bars can be approached directly from the periphery; central bars require a transmetaphyseal approach (Fig. 12–14). If no interposition material is placed in the defect following bar excision, the bony bridge will reform rapidly. A variety of interposition materials have been used; these include autogenous fat [26], methyl methacrylate [41], and Silastic material [9]. The reader is referred to the original articles for the details of these procedures. No clear guidelines exist regarding the need for removal of foreign interposition material. Fat has the disadvantage of weakening the bone if a large bar is excised. Silastic is strong but has the disadvantage of being a substance controlled by the Food and Drug Administration (FDA). Methyl methacrylate is strong and provides excellent hemostasis. Cranioplastic does not contain barium and aids in the detection of postoperative bar reformation. During bar excision, metal markers can be placed within the bone to aid in measuring subsequent growth. Repeat bar formation can be successfully treated by reexcision.

After successful bar excision, growth of the bone varies from 0 to 200% of the normal side, with an average of 94% [41]. Some physes, although they resume active growth, appear to undergo physiologic closure at an earlier age than their contralateral physes. Even when complete growth is not achieved, this technique can prevent further deformity or allow the use of other modalities such as contralateral epiphysiodesis.

Experimental work is being done in the area of microvascular growth plate transfer [7]. Successful revascularization in animals requires restoration of both the epiphyseal and metaphyseal circulation; subsequent growth of the physis continues at a rate 85% of normal. Much work remains to be done before this technique is widely used in humans.

FIGURE 12–14
Technique for excision of central physeal bony bar. *A,* The bar is approached from a transmetaphyseal exposure; a dental mirror is used for visualization. *B,* After resection of the bar, only enough cranioplast is inserted in the defect to bridge the physeal gap. *C,* The remainder of the metaphyseal defect is bone grafted. (From Lovell, D. D., and Winter, D. *Pediatric Orthopaedics.* Philadelphia, J. B. Lippincott, 1986.)

A   B   C

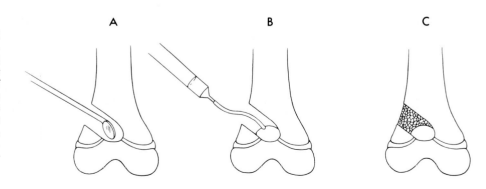

STRESS INJURIES OF THE GROWTH PLATE

In addition to acute physeal injuries in children, the physician caring for young athletes must be aware of chronic stress injuries that can cause physeal damage. As athletes embark on rigorous training programs at younger ages, the number of these injuries is bound to increase. Repetitive stress, and particularly a sudden increase in training, can lead to physeal failure with no history of direct trauma. Stress fractures have been reported in runners through the distal femoral and the proximal tibial physes [12, 19, 65] (Fig. 12–15). These injuries can be misinterpreted as neoplastic or infectious processes. Careful attention to the history, the presence of localized tenderness over the involved physis, and close scrutiny of the radiographs will lead to the correct diagnosis. Treatment is avoidance of running activities for 6 weeks followed by a gradually increasing training program. Most young athletes have been able to return to full sports activity 3 months after treatment is initiated.

In the upper extremity, unilateral bony overgrowth of the entire arm and associated muscle hypertrophy have been seen in high-caliber tennis players [46]. Dotter [16] was the first to describe physeal injuries to the proximal humerus in baseball pitchers, coining the term Little League shoulder. Other authors have reported similar cases involving pitchers and tennis players [21, 22].

These patients have shoulder pain during throwing activities. Radiographs reveal widening of the proximal humeral physeal plate and adjacent osteoporosis. These injuries are thought to represent a Salter I injury due to repetitive rotational stress. The marked irregularity of the proximal humeral physis prevents severe slippage. Treatment is rest from throwing activities, which leads to prompt resolution of the symptoms. It has been recommended that tennis players wait until the next season before resuming their sport; baseball pitchers are advised that until physeal closure has occurred they should play a position other than pitcher.

Perhaps the most common physeal stress injury occurs in the distal radius growth plate in gymnasts. Roy and colleagues [51] reported on 21 young elite gymnasts with wrist pain. Radiographs showed widening of the growth plate with occasional haziness of the physis, cystic changes on the metaphyseal side of the growth plate, and a beaked effect of the distal aspect of the epiphysis on the radial and volar sides pointing toward the physeal plate (Fig. 12–16). They felt that these findings represented stress changes and possibly stress fractures of the distal radial physis. Carter and Aldridge [13] reported similar findings in 21 gymnasts and also noted that the skeletal age of their patients was retarded, increasing the length of time the physis was at risk. Yong-Hing and colleagues [66] found changes on both the distal radial and ulnar growth plates in a gymnast and attributed these changes to a dowel grip worn by the patient during training. Others have noted premature growth arrest of

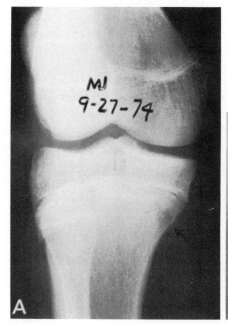
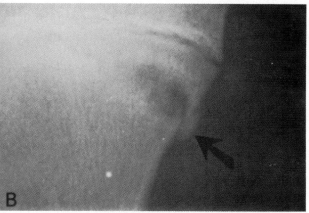

FIGURE 12–15
This 15-year-old long distance runner had gradual onset of right knee pain. He was running 40 to 50 miles/week. Radiographs of the proximal tibia show a small triangular metaphyseal fragment on the medial tibia typical of a Salter-Harris type II fracture (arrow). This represents a stress fracture of the proximal tibial physis. (From Cahill, B. R. Stress fracture of the proximal tibial epiphysis: A case report. *Am J Sports Med* 5:186, 1977.)

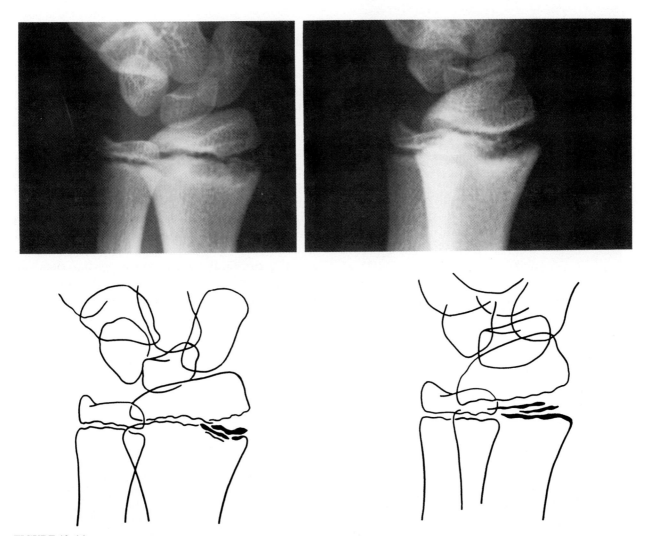

FIGURE 12–16
Radiographs of a young gymnast's wrist illustrating stress injury to the distal radial growth plate. Note the widening of the radial margin of the distal radial physis, and the cystic changes and irregularity of the metaphyseal margin. (From Roy, S., et al. Stress changes of the distal radial epiphysis in young gymnasts. *Am J Sports Med* 13:304, 1985.)

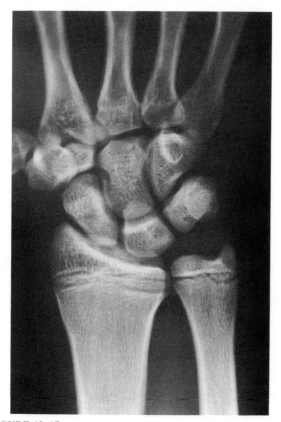

FIGURE 12-17
This 18-year-old UCLA gymnast has been competing for over 10 years. This radiograph of his right wrist demonstrates 5 mm of positive ulnar variance and evidence of premature closure of the distal radial physis. These changes may represent cumulative injury to the distal radial growth plate from overtraining.

lead the physician to recommend avoidance of the offending activity for up to 3 months. Alternative exercises can be prescribed to maintain aerobic conditioning and flexibility and to satisfy the patient's desire for physical activity. If the patient remains asymptomatic, he or she can then begin a graduated training program with the goal of returning to the desired sport. The physician must maintain careful follow-up to guard against any recurrence of physeal injury.

SUMMARY

The physician caring for young athletes frequently encounters physeal injuries. He must comprehend the complex anatomy of the physeal plate and the mechanisms of failure. Although not useful for prognosis, the Salter-Harris classification allows communication between health care providers and has implications for treatment. The majority of physeal fractures can be treated using closed methods; however, open reduction should be used in displaced type III and IV injuries. Fortunately, most physeal injuries heal with no growth arrest or only minor growth disturbances. A variety of options exist for treating premature physeal arrest when it does occur. Finally, the physician needs to be aware of chronic stress injuries that can occur in young athletes who undertake excessive training regimens.

the distal radius in gymnasts [2], and an acquired Madelung-like deformity has been reported (Fig. 12–17). An average 3-mm positive ulnar variance was found in UCLA male gymnasts, possibly representing premature arrest of the distal radial physis [33]. The positive ulnar variance that results can lead to ulnar impingement and may be the cause of the wrist pain reported by many gymnast even after skeletal growth is completed.

Although physical activity is felt to be required for normal bone formation and growth, detrimental effects to the physis undoubtedly occur from repetitive excessive stress [20]. A fine line exists between the beneficial effects of a training regimen and overuse that can cause permanent growth arrest. The exact tolerance of a particular physis in an individual patient is impossible to predict. Education of athletes and coaches can reverse the trend to "play with pain" and will lead to early referral of children with suspected physeal injuries. Young athletes involved in strenuous training programs who develop pain at the end of a long bone should undergo radiologic evaluation of the adjacent physes. Any evidence of physeal widening or other abnormality should

References

1. Aitken, A. P. Fractures of the epiphyses. *Clin Orthop* 41:19–23, 1965.
2. Albanese, S. A., Palmer, A. K., et al. Wrist pain and distal growth plate closure of the radius in gymnasts. *J Pediatr Orthop* 9:23–28, 1989.
3. Aldegheri, R., Trivella, G., and Lavini, F. Epiphyseal distraction, chondrodiatasis and hemichondrodiatasis. *Clin Orthop* 241:117–136, 1989.
4. Arkin, A. M., and Katz, J. F. The effects of pressure on epiphyseal growth. The mechanism of plasticity of growing bone. *J Bone Joint Surg* 38A:1056–1076, 1956.
5. Bertin, K. C., and Goble, E. M. Ligament injuries associated with physeal fractures about the knee. *Clin Orthop* 177:188–195, 1983.
6. Birch, J. G., Herring, J. A., and Wenger, D. R. Surgical anatomy of selected physes. *J Pediatr Orthop* 4:224–231, 1984.
7. Bowen, C. V. A., Ethridge, C. P., et al. Experimental microvascular growth plate transfers. *J Bone Joint Surg* 70B:305–310, 1988.
8. Bright, R. Physeal injuries. *In* Rockwood, C. A., Wilkins, K. E., and King, R. E. (Eds.), *Fractures in Children*. Philadelphia, J. B. Lippincott, 1984.
9. Bright, R. W. Operative correction of partial epiphyseal plate closure by osseous-bridge resection and silicone-rubber implant. An experimental study in dogs. *J Bone Joint Surg* 56A:655–664, 1974.
10. Bright, R. W., Burstein, A. H., and Elmore, S. M. Epiphyseal-plate cartilage. A biomechanical and histological analysis of failure modes. *J Bone Joint Surg* 56A:688–703, 1974.
11. Brighton, C. T. Structure and function of the growth plate. *Clin Orthop* 136:22–32, 1978.

12. Cahill, B. R. Stress fracture of the proximal tibial epiphysis: A case Report. *Am J Sports Med* 5:186–187, 1977.

13. Carter, S. R., and Aldridge, M. J. Stress injury of the distal radial growth plate. *J Bone Joint Surg* 70B:834–846, 1988.

14. Chadwick, C. J., and Bentley, G. The classification and prognosis of epiphyseal injuries. *Injury* 18:157–168, 1987.

15. Chung, S. M. K., Batterman, S. C., and Brighton, C. T. Shear strength of the human femoral capital epiphyseal plate. *J Bone Joint Surg* 58A:94–103, 1976.

16. Dotter, W. E. Little League shoulder. A fracture of the proximal epiphyseal cartilage of the humerus due to baseball pitching. *Guthrie Clin Bull* 23:68–72, 1953.

17. Ertl, J. P., Barrack, R. L., et al. Triplane fracture of the distal tibial epiphysis. Long-term follow-up. *J Bone Joint Surg* 70A:967–976, 1988.

18. Foucher, J. T. E. Separations of the epiphyses. *Clin Orthop* 188:3–9, 1984.

19. Godshall, R. W., Hansen, C. A., and Rising, D. C. Stress fractures through the distal femoral epiphysis in athletes. A previously unreported entity. *Am J Sports Med* 9:114–116, 1981.

20. Greco, F., de Palma, M. D., et al. Growth-plate cartilage metabolic response to mechanical stress. *J Pediatr Orthop* 9:520–524, 1989.

21. Gregg, J. R., and Torg, E. Upper extremity injuries in adolescent tennis players. *Clin Sports Med* 7:371–385, 1988.

22. Hansen, N. M. Epiphyseal changes in the proximal humerus of an adolescent baseball pitcher. *Am J Sports Med* 10:380–384, 1982.

23. Hastings, H., II, and Simmons, B. P. Hand fractures in children. A statistical analysis. *Clin Orthop* 188:120–130, 1984.

24. Hynes, D., and O'Brien, T. Growth disturbance lines after injury of the distal tibial physis. Their significance in prognosis. *J Bone Joint Surg* 70B:231–233, 1988.

25. Johnston, R. M., and Jones, W. W. Fractures through human growth plates. *Orthop Trans* 4:295, 1980.

26. Langenskiold, A. An operation for partial closure of an epiphyseal plate in children and its experimental basis. *J Bone Joint Surg* 57B:325–330, 1975.

27. Langenskiold, A., and Osterman, K. Surgical treatment of partial closure of the epiphysial plate. *Reconstr Surg Traumat* 17:48–64, 1979.

28. Larson, R. L., and McMahan, R. O. The epiphyses and the childhood athlete. *JAMA*, 196:99–104, 1966.

29. Lawson, J. P., Ogden, J. A., et al. Physeal injuries of the cervical spine. *J Pediatr Orthop* 7:428–435, 1987.

30. Light, T. R., and Ogden, J. A. Metacarpal epiphyseal fractures. *J Hand Surg* 12A:460–464, 1987.

31. Lombardo, S. J., and Harvey, J. P. Fractures of the distal femoral epiphyses. Factors influencing prognosis: A Review of thirty-four cases. *J Bone Joint Surg* 59A:742–751, 1977.

32. Makela, E. A., Vainionpaa, S., et al. The effect of trauma to the lower epiphyseal plate. An experimental study in rabbits. *J Bone Joint Surg* 70B:187–191, 1988.

33. Mandelbaum, B. R., Bartolozzi, A. R., et al. Wrist pain syndrome in the gymnast. Pathogenetic, diagnostic, and therapeutic considerations. *Am J Sports Med* 17:305–317, 1989.

34. Markolf, K., Shapiro, M., et al. Wrist loading patterns during pommel horse exercises. Unpublished data.

35. Merloz, P., de Cheveigne, C., et al. Bilateral Salter-Harris type II upper tibial epiphyseal fractures. *J Pediatr Orthop* 7:466–467, 1987.

36. Mizuta, T., et al. Statistical analysis of the incidence of physeal injuries. *J Pediatr Orthop* 7:518–523, 1987.

37. Morscher, E. Strength and morphology of growth cartilage under hormonal influence of puberty. *Reconstr Surg Traumat* 10:1–95, 1968.

38. Neer, C. S., II, and Horwitz, B. S. Fractures of the proximal humeral epiphysial plate. *Clin Orthop* 41:24–35, 1965.

39. Ogden, J. A. Skeletal growth mechanism injury patterns. *J Pediatr Orthop* 2:371–377, 1982.

40. Peltonen, J., Aalto, K., et al. Experimental epiphyseal separation by torsional force. *J Pediatr Orthop* 4:546–549, 1984.

41. Peterson, H. A. Partial growth plate arrest and its treatment. *J Pediatr Orthop* 4:246–258, 1984.

42. Peterson, H., and Burkhart, S. Compression injury of the epiphyseal growth plate: Fact or fiction? *J Pediatr Orthop* 1:377–384, 1981.

43. Peterson, C. A., and Peterson, H. A. Analysis of the incidence of injuries to the epiphyseal growth plate. *J Trauma* 12:275–281, 1972.

44. Poland, J. Traumatic separation of the epiphyses in general. *Clin Orthop* 41:7–18, 1965.

45. Pollen, A. G. Fractures involving the epiphyseal plate. *Reconstr Surg Traumat* 17:25–39, 1979.

46. Priest, J. D., Jones, H. H., et al. Arm and elbow changes in expert tennis players. *Minn Med* 60:399–404, 1977.

47. Rang, M. *Children's Fractures.* Philadelphia, J. B. Lippincott, 1974, pp. 10–25.

48. Rang, M. *The Growth Plate and Its Disorders.* Edinburgh, Churchill Livingstone, 1969.

49. Rogers, L. F., Jones, S., et al. "Clipping injury" fracture of the epiphysis in the adolescent football player: An occult lesion of the knee. *Am J Radiol* 121:69–78, 1974.

50. Rogers, L. F. The radiography of epiphyseal injuries. *Radiology* 96:289–299, 1970.

51. Roy, S., Caine, D., and Singer, K. M. Stress changes of the distal radial epiphysis in young gymnasts. A report of twenty-one cases and a review of the literature. *Am J Sports Med* 13:301–308, 1985.

52. Salter, R. B. Epiphyseal plate injures in the adolescent knee. *In* Kennedy, J. C. (Ed.), *The Injured Adolescent Knee.* Baltimore, Williams & Wilkins, 1979.

53. Salter, R. B., and Harris, W. R. Injuries involving the epiphyseal plate. *J Bone Joint Surg* 45A:587–622, 1963.

54. Selke, A. C. Destruction of phalangeal epiphyses by frostbite. *Radiology,* 93:859–860, 1969.

55. Shapiro, F., Holtrop, M. E., and Glimcher, M. J. Organization and cellular biology of the perichondral ossification groove of Ranvier. 59A:703–723, 1977.

56. Shapiro, F. Epiphyseal disorders. *N Engl J Med* 317:1702–1710, 1987.

57. Shapiro, F. Epiphyseal growth plate fracture-separations. A pathophysiologic approach. *Orthopaedis* 5:720–736, 1982.

58. Siffert, R. S. The effect of staples and longitudinal wires on epiphyseal growth. An experimental study. *J Bone Joint Surg* 38A:1077–1088, 1956.

59. Simon, M. R. The effect of dynamic loading on the growth of epiphyseal cartilage in the rat. *Acta Anat* 102:176–183, 1978.

60. Stark, R. H., Matloub, H. S., et al. Warm ischemic damage to the epiphyseal growth plate: A rabbit model. *J Hand Surg* 12A:54–61, 1987.

61. Torg, J. S., Pavlov, H., and Morris, V. B. Salter-Harris type-III fracture of the medial femoral condyle occurring in the adolescent athlete. *J Bone Joint Surg* 63A:586–591, 1981.

62. Torre, B. A. Epiphyseal injuries in the small joints of the hand. *Hand Clinics* 4:113–121, 1988.

63. Trueta, J., and Morgan, J. D. The vascular contribution of osteogenesis. I. Studies with the injection method. *J Bone Joint Surg* 42B:97–109, 1960.

64. Vender, M. I., and Watson, H. K. Acquired Madelung-like deformity in a gymnast. *J Hand Surg* 13A:19–21, 1988.

65. Weber, P. C. Salter-Harris type II stress fracture in a young athlete. *Orthopedics* 11:309–311, 1988.

66. Yong-Hing, K., Wedge, J. H., and Bowen, C. V. A. Chronic injury to the distal ulnar and radial growth plates in an adolescent gymnast. *J Bone Joint Surg* 70A:1087–1089, 1988.

67. Zionts, L. E., Harcke, H. T., et al. Posttraumatic tibia valga: A case demonstrating asymmetric activity at the proximal growth plate on technetium bone scan. *J Pediatr Orthop* 7:458–462, 1987.

THORACOLUMBAR SPINE INJURIES IN PEDIATRIC SPORTS

Robert A. Yancey, M.D.
Lyle J. Micheli, M.D.

Injuries to the thoracolumbar spine and complaints of back pain comprise a relatively small percentage of sports-related musculoskeletal problems in the child athlete, although the incidence is thought to be increasing [58]. Children rarely complain of back pain unless it is persistent and limits their activities. In contrast, asymptomatic structural anomalies of the thoracolumbar spine are relatively common in the athletic adolescent and young adult population. Most reported series suggest that less than 10% of sports-related complaints involve the spine [76]. Specific sports such as gymnastics [12, 21, 23, 26, 41, 56], dancing [37, 56], football [18, 55, 74], rowing [29, 33], and racquet sports [32, 76] that require repetitive or high-velocity twisting or bending of the thoracolumbar spine have a significantly higher incidence of complaints originating in the spine. This fact is especially relevant to the increasing number of young athletes who pursue rigorous training and intense competition in some of these sports at an early age.

Most injuries to the thoracolumbar spine are associated with symptomatic treatment and relatively short periods of disability and rehabilitation. Serious post-traumatic neurologic damage with permanent sequelae are rare [35, 46]. Nevertheless, persistent complaints related to the thoracolumbar spine in the active adolescent athlete should never be taken lightly, and the differential diagnosis can be quite complex. In our experience, underdiagnosis and delay of diagnosis are common, and all too many "back strains" ultimately turn out to be associated with spondylolysis or apophysitis in this age group.

Injuries to the thoracolumbar spine can generally be traced to two types of patterns of force generation: acute traumatic events involving either contact or noncontact sports, and fatigue injuries secondary to chronic overuse and repetitive microtrauma. Acute and chronic musculotendinous or ligamentous injuries are probably the most common cause of thoracolumbar complaints at all ages, and children may also be subject to these injuries [76]. During the rapid growth spurt in the adolescent period the soft tissues in children fail to keep up with the more rapid growth of the bony elements, resulting in significant decreases in relative flexibility. This is one of the primary intrinsic factors that predispose children to musculotendinous injury. The second intrinsic factor is the increased susceptibility to injury of the vertebral end plates and apophyses in the growing child. Extrinsic factors include the organization of youth sports themselves, in which children of similar ages but varying abilities and sizes may all be grouped in a similar division, increasing the chances of impact overload. Improper training including incorrect technique or a poor understanding of the limitations of the balance between flexibility and strength provide the potential for overuse spinal injuries in this young population.

Although trauma, acute or repetitive, is the major cause of back pain in our young athletic population, the more serious problems related to metabolic, neoplastic, and infectious causes must be entertained in any child with persistent back pain. Any child with this complaint, despite the fact that the pain began in association with sports participation, must have a thorough evaluation by a qualified physician [29, 58].

Hensinger [29] investigated the etiology of low back pain of 2 months duration in skeletally immature patients at the University of Michigan. He noted in his retrospective study that about one-third had a post-traumatic etiology such as an occult fracture or spondylolytic problem, another third had a developmental problem, a category in which he included scoliosis and kyphosis, 18% had pain related to a tumor or infection, and 15% were indeterminate.

Other dilemmas that face the clinician treating a child with pain in the thoracolumbar spine include the need to decide how to optimize the balance between restriction of activity, controlled rehabilitation, and eventual return to competition. The basis of these decisions relies on a careful integrated analysis and understanding of the natural history and mechanism of the disease process, the physical requirements and potential for injury of the particular type of sport, and the specific needs of the young patient or athlete. A useful set of guidelines was recently published by the American Academy of Pediatrics and includes a classification of sports by degree of contact and intensity of exertion [1].

The recovery period for many spine injuries may be relatively prolonged compared to many other sports-related injuries of the axial skeleton. The expectation of the parents, coaches, and the young athletes themselves for a rapid resolution of symptoms and pain-free performance must be integrated into a treatment program that comprise predictably less than optimal compliance. Patient education about the etiology of the pain, the mechanism of injury, and the importance of preventive measures must be coordinated with changes in training regimens and technique.

SCREENING AND DIFFERENTIAL DIAGNOSIS

The primary role of the physician in the preseason evaluation of young athletes involves three primary responsibilities: prevention of injuries, diagnosis and treatment of injuries, and rehabilitation and monitoring of injuries [60, 70]. It is an excellent opportunity to perform a good overall health assessment and carefully reexamine sites of previous injury. The basis for a complete general examination is discussed elsewhere in this text and the literature, and the present discussion is confined to the thoracolumbar spine evaluation.

Whether evaluating an acute problem or performing a routine screening, an accurate and complete medical history is probably the single most important step in the assessment of the spine in the young athlete. A family history is important because there is a genetic predisposition for both scoliosis and spondylolisthesis [29, 84]. The athlete's age, sex, pattern of thoracolumbar complaints, specific location and radiation of pain, and the chronology of the symptoms are all essential facts that must be obtained. Spondylolytic, cartilaginous end-plate

abnormalities, and infectious causes are the most common causes in the 10- to 15-year-old age group, whereas discogenic and mechanical back problems are more common in the older age group. Attention should be directed toward the particular activity or sport that exacerbates the pain. For instance, spondylolytic back pain is seen much more frequently in dancers [37, 56], rowers [29, 33], football [18, 55, 74] and hockey players [34], and female gymnasts [12, 21, 23, 26, 41, 56]. The repetitive overuse demands of flexion and extension of the lumbar spine seen in walkovers in gymnastics, butterfly strokes in swimming, hyperextension maneuvers in diving, and hitting a blocking sled in football all give clues to the cause of the pain. Night pain that is relieved with aspirin use suggests the benign neoplasms of osteoid osteoma and osteoblastoma [27, 47, 54]. Morning stiffness associated with low back pain or sacroiliac pain may be the presenting complaints of juvenile ankylosing spondylitis [29, 72]. More systemic complaints accompanying persistent low back pain in the athlete are more disconcerting. Increasing pain not relieved by rest, fever, malaise, and weight loss are all suggestive of chronic infection [80]. Neurologic complaints of paresthesias, hypesthesias, and bowel or bladder complaints accompanied by neurologic signs demand immediate attention.

The screening physical examination should be thorough and should concentrate on those possibilities that are suggested in the history [60]. The patient should be asked initially to ambulate in the hallway or examination room. Gait should be assessed to evaluate any dynamic asymmetries. As the patient stands, any asymmetry of the pelvis and shoulders should be noted, and one should examine the sagittal and frontal contours of the spine checking for increased lumbar lordosis or thoracic kyphosis. Standing blocks should be used to equilibrate any leg length discrepancy that might accentuate a lumbar scoliosis. Localized areas of tenderness are then elicited by palpating and percussing along the spinous processes, paraspinal muscles, and the lumbosacral junction. The patient is then asked to bend forward and is observed from the front, sides, and back. This allows the scapula to rotate off the rib cage and provides a better assessment of differences in the surface contour of the torso. While the patient is bending forward a gross assessment of the tightness of the lumbodorsal fascia and hamstrings can be made. The patient is then asked to return to an upright posture against slight resistance while the physician examines any splinting or decreases in spinal motion and stresses the posterior structures. The hyperextension test is done next; the patient is asked to hyperextend the back at the lumbosacral junction and then repeat this maneuver while standing on each leg individually to increase the stress on the ipsilateral pars interarticularis. Finally, the patient is asked to lie supine on the examining table. Hip range of motion is recorded.

Thomas tests are performed to assess tightness of the hip flexors, and straight leg raising and Lesague tests are done to determine the relative tightness of the hamstrings and any radicular signs. A Patrick test is then carried out by abducting and externally rotating the hip and compressing the sacroiliac joint in the figure-four position to rule out pathology in the sacroiliac joint. A thorough neurologic examination is then performed to evaluate sensation, muscle strength, and reflexes in the lower extremities.

A thorough preparticipation evaluation of the thoracolumbar spine can be useful not only for evaluating present complaints but also for identifying risk factors that might predispose an athlete to other injuries.

ANATOMY AND PATHOMECHANICS

Multiple anatomic and biomechanical factors distinguish the thoracolumbar spine in children from that in adults. The potential for continued growth and increased elasticity of the soft tissues protects the preadolescent child from the injury patterns seen in the adult [30]. The major anatomic differences in the spine include an initial increased cartilage-to-bone ratio, which reverses over time, and the presence of secondary centers of ossification at the vertebral end plates, which normally fuse with the vertebral bodies by maturity. By the age of 8 to 10 years, the bony thoracolumbar spine has biomechanical properties very similar to those of adults; however, the ring apophysis at the vertebral end plates remains open. Unlike adults who have preexisting degenerative changes in the fibrocartilaginous disc, intervertebral discs in children are generally well hydrated, firm, fibrous, and tightly attached to the cartilaginous plate. The apophyseal ring is thinner in the middle than in the periphery. Increased axial compression of the intervertebral disc combined with forward flexion forces the disc through the end plates into the cancellous bone of the vertebral body—a mechanism not seen in the adult spine except with pathologic structural weakening of the vertebral body secondary to metabolic or neoplastic disease [42]. Whereas in adults preexisting degenerative changes predispose the intervertebral disc to herniation, in the immature skeleton rapid flexion combined with axial compression can fracture the vertebral end plate before the annulus fails and the disc herniates [42, 52, 78].

Repetitive hyperextension, flexion, and torsional forces on the thoracolumbar spine are associated with stress or fatigue injuries [14, 36, 38, 65, 81, 83]. Shear stresses are selectively concentrated across the pars interarticularis of the lumbar spine. They are concentrated across the pars interarticularis, an area calculated to be only 0.75 cm² at the fifth lumbar vertebra [51]. Tensile and shear forces across the pars interarticularis in normal flexion and extension are calculated to be in the range of 400 to 630 Newtons [36]. This mechanism of overuse and stress-induced posterior element failure has been implicated in many sports, including ballet [56], football [18, 55, 74], hockey [34], weight lifting [8, 52, 78], and rowing [29, 33]. Anterior shear across this region has been related to the amount of postural lordosis, accentuated by particular activities [14]. This mechanism correlates with an increased incidence of posterior element injuries in football interior linemen secondary to repeated forced hyperextension and with an increased incidence of spondylytic defects in young female gymnasts.

The pathomechanics of these posterior element injuries of the lumbar spine have been hypothesized; however, it is difficult to pinpoint why one athlete is predisposed to problems whereas another remains without injury. The independent variables that contribute individually or in combination include poor technique, poor conditioning, and abnormal anatomy [34]. Poor technique is reflected in insufficient warm-up periods and inadequate technical supervision. In dance and gymnastics, for instance, poor technique might be reflected in rapid advancement to difficult techniques without concomitant increases in strength and flexibility [56, 57]. Specific selective conditioning is very important in a standard training program, especially with regard to abdominal strengthening. Weak abdominal muscles contribute to the abnormal hyperlordotic posturing of the lumbar spine. The genetic predisposition to development of spondylytic defects has been well documented [19, 68, 84]; however, no definite evidence has proved that there is an increased incidence of pars defects in otherwise healthy individuals due to intrinsic abnormalities of the bone. The susceptibility to injury of growing musculoskeletal tissue is well documented and appears to be a major anatomic factor contributing to the injury patterns of the lumbar spine in the young athlete.

SPONDYLOLYSIS AND SPONDYLOLISTHESIS

Mechanical injury to the pars interarticularis is a common source of discomfort in young athletes involved in competitive sports and is probably the anatomic lesion diagnosed most frequently in the evaluation of young people with back pain. Spondylolysis refers to the condition in which a bony defect exists in the pars interarticularis on one or both sides at a given vertebral level. Spondylolisthesis occurs as translation of a vertebral body on an adjacent vertebral body develops in the coronal plane. In one review 50% of patients with spondylolysis related the onset of their symptoms to competitive sports training [65]. Spondylolytic defects have never been reported in newborn infants and are rarely seen before the age of 5 years. They are seen only in the bipedal human, and studies have shown that spondylolytic defects are not seen in patients who have never assumed a standing posture [68, 71]. The largest series of patients studied reveals that the incidence of spondylolysis in the general population is about 4.4%, increasing to 6% at adulthood [2, 13]. Many patients are asymptomatic unless they place undue stress across the posterior elements of the lumbar spine. The mean age of diagnosis of this problem in the athletic population is between 15 and 16 years of age. Eighty-five percent of the isthmic lesions seen in athletes occur in the pars interarticularis of the L5 vertebral level. LaFond [49] noted that 23% of the patients in his series experienced the onset of symptoms before the age of 20 years; however, only 9% had complaints severe enough to seek medical attention during childhood or adolescence [49]. In Hoshina's series of 177 male high school and college athletes approximately 21% showed radiographic evidence of spondylolysis [32].

Wiltse and colleagues [81, 83] postulated that pars fractures or isthmic spondylolysis represents an acquired ''stress'' or fatigue fracture of the pars interarticularis as a result of repeated microtrauma. This hypothesis is supported by a recent paper by O'Neill and Micheli [64], who noted that 92% of spondylytic defects healed after stabilization of the lumbar segment with an in-situ fusion of the lamina and transverse processes. Biomechanical studies have noted that shear stresses on the pars interarticularis are greater when the spine is extended and accentuated when lateral flexion maneuvers are performed from a hyperlordotic posture [14, 79]. It has been documented in vivo that repetitive sustained stresses can induce fatigue fractures in the lumbar spine [37, 65]. Repetitive traumatic demands on the lumbar spine in contact sports, such as blocking and sled training in football, and specific repetitive lumbar motions such as hurdling, ballet dancing, volleyball spiking, competitive diving, back flips or reverse walkovers in gymnastics, tennis serving, and swimming turns all have been associated with complaints related to pars pathology. In young female gymnasts this defect occurs four times more frequently than in the general female population [41]. Familial studies have suggested a genetic predisposition to these lesions [19, 29, 68, 84].

The history of the onset of pain is very important. The onset of symptoms coincides closely with the adolescent growth spurt. In athletes the initial symptoms are usually complaints of insidious aching back pain that is exacerbated by strenuous activity. Occasionally, there is an associated radiating pain to one or both buttocks. The pain is usually unilateral and is exacerbated by lumbosacral motions of twisting and hyperextension. Initially, the pain is elicited by high activity levels or competitive sports; however, the pain becomes progressively more severe and is associated with activities of daily living. Symptoms are typically relieved by rest. Posterolateral thigh pain radiating to the knee has also been described. The initial symptoms are usually related to the instability of the involved vertebral segment. L5 radicular symptoms secondary to root compression may arise from foraminal encroachment, fibrocartilaginous callus at the healing pars site, or associated disc herniation [4]. L5 root compression may also develop secondary to forward displacement of L5 on S1 as further spondylolisthesis occurs, although this is rare in the athletic population of children and adolescents with isthmic spondylolytic defects.

Physical examination may demonstrate some tenderness to palpation in the lumbar spine, usually well localized to the paraspinous region. The athlete with spondylolysis may have a normal stance. The child sometimes stands with a hyperlordotic posture, splinting and guarding the affected side from excessive motion. Relative hamstring tightness is found in 80% of patients and is associated with limited forward flexion of the hips [67]. ''Relative'' tightness should be emphasized because many gymnasts and dancers may be hyperflexible compared to the range of normal in nonathletes. Occasionally a coach or trainer will be the first to notice the athlete's loss of flexibility. Although forward bending is often painless, rising to an upright posture against resistance may elicit pain. Pain can often be reproduced by asking the patient to actively hyperextend the lumbar spine while standing in a one-legged stance. Hyperextension while standing on the ipsilateral leg produces the pain, whereas the same maneuver with the contralateral leg may be less painful or may result in pain also ipsilaterally. Neurologic examination of the lower extremities is usually unremarkable. Positive Lasègue's and straight leg raising signs may be rarely elicited.

The initial diagnostic work-up includes radiographs of the lumbosacral spine. Anteroposterior, lateral, and both oblique views must be obtained to assess the integrity of the posterior elements adequately. Unilateral defects can be seen in 20% of patients [4]. Acutely, the defect is usually a narrow gap with irregular edges, but over time the edges become rounded and smooth. Oblique views may miss the presence of the defect in 15% of cases. Reactive sclerosis of the opposite pars or lamina can be seen in unilateral lesions and is sometimes confused with osteoid osteomas [29]. Osteoid osteoma can generally be differentiated by the clinical history and the presence of a nidus [27, 29, 47, 54]. Spina bifida occulta is seen in 20% to 50% of patients with pars defects, which is 13 times the incidence noted in the general population [81]. The pars defect or elongation of the pars becomes more apparent with progression of instability, though in our experience symptomatic spondylolysis or grade 1 spondylolisthesis rarely progresses in this patient group. This progression is best followed by taking standing spot lateral radiographs centered on L5 and S1 measuring progression sequentially by measuring the degree of slip.

We believe that spondylolytic lesions in athletes are a reactive response to stress and fatigue fractures secondary to repetitive microtrauma. As with many stress fractures, radiologic changes may not become apparent for weeks to months after the occurrence of an acute pars injury. Radioactive bone scans are very useful in these acute cases and may permit prompt treatment and subsequent healing of these lesions, decreasing the recovery period [13, 66]. It should also be emphasized that an abnormal bone scan in the presence of normal radiographs may indicate early infection or neoplasm as well as a stress reaction of the pars, and these possibilities should be investigated if the clinical picture is suggestive. Negative plain films and bone scans do not rule out spondylolysis as a cause of back pain. Cases have been reported of children with low back pain, normal bone scans, and plain radiographs that were only suggestive of a pars defect who went on to develop further symptoms and obvious pars lesions. Tomography and CT scanning can also be used to assess the integrity of the pars, especially when plain radiographs and bone scans suggest an indeterminate diagnosis. CT scanning is used to evaluate the surrounding soft tissues and the disc for pathology. A useful adjunct at this institution has been single-photon emission computed tomography (SPECT) to help localize painful spondylolytic defects [13].

The management of a symptomatic pars defect in the child athlete is somewhat controversial and must take into account the athlete's age, type of sports activity, and risk of progression and continued symptoms [4, 29, 31, 63, 82]. Some physicians suggest that patients with spondylolysis can be managed symptomatically with limitation or modification of activity combined with an exercise program to strengthen the abdominal musculature while stretching the hamstrings. This philosophy assumes that spondylolysis is a "congenital" lesion that has no potential for healing. In our opinion, this lesion should be managed as a stress fracture and treated by restriction of activities and immobilization. We use a rigid polypropylene lumbosacral brace constructed with 0 degrees of lumbar flexion (antilordosis) to provide some degree of lumbar spinal stability. This is thought to increase the chances of healing by opposing the fractured pars elements, and it keeps the patient comfortable. Once the brace has been satisfactorily fitted, it is worn for 23 of 24 hours a day for 6 months. The 1 hour of freedom from the brace is set aside for bathing and exercises, which include abdominal strengthening, pelvic tilts, and antilordotic and lower extremity flexibility exercises. Brace treatment is reduced in patients whose bone scans, if initially positive, become normal. Braced

patients are allowed to resume limited activities in a modified fashion, usually several weeks after brace wear has been initiated, when most have become asymptomatic. Early termination of brace wear is considered in patients whose bone scans were initially cold on presentation and who have become asymptomatic after resuming activities in the brace for a period of 3 to 4 weeks. If a brace is weaned too early or if the patient is noncompliant with brace wear, symptoms may recur. Patients may need up to 6 months to wean themselves gradually from full-time brace wear. With this type of treatment the results are promising. Thirty-two percent of patients achieved bony healing in our series, and 88% of 75 patients were able to resume previously painful sports activities after the program even if the pars defect had not healed [63]. Bone scans may be helpful in following the status of the lesion [13, 66]. A positive bone scan at the fracture site usually indicates that the defect is healing or has the potential to heal; however, a cold bone scan should not be taken as a contraindication to brace treatment. Bony healing has been noted in patients with initially cold bone scans. Assessment of hamstring tightness has also been suggested as an indicator of the success or failure of a treatment program.

Some patients remain asymptomatic despite the apparent nonunion of the lesion. In these patients most authors agree that there is no need to restrict activities, and full return to vigorous activity including contact sports is allowed. Spondylolysis and grade I spondylolisthesis in this population are rarely if ever mechanically unstable lesions.

Patients who fail to improve with the bracing program or cannot be weaned from the brace without recurrence of symptoms may require surgery. If surgical intervention is indicated for persistent pain, a fusion of the posterolateral transverse process or direct repair of the pars defect can be attempted [4, 6]. The rigid stability provided by a posterolateral spinal fusion accounts for the consistent healing of the pars lesion seen in these patients [65]. Others have described internal fixation with compression wires or direct osteosynthesis of the pars defect [10, 11]. The lumbosacral junction is traditionally immobilized in a cast or brace for up to 6 months following bone grafting, and heavy activities including sports are usually disallowed for 12 months or until the fusion mass matures [61]. Buck describes a return to sports 3 months after direct osteosynthesis and fusion if there is evidence of radiographic union and the patient is asymptomatic [10].

Progression of spondylolisthesis occurs during the adolescent growth spurt, the age of highest risk being 10 to 15 years. The dysplastic type of spondylolysis characterized by dysraphic or malformed posterior elements has a higher incidence of slippage than the isthmic type of defect that is most commonly seen in athletes.

Overall, the incidence of high-grade spondylolisthesis (>75% slip) is twice as high in females as in males [85]. Nonathletic females have the highest propensity for severe spondylolisthesis. These patients develop a classic wide-based gait with a short stride length as increasing lumbosacral kyphosis and postural tilting of the pelvis occur. In severe cases a palpable step-off at the lumbosacral junction may be noted on deep palpation of the spinous processes. These severe grades of spondylolisthesis usually preclude participation in competitive athletics because of associated pain and lack of flexibility.

The treatment of asymptomatic young athletes with spondylolisthesis of less than 50% slip remains controversial. Most authors suggest that patients with 30% slip spondylolisthesis that is asymptomatic should be observed, followed for progression, and allowed to participate in all sports including contact sports. Patients with minimal symptoms of back pain are treated with a conservative program of modification and restriction of activities, physical therapy to institute antilordotic and abdominal strengthening exercises, and possible brace management with a rigid polypropylene lumbosacral brace if initial treatment is not successful. Bracing is generally continued for 3 to 6 months, and patients are allowed to resume their activities in the brace if they are without symptoms [4, 63]. Patients who have 30% to 50% slip spondylolisthesis again fall into a controversial category. Bradford [4] suggests that these patients need surgical management even if they are asymptomatic, whereas at the other extreme, some physicians suggest that conservative management and restriction from contact sports are adequate [76]. If surgical management of the problem is to be undertaken, one should document the progression of the lesion if the patient is within the age of high risk and be certain that the spondylolisthesis is the source of the pain. The athlete must weigh the importance of continuing his or her specific sport against the risk of major spinal surgery with its concomitant possible complications and the possibility of a 1-year rehabilitation program postoperatively.

As vertebral slippage approaches 50% athletic activity predictably becomes more difficult owing to the sacral tilt and tight hip flexors and hamstrings. These patients rarely participate in competitive sports and have an associated waddling gait pattern and an exaggerated lumbar lordosis. It is generally accepted that patients with greater than 50% spondylolisthesis or rapid progression during the high-risk years should have a prophylactic in-situ posterior fusion whether or not symptoms are evident [4, 5, 6]. When solid in-situ fusion is obtained, the patient is generally pain-free; however, a significant lumbosacral kyphosis persists in many patients. Preoperative reduction maneuvers followed by posterior or combined anterior-posterior fusions for severe slips have been discussed extensively by Bradford [5]. He stresses

that these procedures should not be taken lightly and are associated with about a 20% risk of neurologic complications.

DISCOGENIC PROBLEMS

Although much less common in adolescents than in adults, disc herniation can occur in the young adolescent athlete. The true incidence is unknown; however, most reports state that between 0.8% and 3.8% of all disc herniations occur in the pediatric population [17, 22]. This is a very rare cause of pain in the prepubescent child; however, the incidence in athletically active children appears to be increasing, possibly reflecting an increased awareness by health care providers. The natural history of disc disease in this population is not well understood, although some studies have suggested that these patients continue to have back complaints as adults [16]. The diagnosis can be difficult to determine clinically because the presentation can be quite different from the classic radicular symptoms seen in the adult. In the adolescent with an injured disc, low back pain or pain confined to the buttock or hip is predominantly the most frequent complaint. These symptoms are typically exacerbated by increased activity and Valsalva maneuvers like sneezing and coughing. The supine position is usually the best position for relieving the pain. The athlete, coach, or trainer may notice a slight decrease or asymmetry in hamstring flexibility, asymmetrical paravertebral spasm, or the subtle onset of "sciatic" scoliosis. In another presentation pattern, pain is a less prominent feature, and the patient presents with an asymmetrical gait or running pattern.

Only 36% of disc herniations in this age group are associated with an acute episode of trauma, but DeOrio and Bianco [16] suggest that a protruded disc in this age group is more likely to be the result of cumulative trauma than a single event. In contrast to adults with preexisting degenerative changes in the disc, disc tissue in adolescents is usually noted to be firm, well hydrated, fibrous, and firmly attached to the cartilaginous end plate [45, 48, 52, 69]. It is thought that this anatomic difference might predispose the adolescent athlete to vertebral end plate fractures with hingelike displacements of fibrocartilage in the canal rather than the classic extruded or sequestered herniated disc seen in adults. Disc herniations are associated with multiple sporting activities, especially those with repetitive flexion and axial loading on the lumbar spine. Gymnastics, running, football, weight lifting, basketball, soccer, and tennis have all been implicated in the acute exacerbation of discogenic symptoms in the pediatric population [3, 16].

The physical examination is often confirmatory in these patients, although neurologic findings of decreased reflexes, muscle weakness, or atrophy are rare. Examination commonly reveals a positive straight leg raising or Lasègue's sign. Limited motion of the lumbar spine and lumbar scoliosis due to paravertebral and hamstring spasm have been described consistently. Cauda equina due to herniated nucleus pulposus in young patients has been reported [48].

Once the diagnosis of neural entrapment or impingement has been made, appropriate diagnostic studies are performed. Lumbosacral spine films are taken to evaluate the possibility of an underlying osseous injury, especially when the symptoms appear to be initiated by a traumatic incident. Plain radiographs rarely show a narrowed disc space, however, and avulsion fracture of the vertebral end plate is sometimes seen in young patients presenting with radicular symptoms. Noncontrast CT scan and MRI are two noninvasive diagnostic tools that have supplanted the use of myelography in many centers to confirm the presence of a neurocompressive lesion in the canal. As in the adult population, the L4–L5 and L5–S1 levels are the most common sites of the lesion [17, 48]. In cases with severe pain and sciatic symptoms associated with systemic complaints, a complete blood count, sedimentation rate, and bone scan should be performed to rule out an occult disc space infection [80].

Conservative therapy remains the mainstay of treatment. Initial treatment is aimed at resting the back in a neutral position to avoid further sciatic irritation and muscle spasm. This ''relative rest'' period is supplemented with nonsteroidal anti-inflammatory agents. The initial response generally occurs within the first few weeks, and the patient perceives a definite improvement in symptoms. However, this response may not last if the patient returns to sports too quickly. Parents should be advised that vigorous sports activity should be deferred for 6 to 12 months after a documented episode of discogenic back pain and sciatica in a child.

Brace treatment has been a useful adjunct to the management of adolescent athletes with discogenic pain that does not initially respond to conservative measures. A flexible polyethylene brace with 15 degrees of lumbar lordosis is tolerated well, and the patient usually can return to daily activities and a light training program more rapidly. Sitting exacerbates the pain in many of these young patients, and bracing sometimes decreases the number of missed school days. The overall success rate of brace treatment is not as high as that reported for spondylolytic disorders, and only 50% of young athletes return to full sports activity without pain within the first year [62]. In many cases, conservative management is complicated by the unwillingness of these competitive athletes to accept total rest and immobilization for an adequate amount of time.

Jackson has described a program of controlled rest followed by gradual mobilization, pelvic traction, and an exercise program consisting of lumbar flexion exercises and abdominal strengthening [38]. Epidural steroids, chymopapain chemonucleolysis, and percutaneous discectomy are all treatment modalities that have been described in adults, but there are only isolated reports regarding their use in the pediatric population [9, 15, 25, 39, 64].

If symptoms cannot be controlled with conservative management, or if there is an impending cauda equina syndrome with bowel or bladder dysfunction or severe motor loss, operative treatment is indicated. In general, surgical intervention in this age group has had a variable success, ranging from 73% to 98% good to excellent results [3, 16]. The report of DeOria and Bianco stressed that long-term follow-up was essential in these patients because the natural history postlaminectomy is not well understood and half of the patients who required reoperation (24% of the original group) required the procedure) more than 3½ years after the initial discectomy [16]. Some late follow-up examinations revealed herniations at other levels. It should be stressed that if surgery is indicated, every attempt should be made to preserve the facet joints and the interspinous ligaments to prevent segmental instability.

Most orthopedists and neurosurgeons allow patients to participate in sports when they have achieved full return of pain-free mobility and strength [61]. There are no clear guidelines. It is unknown whether a discectomy promotes further degenerative changes at the involved level or whether participating in vigorous contact sports accelerates this degeneration. If this theoretical risk is described to the patient and the parents and is accepted, an unrestricted return to full sports participation may be permitted. In a study of treatment of lumbar disc disease in college football players, Day and associates [15] noted that none of the four players who underwent laminotomy was able to return to football. Whether or not surgery is chosen for treatment of chronic discogenic pain, once nerve root irritation has occurred, the patient may never return to his or her previous performance level even after extensive rehabilitation. Activity modification to avoid the exacerbation of symptoms may be necessary within the sport, or the patient may be forced to change to another sports activity completely.

A condition that is almost indistinguishable from a herniated lumbar disc is a slipped vertebral apophysis or end plate fracture [52, 78]. This condition is usually associated with heavy lifting, and typically the posterior inferior apophysis of L4 is displaced into the vertebral canal along with the apophyseal attachment of its associated disc. Patients present with signs and symptoms of a herniated disc including neurologic findings. Radiographs reveal a small bony fragment pulled off the inferior edge of the vertebral end plate, and CT or MRI images reveal an extradural mass. Treatment consists of excision of both the cartilaginous disc and the bony fragment and provides excellent relief of the symptoms. Postoperative management and rehabilitation are similar to the techniques used after disc excision.

SCOLIOSIS

The incidence of idiopathic scoliotic curves of less than 10 degrees in patients before the age of 16 years old is approximately 2% to 3% [53]. Idiopathic scoliosis does not cause pain and generally does not cause a functional problem that would interfere with sports activities. Congenital scoliosis is often associated with cardiac and renal anomalies, which should be evaluated as part of the preparticipation examination. Patients with congenital vertebral anomalies in the cervical spine at the cervicothoracic junction should be counseled against collision and contact sports. There is a strong familial tendency to the disease, and about 80% of patients with idiopathic scoliosis have a positive family history [29].

Three major medical concerns arise when evaluating the presence of spinal curvature in the young athlete. Initially, sports screening can be used in the early detection process to help isolate patients with congenital curves that might suggest other associated medical problems or idiopathic curves that are likely to progress. Management of moderate curves with bracing and exercise during adolescence is the second task of the physician. Finally, clear guidelines must be defined for limitations of exercise in patients who are braced or have had spinal fusion for curve progression. Unfortunately, historically it has been the concensus of the medical community that all children with scoliosis should refrain from sports activities. In fact, appropriate sports participation offers significant benefits to children with scoliosis including improved strength, flexibility, cardiovascular fitness, self-esteem and body image.

In the skeletally immature child, scoliotic curves are usually detected first by parents or coaches who note an asymmetry in the child's shoulders, a curvature of the spine, or an asymmetry in the thorax resulting in a rib hump. Forward bending accentuates the deformity by allowing the scapula to move off the rib cage. After a thorough history and screening physical examination has been carried out to rule out more serious problems, initial full-length spine radiographs are taken. The curve is then measured by the Cobb method. In the skeletally immature child with an idiopathic curve observation is carried out every 4 to 6 months until the curve reaches 25 to 30 degrees or is noted to progress rapidly. At that point, a bracing program is initiated using a rigid polypropylene corrective Boston brace to control the progression of the curve until the child reaches skeletal maturity. Braces are initially worn 23 hours/day, and the child is allowed to participate in sports with the brace on. One report suggests that bracing for 16 to 18 hours/day gives the same results, and children are allowed to participate in sports while out of the brace [44]. There is no evidence that sports participation increases the risk of progression of curves in these children. As the patient becomes more skeletally mature, brace wear is decreased, and these young athletes are allowed to participate in sports activities without restriction, thus allowing them to maintain strength and flexibility while they are out of the brace 8 hours a day. After growth is complete and bracing has been discontinued, no restrictions are placed on the athlete with idiopathic scoliosis.

Patients with curves of greater than 50 degrees have a high incidence of progression after skeletal maturity, although minimal cardiopulmonary deficit has been noted secondary to scoliosis of this magnitude [85]. Curves of greater than 100 degrees are extremely rare in athletes and have been documented to lead to significant cardiopulmonary compromise [77]. The treatment of choice for these patients is metallic instrumentation to correct the deformity and spinal fusion. This fusion generally involves significant portions of the thoracic and lumbar spine, and because of the loss of spinal mobility and the extensive instrumentation that accompanies the fusion it has been the practice of most spinal surgeons to prohibit contact sports, gymnastics, and diving following fusion for scoliosis. Postoperatively, patients are advised that they may not participate in physical education classes or organized light sports for 1 year after surgery while the fusion mass matures [61]. In this institution most patients who undergo fusion for idiopathic scoliosis are not braced postoperatively and are encouraged to swim when they are comfortable.

In specific lower lumbar deformities that require only the fusion of three segments of spine with anterior instrumentation such as Dwyer or Zeilke, we believe that enough residual flexibility is left above and below the fusion to allow continued participation in light contact sports such as soccer and field hockey, although football and rugby are prohibited. A decreased number of fused segments appears to carry less acute risk of stress concentration above and below the fusion mass, although the chance of chronic long-term acceleration of localized disc degeneration is unknown. Patients who choose to participate in vigorous athletics after a short segment fusion should understand these risks [61].

There have been limited reports of postfusion patients participating in heavy contact sports or gymnastics without problems; however, the potential risks of pseudoarthrosis, hardware failure, and degenerative changes above and below the fusion mass far outweigh the advantages of contact sports for these patients.

A rapidly progressive or painful scoliosis in the child athlete is cause for alarm. Unilateral paraspinal spasm and list associated with disc herniation may cause "sciatic" scoliosis. Other causes of painful scoliosis include osteoid osteoma and osteoblastoma, herniated intervertebral disc, spondylolisthesis, infection, and intraspinal tumors such as astrocytoma. Hairy patches, nevi, and dermal sinuses are associated with congenital anomalies such as diastematomyelia that may present initially with a painful scoliosis in the child athlete. It must be stressed that a very careful patient examination must be completed, and further radiographic and laboratory work-up is essential in the young athlete with painful scoliosis.

SCHEUERMANN'S DISEASE

Some children with tight lumbodorsal fascia and hamstrings subsequently compensate for this tightness by developing a roundback deformity. This happens because of the body's attempt to rebalance the torso over the pelvis. In most cases the deformity is only postural and transient, but some times these patients develop anterior wedging of the vertebral bodies [58]. When three or more consecutive vertebrae are wedged more than 5 degrees, the radiographic criteria for Scheuermann's disease are met [73, 75].

Scheuermann's disease, or juvenile kyphosis, is a common cause of thoracic kyphosis in the adolescent, although it is rarely seen in the athletic population [7, 58, 73]. The radiographic diagnosis can be made at both the thoracic and lumbar levels [28]. In thoracic Scheuermann's disease, the patient usually presents with a main complaint of deformity rather than pain. The presentation is spontaneous without a significant traumatic history, and there is a familial predisposition. The radiographic picture includes irregular vertebral end plates, Schmorl's node formation, narrow disc spaces, and anterior wedging of the vertebral bodies. The etiology is unknown, although the disease is thought by some to fall within the spectrum of repetitive microtrauma and fatigue failure of the thoracic vertebral bodies.

On clinical examination patients with thoracic juvenile kyphosis invariably have a roundback deformity with increased lumbar lordosis in a standing position. Most are unable to reverse this thoracic kyphosis with forced hyperextension. Hip flexors and hamstrings are usually tight.

Initially, treatment of thoracic Scheuermann's disease consists of flexibility exercises to address the tight lumbodorsal fascia and hamstrings. Abdominal strengthening exercises are added to this regimen. Progressive thoracic kyphosis to more than 50 degrees in a skeletally immature child is an indication for brace treatment with a Milwaukee brace or a modified Boston brace with thoracic uprights. Because of the thoracic uprights on

these braces very few sports activities can be pursued while wearing a brace. Patients may be allowed out of the brace for sports activities and usually wear the brace for 16 to 18 hours/day. Further progression of thoracic kyphosis beyond 70 degrees is an indication for anterior-posterior or posterior spinal fusion with instrumentation. Following surgery for thoracic Scheuermann's disease, patients are generally restricted from sports activities except swimming for approximately 1 year while the fusion mass matures [61]. They are then advised to avoid contact sports and gymnastics but are allowed to participate in light noncontact activities.

APOPHYSEAL INJURIES

In contrast to thoracic Scheuermann's disease, the similar radiographic picture seen in the midthoracic to midlumbar spine is less common in the general population but is more frequently seen in athletes. It has frequently been called "atypical" or lumbar Scheuermann's disease because it does not meet the usual radiographic criteria outlined by Sorenson [75]. This phenomenon is usually seen at the thoracolumbar junction but can occur throughout the lumbar spine. Some believe that it is the pediatric equivalent of an adult thoracolumbar compression fracture. These changes in the thoracolumbar spine are frequently accompanied by pain and are thought to be the direct result of microtrauma with resultant multiple growth plate fractures or possible anterior disc herniation through the anterior ring apophysis and secondary bony deformation of the vertebra [69]. It is much more commonly seen in adolescent athletes involved in vigorous training programs involving repetitive flexion-extension activity of the spine such as rowing, gymnastics, and diving. It is almost exclusively noted in patients with relative thoracic hypokyphosis and lumbar hyperlordosis (flat backs). Young athletes may present with transient nondescript pain; radiographs suggest chronic vertebral end plate wedging, irregularities of the end plates, and changes in the disc space. There is typically a period of 2 to 6 months in which the patient complains of moderately severe pain that is accentuated by forward flexion and relieved by rest. On clinical examination generally no appreciable kyphosis is noted at the involved levels. Tight lumbodorsal fasciae and hamstrings are commonly found. Radicular complaints are rare, and the neurologic examination is unremarkable. There is a 2:1 male-to-female predominance, and the peak age incidence is between 15 and 17 years old.

The mechanism of lumbar Scheuermann's disease is thought to be peripheral (usually anterior) disc rupture through the cancellous bone beneath the apophyseal ring. Intradiscal pressure is doubled during heavy lifting, especially when the subject is seated or bending forward and flexing or extending the lumbar spine [42]. Repeated stress fractures secondary to microtrauma weaken the bone of the vertebral body and set up a situation analogous to the formation of Schmorl's nodes in neoplastic and metabolic diseases. The displaced apophyseal fragment at the anterior margin of the vertebral body seldom heals. When vertebral wedging is noted or pain is persistent, a bracing program may be indicated for symptomatic treatment. We suggest the use of a semirigid thermoplastic brace with 15 degrees of lumbar lordosis to immobilize the patient and unload the anterior spine [62]. The brace is worn for 18 to 23 hours/day until sufficient vertebral body remodeling is visible on plain radiographs, which usually requires a 9- to 12-month period. Flexibility exercises and abdominal strengthening exercises are instituted during brace wear, and the athlete may return to sports while wearing the brace when he becomes asymptomatic.

Other injuries involving the vertebral end plates and the apophyseal growth areas of the spine are becoming more frequently diagnosed. Children present with localized nonradicular spinal pain. Repetitive microtrauma involving flexion and extension of the spine is the usual cause. Traction forces on the apophyses of the spinous processes cause injuries very similar to those seen along the iliac crest in the immature pelvis. These stable traction injuries occur most frequently in the low thoracic and thoracolumbar junction, are locally tender, and can be treated symptomatically with rest, nonsteroidal anti-inflammatory drugs, and limitation of activities. Rehabilitation in the form of flexibility exercises combined with abdominal strengthening exercises can be initiated when the pain has subsided, and the patient may return to sports.

FRACTURES

Fractures, dislocations, and fracture-dislocations of the spine in the pediatric population are uncommon, but when associated with neurologic damage they represent the most severe end of the spectrum of spinal injuries in young athletes. Most published series of spinal injuries with neurologic deficits in children report that the cervical spine is the most frequently injured part of the spine; there are very few reports of catastrophic injuries to the thoracic or lumbar spine related to sports [35, 46]. Most of these noncatastrophic fractures of the thoracolumbar spine are displaced fractures of the transverse and spinous processes and occasional compression fractures of the vertebral bodies. These injuries are generally treated symptomatically with limitation of activities until the

pain resolves. Initially, bracing may be necessary to achieve immobilization for 4 to 6 weeks, and the athlete then may undergo conditioning activities in the brace if he or she is comfortable.

The incidence of severe lower spinal injuries with associated acute spinal syndromes is rare in nonvehicular sports. High-risk situations include those in which athletes attain high speeds or are placed at heights. Bicycling, rollerskating, or skateboarding in traffic, skiing, and rock climbing are all athletic endeavors with high-risk scenarios. Organized sports such as gymnastics, wrestling, diving, football, rugby, and equestrian events all have a potential for high risk that is temporized by the organized nature of these sports.

The management of acute spinal trauma in the thoracolumbar spine is beyond the scope of this chapter. Management of the rare unstable thoracolumbar fracture in this young athletic population is well described in standard texts of pediatric fracture management [85]. Although these injuries are extremely rare in the pediatric population, forethought about the possibility of these injuries is necessary, and a health care provider must be familiar with the immobilization and transport techniques needed as well as the availability of acute access to specialized care [50].

Patients who undergo posterior spinal fusion for unstable post-traumatic spine fractures are at special risk of potentially devastating injuries if they return to contact sports. Each case must be decided on an individual basis; however, if the initial event included a neurologic injury, the canal capacity at the level of the fracture may be significantly compromised. We suggest restricting participation in contact sports for these patients [61].

MECHANICAL LOW BACK PAIN

Mechanical back pain secondary to acute or chronic musculoligamentous strains and sprains is rare in the young athlete and should be a diagnosis of exclusion in children with low back pain. Such back pain is commonly thought to be due to overuse or stretch injuries of the soft tissues including the muscle-tendon unit, ligaments, joint capsules, and the facet joints themselves. It is more commonly seen in the older age group and is hypothesized to be related to a transient overgrowth syndrome during the adolescent growth spurt [59]. These young patients have a predisposition to these injuries owing to a weak abdominal musculature and tight lumbodorsal fasciae, hamstrings, and hip flexors, and occasionally thoracic hyperkyphosis [58]. The history usually reveals a picture of poor training methods and conditioning or insufficient preworkout stretching. The pain is often nondescript, is exacerbated by activity, and is relieved by rest. Some authors have suggested that the origin of this pain lies in the facets [40, 76].

Physical examination frequently reveals paraspinous muscle spasm, increased lumbar lordosis, and hamstring tightness as well as asymmetrical truncal motion. Tenderness is generally present off the midline, and occasionally a trigger point can be found with pressure over a particular facet. Tight lumbar fascia is frequently noted. Specific tests such as the hyperextension test and straight leg raising test are inconclusive. The neurologic examination is generally negative. Radiographs and bone scans are taken to rule out other structural causes of pain and are generally normal.

Acutely, the hallmark of treatment is rest. Ice massage, cold spray, and massage over the affected area can be quite helpful during the acute phase [24]. Nonsteroidal anti-inflammatory drugs and buffered aspirin can be added to the treatment regimen, although muscle relaxants are generally reserved for the older athlete. Hydrotherapy, ultrasound, and electrical stimulation can also be used in more mature patients to break up the paraspinal spasm. Facet injections with steroid and local anesthetics have been suggested by some authors [43, 76]. We do not use these. Once the patient is ambulatory and the acute pain has resolved, an early exercise program should be established. An individualized rehabilitation program emphasizing antilordotic posturing, flexibility and abdominal strengthening with pelvic tilts, and stretching of the tight lumbodorsal fascia and hamstrings should be initiated.

After the acute injury phase there may be a 4- to 6-week period of rehabilitation. During this time the patient gradually reenters competition after analysis of the mechanism of injury. If the patient's symptoms do not resolve with exercise and stretching alone the use of a 0- to 15-degree lordotic anterior opening plastic brace has proved useful in relieving symptoms although in refractory cases 3 or 4 months may be needed to wean the patient from the brace [62]. Braced patients continue to participate in a flexibility program, and when weaned from the brace an active exercise program to regain muscular tone is initiated. Changes can then be made in the training schedule or improper technique that will help to prevent recurrence of the vicious cycle of lumbosacral pain. If the pain persists for more than 2 or 3 weeks despite a diligent attempt at conservative management or if the history or clinical examination is suggestive, further diagnostic work-up is indicated. Very few highly motivated young athletes attempt to obtain secondary gain, a pattern that is so clearly evident in adult mechanical back pain.

We must emphasize that this diagnosis is one of exclusion in the young athlete in contrast to that in the adult population. A conscientious search for the cause of thoracolumbar pain in this population must be carried out if pain persists for more than 3 weeks.

References

1. American Academy of Pediatrics. Recommendation for participation in competitive sports. *Pediatrics* 81(5):737–739, 1988.
2. Baker, D. R., and McHolick, W. Spondylolysis and spondylolisthesis in children. *J Bone Joint Surg* 38A(4):933–934, 1956.
3. Borgesen, S. E., and Vang, P. S. Herniation of the lumbar intervertebral disk in children and adolescents. *Acta Orthop Scand* 45(4):540–549, 1974.
4. Bradford, D. S. Spondylolysis and spondylolisthesis in children and adolescents: Current concepts in management. *In* Bradford, D. S., and Hensinger, R. M. (Eds.), *The Pediatric Spine*. New York, Georg Thieme, 1985, pp. 403–23.
5. Bradford, D. S. Treatment of severe spondylolisthesis: A combined approach for reduction and stabilization. *Spine* 4(5):423–429, 1979.
6. Bradford, D. S., and Iza, J. Repair of the defect in spondylolysis or minimal degrees of spondylolisthesis by segmental fixation and bone grafting. *Spine* 10(7):673–679, 1985.
7. Bradford, D. S., Moe, J., Montalvo, J. F., et al. Scheuermann's kyphosis and roundback deformity. *J Bone Joint Surg* 56A(4):740–758, 1974.
8. Brady, T. A., Cahill, B. R., and Bodnar, L. M. Weight training-related injuries in the high school athlete. *Am J Sports Med* 10(1):1–5, 1982.
9. Brown, F. W. Epidurals—management of diskogenic pain using epidural and intrathecal steroids. *Clin Orthop* 129:72–78, 1977.
10. Buck, J. E. Direct repair of the defect in spondylolisthesis. *J Bone Joint Surg* 52B(3):432–443, 1970.
11. Buring, K., and Fredensborg, N. Osteosynthesis of spondylolysis. *Acta Orthop Scand* 44(1):91, 1973.
12. Ciullo, J. V., and Jackson, D. W. Pars interarticularis stress reaction, spondylolysis, and spondylolisthesis in gymnasts. *Clin Sports Med* 4(1):95–110, 1985.
13. Collier, B. D., Johnson, R. P., Carrera, G. F., et al. Painful spondylolysis or spondylolisthesis studied by radiography and single photon emission computed tomography. *Radiology* 154(1):207–211, 1985.
14. Cyron, B. M., and Hutton, W. C. The fatigue strength of the lumbar vertebrae in spondylolysis. *J Bone Joint Surg* 60B(2):234–238, 1984.
15. Day, A. L., Friedman, W. A., and Indelicato, P. A. Observations on the treatment of lumbar disk disease in college football players. *Am J Sports Med* 15(1):72–75, 1987.
16. DeOrio, J. K., and Bianco, A. J. Lumbar disc excision in children and adolescents. *J Bone Joint Surg* 64A(7):991–995, 1982.
17. Epstein, J. A., Epstein, N. E., Marc, J., et al. Lumbar intervertebral disk herniation in teenage children: Recognition and management of associated anomalies. *Spine* 9(4):427–432, 1984.
18. Ferguson, R. H., McMaster, J. F., and Stanitski, C. L. Low back pain in college football linemen. *Am J Sports Med* 2(2):63–69, 1974.
19. Frederickson, B. E., Baker, D. R., McHoluk, W. J., et al. The natural history of spondylolysis and spondylolisthesis. *J Bone Joint Surg* 66A(5):699–707, 1984.
20. Frymoyer, J. W., Pope, M. G., and Kristiansen, T. Skiing and spinal trauma. *Clin Sports Med* 1(2):309–318, 1982.
21. Garrick, J. G., and Requa, R. K. Epidemiology of women's gymnastics injuries. *Am J Sports Med* 8(4):261–264, 1980.
22. Garrido, E., Humphreys, R. P., Hendrick, E. B., et al. Lumbar disc disease in children. *Neurosurgery* 2:22–26, 1978.
23. Goldberg, M. A. Gymnastics injuries. *Orthop Clin North Am* 11:717–724, 1980.
24. Grant, R. E. Massage with ice in the treatment of painful conditions of the musculoskeletal system. *Phys Med Rehabil* 45:223–228, 1964.

25. Green, P., Burke, A., Weiss, C., et al. The role of epidural cortisone injection in the treatment of diskogenic low back pain. *Clin Orthop* 153:121–125, 1980.
26. Hall, S. J. Mechanical contribution to lumbar stress injuries in female gymnasts. *Med Sci Sports Exerc* 18(6):599–602, 1986.
27. Helms, C. A., Hattner, R. S., and Vogler, J. B. Osteoid osteoma: Radionuclide diagnosis. *Radiology* 151(3):779–784, 1984.
28. Hensinger, R. N. Back pain and vertebral changes simulating Scheuermann's disease. *Orthop Trans* 6(1):1–6, 1982.
29. Hensinger, R. N. Back pain in children. *In* Bradford, D. S., and Hensinger, R. N. (Eds.), *The Pediatric Spine.* New York, Georg Thieme, 1985, pp. 41–60.
30. Hensinger, R. N., and Fielding, J. W. Fractures of the spine. *In* Rockwood, C. A., Wilkins, K. E., and King, R. E. (Eds.), *Fractures in Children.* Philadelphia, J.B. Lippincott, 1984, pp. 683–732.
31. Hensinger, R. N., Lang, J. R., and MacEwen, G. D. Surgical management of spondylolisthesis in children and adolescents. *Spine* 1:207–216, 1976.
32. Hoshina, H. Spondylolysis in athletes. *Physician Sportsmed* 8(9):75–78, 1980.
33. Howell, D. W. Musculoskeletal profile and incidence of musculoskeletal injuries in lightweight women rowers. *Am J Sports Med* 12(4):278–281, 1984.
34. Hresko, M. T., and Micheli, L. J. Sports medicine and the lumbar spine. *In* Floman, Y. (Ed.), *Disorders of the Lumbar Spine.* Tel Aviv, Freund, 1989, pp. 879–894.
35. Hubbard, D. D. Injuries of the spine in children and adolescents. *Clin Orthop* 100:56–65, 1974.
36. Hutton, W. C., Stott, J. R. R., and Cyron, B. M. Is spondylolysis a fatigue fracture? *Spine* 2(3):202–229, 1977.
37. Ireland, M. L., and Micheli, L. J. Bilateral stress fracture in the lumbar pedicle in a ballet dancer. *J Bone Joint Surg* 69A(1):140–142, 1987.
38. Jackson, D. W. Low back pain in young athletes: Evaluation of stress reaction and discogenic problems. *Am J Sports Med* 7(6):364–366, 1979.
39. Jackson, D. W., Rettig, A., and Wiltse, L. L. Epidural cortisone injections in the young athletic adult. *Am J Sports Med* 8(4):239–243, 1980.
40. Jackson, D. W., and Wiltse, L. L. Low back pain in young athletes. *Physician Sportsmed* 2(11):53–60, 1974.
41. Jackson, D. W., Wiltse, L. L., and Cirincione, R. J. Spondylolysis in the female gymnast. *Clin Orthop* 117:68–73, 1976.
42. Jayson, M. I. V., Herbert, C. M., and Barks, J. S. Intervertebral discs: Nuclear morphology and bursting pressures. *Ann Rheum Dis* 32:308–315, 1973.
43. Jeremy, E., Fairbank, C. T., Park, W. M., et al. Apophyseal injection of local anesthetic as a diagnostic aid in primary low back syndromes. *Spine* 6(6):598–605, 1981.
44. Kahanovitz, N., Levin, D. B., and Lardon, J. The part time Milwaukee brace treatment of juvenile idiopathic scoliosis. *Clin Orthop* 167:145–151, 1982.
45. Keller, R. H. Traumatic displacement of the cartilaginous vertebral rim. A sign of intervertebral disc prolapse. *Radiology* 110:21–23, 1974.
46. Kewalramani, M. D., and Tori, J. A. Spinal cord trauma in children: Neurological patterns, radiologic features, and pathomechanics of injury. *Spine* 5(1):11–18, 1980.
47. Kirwan, E. O., Hutton, P. A. N., Pozo, J. L., et al. Osteoid osteoma and benign osteoblastoma of the spine. *J Bone Joint Surg* 66B(1):21–26, 1984.
48. Kurihara, A., and Kataoka, O. Lumbar disc herniation in children and adolescents. A review of 70 operated cases and their minimum 5 year follow-up studies. *Spine* 5(5):443–451, 1980.
49. LaFond, G. Surgical treatment of spondylolisthesis. *Clin Orthop* 22:175–179, 1962.
50. Leidholt, J. D. Spinal injuries in athletes: Be prepared. *Orthop Clin North Am* 4(3):691–707, 1973.
51. Letts, M., Smallman, T., Afanasiev, R., et al. Fracture of the pars interarticularis in adolescent athletes: A clinical-biomechanical analysis. *J Pediatr Orthop* 6(1):40–46, 1986.

52. Lippitt, A. B. Fracture of a vertebral body end plate and disk protrusion causing subarachnoid block in an adolescent. *Clin Orthop* 116:112–115, 1976.
53. Lonstein, J. E. Natural history and school screening for scoliosis. *Orthop Clin North Am* 19(2):227–237, 1988.
54. Maclellan, D. I., and Wilson, F. C. Osteoid osteoma of the spine: a review of the literature and report of six new cases. *J Bone Joint Surg* 49A(1):111–121, 1967.
55. McCarroll, J. R., Miller, J. M., and Ritter, M. A. Lumbar spondylolysis and spondylolisthesis in college football players. *Am J Sports Med* 14(5):404–406, 1986.
56. Micheli, L. J. Back injuries in dancers. *Clin Sports Med* 2(3):473–484, 1983.
57. Micheli, L. J. Back injuries in gymnastics. *Clin Sports Med* 4(1):85–93, 1985.
58. Micheli, L. J. Low back pain in the adolescent: Differential diagnosis. *Am J Sports Med* 7(6):362–364, 1979.
59. Micheli, L. J. Overuse injuries in children's sports: The growth factor. *Clin Orthop* 14(2):337–360, 1983.
60. Micheli, L. J. Preparticipation evaluation for sports competition: Musculoskeletal assessment of the young athlete. *In* Kelley, V. C. (Ed.), *Practice of Pediatrics.* Philadelphia, Harper & Row, 1984, pp. 1–9.
61. Micheli, L. J. Sports following spinal surgery in the young athlete. *Clin Orthop* 198:152–157, 1985.
62. Micheli, L. J. Hall, J. E., and Miller, M. E. Use of modified Boston back brace for back injuries in athletes. *Am J Sports Med* 8(5):351–356, 1980.
63. Micheli, L. J., and Steiner, E. M. Treatment of symptomatic spondylolysis and spondylolisthesis with the modified Boston brace. *Spine* 10:937–943, 1985.
64. Nordby, E. J. Chymopapain in intradiscal therapy. *J Bone Joint Surg* 65A:1350–1353, 1983.
65. O'Neill, D. B., and Micheli, L. J. Post-operative radiographic evidence for fatigue fracture as the etiology of spondylolysis. *Am J Sports Med* 17:196, 1989.
66. Papanicolaou, N., Wilkinson, R. H., Emans, J. B., et al. Bone scintigraphy and radiography in young athletes with low back pain. *Am J Roentgenol* 145:1039–1044, 1985.
67. Phalen, G. S., and Dickson, J. A. Spondylolisthesis and tight hamstrings. *J Bone Joint Surg* 43A(4):505–512, 1961.
68. Pizzutillo, P. D. Spondylolisthesis: Etiology and natural history. *In* Bradford, D. S., and Hensinger, R. N. (Eds.), *The Pediatric Spine.* New York, Georg Thieme, 1985, pp. 395–402.
69. Resnick, D., and Niwayama, G. Intravertebral disk herniation: cartilaginous (Schmorl's nodes). *Radiology* 126:57–65, 1978.
70. Rooks, D. S., and Micheli, L. J. Musculoskeletal assessment and training: The young athlete. *Clin Sports Med* 7:641–677, 1988.
71. Rosenberg, N. J. U., Bargar, W. L., and Friedman, B. The incidence of spondylolysis and spondylolistheses in nonambulatory patients. *Spine* 6(1):35–38, 1981.
72. Schaller, J. G. Ankylosing spondylitis of childhood onset. *Arthritis Rheum* 20:398, 1977.
73. Scheuermann, H. W. Kyphosis dorsalis juvenilis. *Ugeskr Laeger* 82:385, 1920.
74. Semon, R. L., and Spengler, D. Significance of lumbar spondylolysis in college football players. *Spine* 6(2):172–174, 1981.
75. Sorenson, H. K. *Scheuermann's Juvenile Kyphosis.* Copenhagen, Munksgaard, 1964.
76. Spencer, G. W., and Jackson, D. W. Back injuries in the athlete. *Clin Sports Med* 2(1):191–216, 1983.
77. Swank, S. M., Winter, R. B., and Moe, J. H. Scoliosis and cor pulmonale. *Spine* 7(4):343–353, 1982.
78. Techakapuch, S. Rupture of the lumbar cartilage plate into the spinal canal in an adolescent. A case report. *J Bone Joint Surg* 63A(3):481–482, 1981.
79. Troup, J. D. G. Mechanical factors in spondylolisthesis and spondylolysis. *Clin Orthop* 147:59–67, 1976.
80. Wenger, D. R., Bobechko, W. P., and Gilday, D. L. The spectrum of intervertebral disc space infection in children. *J Bone Joint Surg* 60A(1):100–108, 1978.

81. Wiltse, L. L. The etiology of spondylolisthesis. *J Bone Joint Surg* 44A(3):539–560, 1962.

82. Wiltse, L. L., and Jackson, D. W. Treatment of spondylolisthesis and spondylolysis in children. *Clin Orthop* 117:92–100, 1976.

83. Wiltse, L. L., Widell, E. H., and Jackson, D. W. Fatigue fracture: The basic lesion in isthmic spondylolisthesis. *J Bone Joint Surg* 57A(1):17–22, 1975.

84. Winney-Davies, R., and Scott, J. H. S. Inheritance and spondylolisthesis—a radiographic family survey. *J Bone Joint Surg* 61B(3):301–305, 1979.

85. Winter, R. B. Spinal problems in pediatric orthopedics. *In* Lovell, W. W., and Winter, R. B. (Eds.), *Pediatric Orthopedics.* Philadelphia, J.B. Lippincott, 1986, pp. 569–648.

SHOULDER INJURIES

Kaye E. Wilkins, M.D.

S E C T I O N A

Epidemiology

Kaye E. Wilkins, M.D.

Shoulder injuries are relatively uncommon in the overall picture of injuries to the pediatric musculoskeletal system. Although fractures to the upper extremities per se are the most common injuries seen in the pediatric age group, most are distal rather than proximal. In his study of 8682 fractures in children Landin [32] found that 22.7% involved the distal forearm, 8.1% involved the clavicle, and only 2.2% involved the proximal end of the humerus. In clavicular fractures occurring after the age of 10 most were in boys and occurred in ball or contact sports. The sporting event that produced the highest percentage of shoulder injuries was horseback riding (Fig. 14–1). Twenty-eight per cent of the injuries sustained from horseback riding involved the proximal humerus, and another 9% involved the clavicle. In Landin's overall global review of all pediatric fractures, only 21% occurred in organized sporting events. Most pediatric fractures (24%) occur in unorganized recreational or play activities.

SOCIAL FACTORS

Sporting events for children have become very popular. There have been increases not only in participation but also in the number of injuries. Landin [32] found that in the three decades from 1950 to 1980 there was a fivefold increase in the incidence of injuries to children from sporting activities.

In the pediatric age group most sports activity occurs outside the organized educational setting. This has been a popular trend in the last 20 years. It was estimated in 1980 that nearly 30 million young people aged 6 to 21 were involved in nonscholastic athletic programs [12]. On the other hand, in organized interscholastic sports in 1981 [36], only 5.35 million young people were active participants. In the same study the most popular sport reported for boys was football. For girls, basketball was the leader.

Sports injuries necessitate visits to emergency rooms. In 1981 [37], among organized sports, football was the leading cause of such injuries, with 453.9 visits per 100,000 participants in the 5- to 14-year age group. The greatest number of emergency room visits (906.7/100,000) were related to bicycling [14].

Age is a factor in the overall incidence of athletic injuries in the pediatric age group. In 1956 the American Medical Association published a statement warning against the participation of skeletally immature individuals in organized athletic events [13]. The AMA stated categorically that such participation was unsafe because of the large number of physeal or growth injuries that could occur. Subsequent follow-up studies showed that this fear of so-called "crippling injuries" was unfounded [33]. In fact, injuries to the physes accounted for less than 5% of all sports injuries. Other studies [16, 25, 32] showed that far more injuries occur in unorgan-

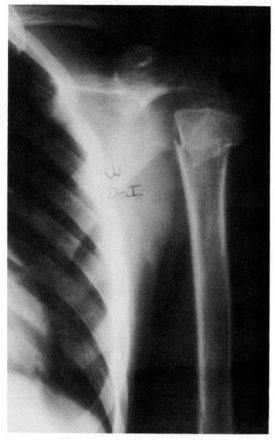

FIGURE 14–1
Proximal humeral metaphyseal greenstick fracture in an 11-year-old girl who fell off a horse.

ized play than in organized activities. These and other studies [54] showed that in organized athletic events the injury rate is age-related. In grade school athletes the injury rate is very low. It increases steadily with age so that the maximum rates are seen in the high school age group [35].

In summary, the overall risk of injury to the pediatric athlete is related to the nature of the sporting event, the age of the participant, and the method by which the players are grouped. There appears to be a greater risk of injury in the skeletally immature individual and in participants in the nonorganized recreational or play activities than in players who are under some type of adult supervision.

PHYSICAL FACTORS

Effects of Growth

The presence of the physeal plates about the shoulder provides matrices of lesser strength than those provided by the adjacent capsules and ligaments or even in some

cases by the periosteum. The physes have an age-related variability in strength. Apparently the physis and its perichondrial ring weaken just prior to maturity [11]. This fact is borne out clinically in the classic study by Peterson and Peterson [39], who found that physeal injuries occurred between 11 and 12 years in girls and between 13 and 14 years in boys.

Weakness of metaphyseal bone results in minimally displaced greenstick-type fractures (see Fig. 14–1). The proximal humerus is one of the most common locations for unicameral bone cysts. Because of the weakened cortex, fractures can occur in this location with simple throwing activities (Fig. 14–2).

SPECIFIC SPORTING EVENTS

Macrotrauma

In 1978 Garrick and Requa [22] surveyed the overall incidence of injuries in a 2-year period in high school sports. They mainly looked at macrotrauma injuries. Predictably, football and wrestling produced the greatest number of injuries overall (Fig. 14–3), whereas swimming and tennis had the lowest injury rates.

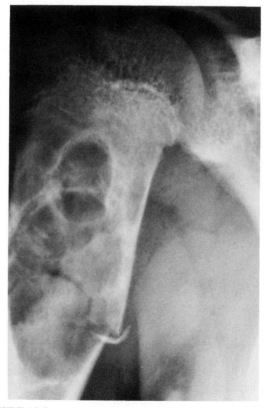

FIGURE 14–2
Fracture through a large unicameral bone cyst. This developmental defect greatly weakens the bone, making it susceptible to pathologic fractures.

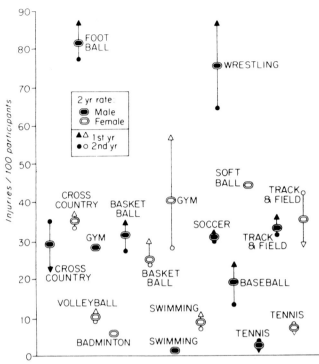

FIGURE 14–3
Injury rates for macrotrauma in the various athletic events in high school sports. (From Garrick, J. G., and Requa, R. K. Injuries in high school sports. Reproduced by permission of *Pediatrics,* Vol. 61, page 465, Copyright 1978.)

Football. Most injuries to the shoulder in football result in macrotrauma (i.e., fracture of the clavicle or glenohumeral dislocation). The overall injury rate increases with age. In the Little League age group the rate of football injuries overall was only 7.8% versus 17% in high school players [24]. When specific body areas are examined the percentage of football injuries involving the shoulder is fairly consistent, ranging from 8% to 12% [7, 17, 24, 38]. The shoulder ranks second after the knee in overall injuries sustained in football. There does appear to be an increased incidence of shoulder injuries in more recent years. Culpepper and Niemann [17] theorized that this was due to the outlawing of spearing, which brought a return of shoulder-body contact to tackling.

In one study of recurrent anterior shoulder dislocations requiring surgical correction, 49% of the patients sustained their initial injury in football [28]. In another study of acromioclavicular injuries 41% of patients sustained their initial injury in football [15].

Bicycling. Although bicycling is usually a recreational activity, it is becoming increasingly popular as an organized sport. Most bicycle injuries in the pediatric age group occur during idle play. Sixty per cent of all bicycle injuries occur in children between 5 and 14 years of age [14, 37]. In bicycle injuries 85% involve the upper extremity [31]. One unique injury is the so-called

bicycle shoulder [23]. This occurs when the cyclist is thrown over the front of the cycle when it is suddenly stopped. Failure to stay with the bicycle causes the cyclist to be thrown forward, landing directly on the shoulder. This forward propulsion over the wheels produces a direct injury to the acromioclavicular area (fracture of the distal clavicle or acromioclavicular separation) (Fig. 14–4). Bicycle shoulder injuries can be prevented by teaching the cyclist to maintain a tight grip on the handlebar and roll with the cycle, allowing the body to absorb some of the forces of the fall (Fig. 14–4*B*).

Basketball. There are no published data on high school basketball shoulder injuries. In a review of professional players by Henry and colleagues [27], shoulder injuries accounted for only 3% of all injuries and 1% of the games missed.

Skiing. In a study of skiing injuries by Carr and co-workers [10], only 25% involved the upper extremity. Forty per cent of these involved the hand (specifically

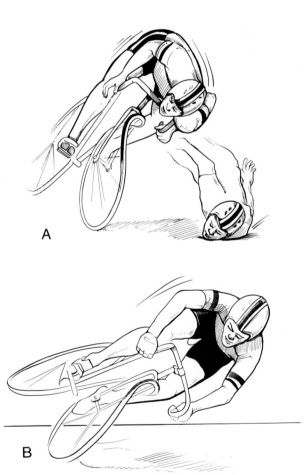

FIGURE 14–4
Bicycle shoulder. *A,* If the bicyclist maintains his grip on the handle bars and is thrown forward, he often lands directly on his shoulder, sustaining a disruption of the acromioclavicular joint. *B,* The proper way of falling is to stay with the bicycle and roll, so that the pressure is distributed evenly throughout the body rather than on the shoulder alone.

the thumb). The shoulder was next with dislocations and severe sprains occurring in almost 30% of the upper extremity injuries. It was surmised that conditions that increased the speed of the skier (i.e., ability and snow pack) increased the chances of sustaining an injury to the upper extremity.

Wrestling. During the average high school season as many as 75% of participants in wrestling sustain some type of injury [41]. Twenty-nine per cent of these injuries involve the upper extremity, of which almost all involve the shoulder. In looking at shoulder injuries occurring in wrestling specifically, Snook [47] found that almost 78% involved the acromioclavicular joint. Such injuries are probably the result of a direct blow when the shoulder hits the mat. Since the object of wrestling is often to put leverage about the shoulder, one might expect a high incidence of glenohumeral dislocations. The incidence of glenohumeral dislocations, however, is quite low (less than 10% of all shoulder injuries and less than 2% of injuries overall). This fact can probably be explained by the fact that the leverage forces applied to the shoulder are gradual and are strongly resisted by the muscular forces of the opponent.

Horseback Riding. Trauma sustained by young horseback riders most frequently involves head and neck injuries. Next to head injuries, however, is skeletal trauma, with two-thirds of the fractures occurring in the upper extremity [5]. In Sweden the major cause of fractures of the proximal humerus in girls (see Fig. 14–1) is falling off a horse [32].

Microtrauma

Injuries due to microtrauma are especially prevalent in the shoulder region. Hill [29] divided these microtrauma or overuse forces into three categories. The first is *explosive* force such as that occurring in pitching a baseball, which is thrown repetitively at maximum force but for relatively short periods of time. The second or *dynamic* force is gentler but is sustained for more repetitions and for longer periods of time. The classic example of this dynamic force is swimming. The third type is a *static* force in which isometric contractions are maintained across the shoulder for various periods of time. Examples of this type of force are seen in the weight lifter or gymnast who suspends his trunk with his upper extremities.

Baseball. In the shoulder, baseball is the sport that produces little macrotrauma but a great deal of microtrauma. Tullos and King [51] divided the pitching activity into three phases (Fig. 14–5). First is the *cocking* phase, in which the shoulder is markedly externally rotated. This tightens the triceps and biceps as well as both the internal and external rotators across the shoulder. This part of the throwing act in the adolescent pitcher

results in increased external and decreased internal rotation arcs in the shoulder. Richardson [43] pointed out that during this phase the internal rotators and adductors are at maximum stretch. If the body or shoulder moves forward too soon, the arm has to catch up by putting an excessive load on these structures, creating an inflammatory tendinitis that is the most common cause of anterior shoulder pain in adolescent pitchers.

The second or *acceleration* phase consists of two parts. First, the shoulder is brought forward with the forearm behind. Next, the forearm and hand are whipped forward, owing in large part to forces generated by the pectoralis major and latissimus dorsi.

The final or *follow-through* phase involves coordination of the forearm muscles to release the ball at the proper time and with the proper spin. The deceleration forces generated in this phase are unique to baseball and tennis [43]. This phase puts stretch on the posterior capsule and external rotators that can be a source of the posterior shoulder pain syndrome. Richardson [43] found that during this phase there may also be stress on the rhomboids and levator scapular insertions, producing pain along the medial scapular border.

Tullos and King [51] found that the pitching patterns in adolescents and adults were remarkably similar. The forces generated during pitching are very large, especially when rotation is considered. Gainor and his coworkers [21] pointed out that pitching involves both rotational forces from the internal and external rotators of the shoulder and compressive forces from the flexors and extensors of the elbow. They calculated that internal rotational torque is 14,000 inch-pounds just prior to release of the ball. The kinetic energy produced is 27,000 inch-pounds during the throw. These forces are four times greater than those generated in the lower extremity when kicking a ball. In addition, they are greater than the forces required to fracture an isolated cadaver humerus.

In baseball, however, elbow problems predominate in immature players. Shoulder pain and chronic problems do not develop until adolescents are in their late teens [2, 3, 29, 45]. Some authors have speculated that the late incidence of shoulder problems is related to abnormal pitching patterns due to chronic elbow conditions that have developed during the earlier years [2, 45].

One area of skeletal weakness that can fail with repeated microtrauma is the proximal humeral physeal plate. Failure usually occurs as a stress fracture of the proximal humeral physis. This entity was first described as Little League shoulder by Dotter in 1953 [19]. Since then numerous cases have been described in the literature [1, 4, 9, 34, 49, 50, 52]. All of these cases occurred in high-performance male pitchers who were 11 to 13 years old. The common radiographic finding is a widening of the proximal humeral physeal plate (Fig. 14–6). In the cases presented, all except one responded to rest

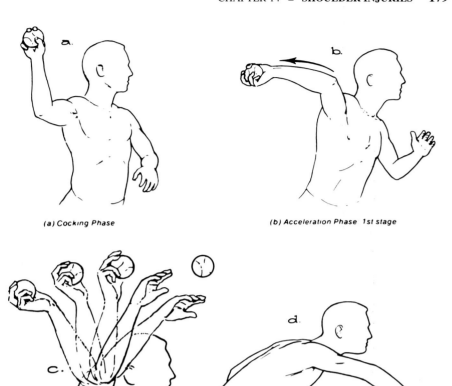

FIGURE 14–5
The three phases of pitching. *a*, Cocking phase. *b–c*, Acceleration phase. *d*, Follow-through phase. (Reprinted with permission from Woods, G. W., Tullos, H. S., and King, J. W.: The throwing arm: Elbow joint injuries. *J Sports Med* 1(Suppl 4):45, 1973.)

(a) Cocking Phase

(b) Acceleration Phase 1st stage

(c) Acceleration Phase 2nd stage

(d) Follow-through Phase

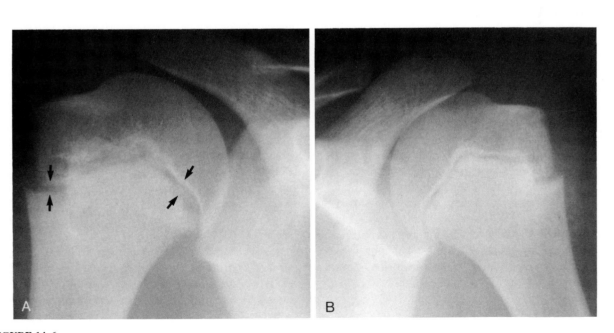

FIGURE 14–6
"Baseball shoulder." *A*, A 13-year-old high-performance Little League pitcher who experienced pain toward the end of the season while throwing. These x-rays demonstrate widening of the physis (arrows), which is indicative of a stress fracture through the physis of so-called baseball shoulder. *B*, Normal left side for comparison.

for the remainder of the season plus a vigorous preseason conditioning program the following year [48]. In only one case was operative intervention necessary. This was an individual described by Lipscomb [34] in whom a localized avascular necrosis of the epiphysis per se developed, producing a loose body that had to be removed surgically.

In addition to chronic repetitive rotational and compressive forces across the shoulder, there appear to be other factors that may create microtrauma in young, skeletally immature pitchers. Albright [2] found in an extensive study of Little League pitchers that the incidence of symptoms reflected the form of pitching rather than the age of the pitcher. Those who had poor pitching skills were more likely to become symptomatic. For this reason, Slager [45] advised that the first emphasis of immature pitchers should be on the development of skills and control; as they mature, emphasis can be placed on increasing the speed of pitching. Social tensions can also be a factor. Torg and associates [50] found that in comparable age groups, those who performed in a less competitive environment were less likely to develop symptoms in the throwing arm than those who were subjected to high competitive pressures.

Fractures of the humeral shaft in the pediatric age group are relatively rare but do occur [30]. Usually they are related to some inherent defect in the bony structures (Fig. 14–7). Ireland and Andrews [30] have described a case in a young pitcher with an acute avulsion of the coracoid epiphysis. By and large, most of the trauma to the shoulder region that occurs in baseball is microtrauma due to pitching.

Swimming. The most common orthopedic problem in competitive swimmers involves the shoulder and is almost exclusively seen in high-performance swimmers. In Dominquez' [18] study shoulder problems were rare in athletes under the age of 10 but increased dramatically after that age.

Swimming is a sport that involves a tremendous amount of repetition. It has been calculated that the average male free-style swimmer performs almost 400,000 strokes per arm per year [42]. Women, who require more strokes to swim the same distance, may perform as many as 660,000 strokes per year. Richardson and colleagues [42], in their classic review of swimming injuries, found consistent patterns in swimmers who had shoulder problems. Symptoms increased with the caliber of the athlete, were more common in men, and were more frequent in sprint than in long-distance swimmers. Symptoms were more common in the early and middle portions of the season and were often exacerbated by the use of hand paddles during training.

The major cause of shoulder pain in swimming is repeated friction of the humeral head and rotator cuff on the coracoacromial arch during abduction of the shoul-

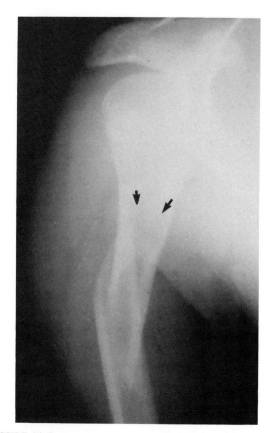

FIGURE 14–7
This 12-year-old sustained a acute fracture while throwing in a simple practice. The fracture occurred through a cystic osseous defect in the proximal humeral diaphysis (arrows).

der. This produces what Richardson terms an "impingement syndrome" [42, 43]. The maximum amount of impingement occurs at the beginning of the pull-through phase of the swimming stroke (Fig. 14–8). In the backstroke the greatest stress is on the anterior capsule during the pull-through phase (Fig. 14–8*B*). In addition, backstroke swimmers often stretch the capsule to the point where they develop anterior subluxation [42].

Gymnastics. Gymnastic events produce unique forces across the shoulder. Rather than performing motions repetitively, the gymnast often has to maintain one position for relatively prolonged periods of time [43]. In male gymnasts who perform extensively on the rings, which produce a great deal of stress across the shoulder, a benign cortical hypertrophy often develops at the insertion of the pectoralis major muscle into the proximal humerus. This has been termed by Fulton and his coworkers [20] the "ringman's shoulder lesion." In a study of female gymnasts by Snook [46], the second most common injury was a supraspinatus tendinitis, which emphasizes the great degree of tension and compressive forces about the shoulder that occurs with gymnastics.

Tennis. In tennis the forces placed on the upper ex-

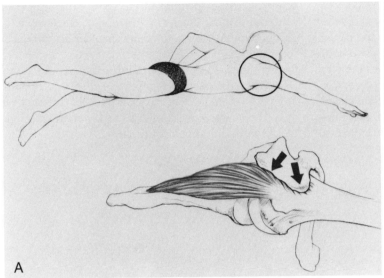

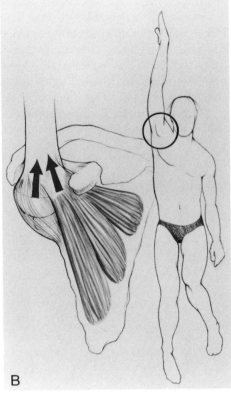

FIGURE 14–8
Swimmers shoulder. *A,* During the beginning of the pull-through phase, the humeral head forces the rotator cuff against the acromion (arrows), creating an impingement in this area. *B,* In the backstroke, with initiation of the pull-through phase, there is a tendency to place tension on the anterior portion of the glenohumeral capsule (arrows).

tremity in the forearm stroke and the serve are very similar to those characteristic of baseball pitching. Cocking, acceleration, and follow-through phases occur. The only difference is that the racquet, which serves as an extension of the extremity, increases the forces applied to this extremity. In the backhand stroke there is a reverse mechanism. Here the internal rotators are the decelerators, and the weaker external rotators must provide the acceleration force. Because of this, many players use a two-handed stroke, which allows the twisting motion of the body to add some power to the stroke [43].

FIGURE 14–9
Tennis shoulder results from stretching of the shoulder elevator muscles during both the acceleration and follow-through phases of overhead serve. (From Priest, J. D., and Nagel, D. A. Tennis shoulder. *Am J Sports Med* 4:28–42, 1976.)

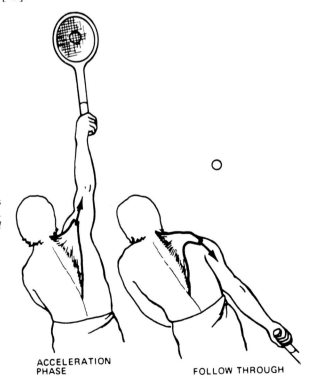

ACCELERATION
PHASE

FOLLOW THROUGH

Priest and Nagel [40] described a characteristic posture of young tennis players called the tennis shoulder. It is a depression or drooping of the shoulder associated with a postural scoliosis. They ascribed this to two etiologic factors. First, the service motion stretches the elevators of the shoulders (trapezius, levator scapulae, and rhomboids) (Fig. 14–9). This stretching makes the player less able to maintain the normal postural elevation of the shoulder. Second, a documented hypertrophy occurs that simply increases the mass of the upper extremity. It was surmised that the downward rotation of the scapula that occurs with the drooping of the shoulder can produce a rotator cuff irritation by decreasing the distance between the acromion and the greater tuberosity. These authors also described cases of this phenomenon (i.e., shoulder drooping) in adolescent baseball pitchers and shot putters. Treatment consists of selective exercises designed to strengthen the shoulder elevators.

Anatomy, Biomechanics and Physiology

Ralph J. Curtis, Jr., M.D.

ANATOMY

Developmental Anatomy

The limb buds appear and differentiate toward an adult form during the first 8 prenatal weeks (embryonic period). By the fetal period (8 weeks of gestation), the components of the shoulder region are adultlike in configuration, and they progressively enlarge and mature throughout this phase until birth. At birth the diaphyseal and metaphyseal portions of the humerus are completely ossified. The primary ossification center proximally is rarely ossified until after the first 6 postnatal months. Additional ossification centers develop for the greater tuberosity between 7 months and 3 years of age and 2 years later for the lesser tuberosity. By age 5 to 7 years, these three proximal ossification centers coalesce to become a single center. The proximal humeral physis usually closes between 19 and 22 years of age. The proximal humeral physis contributes approximately 80% of the longitudinal growth of the humerus [59, 60, 65, 66].

The clavicle, one of the first bones in the human to ossify, does so by the fifth gestational week, forming intramembranous ossification at two different areas in its central portion. By 45 days in utero these two centers fuse to form a single center for the clavicular shaft [55, 56, 64]. The medial secondary ossification center or physis provides up to 80% of the remaining longitudinal growth of the clavicle. It is one of the last to ossify (between the ages of 12 and 19 years), and fusion of the shaft does not occur until the age of 22 to 25 years. The lateral or acromial epiphysis is usually very inapparent radiographically because it appears, ossifies, and then fuses over a period of a very few months at about age 19 [64, 71].

The scapula first appears as a chondrified anlagen in the fifth gestational week. It begins at the level of C4–C5 and then migrates to occupy a position extending from C4 to C7 during the sixth and seventh gestational weeks. After formation of the shoulder joint at about the seventh week, the scapula descends from the cervical area to its more adultlike position overlying the first through fifth ribs [66]. Failure of the scapula to descend results in Sprengel's deformity [58]. The scapula forms by intramembranous ossification throughout its primary center. This area is usually completely ossified by birth. The remaining multiple ossification centers are highly variable in terms of number and position. At approximately 1 year, an ossification center for the coracoid process appears. By age 10 a common physis appears for the base of the coracoid and upper glenoid. A third, somewhat variable ossification center can appear at puberty at the tip of the coracoid and may be misidentified as an avulsion fracture. By age 15 to 16, these three centers usually coalesce. The acromion ossifies by forming between two and five ossification centers. These usually appear at puberty and are completely fused by age 22 years. Failure of fusion of one of the acromial physes results in an unfused "os acromiale" [58, 69]. At puberty the center for the vertebral border and inferior angle of the scapula as well as a horseshoe-shaped epiphysis for the lower three-quarters of the glenoid appear. They fuse to the remaining scapula by the twenty-second year. Due to the multitude of centers of maturation, many anomalies of the scapula have been described, including a bipartite coracoid, duplication of the acromion process, dysplasia of the glenoid, and scapular clefts [58].

Surgical Anatomy

Clavicle

The clavicle, a subcutaneous bone that extends from the sternum, provides the only bony articulation with the upper extremity at the acromioclavicular joint. This S-shaped bone has a double curve with the anterior convexity medial and the posterior convexity lateral. Medially, the clavicle provides attachment to the axial skeleton through the sternoclavicular joint. Laterally, its attachment at the acromioclavicular joint is supported by the acromioclavicular and coracoclavicular ligaments. The clavicle provides attachment for many of the major shoulder girdle muscles including the trapezius, deltoid, sternocleidomastoid, and pectoralis major muscles. It provides a bony protective roof over the thoracic outlet through which pass the axillary vessels and brachial plexus [59, 60, 66].

The clavicle is capable of motion in multiple planes. Most of this motion occurs through the sternoclavicular joint and includes rotation, translation, and an ability to pivot anterior to posterior as well as superior to inferior. When the shoulder is taken through a full range of motion, the clavicle rotates about its long axis approximately 50 degrees and is elevated upward approximately 30 degrees. A small amount of motion also occurs through the acromioclavicular joint [57].

The medial clavicular physis provides approximately 80% of the longitudinal growth of the developing clavicle. Unlike the medial epiphysis, the lateral clavicular epiphysis is quite small and provides very little longitudinal growth.

Acromioclavicular Joint

The lateral end of the clavicle and acromioclavicular joint is relatively well protected by muscular and ligamentous attachments. The clavicle becomes more flattened in its outer third and is surrounded by an extremely thick periosteal tube. This periosteal tube is continuous with both the acromioclavicular ligaments that span the acromioclavicular joint and the coracoclavicular liga-

ments inferiorly that provide stability for the distal clavicle (Fig. 14–10). The diarthrodial acromioclavicular joint is stabilized primarily by the strong coracoclavicular ligaments that extend from the coracoid to the undersurface of the distal third of the clavicle. The two coracoclavicular ligaments (conoid and trapezoid) extend medially and laterally on the underside of the distal clavicle almost completely out to the acromioclavicular joint. In addition, the joint capsule is reinforced by the acromioclavicular ligaments. In the mature individual an intra-articular disc covers the end of the distal clavicle and ameliorates some of the incongruity that normally exists in this joint [60, 66, 67, 71].

The deltoid attaches all along the anterior aspect of the distal clavicle and anterior acromion. Posteriorly on the distal clavicle is the strong insertion of the trapezius muscle. These multiple muscular and ligamentous attachments surrounding the distal clavicle provide relative protection compared to the clavicular shaft. In children, injury to this region commonly consists of a fracture through the distal physis that splits the periosteal tube, forcing the clavicle to herniate superiorly, rather than a true acromioclavicular dislocation.

Sternoclavicular Joint

The sternoclavicular joint is a diarthrodial joint composed of the large medial end of the clavicle, the sternum, and the first rib. The medial clavicle becomes somewhat bulbous lateral to the epiphysis at the medial end of the clavicle. The articulating portion of the sternum and first rib form a relatively flat and shallow surface for the articulation of the medial clavicle. This joint is extremely incongruous and has very little inherent bony stability. A fibrocartilaginous disc provides further

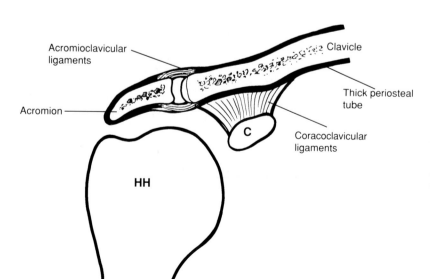

FIGURE 14–10

Anatomy of the distal clavicle and acromioclavicular joint in children. Note the thickened periosteal tube surrounding the distal clavicle that is continuous with the acromioclavicular and coracoclavicular ligaments.

cushioning and stability for this joint, which is surrounded by a very strong series of ligaments [57]. The anterior and posterior capsular ligaments provide the major support. The anterior portion of the capsular ligaments is stronger and heavier and provides the primary support against both upward and anterior displacement of the medial clavicle. These ligaments attach primarily to the epiphysis of the medial clavicle, helping to explain why medial clavicular physeal injuries in children are more common than true sternoclavicular dislocations. In addition, the intra-articular disc ligament is a very dense fibrous structure extending from the first rib through the joint and attaching both anteriorly and posteriorly to the strong capsular ligaments. Further stability for the joint is provided by the interclavicular ligament and costoclavicular ligaments. The interclavicular ligament runs from clavicle to clavicle, attaching to the superior aspect of the manubrium. The costoclavicular ligaments run from the first rib to the inferior surface of the medial clavicle. They help to suspend the clavicle much like the boom of a crane [57, 67] (Fig. 14–11).

The medial clavicular epiphysis is the last epiphysis of the long bones to appear and the last to close. This epiphysis ossifies between the eighteenth and twentieth years, and fusion to the shaft occurs between the twenty-third and twenty-fifth years [66, 71].

Most clavicular motion occurs through the sternoclavicular joint. This joint has the capability of allowing 30 to 35 degrees of upward clavicular elevation (pivot), 35 degrees of anterior to posterior glide (translation), and 45 to 50 degrees of rotation about the long axis of the clavicle. This motion is extremely important for normal shoulder function as the scapula rotates to allow normal abduction and elevation [59, 60, 67].

In addition to its important function of mobility, this joint provides the only true bony articulation between the upper extremity and the axial skeleton. Its position anterior to the mediastinum also gives it a protective

function. In posteriorly displaced fractures and dislocations about the medial clavicle and sternoclavicular joint, injury can occur to some major neurovascular structures exiting the aortic arch and brachial plexus, the trachea, and the esophagus.

Glenohumeral Joint

The articulation between the humerus and the scapula at the glenohumeral joint is the most mobile major joint in the body. The unique anatomic configuration of this joint accommodates motion while sacrificing inherent stability.

The proximal humerus is composed of the head of the humerus with its articular surface, the greater and lesser tuberosities, and the complex proximal humeral physis. The articular surface of the humerus at the shoulder is a sphere with a radius of curvature of about 2.25 cm in the adult. By comparison, the relatively flat glenoid articular surface has a radius of curvature of approximately one-third that of the humeral head. This mismatch allows an inherent translation of the humeral head on the glenoid with motion [63, 66].

The capsule of the glenohumeral joint along with the reinforced, thickened areas known as the glenohumeral ligaments provide the primary stability for the joint. These ligaments attach through the glenoid labrum at the edges of the glenoid surface. The humeral attachment of the capsular ligaments occurs along the region of the anatomic neck except medially, where the attachment extends distally along the shaft. The physis lies in an extracapsular position except along this medial side, where it is intra-articular (Fig. 14–12). The glenoid labrum very slightly deepens the glenoid, and its main function is to provide an area of strong attachment for the capsular ligaments. The capsular ligamentous complex at the glenohumeral joint is a very complex functional unit. With the arm at the side, the inferior capsule and ligaments are highly redundant. This allows the arm to be taken through a range of abduction, elevation, and extension with free motion. As the arm reaches the limit of abduction or is combined with abduction and rotation, the anterior or posterior inferior capsule tightens to limit translation of the humeral head on the glenoid [59, 60, 66, 70]. Shoulder arthroscopy has allowed us to define the capsular ligamentous complex more precisely, demonstrating succinct bands within the anterior capsule including the superior, middle, and inferior glenohumeral ligaments [62].

With the arm in the anatomic position, the intertubercular groove between the greater and lesser tuberosities lies approximately 1 cm lateral to the midline. This groove is covered by a transverse ligament, and through it the long head of the biceps gains access to the joint.

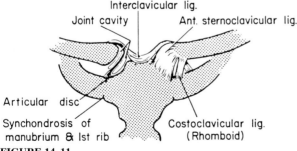

FIGURE 14–11
Medial clavicle and sternoclavicular joint anatomy. The medial physis lies in an extra-articular position while the epiphysis is bound by the heavy ligamentous structures surrounding the sternoclavicular joint. (Reproduced with permission from Rockwood, C. A., and Green, D. P. [Eds.], *Fractures* (3 vols.). 2nd ed. Philadelphia, J. B. Lippincott, 1984.)

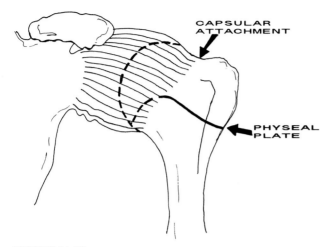

FIGURE 14-12
Glenohumeral joint anatomy. Note that the capsule of the glenohumeral joint attaches along a line consistent with the surgical neck of the humerus. The physeal plate extends from an extra-articular position laterally to an intra-articular position on the medial cortex.

The long head of the biceps attaches superiorly to the glenoid rim and labrum as a prominent intra-articular structure. The rotator cuff tendons form a sleeve of thickened tissue that covers the joint anteriorly, posteriorly, and superiorly. The tendinous contributions from the subscapularis muscle, supraspinatus muscle, infraspinatus muscle, and teres minor coalesce to form the major dynamic stabilizers of the glenohumeral joint. The rotator cuff inserts immediately adjacent to the insertion of the capsular ligaments. The subscapularis tendon inserts into the lesser tuberosity, while the supraspinatus, infraspinatus, and teres minor insert into the region of the greater tuberosity [66]. The blood supply to the proximal humerus enters the bone at the level of the capsular and cuff attachments and receives a major contribution from the anterior humeral circumflex artery [68].

Scapula

The scapula is positioned at the posterior lateral aspect of the bony thorax approximately between the third and ninth ribs. Its two main functions are to provide a major attachment site for many of the stabilizing muscles and a mobile base for the upper extremity. The bone is completely encased in muscle, and this fact, along with its position on the posterior lateral aspect of the thorax, protects it from injury [59, 60].

Of clinical importance are the multiple ossification centers that form within the scapula (Fig. 14–13). Multiple physes within the coracoid, the upper quarter of the glenoid, and the acromion can be confused radiographically with fractures. They can, however, also be the sites of avulsion injuries, for which clinical confirmation is required [58, 66, 69].

BIOMECHANICS OF THE SHOULDER

The demands on the shoulder in sports are rigorous. The main function of the shoulder is to position the arm and hand in space to carry out the desired activity. A multiplanar range of motion is required to accomplish this task, and stability is sacrificed somewhat to allow mobility.

Normal Biomechanics

When the arm is elevated, motion occurs at both the glenohumeral and scapulothoracic articulations. Secondary supportive motion occurs at the sternoclavicular joint and to a lesser degree at the acromioclavicular joint. Approximately one-third of the total 180 degrees

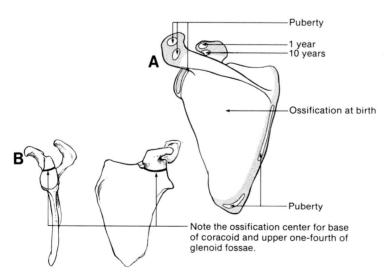

FIGURE 14-13
Note the multiple ossification centers present in the scapula. These multiple physes can be confused radiographically in cases of trauma with fracture. (From Curtis, R. J., Jr., and Rockwood, C. A. Jr. Fractures and dislocations of the shoulder in children. *In* Rockwood, C. A., Jr., and Matsen, F. A. III [Eds.], *The Shoulder.* Phildelphia, W.B. Saunders, 1990.)

of elevation of the arm occurs through the scapulothoracic articulation [74, 80, 82, 93].

Stability of the glenohumeral joint has both static and dynamic components. The primary static stabilizers of the joint are the glenohumeral ligaments within the joint capsule [80, 91, 99, 100]. There is considerable capsular redundancy inferiorly, resulting in a capsular surface area that is about twice that of the humeral head. The anterior capsule is reinforced by several thick folds along its inner surface called the glenohumeral ligaments (Fig. 14–14). The inferior glenohumeral ligament complex appears to serve as a hammock or sling inferiorly that protects the joint against both anterior and posterior instability when it is abducted or rotated internally or externally.

The primary source of dynamic stability for the glenohumeral joint is provided by the musculotendinous units of the rotator cuff muscles: the subscapularis, supraspinatus, infraspinatus, and teres minor. The combined effect of these muscles is to increase joint compression and therefore resist the sheer forces exerted on the joint by the forces of the other larger muscles such as the deltoid, pectoralis major, and latissimus dorsi [73, 80, 86, 88, 93, 94, 99] (Fig. 14–15). Dynamic anterior control is provided primarily by the subscapularis tendon, which is closely approximated to the anterior capsule [78]. With the arm at the side, this tendon is a primary dynamic stabilizer for anterior instability. When the arm is abducted more than 90 degrees, the subscapularis tendon rotates into a more superior position, and its effec-

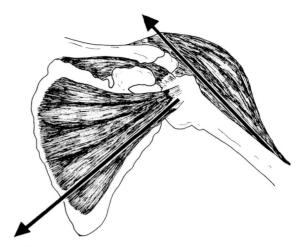

FIGURE 14–15
The tendons of the rotator cuff act as a dynamic stabilization mechanism to resist the sheer forces exerted on the joint by the larger muscles such as the deltoid, pectoralis major, and latissimus dorsi.

tiveness in providing stability is decreased. The supraspinatus, infraspinatus, and teres minor make up the stronger superior and posterior portions of the rotator cuff. These muscle-tendon units serve as strong dynamic stabilizers of the glenohumeral joint, protecting it against excessive superior, posterior, and anterior translation. The three components of the deltoid, pectoralis major, and latissimus dorsi muscles provide additional stability when the arm is in a relatively adducted position or is extremely abducted.

Synergy between the rotator cuff and the deltoid is a key to normal function at the shoulder. Freedman and associates and Inman and colleagues described in detail the synergistic force-couple that is necessary for normal shoulder function [81, 87]. The deltoid has a mobile point of origin on the acromion, clavicle, and scapula. At the initiation of abduction, the long lever arm of the deltoid leads to inefficient function with a tendency to cause upward displacement or sheer of the humeral head into the coracoacromial arch. This force exerted by the deltoid becomes a compressive force once the shoulder is abducted more than approximately 45 degrees, when the deltoid becomes much more effective. All four components of the rotator cuff work to help improve deltoid function by serving as a humeral head depressor and stabilizer against the superior sheer force created by the deltoid. The rotator cuff is therefore extremely important in providing dynamic stability in its force-couple relationship with the deltoid [75, 76, 77, 79, 85, 95, 98].

Biomechanics of Throwing

The demand on the shoulder during throwing is to position the arm so that a ball can be propelled through

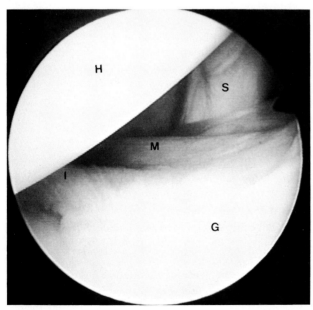

FIGURE 14–14
Arthroscopic view of the glenohumeral ligaments. (I, inferior glenohumeral ligament; M, middle glenohumeral ligaments; G, glenoid; H, humeral head; S, subscapularis tendon.)

space at variable speeds. The pitch has been broken down into three major phases of action: (1) cocking phase (wind-up), (2) acceleration phase, and (3) follow-through phase [72, 83, 84, 89, 93].

The cocking phase begins as the arm is elevated to approximately 90 degrees and then is horizontally extended. With these motions, the shoulder is externally rotated, tightening the anterior capsule in much the same way as a washcloth that is being wrung (Fig. 14–16). The anterior-inferior glenohumeral ligament complex is maximally tightened as a dense band across the anterior-inferior surface of the joint. The subscapularis tendon is elevated into a more superior position, decreasing its effect as an anterior stabilizer. In the baseball pitching motion, this cocking phase takes place in about 0.14 second. This phase is complete when the shoulder reaches its maximal external rotation. Electromyographic (EMG) studies have shown that deltoid activity is quite high during this phase [79, 84, 89]. The posterior deltoid serves as the prime source of extension while the anterior and lateral components of the deltoid provide elevation and some external rotation. The supraspinatus, infraspinatus, and teres minor are active throughout external rotation. With their posterior pull, they provide some relief from stress across the anterior capsular structures. Adequate strength in the posterior cuff musculature in this phase is of critical importance.

The acceleration phase can be looked on as a rapid unwinding of the potential energy stored in the soft tissues as they are positioned in the cocking phase. Initiation of the acceleration phase occurs as the subscapularis and pectoralis major begin internal rotation. This phase is very short, lasting only 0.01 second. Peak rates of internal rotation of up to 7000 degrees/second have been measured. This relatively passive activity imparts

tremendous stress across the glenohumeral joint in multiple planes.

The follow-through phase consists of the shoulder's final continuation of internal rotation and horizontal adduction after the ball leaves the hand. Many muscle groups are active including the deltoid, rotator cuff, latissimus dorsi, and pectoralis major in the attempt to decelerate the arm. Stress occurs across the posterior capsule and is at a peak during this phase.

As an individual moves from a side-arm throw to a more overhand position, the amount of true arm abduction of the shoulder changes very little. In the more overhand throw, the trunk deviates away from the throwing arm to a greater degree. During the follow-through phase, less stress is exerted across the posterior capsule. Apparently the increase in trunk flexion and rotation reduces the need to decelerate the arm.

Biomechanics of the Tennis Serve

The serve in tennis has a biomechanical pattern of motion very similar to that of the overhand throw [93]. Some very specific differences exist. Again, the activity can be categorized into cocking, acceleration, and follow-through phases. During the cocking phase, the shoulder first extends, then abducts and externally rotates. Posterior deltoid activity is decreased by a backward lean of the trunk. Anterior and lateral deltoid activity is increased for abduction. The participation of the infraspinatus is important in external rotation throughout this phase.

Acceleration combines a quick, passive overhead reach with internal rotation and forceful depression. During follow-through, deceleration is prominent with strong posterior deltoid, infraspinatus, and anterior deltoid activity. Most of the differences between the tennis serve and the overhand throw can be expected with the differences in body position.

Biomechanics of Swimming

The four major swimming strokes can be broken down into two major phases of action: pull and recovery. In swimming the shoulder positions the hand so that the upper extremity can be used as a paddle, pulling through the water to propel the body forward. The shoulder is stressed in swimming by the extreme range of motion used, the tremendous force required to sustain a propulsive effort, and the high rate of repetition. Competitive swimmers may routinely swim 8000 to 10,000 meters daily [92, 93, 96, 97].

The pull phase in the swimming stroke is equivalent to the acceleration phase in throwing sports. Except for

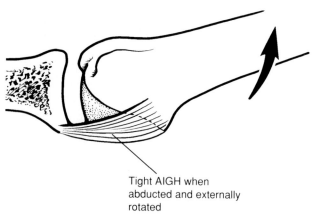

Tight AIGH when abducted and externally rotated

FIGURE 14–16
Although the cocking phase of the baseball throw is the prototype of abduction, external rotation stress across the glenohumeral joint, the tennis serve and free-style swimming stroke are similar biomechanically. The anterior-inferior glenohumeral ligament complex is maximally tightened when the arm is abducted and externally rotated.

the breaststroke, this phase begins as the hand enters the water. The shoulder begins in maximal abduction and elevation and then is forcefully adducted to the side of the body. The course of the hand and upper extremity through the water is performed in a different way for each of the various strokes.

In the crawl and butterfly, the shoulder is abducted and externally rotated as the hand enters the water, and an extension maneuver is used for propulsion. The difference between these strokes is the reciprocal arm motion in the crawl and simultaneous motion in the butterfly. For the backstroke, the arm is maximally abducted and internally rotated. Forceful depression moves the shoulder into an adducted, neutrally rotated position. Body roll from side to side reduces the amount of extension necessary. For the breaststroke, the arm motion begins with the shoulders elevated and internally rotated. Propulsion is by sustained lateral adduction with slight flexion in relation to the scapula.

The recovery phase is the period in which the arm is repositioned for the next pull phase. In the crawl and butterfly strokes, recovery begins with shoulder extension and abduction and elbow flexion. The shoulder is initially rotated internally and then rotates progressively externally as the hand exits from the water. The backstroke utilizes less elbow function, and therefore recovery consists of rapid flexion or elevation to the overhead position. The breaststroke is the only stroke in which recovery occurs beneath the surface of the water. Recovery consists of midline adduction and elevation.

Maximal muscle force is exerted at the hands' deepest position in the water at about 90 degrees of shoulder flexion. Hand propulsion provides approximately 70% to 85% of total thrust. Elbow flexion reduces work at the shoulder and therefore decreases stress on the joint structures and improves joint stability.

EMG studies demonstrate that the pectoralis major is the dominant muscle during the pull phase. The primary source of propulsion in swimming is the musculature between the trunk and the arm, specifically the pectoralis major and the latissimus dorsi. EMG recordings indicate, however, that participation by the latissimus dorsi is poor. Subscapularis activity is important for resisting the anterior thrust of the humeral head. In the recovery phase, the anterior deltoid as well as the posterior deltoid are actively involved.

Pathologic Biomechanics with Injury About the Shoulder

After injury, the force-couple between the deltoid and the rotator cuff is often disrupted. When weakness of the rotator cuff occurs, the sheer stress imparted to the joint by the action of the deltoid, pectoralis major, and latis-

simus dorsi is not well counterbalanced. This leads to excessive joint translation in both the anterior-posterior and superior-inferior planes. This pathologic state can lead to impingement as the humeral head glides superiorly into the coracoacromial arch as well as to painful anterior subluxation. This abnormal biomechanical state can affect both active participation in sports and rehabilitation. Attempting to strengthen a weak rotator cuff with long lever arm abduction exercises leads to sheer stress that forces the humeral head up into the impingement zone. This could lead to increasing pain from impingement rather than appropriate rehabilitation.

PHYSIOLOGY

Demands on the shoulder in sports are related to either the mechanics involved in creating a range of motion or the structural strength involved in absorbing a blow. Injury in the pediatric athlete can result from either a single highly stressful event or from repeated performance of a highly stressful activity that requires the shoulder to extend itself beyond its physiologic and anatomic limits.

Although musculoskeletal tissues do respond to the applied stresses encountered in sports along accepted physical and biomechanical principles, living tissues have the characteristics of other organ systems whereby they can alter or heal themselves in response to demand [103, 111, 112]. Pediatric patients are even more able than adults to meet applied demands at the tissue level due to the tremendous active growth potential of the physis.

Physiologic Response to Demand

Wolff's law was formulated for bone but can be used to describe the response of all connective tissue to applied demands. Ligaments and tendons as well as bone respond by varying strength and dimensions in a direct relationship to applied stress [103, 109, 111, 112]. They can become thicker with repeated stresses, and their internal fibers become oriented to withstand stress loading in a certain direction. Wolff's law can also apply to disuse in that structures can lose their internal orientation if inadequate stress is applied [101, 102, 106].

An important physiologic response is the ability of musculoskeletal tissues to heal themselves by replacing damaged tissue with tissue of similar properties. Tendons and ligaments heal over a prolonged time [103]. During this remodeling period significant alterations can occur in the ability of the tissue to respond to stress according to whether healing has occurred by scar or granulation tissue. This leads to stress risers within the tissue that can increase its vulnerability to injury.

In the pediatric age group the anatomy and physiology of the physis are unique. The physis is the anatomic center of rapid cellular multiplication and longitudinal bony growth. The area immediately adjacent to the physis is a region of transition between the unstructured and weak physis and the mature orientation of the diaphysis of the bone. It is this transition area adjacent to the physis that is the most vulnerable to injury.

Pathologic Response to Demand

The cumulative effect of athletic performance of repetitive activities can sometimes lead to microstresses that are applied at a rate faster than the body can heal [104, 107, 108]. This can lead to microfailures, and eventually to the cumulative effect of macrofailure. This effect is commonly seen in bone as a stress fracture and in ligaments, tendons, and muscles as sprains, strains, and ruptures.

Treatment

In allowing the body to heal in a situation in which repetitive stress has caused injury, rest is of paramount importance. It alleviates further damaging stresses and allows time for the body's natural healing processes to take effect. A certain amount of physiologic stress is necessary to stimulate the body to heal. By controlling the timed course of the application of stress as well as the magnitude of the stress applied, a program of exercise can be prescribed during the rest and healing phase [106, 111, 112] (see Chap. 8).

Skeletal Injuries

Ralph J. Curtis, Jr., M.D.

CLAVICULAR SHAFT FRACTURES

Due to its prominence and superficial position, the clavicular shaft is vulnerable to injury in contact and collision sports. The prominent use of the shoulder girdle during blocking and tackling in football as well as its use as a battering ram in hockey or rugby can lead to fracture caused by direct blows to the clavicular shaft [144]. The clavicle can also be injured indirectly during sports, for example, during a fall on the outstretched hand while running. The clavicular shaft is fractured more commonly than either the medial or lateral ends, and shaft fractures represent more than 80% of all clavicular fractures [141]. In addition to a relatively unprotected anatomic position, the shaft has a biomechanically weak area at the junction of the S curve in its midshaft portion. These factors contribute to the relative frequency of clavicular shaft fractures that occur in sports [113, 130, 134].

Clinical Evaluation

The pediatric athlete usually has a distinct history of injury when a fracture of the clavicular shaft is present. The athlete complains of pain and in many cases is unable to move the upper extremity without discomfort. Two major mechanisms of injury have been described. Classically, the indirect mechanism was thought to be the most frequent. The athlete sustains a fall on the outstretched hand in which the forces of the fall are transmitted through the upper extremity to the shoulder joint. Because of the strong ligamentous bindings medially and laterally, the weak link in the system is the clavicular shaft, and fracture therefore occurs by this indirect mechanism [114, 118, 119, 127, 129, 141]. Most recently, however, Stanley and colleagues [146] noted that 94% of clavicular fractures in their series resulted from a direct blow, which reflected the types of sports their patients were playing.

Fractures of the clavicular shaft can be classified by degree of displacement, angulation, and comminution. They can also be classified as open or closed [114, 119, 140]. The younger the child, the more likely that the fracture will be of the greenstick variety, angulated without significant displacement. Plastic bowing without an overt fracture line has been described [117]. Fractures of the indirect variety are also more likely to be greenstick. Direct fractures are more likely to be of the higher energy variety with displacement and comminution. These fractures are also more likely to be open and have a higher incidence of complications such as neurovascular injury, pneumothorax, and nonunion [135, 138].

In fractures of the clavicular shaft, typical signs of fracture are usually apparent clinically, but the severity varies with the degree of displacement [114, 116, 119, 140–142] (Fig. 14–17). There is often swelling with tenderness at the fracture site. In displaced fractures, deformity is obvious. Many times the patient is unable to move the ipsilateral arm and holds it bound to the side. Due to spasm of the sternocleidomastoid muscle, the head is often turned toward the affected side. Spasm in both the sternocleidomastoid and trapezius can result in a superior displacement of the proximal fragment that becomes apparent clinically. In greenstick or minimally displaced fractures, range of motion of the shoulder can be accomplished but is painful. As displacement increases, the ability to take the arm through a range of motion decreases. Some fractures with comminution and displacement may be very prominent in the subcutaneous area. It is important to observe and test the neurovascular status because both brachial plexus and subclavian vascular injuries have been cited [124, 132, 133, 138, 147]. Venous distention and expanding hematoma, absence of pulses, and subjective complaints of numbness in the shoulder and arm must be taken seriously and rapid treatment initiated.

191

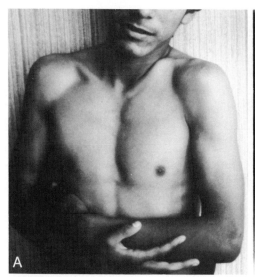
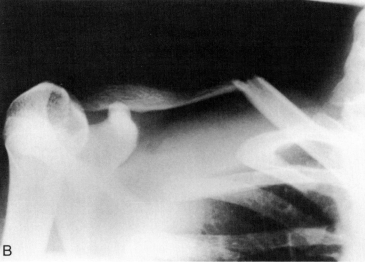

FIGURE 14–17
Fracture of the shaft of the clavicle. *A*, This 14-year-old football player had a direct blow to his clavicle, sustaining a displaced fracture. Clinically, note that he splints the arm to his body and supports it with the opposite hand. *B*, Radiographic view of the same fracture showing displaced and angulated fracture of the clavicular shaft. (From Curtis, R. J., Jr., and Rockwood, C. A., Jr. Fractures and dislocations of the shoulder in children. *In* Rockwood, C. A., Jr., and Matsen, F. A. III [Eds.], *The Shoulder*. Philadelphia, W.B. Saunders, 1990.)

Radiographic Examination

Plain radiographs of the clavicle are usually adequate for diagnosis [118, 121, 137, 140]. A single anteroposterior view supplemented by a 30-degree cephalic view is successful in making the diagnosis in the great majority of cases. In the younger child with a nondisplaced greenstick fracture, a soft tissue technique is often helpful for outlining the subcutaneous soft tissue shadows overlying the clavicle (Fig. 14–18). In a patient with an inapparent fracture, the subcutaneous tissues are often elevated by hematoma before the fracture is clearly seen radiographically [145]. When the fracture is somewhat inapparent, repeat films 7 to 10 days postinjury will usually demonstrate a healing callus about the fracture site. Care should be taken not to confuse radiographically a case of congenital pseudarthrosis of the clavicle with a true clavicular shaft fracture. Congenital pseudarthrosis is characterized radiographically by a large defect between smoothed-off, hypertrophic bony ends, almost always right-sided (Fig. 14–19). In addition, congenital pseudarthrosis is usually not associated with a recent history of trauma [118, 148, 150].

Treatment Options

The reported results of treatment of clavicular shaft fractures in children are excellent [114, 118, 119, 128,

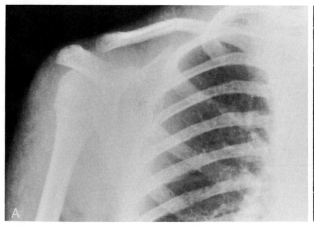
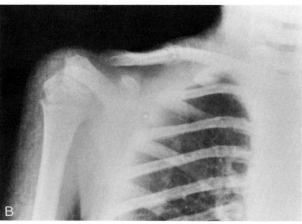

FIGURE 14–18
A, In the younger child with minimally displaced fractures of the shaft of the clavicle, a "soft tissue" technique is often helpful in outlining subcutaneous swelling around an otherwise inapparent fracture. *B*, Note the callus formation at the fracture site two weeks after injury.

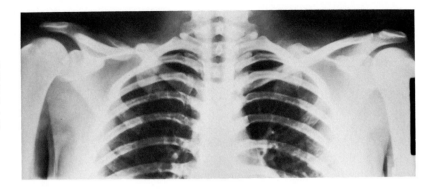

FIGURE 14–19
Congenital pseudoarthrosis of the clavicle can be confused with traumatic fracture. This 15-year-old gymnast had had no symptoms prior to a fall approximately two weeks before this radiograph was taken. Note the relatively large defect between smoothed-off, hypertrophic bony ends, and lack of soft tissue swelling.

142, 148]. It is uniformly accepted that nonoperative treatment is best [116, 127, 129, 139, 140, 141]. Nonunion has been reported but is extremely rare. Clinically significant malunion is also unusual except for an occasional mild cosmetic deformity. Anatomic reduction is not required for successful treatment. The mainstay of treatment is the use of nonoperative supportive measures to help obtain comfort early, followed by progressive healing and rehabilitation.

Numerous devices to ensure immobilization in clavicular shaft fractures have been described [115, 118, 143]. In addition to soft bandages, shoulder plaster spica casts have been used. The figure-of-eight sling, either the commercial variety or one made with stockinette and felt padding, is the most commonly used form of immobilization (Fig. 14–20). Either of these devices allows gentle immobilization while exerting posteriorly directed pressure against the shoulders, helping to reduce the fracture and maintain a position of comfort.

For children under age 12, most authors agree that attempts to reduce the fracture, even if it is displaced, are not needed [118, 140, 142]. Immobilization is accomplished by any of the previously described devices and is usually necessary for 3 to 6 weeks for clinical union. A prominent "bump" of healing callus will remodel almost completely over a period of 6 to 12 months and should be explained to the parents during initiation of treatment.

There is more controversy about treatment in the older adolescent child with a displaced fracture [118, 127, 135, 140, 142]. For displaced fractures, many authors prefer a more vigorous attempt at closed reduction, followed by maintenance of this reduction either in a plaster shoulder spica cast or in a figure-of-eight dressing reinforced by plaster. Gross displacement and severe angulation can be reduced under a local anesthetic hematoma block or intravenous sedation. Gentle manipulation is accomplished with the patient in the supine position, using a bolster placed longitudinally between the scapulae. Gentle upward and backward pressure is placed against the ipsilateral shoulder while the fracture site is manipulated. Aggressive attempts at manipulation

are unwarranted and may only lead to damage of the underlying neurovascular structures. Following manipulation, the figure-of-eight device can be used, although some authors advocate the use of a plaster shoulder spica cast [140]. Serial radiographs are required to document healing. Clinical union often requires 6 to 12 weeks depending on the age of the patient and the severity of displacement.

In open fractures, irrigation and debridement are carried out consistent with standard treatment for open fractures. The use of internal fixation for treatment of these fractures in children or adolescents is contraindicated.

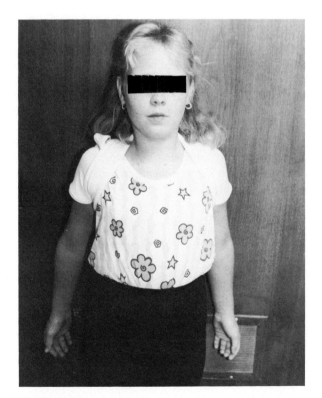

FIGURE 14–20
The figure-of-eight bandage is the most popular for treatment of clavicle fractures in children. (From Curtis, R. J., Jr., and Rockwood, C. A., Jr. Fractures and dislocations of the shoulder in children. *In* Rockwood, C. A., Jr., and Matsen, F. A. III [Eds.], *The Shoulder*. Philadelphia, W.B. Saunders, 1990.)

Open reduction and internal fixation have been described in cases in which vascular compromise has resulted from a displaced clavicular fracture [124, 138]. Most authors recommend rigid internal fixation using an intramedullary device such as a threaded Steinmann pin or Hagie pin [126, 151]. Jablon and colleagues [125] described a case of severe subcutaneous displacement in an adolescent that required open reduction and fixation with suture technique. In this case, the proximal fragment had penetrated the trapezius and platysma and was held in a severely displaced position, compromising the overlying skin.

Complications

Malunion of clavicular shaft fractures in children is not unusual. Displaced fractures are virtually always allowed to heal in a malunited position with the development of prominent callus. In these fractures, the rule is that they will remodel successfully over a period of 6 to 12 months. Significant clinical malunion is virtually never documented, and malunited clavicular shaft fractures that compromise function have not been reported.

Nonunion of the clavicular shaft is a rare entity [122, 123, 149]. Most series describe a 1% to 3% incidence in all age groups. The incidence of clavicular nonunion in children and adolescents has not been specifically reported. Manske and Szabo [131] recently described two cases of clavicular shaft nonunion during adolescence that were treated by open reduction and internal fixation.

Neurologic, vascular, and pulmonary injuries have been described after closed fracture of the clavicle [120, 124, 132, 133, 138, 147]. The incidence is low; however, close attention to a detailed neurovascular and pulmonary examination is recommended to allow early recognition and treatment.

Criteria for Return to Sports Participation

Essentially all athletes who sustain fractures of the clavicular shaft are at some point able to return to athletic endeavor. The fracture should be clinically nontender, and radiographic union should be documented before return to play is permitted. Additionally, the patient should have regained a full range of shoulder motion and good protective strength including a strong rotator cuff musculature. In the younger child, this often requires 4 to 6 weeks, whereas in the adolescent 6 to 12 weeks may be needed.

Author's Preferred Method of Treatment

I prefer to treat all clavicular shaft fractures in children nonoperatively if possible. For minimally displaced and angulated fractures in all age groups, I use a figure-of-eight bandage or a sling initially for comfort, along with ice and analgesics. The patient begins active motion of the shoulder and upper extremity as comfort allows. The parents are counseled about acceptance of the deformity and the normal delayed appearance of a "bump" of healing callus in treatment of this fracture.

For displaced fractures in children younger than age 12, I still make no attempt to reduce the fracture unless vascular compromise is present. The great propensity in children for healing and remodeling even in the presence of large degrees of displacement does not warrant overly aggressive treatment of this type of fracture. These fractures are treated in the same way as minimally displaced or angulated fractures.

Even in the adolescent older than 12 years, I adhere to a conservative philosophy. Most of these fractures, even if displaced, are treated by progressive tightening of a figure-of-eight bandage and early active functional use of the extremity. If gross displacement of a fracture occurs, compromising the overlying skin by penetration of the trapezius fascia or a 90-degree rotation of a butterfly fragment, an attempt at gentle manipulation is made under a hematoma block. I do not use a plaster shoulder spica cast even after manipulation owing to the discomfort it causes. These fractures are maintained in a figure-of-eight splint like nondisplaced fractures.

In open fractures of the clavicular shaft, surgical irrigation and debridement is undertaken. Internal fixation is avoided. In my practice the only indication for open reduction and internal fixation is an unstable fracture associated with vascular compromise. If a fracture can be manipulated closed to regain normal vascular status, this would be preferable.

INJURIES TO THE LATERAL END OF THE CLAVICLE

Fractures of the distal clavicle are much more common than fractures of the medial end and represent approximately 10% to 12% of all clavicular fractures according to Neer [175] and Rowe [180]. No specific incidence data is available for these fractures in children [152, 153]. A fall on the point of the shoulder that drives the scapula downward usually causes an acromioclavicular dislocation in the older adolescent and adult, but fractures of the distal clavicle are much more common in children with the same mechanism. These fractures represent "pseudodislocations" because the distal shaft is herniated upward through a rupture of the thick periosteal tube that surrounds the distal clavicle. The coracoclavicular and acromioclavicular ligaments remain intact to the periosteal tube along with the usually inapparent distal clavicular physis. This injury, therefore, is the childhood version of the true acromioclavicular joint dislocation of the adult [178].

Clinical Evaluation

As just mentioned, the mechanism of injury for distal clavicular fractures in children is similar to that causing acromioclavicular dislocation in older patients. This injury is not uncommon in collision and contact sports when the patient falls on the point of the shoulder. The acromion and scapula along with the arm are driven downward while the clavicle maintains its position. The injury represents a herniation of the distal clavicle superiorly through the thickened surrounding periosteal tube. Fracture can occur through the physis, which is clinically inapparent in most patients, or through the distal metaphysis. The coracoclavicular and acromioclavicular ligaments remain intact to the periosteal tube, thus producing a fracture or pseudodislocation rather than a true acromioclavicular dislocation.

In the history the patient describes a fall on the point of the shoulder. There is immediate pain, often deformity, and decreased ability to move the arm. The patient usually seeks medical attention promptly. Clinically, the examiner is unable to differentiate a true dislocation of the acromioclavicular joint from a pseudodislocation. The clavicle is usually prominent, and swelling, tenderness, and pain are evident with range of motion.

A classification scheme for these fractures has been described by Rockwood [161, 178]. The classification of injuries of the distal clavicle is similar to that used in adults for acromioclavicular dislocations. Children who are older than approximately 13 years of age may have a true adult type of acromioclavicular dislocation. However, in children less than this age, the injury is more likely to be a fracture of the distal clavicle or pseudodislocation. The classification in children is based on the position of the distal clavicle and the accompanying injury to the periosteal tube rather than on injury of the ligaments as occurs in a true dislocation. The Rockwood classification of injuries of the distal clavicle in children is as follows (Fig. 14–21).

Type I. Mild ligamentous sprain of the acromioclavicular ligaments without disruption of the periosteal tube. The distal clavicle is stable on examination, and x-rays are normal compared to the opposite shoulder.

Type II. There is partial disruption of the dorsal periosteal tube with some instability at the distal clavicle on examination. Radiographically, there is a slight widening of the acromioclavicular joint but no change in the coracoclavicular interval.

Type III. There is a large dorsal longitudinal split in the periosteal tube with gross instability of the distal clavicle. Radiographs reveal superior displacement of the clavicle in relation to the coracoid and acromion. The coracoclavicular interval is 25% to 100% greater than that on the normal shoulder.

Type IV. This injury is similar to a type III injury, but the distal clavicle is displaced posteriorly and is buttonholed through the trapezius muscle fibers with the distal end completely buried in muscle [154]. On an anteroposterior (AP) radiograph, there is widening of the acromioclavicular joint but little superior migration, similar to a type II injury. The axillary radiograph reveals posterior displacement of the distal clavicle in relation to the acromion.

Type V. There is a complete dorsal periosteal split with superior subcutaneous displacement of the clavicle. This is often associated with a split of the deltoid and trapezius attachments. On radiographs the coracoclavicular distance is greater than 100% compared to the normal shoulder.

Type VI. An inferior dislocation of the distal clavicle occurs with the distal clavicle lodged beneath the coracoid process [165].

Fractures of the coracoid, through the tip or at the base, can mimic distal clavicular fractures [155, 174, 183]. Clinically, these fractures are similar to type II distal clavicular injuries, but radiographically there is no widening of the acromioclavicular joint or the coracoclavicular distance. These fractures can be easily diagnosed on the Stryker notch x-ray view.

Radiographic Examination

As is evident from this classification, adequate radiographic views are necessary to classify injuries of the distal clavicle and acromioclavicular joint in children and adolescents [161, 168, 171]. Routine radiographic views of the shoulder are often well centered on the glenohumeral joint and therefore allow too much penetration to visualize the distal clavicle and acromioclavicular joint adequately. Films using a soft tissue technique allow adequate visualization and should be requested. The axillary lateral view and a 20-degree cephalic tilt view can further demonstrate the displacement involved in fractures in the distal clavicle region. As previously mentioned, the Stryker notch view should be used to rule out fractures involving the coracoid base or tip.

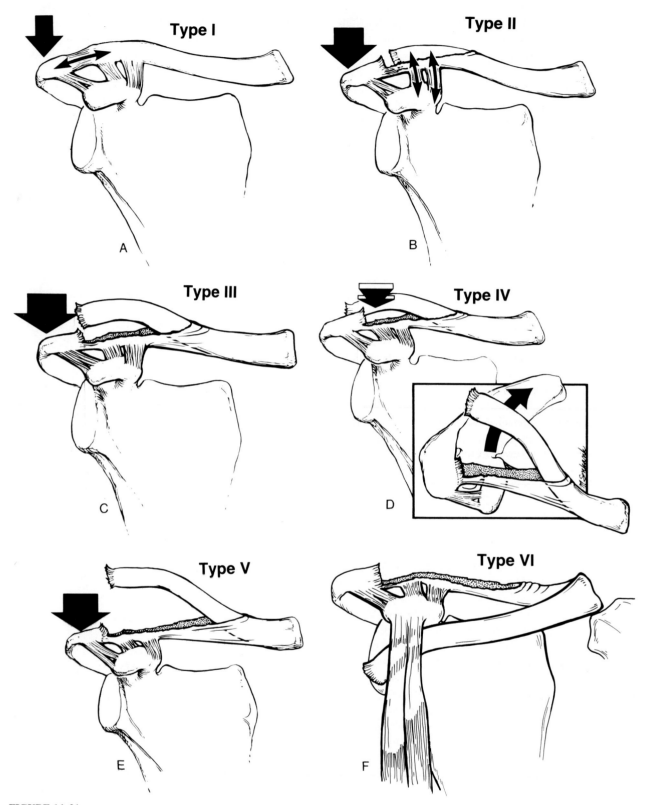

FIGURE 14–21
The Rockwood Classification for distal clavicle injuries in children. Refer to the text for a complete description of this classification system. (Reproduced with permission from Rockwood, C. A., Jr., and Green, D. P. [Eds.], *Fractures* (3 vols.). 2nd ed. Philadelphia, J. B. Lippincott, 1984.)

When injury to the distal clavicle is suspected but not well defined on routine views, "stress" radiographs can be requested. Stress radiographs using an AP soft tissue technique of both acromioclavicular joint regions are taken simultaneously on the same x-ray cassette. The first view is taken without weights, and the second stress view is taken with weights suspended from the wrists. Five to ten pounds of traction are applied longitudinally by looping stockinette around the patient's wrists. Measurements of the coracoclavicular distance on the affected side can then be compared to the normal side to help classify the distal clavicular injury. A type I injury demonstrates no difference on comparison views. In type II injuries, the coracoclavicular distance is increased less than 25% from side to side. In type III injuries, the displacement is 25% to 100%, and in type V injuries the coracoclavicular distance is increased by more than 100%. A type IV injury is best demonstrated on the axillary lateral view, which shows the clavicle displaced posteriorly in its relationship to the acromion.

Treatment Options

Most current authors agree that distal clavicular injuries in children and adolescents represent fractures through the distal physis or pseudodislocations rather than true adultlike acromioclavicular separations [157, 161–163, 169, 173, 176, 178]. The medial clavicular fragment herniates through the periosteal tube that remains in continuity with the distal epiphyseal fragment and the coracoclavicular ligaments below. There is tremendous potential for fracture healing and remodeling in this region (Fig. 14–22). Rockwood, who described the classification system in this chapter, indicated that open reduction and internal fixation was reserved for type IV, V, and VI injuries that show fixed deformity or gross displacement. He and his associates believe that type I, II, and III injuries all are expected to heal solidly and to remodel without long-term sequelae [161, 180].

Falstie-Jensen and Mikkelsen [163] reported two cases of pseudodislocation of the distal clavicle that were treated surgically with good results. They argued that failure to address the injury surgically led to permanent deformity and dysfunction. Ogden [176] recognized in a series of 14 cases that this injury did represent a true physeal fracture rather than a true acromioclavicular dislocation in patients younger than 13 years old. He recommended closed reduction or nonoperative treatment for most cases but pin fixation if instability was present. He presented an example of clavicular reduplication that resulted from formation of bone in the periosteal tube and argued that this was an indication for open reduction and internal fixation.

Eidman and colleagues [162] concluded from their series of 25 children that true acromioclavicular dislocation does not occur in children under the age of 13 years. Although all patients in their series were treated surgically, these investigators concluded that nonoperative treatment could be utilized in children less than 13 years old and should produce good or excellent results.

Havranek [169] found that in all children in his series, distal clavicular physeal injuries healed without functional sequelae regardless of the type of treatment. However, in cases with great displacement, he recommended surgical reduction with internal fixation for cosmetic reasons. More recently, Black and colleagues [157] reported 48 cases of distal clavicular injury in children under 16 years old who were treated nonoperatively; all patients resumed full activity and regained full motion without major complaints at follow-up.

Reports from the adult literature seem to agree that nonoperative treatment for types I, II, and III acromioclavicular joint dislocations leads to acceptable results in terms of motion, strength, and function [156, 160, 164, 166, 170, 172, 179, 181, 182]. Although cosmetic results leave a residual deformity, if the shoulder is accurately rehabilitated several series have shown that return of strength, motion, and function is complete [172, 184]. Only rarely do type III injuries leave residual pain and dysfunction [159, 177]. It appears, therefore, from both the pediatric and adult literature that surgical treatment for these injuries involving the distal clavicle is limited to fractures with gross displacement such as types IV, V, and VI.

Complications

Few complications have been associated with this injury. Cosmetic deformity such as prominence or reduplication of the clavicle can occur but rarely causes a functional deficit.

Author's Preferred Method of Treatment

For all children up through the age of 13 years and for older adolescents who are skeletally immature, I believe that most injuries of the distal clavicle can be treated in a nonoperative fashion. This reservation certainly applies to all Rockwood type I, II, and III injuries.

In children with type IV, V, and VI injuries surgical treatment is carried out to accomplish reduction and stable fixation. In the older adolescent athlete who participates in sports requiring repetitive overhead activity such as throwing, tennis, or swimming, I believe that surgical treatment is also indicated.

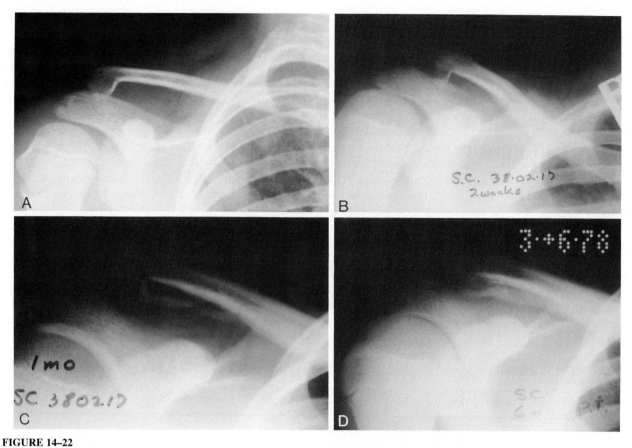

FIGURE 14–22

This 12-year-old soccer player fell on the point of his right shoulder, sustaining a fracture of the distal clavicle. *A,* X-ray film taken shortly after injury. *B,* At 2 weeks, x-ray film demonstrates some early periosteal new bone formation. *C,* At 1 month, the periosteal tube is evident inferiorly as it fills with periosteal new bone. *D,* At 6 months, the fracture has completely healed clinically and the periosteal tube has filled in.

Conservative care consists of a short period of immobilization followed by progressive range of motion and strengthening exercises. Most fractures will heal and function will be regained within 4 to 6 weeks. Return to sports is delayed until full shoulder motion and strength are obtained. Residual bony prominence is not a contraindication to return to sports.

Surgical treatment is carried out through a superior strap-type incision overlying a point 2 cm medial to the acromioclavicular joint. Reduction is accomplished, and repair of the periosteal tube is carried out using heavy suture. In the older patient, supplemental temporary fixation is accomplished with a coracoclavicular screw [7]. This screw is removed in 6 weeks when rehabilitation is begun.

INJURIES TO THE MEDIAL END OF THE CLAVICLE

The sternoclavicular joint in children is much less commonly affected by injuries than the physis or medial metaphysis. Most injuries about the medial end of the

clavicle involve the medial physeal plate and occur as Salter-Harris type I or type II fractures. True dislocations of the sternoclavicular joint in children are reported but are extremely rare. Injuries in this region constitute less than 1% of all fractures of the clavicle and account for only 6% of clavicular fractures in all age groups [208]. Injuries to the medial clavicle can occur in athletic events, predominantly in contact or collision sports. The most common mechanism is an indirect blow applied to the lateral aspect of the shoulder that transmits force along the clavicle, resulting in a fracture in the region of the physis medially. This can occur in a pile-up when the affected shoulder contacts the ground as the weight of other players lands on the contralateral shoulder. If the shoulder is compressed and rolls forward, a posterior displacement at the medial end occurs. If the shoulder is compressed and forced posteriorly, anterior displacement occurs at the medial clavicle [189, 193, 208]. Direct blows to the medial clavicle may also result in fracture. These forces are commonly applied directly and can produce either nondisplaced or posteriorly displaced fractures.

Since the most common injury in this region is a

fracture involving the medial physeal plate, the Salter-Harris classification is best utilized to describe these fractures [208]. Type I and type II injuries are the most common. These injuries are further classified according to the direction of displacement of the shaft fragment. The epiphysis commonly stays attached to the sternoclavicular joint at the sternum while the shaft is displaced either anteriorly or posteriorly. The direction of displacement is somewhat difficult to determine because of the swelling that occurs in the area. Certainly, posterior displacement can be a life-threatening emergency, and rapid diagnosis is important. Extraphyseal fractures involving the metaphysis can also occur but are much less common. Sternoclavicular dislocations have been reported as well, but most of these were probably unrecognized injuries to the epiphyseal plate.

Clinical Evaluation

The patient commonly describes an indirect injury that causes immediate pain and often a feeling of a "pop" in the region of the medial clavicle (Fig. 14–23).

The ipsilateral arm is supported across the chest by the opposite hand. Swelling can be substantial. Tenderness to palpation is notable, and crepitus may be present. The head is often tilted toward the side of the injury owing to the spasm within the sternocleidomastoid muscle. Deformity is commonly present, but the direction of displacement of the shaft fragment can be masked by swelling in the region of the injury. Careful palpation along the superior aspect of the sternum and along the shaft fragment can help to determine the relative position of the clavicular shaft to the remaining sternoclavicular joint. Nondisplaced fractures or minimally displaced fractures in this region in the younger child often present late as a mass effect when callus builds up around the healing fracture. If it is determined that posterior displacement of the shaft fragment exists, this may become a medical emergency [188, 202, 214, 215]. The posteriorly displaced fragment can impinge on structures within the mediastinum including the innominate vessels, trachea, or esophagus. Ipsilateral venous congestion, diminished pulses, difficulty in breathing, or a sensation of choking and difficulty in swallowing should all be recognized as possible signs of impingement.

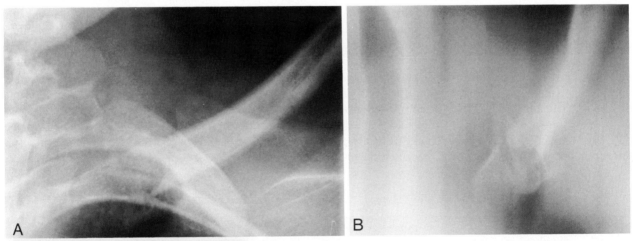

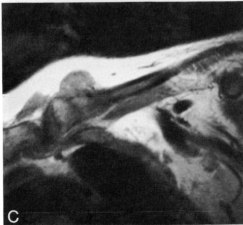

FIGURE 14–23
This 13-year-old football player complained of pain in the medial clavicular region after a pile-up. *A*, Anteroposterior (AP) radiograph shows indistinct fracture of the medial clavicle. *B*, Tomographic view more clearly defines the fracture line. *C*, MRI scan of this same region demonstrates early fracture callus.

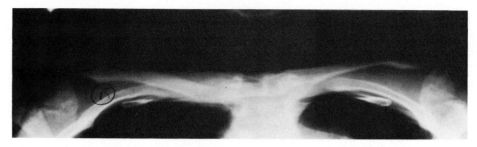

FIGURE 14–24
Serendipity view. This patient has sustained a posteriorly displaced injury to the medial clavicle. The medial clavicle can be compared side to side on this film to help determine relative displacement.

Radiographic Examination

Adding to the difficulty of diagnosis of fractures about the medial clavicle is the fact that radiographic visualization in this area is difficult. Standard anteroposterior views are confusing because the medial clavicle overlaps with structures in the mediastinum and spine. Additionally, x-ray views that are angled 90 degrees to each other to confirm displacement of fragments are virtually impossible to obtain in this region. Today, a simple and effective technique using a tangential x-ray view as described by Rockwood is the first step in visualizing fractures in this region [208]. The so-called *serendipity view* is a 40-degree cephalad-directed x-ray beam on a chest cassette that projects the medial clavicles bilaterally above the rib cage and other structures that overlap in this area (Fig. 14–24). The relative positions of the medial clavicle can be compared side to side on the same x-ray film. Although this view is helpful in distinguishing between a fracture of the medial clavicle and an injury to the epiphyseal plate, it is still difficult to view this area accurately. The CT scan has revolutionized x-ray visualization of this difficult anatomic area [194, 195, 201, 203]. CT scans can accurately distinguish fractures from dislocations involving the medial clavicle and can demonstrate displacement of the fragments either anteriorly or posteriorly (Fig. 14–25).

Treatment Options

As with most fractures in children involving the epiphyseal plate, fractures of the medial clavicle are characterized by rapid healing and vigorous remodeling. Nonunion and significant malunion in this fracture have not been reported. Anteriorly displaced fractures that most commonly mimic sternoclavicular joint dislocations can be treated expectantly [190, 200, 210]. A gentle attempt at closed reduction can be performed under local or general anesthesia. The patient is placed supine on a table with a bolster lying vertically between the scapulae. The arm is abducted to 90 degrees and then extended while direct pressure is placed on the anteriorly displaced shaft fragment. After reduction, immobilization is accomplished in a well-padded figure-of-eight dressing or spica cast. These fractures become stable rapidly during the first 2 to 4 weeks. Many of these fractures, however, are unstable after reduction despite the limited immobilization described. Despite this instability, these fractures heal and remodel rapidly. There is

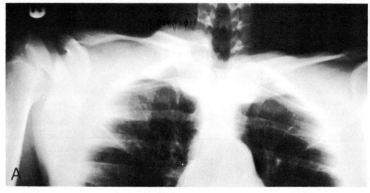
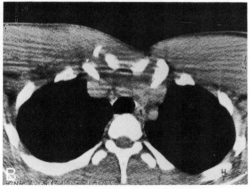

FIGURE 14–25
This 15-year-old football quarterback was hit from the left side while his right shoulder was on the ground. He sustained an anterior injury to the medial clavicle. *A,* This plain radiograph demonstrates obvious displacement in this region. *B,* On the coronal CT scan, the anterior Salter-Harris Type II injury is apparent and anteriorly displaced.

no indication for open reduction and internal fixation in an anteriorly displaced fracture. The hazards of internal fixation at the medial clavicle or across the sternoclavicular joint have been well described, including broken and migrating pins that have penetrated the lung, heart, or great vessels [192, 204, 205]. Due to the tremendous potential for remodeling at the medial physis, even substantial residual displacement can be expected to heal and remodel quite well.

Fractures of the medial clavicle with posterior displacement can require emergency reduction if structures within the mediastinum are thought to be compromised [191, 196, 197, 199, 206, 207, 211–213]. Compromise of mediastinal structures after posterior displacement is rare and probably is more rare in children than in adults. If the examination reveals ipsilateral diminished pulses, venous engorgement, or evidence of impingement on the trachea or esophagus, emergency reduction is required. Under general anesthesia, the patient is placed supine with a bolster placed between the shoulders posteriorly. Traction is applied to the arm while the medial clavicular area is sterilely prepared and a towel clip is used percutaneously to exert lateral and anterior traction on the displaced medial clavicular shaft fragment. This fragment is usually delivered anteriorly without difficulty, but open reduction may be required in some cases. After reduction is accomplished, the shoulder is usually stable. Limited immobilization with a figure-of-eight dressing is used for 3 to 4 weeks. Rapid healing and remodeling are expected.

Author's Preferred Method of Treatment

Fractures of the medial clavicle in children with anterior displacement are confirmed by CT scan. When marked displacement and clinical deformity are present, a gentle attempt at closed reduction is made. A figure-of-eight strap is used after reduction. There is no indication for open reduction and internal fixation in this injury. Gentle motion exercises are started as pain allows. Most fractures become stable in 3 to 4 weeks, at which time a vigorous rehabilitation program can be started. Return to sports participation requires full shoulder motion without pain or instability and shoulder strength equal to that in the opposite arm.

In cases of posterior displacement, an appropriate physical examination to assess possible impingement on the mediastinal structures is carried out. If the patient is stable, a CT scan is performed to assess the position of the displaced fragment. An attempt at reduction is made in every case with the patient under general anesthesia. Closed reduction applying percutaneous traction with a towel clip is usually successful, but open reduction is

accomplished if necessary. Bony healing requires 4 to 6 weeks, and rehabilitation parallels that described for anterior displacement. Return to contact sports should be delayed at least 8 weeks to confirm stability at the fracture site.

FRACTURES OF THE SCAPULA

Fractures of the scapula represent approximately 1% of all fractures in children and adolescents [223, 224, 240]. These injuries are most commonly a result of direct trauma in collision sports such as football and rugby. Avulsion fractures of the coracoid and glenoid can also result from indirect trauma, and stress fractures from repetitive activity have also been reported [218, 220, 230].

Most of the available articles on scapular fractures include pediatric and adolescent patients but do not differentiate between diagnostic and therapeutic differences [217, 219, 229, 231, 232, 237, 242, 244]. Scapular fractures as a result of direct high-energy injuries in vehicular trauma are associated with other injuries, even life-threatening injuries, in 80% to 95% of cases. Sports injuries commonly result from lower energy trauma and are rarely associated with other severe injuries.

The scapula develops from many ossification centers that are quite variable in both number and time of appearance and fusion. This variability can make radiographic diagnosis in children's scapular fractures confusing and difficult [222, 233, 236, 239, 243].

Scapular fractures in children are sufficiently uncommon that no classification scheme has been described in the literature. Therefore, scapular fractures will be discussed here based on the specific anatomic location of the fracture in the scapula including fractures of the scapular body and neck, glenoid, acromion, and coracoid.

Fractures of the Body and Neck of the Scapula

Fractures of the body and the neck of the scapula result from a severe direct blow (Fig. 14–26). This fracture can occur when a player is fully extended and unprotected and receives a direct blow or else is upended, landing on the posterior aspect of the shoulder. Although these fractures are associated with significant other systemic injuries in 35% to 90% of cases, these cases are associated with polytrauma, usually vehicular, and this high incidence has not been reported in scapular fractures in sports. Ipsilateral rib fractures with pneumothorax or pulmonary contusion can occur in up to 50% of cases [224, 232, 237]. Fractures of the cervical spine

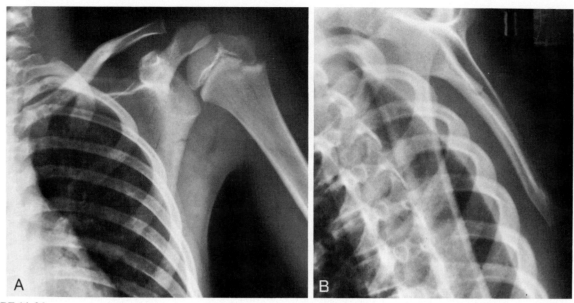

FIGURE 14–26
AP *(A)* and true scapular *(B)* radiographs of the scapula demonstrate a nondisplaced fracture through the body. This patient had been tackled and slammed to the turf directly on the posterior aspect of the shoulder.

and clavicle and brachial plexus injuries are also reported and should be diligently excluded in the evaluation.

Clinically, swelling, pain, and tenderness to palpation are present. The arm is usually supported by the other arm, and motion is avoided. Deformity is occasionally present. Careful evaluation of the pulmonary and neurovascular status should be carried out. These patients commonly are unable to initiate contraction in the rotator cuff musculature and present with a "pseudoparalysis" or "pseudorupture." The pathogenesis of this pseudorupture is hemorrhage from the fracture within the muscle bellies of the supraspinatus, infraspinatus, subscapularis, and teres minor that causes enough pain to inhibit muscular contraction reflexively.

Radiographs are diagnostic in cases of fracture of the body and neck of the scapula. It is important to visualize the scapula in two planes, using a *true AP view* of the shoulder as well as a *true scapular lateral* view. For further detail, a CT scan can also be helpful to rule out extension of the fracture into the base of the coracoid or glenoid.

The literature does not clearly describe specific treatment for children with fractures of the scapular body. In general, however, most authors agree that these fractures can be treated without surgery in most cases [217, 242, 244]. Ada and Miller [216] recently concluded that residual pain and weakness with exertion are associated with significantly displaced fractures and that open reduction and internal fixation is indicated.

Scapular body fractures can be treated symptomati-

cally with rest, analgesics, ice, and immobilization initially. Pain and swelling usually begin to subside during the first 5 to 7 days, and this increased comfort can be followed by a progressive program of exercises including shoulder range of motion and rotator cuff strengthening exercises. With a fracture of the body of the scapula, often a pseudoparalysis or pseudorupture of the rotator cuff occurs and should be expected. This pseudoparalysis usually resolves during the first 2 weeks after injury. These fractures heal in 4 to 6 weeks. As with other children's fractures, considerable remodeling can be expected, even with displaced fractures. Excellent functional results can be obtained, even in fractures with substantial overlap and shortening of the scapular neck. There is no indication for open reduction and internal fixation of scapular fractures in children and adolescents [229].

The patient with a scapular body or neck fracture can be allowed to return to sports participation after full range of shoulder motion and shoulder girdle strength equal to that of the opposite side are regained.

Fractures of the Glenoid

Fractures of the glenoid represent approximately 10% of all scapular fractures [219, 226, 227]. Although Ideberg [231] has classified fractures of the glenoid into five separate groups in the adult, in children we can separate these intra-articular fractures into just two types: (1) glenoid rim fractures, which are associated

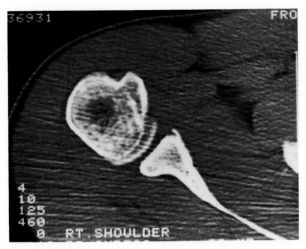

FIGURE 14–27
This CT scan of the shoulder demonstrates an anterior glenoid rim fracture after recurrent dislocation.

with residual instability of the glenohumeral joint, and (2) glenoid fossa fractures, which extend into the scapular body and neck.

Fractures involving the glenoid rim can occur on the anterior or posterior surface (Fig. 14–27). Smaller avulsion-type fractures are associated with glenohumeral dislocations and are of little consequence [228, 230]. Larger rim fractures occur when a lateral force drives the humeral head directly against the glenoid rim, shearing a bony fragment. This can happen when a player is tackled and lands directly on the shoulder. The second group of fractures, which extend across the glenoid fossa back into the neck and body of the scapula, also result from a direct blow to the lateral aspect of the shoulder. Usually the fracture involves the common physis for the upper fourth of the glenoid and the base of the coracoid. Severe displacement of these intra-articular fractures is extremely rare.

Avulsion fractures of the rim of the glenoid associated with dislocations of the glenohumeral joint are the most common type. These fractures can be treated as if for a dislocation. Large glenoid rim fragments that render the joint unstable may require open reduction and internal fixation. This must be an uncommon entity in children and adolescents, because there are no reports of it in the literature [218, 226].

Fractures that occur through the glenoid fossa and extend into the body of the scapula are rarely substantially displaced. These fractures heal quite rapidly, and remodeling of the glenoid occurs even with displacement. After an initial period of immobilization, rest, analgesics, and ice, an early program of motion designed to help the intact humeral head mold the glenoid to a congruent surface is begun. Healing is expected in 4 to 6 weeks. Return to competitive sports is allowed when a full range of motion and strength equal to that of the opposite side are regained.

Fractures of the Acromion

Even though the acromion is quite prominent, it is rarely fractured in any age group. A severe direct blow to the point of the acromion is more likely to result in a distal clavicle fracture-dislocation or an acromioclavicular joint injury rather than a fracture of the acromion.

Failure of one of the multiple acromial epiphyses to fuse can lead to the *unfused os acromiale* variant [234, 241] (Fig. 14–28). This entity should not be mistaken for a fracture on routine radiographs. It is associated with problems of impingement in the older adolescent athlete who uses the arm for overhead sports such as pitching, swimming, or tennis.

Fractures of the acromion are rarely displaced, and most can be treated symptomatically with 5 to 7 days of rest and immobilization followed by an aggressive rehabilitation program. As in other fractures of the scapula, the requirement for return to play should include a full range of motion of the shoulder and protective strength equal to that of the opposite side.

Fractures of the Coracoid

Fractures of the coracoid occur at the base through the common physis for the coracoid and the superior portion

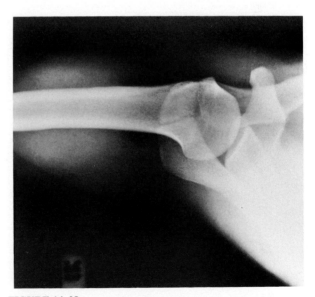

FIGURE 14–28
Axillary radiograph of the shoulder demonstrates an unfused os acromiale in an 18-year-old baseball pitcher. This can lead to impingement in the older adolescent athlete who uses the arm for overhead sports such as pitching, swimming, or tennis.

of the glenoid [225, 238]. These fractures are the result of an avulsion mechanism when the point of the acromion and scapula are driven inferiorly in a fall on the point of the shoulder. The coracoclavicular ligaments maintain their integrity and avulse the coracoid through its common physis (Fig. 14–29). This fracture can mimic an injury to the acromioclavicular joint region or distal clavicle [235]. Clinically the ipsilateral arm is supported, and the acromioclavicular joint region may be tender and slightly prominent. There is anterior pain in response to direct palpation over the coracoid and occasionally ecchymosis. Motion is restricted. Radiographic diagnosis can be difficult on routine views. The axillary lateral view shows the tip of the coracoid, but often the base is obscured by bony overlap. The *Stryker notch view* is used to demonstrate the coracoid in profile. A fracture at the base is quite evident on this view. Significant displacement is rare. Treatment is nonoperative using supportive measures including a sling until the acute pain and swelling have diminished. A progressive range of motion and strengthening program then follows. Healing and return to sports usually require 6 weeks.

GLENOHUMERAL JOINT SUBLUXATION AND DISLOCATION

The shoulder joint is the most commonly dislocated major joint in adolescents and adults but is less commonly involved in children before they reach skeletal

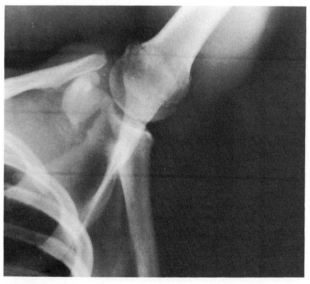

FIGURE 14–29
A Stryker notch x-ray view of the shoulder demonstrates a fracture through the base of the coracoid. Note the callus that is present on the medial aspect of the fracture. These injuries can be missed on initial examination and x-ray without the appropriate Stryker notch view.

maturity. The incidence figures for instability of the shoulder in skeletally immature patients demonstrate a range of from 1% to 5% based on the age criteria used for classification [249, 282, 298]. In Rowe's classic series in 1956 [298], a review of 500 dislocated shoulders found that only eight patients were less than 10 years old, whereas 99 patients were between 10 and 20 years old. Wagner and Lyne [307] presented a series of 9 children with open epiphyses out of 212 patients with traumatic glenohumeral dislocations, which represents a 4.7% incidence rate. Heck [268] and Foster and colleagues [263] reported cases of true glenohumeral dislocation due to trauma in children less than 10 years of age. Many reports in the literature on shoulder instability include patients between the ages of 11 and 20 years, but no attempt is made to identify patients who are skeletally immature [249, 252, 258, 260, 270, 272, 273, 278, 286, 291, 294]. Shoulder instability in children less than 10 years old is thought to be relatively rare. Although shoulder instability in the adolescent is much more common, true incidence data for shoulder instability in skeletally immature patients in the age group from 11 to 16 years is difficult to determine from the literature.

Classification

Shoulder instability can be classified by degree of instability, direction of instability, and the etiology of the dislocation. The etiologic classification is the most important when formulating treatment options and when predicting prognosis.

Degree of Instability
    Subluxation
    Dislocation
Direction of Instability
    Anterior
    Posterior
    Inferior (luxatio erecta)
    Multidirectional

Anterior dislocations of the glenohumeral joint in children are the most common of these injuries, constituting greater than 90%. Isolated cases of posterior dislocation in children and adolescents have been reported, but true traumatic posterior instability of the shoulder is as rare in this age group as it is in adults. Luxatio erecta due to extreme trauma has been described in children and has been reported in at least two cases [19]. As more is learned about multidirectional shoulder instability, this common and important form of shoulder instability is being more readily appreciated so that proper treatment can be instituted.

Etiology of Instability
   Traumatic instability
   Atraumatic instability
      Voluntary
      Involuntary
   Recurrent instability

To be classified as a case of traumatic instability, a history of significant high-energy trauma and an appropriate mechanism should exist. Atraumatic instability of the glenohumeral joint occurs only in the presence of multidirectional laxity of the shoulder. Recurrent instability can exist after either traumatic or atraumatic primary instability.

Traumatic Instability

Clinical Evaluation

Anterior instability of the glenohumeral joint is the most common form of this injury. To qualify as a traumatic dislocation, a history of significant trauma should exist [13, 22, 48, 49]. A fall on an outstretched hand that forces the arm into excessive abduction and external rotation is the primary mechanism of injury. The humeral head is levered anteriorly, tearing the anterior glenohumeral ligament complex and eventually dislocating, with the humeral head lodging against the anterior neck of the glenoid. Quite commonly, this results in the Bankart-type injury, in which the glenohumeral ligament attachment is stripped off the anterior neck of the glenoid (Fig. 14–30). Traumatic dislocations of the shoulder are seen frequently in all collision and contact sports.

Traumatic posterior dislocations are not commonly reported in children but would be expected in the same proportion relative to anterior dislocation as seen in adults [16, 17, 21, 39, 47, 56, 61]. If all age groups are included, 2% to 4% of all dislocations of the shoulder can be expected to occur posteriorly. Both direct and indirect mechanisms can result in posterior instability. A blow to the outstretched arm when the shoulder is adducted, internally rotated, and flexed can drive the shoulder out posteriorly. Also, a direct blow to the anterior aspect of the shoulder can force the humeral head out posteriorly. Both mechanisms occur in contact sports. We must not forget that it is not uncommon to see posterior dislocations associated with convulsions. The humerus is dislocated posteriorly by a violent contraction of the strong shoulder internal rotators during seizure activity. Any complaint of shoulder pain in an athlete who has suffered a convulsion should be taken seriously, and a posterior dislocation should be suspected.

The patient with a traumatic glenohumeral anterior dislocation presents with obvious deformity, often with swelling, and always with pain. The deformity consists of a very prominent acromion with an area below the acromion that is void of the usual fullness associated with a normally positioned humeral head. The humeral head is located anteriorly and sometimes can be visualized or palpated in the axilla. The arm is commonly held in a slightly abducted, externally rotated position, usually supported by the opposite hand. There is pain with attempted motion. Careful examination should be carried out to assess the neurologic and vascular status because reports of both nerve and vessel injury have been cited. The axillary nerve is the nerve most commonly injured with anterior dislocation, but the entire brachial plexus can be involved. Careful examination of the axillary nerve can be accomplished quite easily. The sensory distribution of the axillary nerve is along the upper lateral arm and can be tested by light touch or pinprick. The axillary nerve innervates the deltoid and teres minor muscles. By supporting the elbow with one hand and grasping the deltoid lightly with the other hand, motor

FIGURE 14–30
Schematic diagram in the coronal plane of the humeral head and glenoid in anterior traumatic dislocation. Note the Perthe's or Bankart lesion, stripping of the anterior ligaments off the glenoid rim, and the Hill-Sachs compression fracture on the posterior aspect of the humeral head.

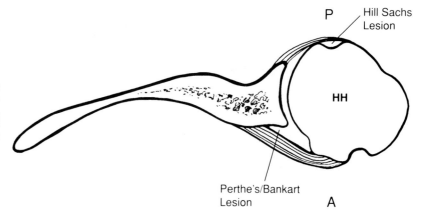

innervation can be tested by having the patient voluntarily contract the deltoid in an attempt to lightly abduct the elbow (Fig. 14–31). This can be accomplished without undue pain to the patient.

Traumatic posterior dislocation is less apparent on clinical examination and may be easily missed. Many times a quick review of the patient reveals no deformity. On closer inspection, looking at the shoulder from above, flattening of the anterior aspect of the shoulder is noted with fullness posteriorly. The arm is held internally rotated with the hand across the abdomen. The coracoid is usually slightly prominent. The shoulder is painful, and the patient resists any motion. The hallmark of diagnosis of posterior dislocation is the lack of shoul-

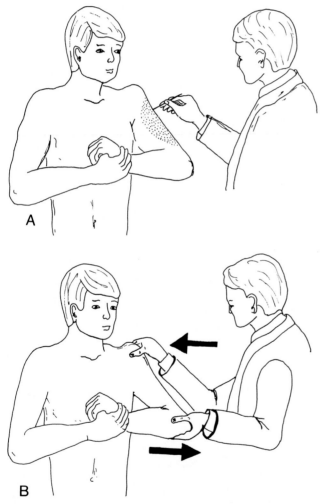

FIGURE 14–31
Clinical examination of axillary nerve function should be carried out in every patient with anterior dislocation. *A*, Sensory examination to light touch and pinprick can be carried out in the area on the upper lateral arm. *B*, Motor testing for deltoid function can be carried out by grasping the deltoid in one hand, while resisting abduction with the other. Any ability to contract in this position would mean that the axillary nerve is intact.

der external rotation and an inability to supinate the forearm. These findings are difficult to elicit in the acute situation, and the lack of clinical physical findings can lead the examiner into a false sense of security.

Radiographic Findings

In anterior glenohumeral instability, the radiographic diagnosis is usually quite clear. On an AP view the humeral head is situated anterior and inferior to its usual position in the glenoid. There is overlapping of the humeral head adjacent to the glenoid. A lateral radiograph is important to confirm the position of the humeral head, and this can be accomplished with either an axillary lateral view or a true scapular lateral view. Postreduction films are important in both the AP and lateral planes to confirm the position of reduction. Common radiographic lesions present in patients with anterior instability include a posterolateral humeral head indentation fracture (Hill-Sachs lesion) (Fig. 14–32). Anterior glenoid rim fractures or deficiencies should also be noted on the postreduction anteroposterior and lateral views [13, 48, 49, 59].

Historically, posterior glenohumeral dislocations are commonly misdiagnosed on initial radiographs. In adults, up to 60% of these injuries are missed on initial radiographs owing to inadequate study. The glenohumeral joint must be visualized in two planes oriented at 90 degrees to each other to adequately eliminate posterior dislocation as a diagnosis. The *trauma series* is recommended; this includes an *AP view* of the glenohumeral joint as well as a *true scapular lateral view* and an *axillary lateral view*. With appropriate lateral radiographs, this diagnosis should easily be made. On the AP view, the findings are often quite subtle. The "empty glenoid sign," in which the articular surface of the humeral head does not seem to fit appropriately into the glenoid fossa, is often present. On the axillary lateral view, the humeral head can easily be seen posterior to the glenoid fossa, and many times a "reversed" Hill-Sachs lesion is present on the anterior surface of the humeral head. On the true scapular lateral view, the humeral head can also be seen posterior to the glenoid. After reduction, fractures of the glenoid rim can be assessed, and the reversed Hill-Sachs lesion is also noted.

Treatment

The literature on specific treatment for traumatic glenohumeral instability in the skeletally immature patient is extremely limited [4, 13, 23, 37, 62]. In the acute situation, the humerus should undergo closed reduction by one of the standard and accepted techniques. Light

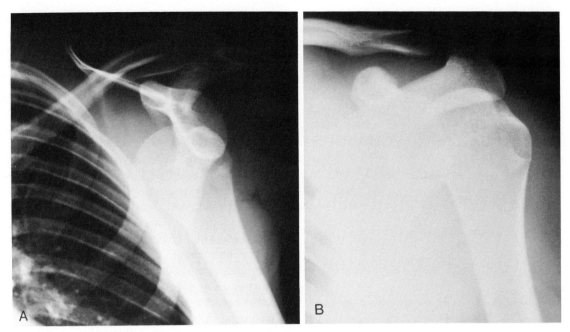

FIGURE 14–32
Anterior dislocation of the shoulder. *A*, AP radiograph demonstrates anteroinferior dislocation of the left shoulder. *B*, After reduction, this x-ray film demonstrates the posterolateral compression fracture known as the Hill-Sachs lesion.

sedation with either an intravenous or intramuscular technique is usually adequate for reduction. Several methods have been described including the traction-countertraction technique, the Stimson maneuver, and the abduction maneuver. Any maneuver that gently and carefully reduces the joint is acceptable.

The traction-countertraction technique is accomplished with the patient in the supine position. Longitudinal traction is applied to the arm on a continuous basis while countertraction is applied to the thorax by means of a sheet passed around the patient. The humeral head is disengaged from the anterior glenoid rim and reduces once the shoulder musculature is fatigued by traction (Fig. 14–33).

The Stimson maneuver is carried out with the patient lying prone and the dislocated arm hanging off the edge of the table. Weights up to 10 pounds are suspended from the patient's wrist. Spontaneous reduction occurs as the shoulder musculature is relaxed by the traction (Fig. 14–34).

Closed reduction by the abduction maneuver is performed with the patient in the supine position. The arm is gently abducted and externally rotated into an overhead position. The arm is then adducted while external rotation is maintained; the surgeon then gently brings the arm in front of the patient while rotating it internally. This very gentle technique is best used by the experienced surgeon.

Postreduction care is a highly controversial point. In the limited literature available on this injury in the child,

it is inconclusive whether immobilization after reduction truly alters the prognosis [2, 4, 10, 13, 26, 37, 49, 52, 58, 62, 63]. After a period of immobilization, an aggressive rehabilitation program that focuses on strengthening the rotator cuff and deltoid should be instituted. The most common problem associated with traumatic anterior dislocation of the shoulder is recurrent instability.

Posterior glenohumeral dislocation is reduced with traction in line with the deformity. Counteraction is applied to the chest while simultaneously applying a direct

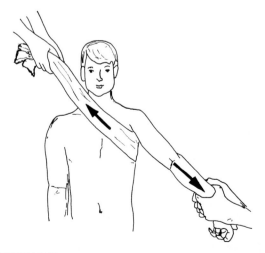

FIGURE 14–33
Traction–countertraction maneuver for reduction of anterior dislocation of the shoulder.

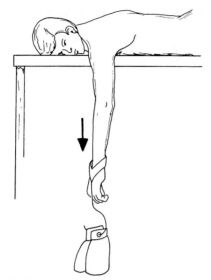

FIGURE 14–34
Stimson maneuver for reduction of anterior dislocation of the shoulder.

anterior pull. The arm is immobilized in neutral or slight external rotation with the arm at the side. This may require a modified spica cast or custom-made brace.

Atraumatic Dislocations

This is probably the most common type of instability in children and adolescents, but it is often not recognized on initial presentation. An underlying multidirectional laxity of the shoulder is a prerequisite for atraumatic instability. Although multidirectional laxity may be associated with true syndromes of collagen deficiency such as Marfan's syndrome and Ehlers-Danlos syndrome, in most patients this excessive joint laxity is just an extreme variant of normal [11, 31, 45, 46, 60].

Clinical Evaluation

A shoulder "dislocation" in a child without a clear-cut significant history of trauma should arouse suspicion that this may be an instance of atraumatic instability. These patients have inherent joint laxity, and the glenohumeral joint can be dislocated either voluntarily or involuntarily as a result of minimal trauma (Fig. 14–35). Episodes such as this may occur with throwing, hitting an overhead serve in tennis or volleyball, or just pushing the body up from the prone position. These episodes do not constitute significant trauma, and a high index of suspicion should be maintained in such cases for atraumatic instability. Voluntary instability is accomplished by the consciously firing certain muscle groups while inhibiting their antagonists. Combining this motor manipulation with certain arm positions allows the glenohumeral joint to dislocate. Voluntary instability is often associated with psychological instability [32, 36, 55, 57].

The most notable finding in these cases is the lack of pain associated with the subluxation or dislocation. In most cases a reduction is not required because spontaneous reduction occurs. Clinical examination shows evidence of multiple joint laxity, which may include hyperextensibility at the elbows, knees, and metacarpophalangeal joints. Skin hyperelasticity and striae may be present. In cases of acute trauma, the opposite shoulder should be examined for findings of multidirectional laxity because the affected shoulder may be too painful to undergo complete examination. These signs of multidirectional laxity at the glenohumeral joint include a positive sulcus sign and significant humeral head translation on anterior and posterior drawer tests [13, 20, 22]. The sulcus sign, a dimpling of the skin below the acromion when manual longitudinal traction is applied to the arm (Fig. 14–36), is due to inferior subluxation of the humeral head within the glenohumeral joint. The drawer test is performed with the examiner seated at the side of the patient. The scapula is stabilized with one hand while the opposite hand manually translates the humeral head anteriorly and posteriorly (Fig. 14–37). In patients with atraumatic instability these tests are all painless. With atraumatic instability, the glenohumeral joint is unstable anteriorly, posteriorly, and inferiorly, but the relative proportion of both posterior and inferior instability is much higher.

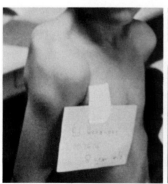
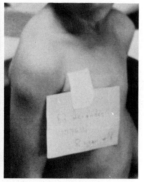

A   B

FIGURE 14–35
This 9-year-old boy complained of a dislocated shoulder after throwing a baseball. On close examination in the office, he can demonstrate voluntary ability to anteriorly and inferiorly dislocate his shoulder. (Reproduced with permission from Rockwood, C. A., and Green, D. P. [Eds.], *Fractures* (3 vols.). 2nd ed. Philadelphia, J. B. Lippincott, 1984.)

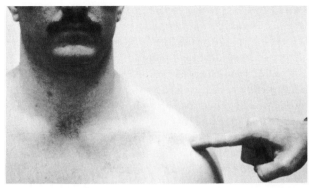

FIGURE 14–36
Sulcus sign. While longitudinal traction is applied to the arm, the humeral head subluxates inferiorly, causing a dimpling of the skin or sulcus sign below the acromion.

Radiographic Examination

In patients with atraumatic instability, radiographic evaluation is usually normal. Stress x-rays can be used to supplement the clinical examination to demonstrate instability in anterior, posterior, and inferior directions. The inferior component of multidirectional instability can be demonstrated by applying weights to the arm during an anteroposterior radiographic film. The Hill-Sachs lesion and anterior glenoid lesions are not characteristic of atraumatic instability.

Treatment Options

Treatment of patients with atraumatic instability should emphasize careful diagnosis, since the approach to treatment differs from treatment for true traumatic instability. A nonoperative approach emphasizing a vigorous rehabilitation program involving strengthening of the rotator cuff has been described for these patients [10, 45]. Most patients who do not have significant emotional or psychiatric problems successfully improve their shoulder stability with this program. Neer and Foster [291], in the classic description of multidirectional laxity, restricted surgical intervention to patients who failed a 12-month rehabilitation program. Burkhead and Rockwood [255] reported an 80% success rate in treatment of atraumatic instability with a vigorous rehabilitation program.

For patients with multidirectional laxity who fail to improve after a thorough rehabilitation program, capsular-type reconstruction has been recommended. The inferior capsular shift reconstruction was described by Neer and Foster specifically for patients with atraumatic instability due to multidirectional laxity who had failed a rehabilitation program [291].

Recurrent Dislocation of the Shoulder

The literature on the natural history of glenohumeral dislocation in adolescents and young adults demonstrates recurrence rates of 25% to 90% depending on the treatment program used after the initial dislocation [247, 253, 255]. The true incidence of recurrent dislocation of the glenohumeral joint after traumatic dislocation in a child is difficult to assess because of both the rarity of the injury and the variation in reports in the literature. Rowe [297], in 1963, reported a 100% incidence of recurrence in children with anterior dislocation who were less than 10 years of age. He reported a 94% incidence of recurrence in adolescent and young adult patients from 11 to 20 years old. Rockwood [258] reported in 1975 a recurrence rate of 50% in a series of adolescent patients between 13.8 and 15.8 years of age. Heck [268] reported a case of traumatic anterior dislocation in a 7-year-old boy who remained stable at 5-year follow-up. Wagner and Lyne [307] reported an 80% recurrence rate in 10

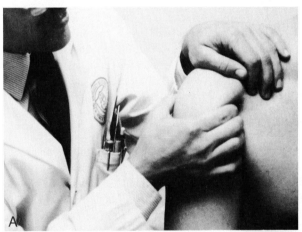

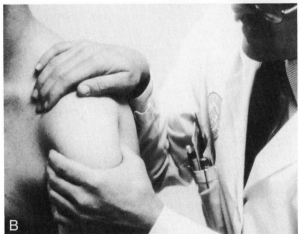

FIGURE 14–37
Drawer test. The examiner is seated beside the patient, who is comfortably relaxed. The examiner places one hand for stability on the scapula while grasping the humeral head and balloting anteriorly and posteriorly with the other hand.

patients with clearly open proximal humeral epiphyses. Most recently, Marans and associates [282] reported on the fate of 21 children between the ages of 4 and 15 years with open physes at the time of initial dislocation. They found a 100% recurrence rate no matter what post-reduction treatment program was used.

Treatment of the patient who has demonstrated recurrent anterior dislocation of the shoulder should begin with an attempt to confirm the cause of the dislocation. If it is determined that the patient has an atraumatic dislocation, a continued nonoperative approach is recommended. If it is determined that a recurrent dislocation has a true traumatic cause, treatment is surgical. Many series of shoulder reconstructions for recurrent anterior instability have included adolescent patients and the results of surgery are reasonably well documented [246, 252, 260, 269, 272, 273, 275, 279, 283, 286, 288, 289, 295, 299]. For patients with open epiphyses, little has been written about assessing the long-term results of surgical treatment. Because of the open nature of the physis in the proximal humerus, it seems prudent to consider soft tissue procedures about the shoulder for reconstruction. Subscapularis shortening procedures (Putti-Platt, Magnuson-Stack) are commonly done. Bone block procedures (Bristow, Dutoit) have been successful in adolescent athletes. Capsular procedures similar to the Bankart repair are becoming more popular.

Complications

Complications of glenohumeral instability can be divided into two categories: (1) problems associated with the injury itself, and (2) problems associated with treatment. The biggest single problem with shoulder instability is the tendency toward recurrent instability. Other complications of the original injury are rare and involve injury to the neurovascular structures. Injuries to the brachial plexus and axillary artery have been reported. Axillary nerve injury is the most common after anterior dislocation of the shoulder [251, 257, 280].

Complications after surgical treatment of the dislocation include neurovascular injury, recurrence of dislocation, painful restricted motion, painful metal loosening or impingement, and degenerative arthritis [248, 250, 274, 296, 309]. Although these complications have been reported after all types of anterior reconstruction, procedures utilizing metallic internal fixation such as the Bristow procedure, Dutoit stapling, and arthroscopic stapling apparently have the highest incidence of such problems.

Author's Preferred Method of Treatment

Careful history of the mechanism of injury, thorough physical examination to elicit signs of multidirectional

laxity, and appropriate radiographs should elucidate whether instability is traumatic or atraumatic in nature. Once the etiology of the instability has been determined, a more rational treatment program can be outlined.

In acute traumatic dislocations, either anterior or posterior, gentle closed reduction should be performed. Before and after reduction the neurologic status of the axillary nerve and brachial plexus is carefully evaluated, and radiographic evaluation of the trauma series is performed. We believe that immobilization for 3 to 4 weeks followed by a vigorous rehabilitation program and abstention from provocative sports for 3 months may reduce the rate of recurrence. A sling is used for anterior dislocations, but in posterior dislocation a modified spica cast to hold the joint in neutral or slight external rotation is used.

The rehabilitation program begins with five exercises performed with the arm at the side that isolate and strengthen the rotator cuff and three components of the deltoid muscle (Fig. 14–38). Light resistance is used early with a steady progression of isometric-isotonic exercises. At 4 to 6 weeks, additional exercises are added including dips, bent-over rowing, push-ups, and lattisimus pull-downs. After basic strengthening has been obtained, controlled isokinetic exercises within acceptable range of motion limits are performed.

In the skeletally immature patient with a traumatic shoulder dislocation who has developed recurrent instability, surgical reconstruction is indicated. We prefer the capsular reconstruction described by Rockwood along with direct repair of the Bankart lesion if present. A vigorous 6- to 9-month rehabilitation program then follows prior to return to competitive sports.

Diligent examination should confirm the presence of multidirectional shoulder laxity in the patient who presents with a suspicious atraumatic history after dislocation. Reduction is accomplished by one of the standard methods. The key to long-term care of these patients is to institute and maintain a strict rehabilitation program for 9 to 12 months before considering any more aggressive intervention. In the atraumatic dislocator who has failed to improve with a rehabilitation program, voluntary dislocation should be carefully ruled out. If surgical reconstruction does become necessary, a capsular reconstruction is performed to accomplish a global tightening of the redundant capsule.

IMPINGEMENT SYNDROME

Although much less common than in adults, impingement of the rotator cuff and subacromial bursa underneath the coracoacromial arch can be a cause of symptoms in the pediatric athlete [313, 323]. Impingement syndrome was clearly described by Neer in the 1970s [324]. Classically, impingement occurs as the structures

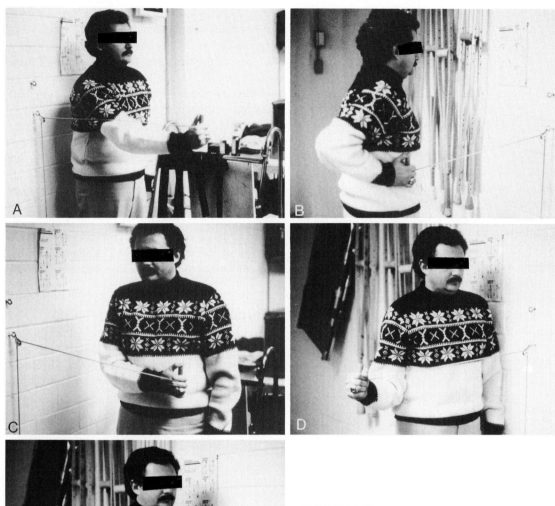

FIGURE 14–38
Rehabilitation program, using five exercises with the arm at the side to strengthen the rotator cuff and three components of the deltoid muscle. These can be performed with Theraband, surgical tubing, or a pulley and weight set as demonstrated here.

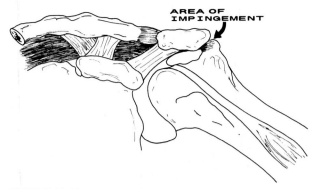

FIGURE 14–39
This diagram demonstrates the concept of impingement of the bursa, supraspinatus tendon, and greater tuberosity underneath the coracoacromial arch.

(greater tuberosity, supraspinatus tendon, long head of the biceps, and subacromial bursa) pass beneath the anterior and inferior surfaces of the coracoacromial arch composed of the coracoid, acromion, and coracoacromial ligament (Fig. 14–39). This mechanical contact on a repetitive basis leads to acute and chronic inflammation and the changes and clinical symptoms that we describe as the impingement syndrome. Neer described impingement as a continuum; if left untreated, the process can progress from stage I, which includes acute inflammation and swelling, to stage II, a more chronic phase of inflammation, chronic scarring, and tendinitis, through to stage III, which is defined as a rotator cuff tear [325, 326]. Bigliani and Morrison [312] as well as Neer [324] described the prominent anterior and inferior acromion as a common cause of a tight coracoacromial arch that can lead to impingement syndrome. This mechanical decrease in space under the coracoacromial arch may be due to congenital differences in the shape and slope of the acromion as well as to the development of pathologic spurring in this area with aging.

As our understanding of impingement syndrome has expanded, we have recognized that the athlete's shoulder can be afflicted with this problem despite the normal architecture of the coracoacromial arch. Most athletes in sports such as swimming, baseball, and tennis that require overhand repetitive shoulder function perform at a high level just below maximum stress. This repetitive microtrauma as described by Jobe and colleagues [319, 320] can lead to structural changes in the tendon, ligament, and capsule. An intrinsic overload in the rotator cuff tendons can lead to tendinitis, secondary muscle weakness and biomechanical imbalance. As weakness in the rotator cuff develops, subtle upward migration of the humeral head can create impingement as a secondary problem. If weakness of the rotator cuff is allowed to persist, repetitive anterior thrust of the humeral head against the anterior capsular ligaments can lead to atten-

uation of these ligaments and anterior subluxation. In older athletes, secondary impingement symptoms may occur as a result of this repetitive anterior subluxation [319, 320, 322].

Younger patients, both pediatric and adolescent, have a higher incidence of inherent multidirectional laxity of the shoulder and generalized joint laxity. In sports activities requiring repetitive stress on the shoulder, these patients require greater dynamic stability by the rotator cuff musculature. As the rate of stress increases and the rotator cuff becomes fatigued, impingement results secondary to the multidirectional instability. Treatment is directed toward improving joint stability rather than primarily toward the impingement phenomenon [320, 326, 327].

Impingement, therefore, is a multifactorial problem in the pediatric and adolescent age group. It is more commonly seen in athletes who spend a great number of hours in sports that require repetitive overhead elevation. Swimming, overhand throwing sports, and racquet sports are particularly stressful on the shoulder. In swimmers, the incidence of shoulder problems increases with the ability of the swimmer, with as many as 57% of elite swimmers complaining of shoulder problems [316].

Clinical Evaluation

Classification of impingement syndrome is based on the underlying etiology of the process. The classification used is modified from the system described by Jobe and Jobe [320].

Type I. Pure impingement (no instability)
    A. Mechanical—tight coracoacromial arch
    B. Microtrauma—overuse
Type II. Secondary impingement (instability)
    A. Microtrauma with structural changes
    B. Multidirectional shoulder laxity

The presenting symptom in all patients is pain. In mild disease, pain occurs only with specific activities, but as severity increases, the pain can become constant. Night pain is a hallmark symptom of rotator cuff pathology. The pain is usually described as deep or anterior and commonly radiates down the arm laterally to the area of deltoid insertion. As the process becomes more severe, range of motion and strength can be diminished. Deficits in elevation and internal rotation are usually the first signs noted by the patient. Patients who participate in overhand sports often complain of lost power in the serve, stroke, or pitch [313, 317, 327].

The gross appearance of the shoulder is usually normal. Only in advanced disease does atrophy of the deltoid and supraspinatus appear. There is tenderness over the anterior edge of the acromion, coracoacromial ligament, and cuff insertion. Range of motion is often normal, but subtle decreases in elevation and internal rotation should be tested. Strength can be affected by pain, most often in abduction and external rotation. The impingement sign is always positive in patients with pure impingement (Fig. 14–40). It is elicited by stabilizing the scapula while forcing the arm up into forward elevation. This maneuver compresses the subacromial space and causes pain in patients with impingement. The impingement reinforcement test can also be performed by positioning the arm at approximately 90 degrees of forward flexion and then forcibly rotating the shoulder internally (Fig. 14–41). This maneuver brings the greater tuberosity and supraspinatus under the subacromial arch, reproducing mechanical impingement. The impingement test is used to confirm the diagnosis of impingement syndrome in the absence of instability. Substantial relief of symptoms occurring after injection of 10 ml of 1% lidocaine (Xylocaine) into the subacromial space indicates a positive test result [312, 317, 325].

Great care should be taken to elicit signs of instability and generalized laxity on examination to confirm a diagnosis of secondary impingement. Generalized ligamentous laxity is demonstrated by hyperextensibility at the knees, elbows, and metacarpophalangeal joints. The opposite shoulder as well as the painful shoulder should be examined for signs of multidirectional laxity because guarding in a painful shoulder can mask these signs. A positive sulcus sign and translation of the humeral head of more than 1 cm on the drawer test are characteristic of multidirectional shoulder laxity. The anterior apprehension maneuver should also be done to rule out anterior subluxation as a primary cause of secondary impingement [317, 319, 325, 329].

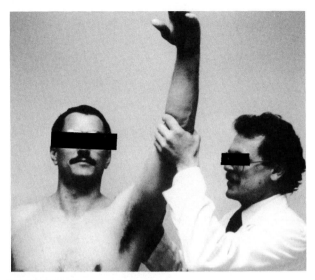

FIGURE 14–40
The impingement sign. The arm is elevated into extreme flexion at the shoulder, causing pain as the bursa and tendons are compressed into the coracoacromial arch.

Radiographic Evaluation

The routine radiographic evaluation of the shoulder with impingement syndrome is often normal. In more advanced stages of the process, degenerative changes about the acromioclavicular joint, anterior acromion, and greater tuberosity can be noted.

Bigliani and Morrison [312] noted variability in the shape and slope of the acromion in adult cadaver and radiographic studies. Specific radiographic views such as the 30-degree caudal tilt view and the supraspinatus

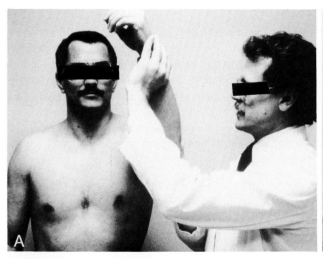

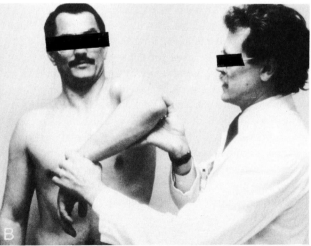

FIGURE 14–41
Impingement reinforcement test. With the elbow flexed at 90 degrees and the shoulder elevated 90 degrees, the shoulder is internally rotated, bringing the bursa and greater tuberosity structures beneath the coracoacromial arch.

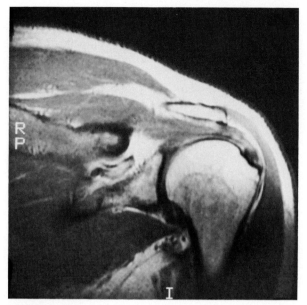

FIGURE 14–42
This MRI scan demonstrates increased signal intensity within the supraspinatus tendon. There is a small effusion within the subacromial bursa but no discontinuity of the tendon consistent with impingement syndrome.

outlet view have been developed to assess the shape and slope of the anterior acromion.

Arthrography and, more recently, magnetic resonance imaging (MRI) are used to assess the status of the rotator cuff (Fig. 14–42). Fortunately, full-thickness rotator cuff pathology in pediatric and adolescent athletes is extremely rare, and the need for MRI is uncommon.

Treatment Options

The differential diagnosis of a painful shoulder in the throwing athlete includes stress fractures of the proximal humerus, epiphyseolysis, instability, and primary and secondary impingement [317, 323]. Careful physical examination should be used for appropriate assessment of potential multidirectional laxity or anterior instability in a child or adolescent who presents with impingement symptoms in the shoulder. Treatment for mild to moderate impingement of any cause should consist of rest, ice, immobilization if the shoulder is acutely painful, and nonsteroidal anti-inflammatory medications. Once pain at rest has subsided, rehabilitation should be directed toward regaining a full range of motion with flexibility exercises plus strengthening of the rotator cuff musculature to regain dynamic stability. Changes in training regimen and technique are necessary to prevent recurrence and should be part of the overall treatment plan for the athlete. Inappropriately sized or resistance equipment (racquets, swimming paddles, gymnastic

dowel grips) may be an important disuse factor. In almost all cases, pediatric and adolescent athletes respond to nonoperative treatment for impingement syndrome [313, 317, 327, 329].

Very little has been written about failure of noninvasive treatment in pediatric and adolescent patients with shoulder impingement. In the 1970s, a few cases were described of older adolescents who required surgical treatment by resection of the coracoacromial ligament. Jackson [318] reported only 50% satisfactory results in throwing athletes, however, Tibone and colleagues [328] presented a series of young athletes (adolescent and young adults) with rotator cuff impingement that was treated by open acromioplasty and cuff repair. Improvement was noted in more than 80%, but only 41% returned to throwing sports. Bigliani and colleagues [311] also presented a series of young adult patients treated by open acromioplasty and reported more than 81% excellent and good results. The use of arthroscopic acromioplasty has become an increasingly popular option for the treatment of refractory impingement syndrome. Although pediatric and adolescent patients have not been specifically mentioned, series by Altchek and associates [310], Ellman [314], Ellman and Kay [315], and Gartsman [316] have reported results with this technique comparable to those achieved with open procedures while requiring shorter postoperative rehabilitation times. Use of such techniques seems to have a limited role in the young athlete.

Since impingement symptoms in the young athlete are usually secondary to instability, great care in making this diagnosis is extremely important. Early reports on capsular reconstructions in the overhand athlete have been encouraging [319].

Criteria for Return to Sports

The young athlete with impingement syndrome should be made to realize that "overuse" is the common denominator in this problem, no matter how it is classified. The overhand athlete should be pain-free and actively involved in the rehabilitation program before he is allowed to return to specific sports. Most recurrences are due to insufficient rotator cuff strength and secondary dynamic instability in patients with secondary impingement.

Author's Preferred Treatment

Most young athletes present with mild symptoms during specific sports activities only. I allow these patients to continue to participate while beginning treatment with nonsteroidal oral anti-inflammatory medications and rehabilitation. These patients are asked to use a moist heat-to-ice contrast treatment, along with a program of flexibility and rotator cuff strengthening exercises on a daily basis.

In moderately severe cases when the patient has pain at rest after athletic activities, the athlete is removed from the activity. Nonsteroidal anti-inflammatory medications and modality treatments such as hydroculator and ultrasound are initiated. When pain at rest subsides, the athlete begins the usual rehabilitation program including flexibility, strengthening, and sport-specific exercises.

In severe cases that have persisted for more than 3 months despite a supervised treatment program, further work-up with shoulder MRI is performed to determine the degree of rotator cuff involvement. If the diagnosis of impingement is confirmed, injection of the subacromial space with steroid followed by continued rehabilitation is carried out. Rarely, in older adolescent patients surgical treatment may be necessary. A specific diagnosis is mandatory for successful treatment. In cases of primary impingement, arthroscopic decompression is performed. If instability is the primary cause, capsular shift reconstruction is the treatment of choice.

Fractures of the Proximal Humerus

Kaye E. Wilkins, M.D.

Fractures of the proximal humerus include both pure metaphyseal fractures and fractures involving the physeal plate. Because this is the area where growth and remodeling occur, the incidence and patterns of fractures are much different from those in the shaft. Because of the increased remodeling potential there is more leeway in accepting the position of the fracture fragment. This metaphysis is also the most common location for a unicameral bone cyst. As a result, there is a high incidence of pathologic fractures in this area (see Fig. 14–2).

STRUCTURE

The proximal humerus is composed of the epiphysis, the physeal plate, and the metaphysis, all of which have unique biomechanical properties. These properties contribute to the specific injury patterns seen in this area. A review of the unique structural anatomy of this area will give the reader a better understanding of both the mechanism and the treatment of injuries that occur in the proximal humerus.

Proximal Humeral Physis

The proximal humeral epiphysis is a hemispherical structure with a cone-shaped physeal plate. The physis is more proximally directed posteriorly, which provides some intrinsic stability (Fig. 14–43). The hemispherical epiphysis contains the articular surface and the greater and lesser tuberosities. The epiphyseal mass is formed by two separate ossification centers, which fuse to form a single center by about 7 years of age and are completely fused to the proximal humerus by 17 or 18 years of age [332].

This serial development of the proximal humeral epiphysis has been studied in great detail by Ogden and his co-workers [334]. The initial contour of the physis is transversely oriented. At birth there is usually no radiographically discernible ossification center. The first center develops as the capital or articular center at about 2 months of age (Fig. 14–44). By 7 months of age a second center develops in the area of the greater tuberosity. By 3 years these centers have enlarged and matured, and the physis is assuming its conical shape. By 7 years there is complete fusion of these two centers, and the physis becomes more conical in shape. In addition, at this stage the lateral metaphyseal cortex is thicker, composed almost entirely of cortex up to the physis, whereas the cortex on the medial metaphysis remains thin with a trabecular structure. This is thought to be one of the reasons why the metaphyseal fragment in the Salter-Harris II fracture occurs on that site.

From 10 to 13 years of age the greater tuberosity ossification center expands until it completely fills the cartilaginous space on the lateral portion of the epiphysis. Concurrently, the medial metaphyseal cortex is increasing in density. By 14 years the physis is beginning to close, starting in the center and extending peripherally. The cortex on the medial side, although still thicker, has developed some trabecular pattern next to the physis. This indicates an inherent weakness on the medial side of the proximal humerus.

The Periosteum

In laboratory studies on humerii obtained from stillborn infants, Dameron and Reibel [330] found that displacement of the metaphysis was extremely difficult to accomplish. They attributed this to the fact that the periosteum of the metaphysis was considerably thicker posteromedially. Anterior displacement of the metaphysis was relatively easy to achieve because of the thinner periosteum on the anterolateral surface. If it remains intact, the periosteal sleeve can also stabilize an undisplaced fracture. Once the metaphyseal fragment has torn

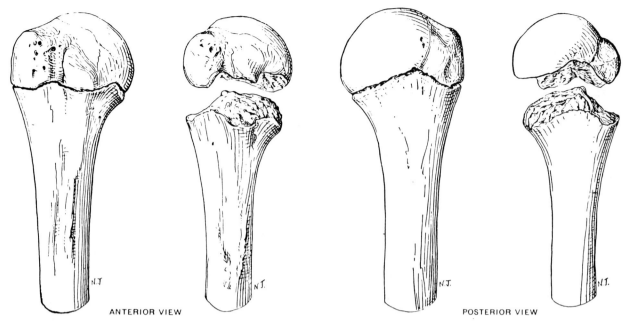

FIGURE 14–43
The proximal epiphysis and physis of the humerus form a conical configuration. (From Grant, J. C. B. *An Atlas of Anatomy*, 5th ed. © 1962, The Williams & Wilkins Co., Baltimore.)

the periosteum, all of its intrinsic stability is lost. When the periosteum disrupts, it tends to displace laterally to the intertubercular groove under the long head of the biceps [335].

Muscle and Capsule Attachments

The proximal humeral epiphysis has four muscles attached to it. In the greater tuberosity posterolaterally are the teres minor, infraspinatus, and supraspinatus (Fig.

14–45). The subscapularis inserts into the lesser tuberosity anteriorly. The pectoralis major attaches distally to the anterior metaphysis. When the proximal epiphysis becomes disrupted from the metaphysis, the unopposed action of the muscles on the epiphysis tends to pull this fragment into flexion, abduction, and external rotation [330]. The pectoralis major muscle pulls the metaphyseal fragment anteriorly (see Fig. 14–45).

The glenohumeral joint capsule on the medial side attaches distally past the edge of the articular surface to the metaphysis. Thus, the fracture line, when it passes

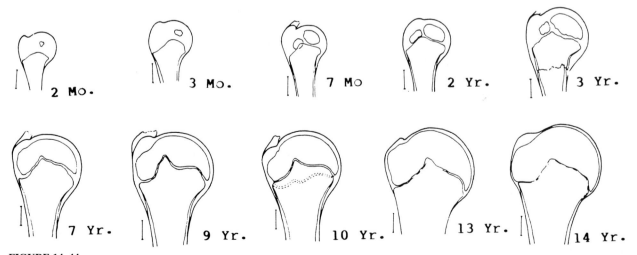

FIGURE 14–44
The schematic development of the proximal humeral epiphysis and metaphysis from age 2 months to 14 years. (From Ogden, J. A., Conlogue, G. J., and Jensen, P. Radiology of postnatal skeletal development: The proximal humerus. *Skel Radiol* 2:153–160, 1978.)

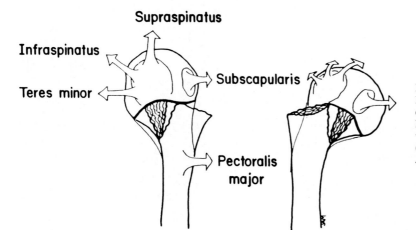

FIGURE 14–45
Effect of muscle forces on the proximal humeral epiphysis and metaphysis. (From Dameron, T. B. Fractures and dislocations of the shoulder. *In* Rockwood, C. A., Jr., Wilkins, K. E., and King, R. E. (Eds.), *Fractures in Children*, Vol. 3. Philadelphia, J. B. Lippincott, 1984.)

through the medial physeal plate, creates a line that is intra-articular in location [331] (Fig. 14–46).

Blood Supply

With the exception of the suprascapular artery, the blood supply to the shoulder arises from the second and third parts of the axillary artery (Fig. 14–47). The major supply to the proximal humerus comes from the anterior and posterior circumflex humeral arteries, which arise from the third part of the axillary artery. Most of the blood supply to the osseous humeral head comes from the anterior ascending branch of the anterior circumflex artery [333]. This artery ascends proximally along the upper end of the bicipital groove and then enters the head by branches that pierce the greater and lesser tuberosities. Once inside the humeral head, this artery as-

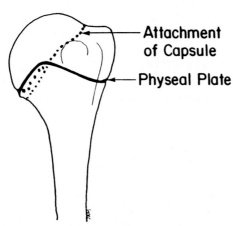

FIGURE 14–46
The relationship of the physeal plate and the glenohumeral capsular attachment to the proximal humerus. The medial end of the physeal plate extends across an area covered by articular cartilage in the area noted by stippling. This area of metaphysis is intra-articular. (From Dameron, T. B. Fractures and dislocations of the shoulder. *In* Rockwood, C. A., Jr., Wilkins, K. E., and King, R. E. (Eds.), *Fractures in Children*, Vol. 3. Philadelphia, J. B. Lippincott, 1984.)

sumes a form like that of the lateral epiphyseal artery of the femoral head—that is, it forms an arcuate system from which branches radiate at right angles to the periphery of the epiphysis.

A small amount of blood is also supplied from the posterior humeral circumflex artery. This artery enters the epiphysis through a small portion on the posteromedial surface of the humeral head and corresponds to the medial epiphyseal arteries of the femoral head. A part of the blood supply also arises anterolaterally through the rotator cuff into the greater tuberosity. Because much of the blood supply enters through the muscular attachments to the proximal humeral epiphysis, avascular necrosis of the humeral head is extremely rare after a fracture through the proximal humeral physis.

INCIDENCE

In Landin's study [344] fractures of the proximal humerus comprised only 2.2% of all fractures in children. More of these fractures occurred in girls. In his series of children between the ages of 9 and 10 years in Sweden, fully 50% of the fractures resulted from falls that occurred with horseback riding, and almost all of these patients were girls. Even when horseback riding injuries were removed from the overall group, there was still a preponderance of girls. In this same study Landin found that the incidence of females sustaining fractures of the proximal humerus increased dramatically since 1970. This large preponderance of girls sustaining fractures of the proximal humerus was also found in another study from Sweden [341]. In still another study that looked only at fractures of the proximal humerus per se, Kohler and Trilland [343] found that 22% of 136 fractures occurred in sporting events. In their series 60% of patients were males. The peak age incidence was 10 to 14 years old. Two-thirds of the fractures involved the proximal metaphysis, and the other third involved the physeal

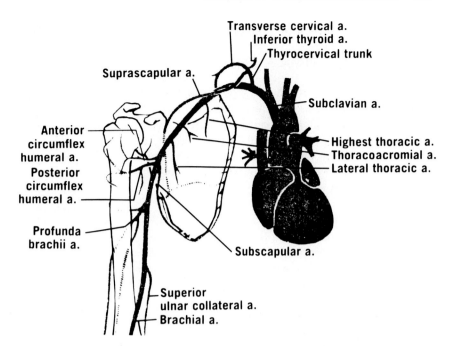

FIGURE 14-47
The arteries of the shoulder region. (From O'Rahilly, R. *Gardner-Gray-O'Rahilly: Anatomy*, 5th ed. Philadelphia, W. B. Saunders, 1986.)

plate. During their review period of 20 years, one-fourth of the metaphyseal fractures occurred through unicameral bone cysts.

In examining the incidence of physeal humeral fractures in relation to the incidence of all physeal fractures the classic work by Peterson and Peterson [350] is important. They combined previous reviews in the literature of series of physeal fractures. In this combined series the incidence of fractures of the proximal humerus was 3%. Neer and Horowitz [346], in their review of over 2500 physeal injuries, found the same incidence (3%) of fractures involving the proximal humerus. However, the Petersons' review of their own series from the Mayo Clinic showed a higher incidence (6.7%). Almost all physeal fractures in this area are either Salter-Harris type I, or II [337, 339, 343]. Type I fractures are less common and occur usually in younger children (i.e., below the age of 10 years). Almost all fractures in individuals over the age of 10 are Salter-Harris type II lesions [339, 343]. Because of the flexibility of the shoulder, forces applied directly against the articular surface or perpendicular to the physis are rarely applied to the proximal humerus. As a result, Salter-Harris type III and IV fracture patterns are almost unheard of [336, 337, 349]. Type V lesions, which involve the development of a humerus varus, are usually the result of injuries that occur in early infancy or childhood and usually do not occur in athletic events.

MECHANISM OF INJURY

Proximal metaphyseal fractures are characteristically more predominant in children under 10 years old. The mechanism of the fracture probably is the same as that

causing proximal humeral physeal fractures. The combination of a weaker metaphysis and a stronger perichondrial physeal ring probably accounts for the fracture occurring in the metaphysis rather than the physis in this younger age group.

The exact mechanism of proximal humeral physeal injuries is not completely clear. In past reports a theory of the mechanism was developed based on the patient's history and the position of the fracture fragments [353]. The periosteum is weaker on the anterolateral aspect of the proximal humerus. In fractures involving the humeral physis the distal fragment usually is forced anteriorly and laterally through this weakened area. Neer and Horowitz [346] thought that this force resulted from a direct blow on the shoulder from a posterolateral shearing force that adducted the humeral shaft and forced it anteriorly. Dameron [340], on the other hand, believed that the force was directed longitudinally up the upper extremity as it was used to break a fall in a backward direction. The force originating as the hand hits the ground is transmitted proximally through the humeral shaft with the shoulder extended and adducted. This forces the metaphysis anteriorly, laterally, and cephalad. The horizontal alignment of the physis in the anterolateral portion of the proximal humerus augments the displacement occurring in an anterolateral direction. The combination of a stronger intact medial periosteum and compressive posteromedial forces creates the triangular metaphyseal fracture fragment in this area.

CLASSIFICATION

Ogden [349] classifies metaphyseal fractures into two types. In the first type the cortex remains intact. These are usually torus or greenstick compressive fractures (see Fig. 14–1). In the other type there is loss of cortical integrity with either angular or translocation displacement (Fig. 14–48).

Fractures of the proximal humeral physis can be classified by location, degree of displacement, and stability. The degree of stability usually depends on the degree of initial displacement and the magnitude of the injury. The most commonly accepted classification of displacement is that proposed by Neer and Horowitz [346]. They separated displacement into four grades:

Grade I, Less than 5 mm.
Grade II, Up to one-third of the width of the physis.
Grade III, Up to one-third of the width of the physis.
Grade IV, Greater than two-thirds of the width of the physis including total displacement.

It should be noted that Neer and Horowitz in their original article used the term ''width of shaft'' instead of ''width of physis'' to denote the degree of displacement. In their illustrative cases, however, they demonstrated displacement of the physis. Thus we have taken the license to correct this anatomic inaccuracy because the actual displacement is measured by the amount of physeal displacement, not by the amount of displacement of the more distal shaft.

SIGNS AND SYMPTOMS

In undisplaced metaphyseal fractures, especially those in which cortical integrity is maintained, there may be only minimal swelling. The tenderness is usually localized over the proximal humerus. In physeal fractures and metaphyseal fractures with displacement there is usually considerable bleeding into the soft tissues of the deltoid area with marked swelling. The athlete with this type of fracture is usually uncomfortable and holds the extremity adducted to the chest. The weight of the extremity is often supported at the elbow and forearm with the opposite hand.

It is important to assess all of the nerves of the upper extremity to rule out a concomitant injury of any of the brachial plexus peripheral nerves. The vascular status of the upper extremity needs to be evaluated. Since the force was transmitted from the hand longitudinally, the entire extremity must be checked for the occurrence of less obvious ipsilateral fractures, especially in the distal radial metaphysis.

DIAGNOSTIC STUDIES

Usually routine roentgenograms are enough to demonstrate the presence of the fracture. The proximal and

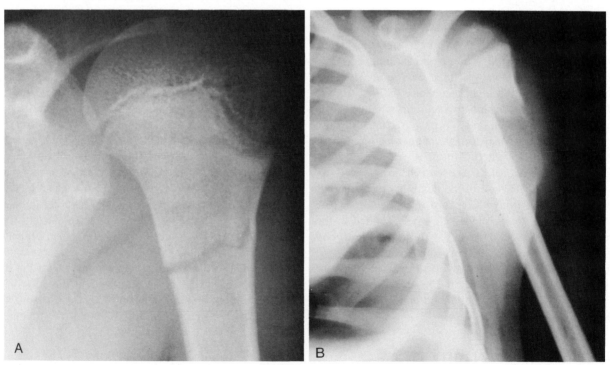

FIGURE 14–48

A, Angulated fracture of the proximal humeral metaphysis in a 12-year-old basketball player in which there is loss of the integrity of the medial cortex. *B,* Completely translocated fracture of the proximal humeral metaphysis in a 7-year-old gymnast. The proximal fragment has not angulated because it is partially attached to the shoulder adductors.

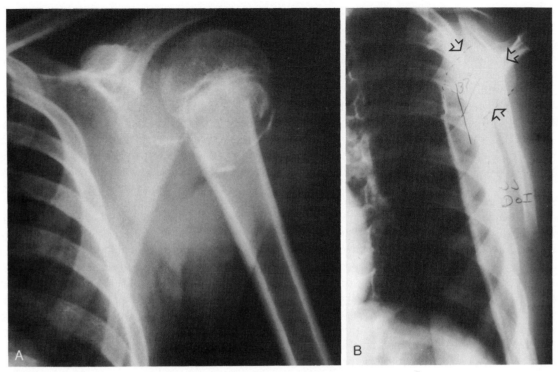

FIGURE 14–49
A, AP view of a swimmer who injured her proximal humerus when she fell from a diving board. Anterior angulation cannot be determined from this view. *B*, The degree of anterior angulation is determined by using the oblique transscapular view (arrows).

lateral displacement of the metaphyseal portion is usually obvious on routine anteroposterior views of the shoulder. It may be necessary to use transthoracic lateral or oblique scapular views to determine the degree of anterior displacement (Fig. 14–49). In some cases when there may be complex fragment patterns, a CT scan with horizontal cuts or coronal reconstruction may be helpful in determining the fracture patterns and degree of displacement.

TREATMENT

Simple metaphyseal fractures that are undisplaced or only minimally angulated can usually be treated quite adequately with a collar and cuff. Initial added comfort may be achieved by binding the arm to the chest with a circular Ace bandage. Since most of these fractures are usually intrinsically stable, shoulder motion can be initiated early, in some cases within a few days. In the pediatric athlete it is extremely important to regain shoulder motion as soon as possible to achieve maximum rehabilitation.

In the completely displaced metaphyseal fracture very little abduction of the proximal fragment is usually present because some adduction force is maintained by both the pectoralis major and the latissimus dorsi on the proximal metaphysis. As a result, these fractures often develop a true bayonet opposition (see Fig. 14–48*B*). Although shortening occurs because of the longitudinal pull of the triceps and biceps as in shaft fractures, it is usually not sufficient to cause any functional or cosmetic residuae. These fractures can usually be treated quite well using a collar and cuff plus a thoracic elastic bandage. Healing with the bayonet opposition (although it may concern the parents) usually results in an acceptable cosmetic and functional result even in the adolescent patient.

If there is an extremely marked displacement of the proximal metaphysis and concern exists that the bayonet opposition may restrict shoulder motion, especially in an athlete who performs throwing activity, the patient can be placed in overhead olecranon pin traction to alleviate the shortening. Usually these fractures stabilize rapidly, and the skeletal traction can be converted to a hanging arm cast or simple collar and cuff after 10 to 14 days when callus first appears at the fracture site.

In displaced fractures of the proximal humeral physis, rotation of the proximal fragment often occurs because there is an absence of adductor forces on this fragment. The adductor forces act entirely on the distal metaphyseal fragment (see Fig. 14–45). At no other physis in the body is there a larger proportional contribution to longitudinal growth than at the proximal humeral physis. Approximately 80% of the longitudinal growth occurs in this area [337, 342, 348]. As a result, the remodeling potential in this area is tremendous. The younger the athlete, the greater the potential for remodeling. Because of the wide range of motion of the glenohumeral joint, the residual varus that may occur usually does not result in any functional limitation [337]. Shortening of these fractures is also well tolerated because of the independent function and weight-bearing status of the upper extremity.

Closed Methods

The argument for reduction of the fragments is that it decreases the degree of shortening that can develop if the displacement is allowed to remain [338, 340]. Various closed methods have been advocated to realign the fracture fragments into a more anatomic position. In some cases a primary closed reduction is performed, either with sedation or under general anesthesia, and then the reduction is maintained by external support. The reduction per se is usually achieved by bringing the distal shaft fragment into flexion and some abduction and external rotation to align it with the flexed, abducted, and externally rotated proximal fragment [340]. If the fracture is stable after the reduction, it can be immobilized alongside the chest. If it is not stable, this position of flexed abduction and external rotation must be maintained with either a shoulder spica cast in the salute position or a commercial splint, neither of which are well tolerated by the athlete or the parents. The "statue of liberty" position with a spica cast should be avoided because of its potential to cause injury to the brachial plexus or to lead to development of vascular compromise to the upper extremity [349, 351]. Some [347] have used the traction produced by the hanging arm cast to achieve a reduction or to improve the position of the proximal fragment. Others [339, 343, 352] have not found this method successful, especially if the cast was applied after the fracture clot had congealed.

Overhead skeletal olecranon traction can be used in patients in whom the usual external immobilization techniques cannot be utilized. It is a good method of achieving and maintaining a reduction, but it requires expensive and extensive hospitalization and has all the problems associated with the management and care of the skeletal pin or screw.

The real question concerns whether an anatomic reduction is necessary. Many series [337, 343, 347] have shown that for most individuals, even those who have considerable initial displacement, simple immobilization often produces satisfactory results. Baxter and Wiley [337] found in their retrospective review that the manipulative process improved the arm's position in only a third of the patients in whom it was attempted. When there was an improvement in position the final result was no better than that seen in patients in whom the equal displacement had been accepted. These authors questioned whether active manipulation had any effect on the final outcome.

It must be remembered, however, that these series concern individuals with normal activity. What about the high-performance athlete? Is there a greater need to achieve a more anatomic reduction in athletes? The only item in the literature that relates to this is a case described by Dameron and Rockwood [340] in which a 14-year-old track star sustained a displaced Salter-Harris type II fracture of the proximal humerus while pole vaulting. At the time of healing there was a small proximal lateral spur on the anterolateral aspect of the metaphysis due to proximal migration of the distal fragment. When the patient had fully recovered he was able to play football but was unable to participate in throwing sports because of a restriction of about 20 degrees in flexion and abduction. Thus, in the high-performance throwing athlete a more aggressive approach may be necessary to obtain an anatomic reduction.

Operative Intervention

There appear to be very few indications for operative intervention. A semiclosed method of operative management involves reducing the fracture by closed methods first and then stabilizing it with pins placed across the fracture site percutaneously under image intensifier guidance. This technique has the advantage of maintaining fracture alignment with the arm in the normal position supported only with a splint or collar and cuff. The pins can be removed in 3 to 4 weeks.

Primary open operative reduction just to improve the position has almost no role in treatment of this fracture. The major absolute indications are the rare open fractures and fractures with vascular injuries. Other relative indications include comminuted intra-articular Salter-Harris type III and IV injuries or cases in which large amounts of periosteum or the biceps tendon have become interposed in the fracture site.

In general, open reduction of these fractures has produced poor results, worse than the results of comparable fractures managed closed [345]. Nilsson and Svartholm [347] believed that the poor outcomes seen after an open reduction were the result of the surgical intervention and not the fracture per se. This conclusion was echoed 20 years later by Baxter and Wiley [337], who stated that "open reduction improved the displacement in only three of seven patients, inflicting a cosmetically unattractive scar for no obvious advantage."

AUTHOR'S PREFERRED METHOD OF TREATMENT

For undisplaced or minimally displaced fractures of the proximal humeral metaphysis or Neer type I or II proximal humeral physeal fractures we use a collar and cuff supplemented with an elastic bandage, strapping the extremity to the chest wall. In a few days the elastic bandage strap is discontinued, and the cuff is gradually lowered until the elbow is at 90 degrees. At this time, circumduction exercises of the shoulder are begun. By 3 weeks after the injury when early callus has formed, active abduction exercises can be initiated, and usually the arm can then be supported with a simple sling. Usually after 6 weeks there is sufficient stability to initiate a formal rehabilitation program that includes strengthening all the muscles about the shoulder girdle in addition to the biceps, triceps, and forearm muscles. In noncollision sports the athlete can return to participation when muscle strength and range of motion in the affected extremity are equal to those in the uninjured extremity. In collision sports there must be in addition sufficient bony healing to have reestablished good cortical margins at the fracture site.

In markedly displaced physeal fractures one must be sure that sufficient reduction exists to ensure uninhibited motion of the glenohumeral joint. This is especially true of those athletes who need full glenohumeral motion for throwing, gymnastic, or swimming activities. In such cases an anatomic reduction is achieved first by manipulation. This reduction is stabilized with percutaneous pins (Fig. 14–50). We have found that external immobilization methods are cumbersome and uncomfortable and are not well accepted by the patient in addition to being unreliable in maintaining the position of the fragments.

In most displaced metaphyseal fractures there is usually no concern about impingement of shoulder motion. These fractures can be treated in the same way as undisplaced fractures (i.e., with collar and cuff and Ace bandage strapping) (Fig. 14–51). The major problem initially is severe swelling and pain. Considerable analgesic and psychological support and reassurance must be given to both the patient and the family during this initial phase. The same program of initial early motion is used for treatment of these fractures except that progression to the various stages is usually slower.

If there is marked displacement of the metaphyseal fracture and the distal fragment is displaced proximally, creating danger of compromising shoulder motion, we usually treat these injuries with overhead olecranon pin skeletal traction (Fig. 14–52). We usually try to avoid violating the shoulder muscles with an open reduction because this runs the risk of compromising function later on. Although overhead skeletal traction is costly and troublesome, it is the best way to reestablish length noninvasively and in many cases provides a satisfactory reduction. Elevation of the extremity with traction also hastens the loss of swelling, which can facilitate the rehabilitation phase later.

In our experience we have found no indications for an open reduction. In these very rare open fractures or fractures with vascular compromise we would not hesitate to perform an open reduction. In an athlete in whom

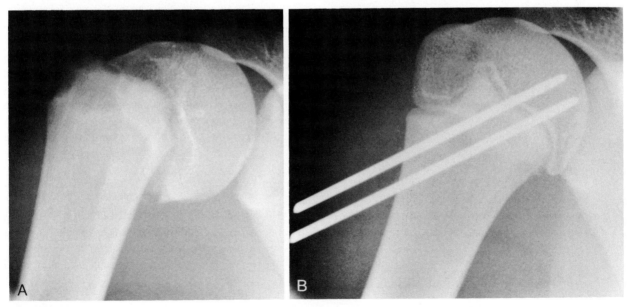

FIGURE 14–50
A, Displaced proximal humeral physeal injury in the dominant extremity of a 13-year-old high-performance quarterback. *B*, Anatomic reduction was achieved by closed reduction and was maintained by percutaneous pin fixation. Pins were removed 4 weeks postinjury, and shoulder motion was initiated.

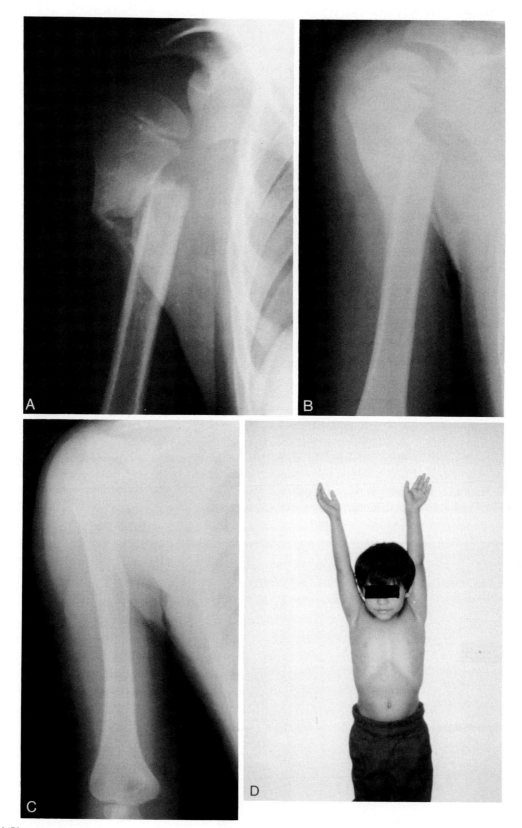

FIGURE 14–51
A, Radiograph taken 2 weeks postinjury in a 6-year-old male soccer player. The fracture is healing with early callus and bayonet apposition. *B,* Radiograph taken 6 weeks postinjury. *C,* Fracture 9 months postinjury shows almost complete remodeling. *D,* Nine months postinjury the shoulder has a full range of motion and no cosmetic deformity.

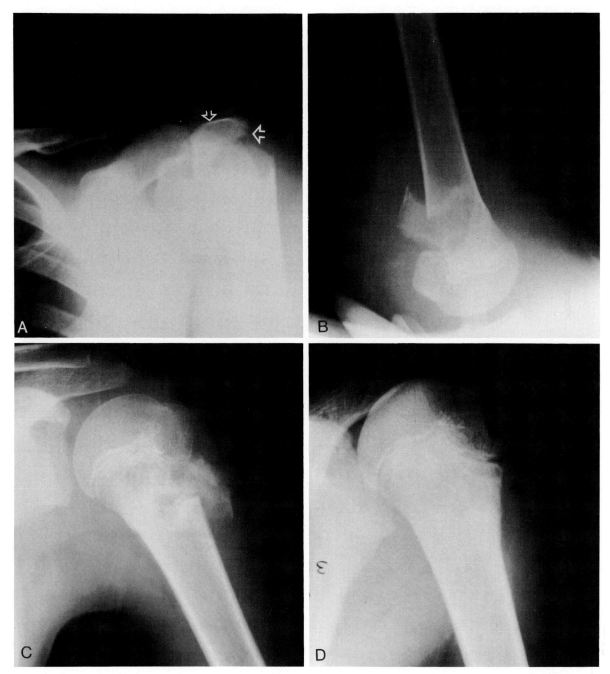

FIGURE 14–52
A, Initial view of a fracture of the proximal humerus in a 15-year-old quarterback. There is marked displacement of the proximal fragment with some comminution (arrows). *B*, Because of the comminution, the fracture was treated with overhead skeletal traction. A good linear alignment was maintained, but there was some concern about the small metaphyseal fragment. *C*, Roentgenograms taken 6 weeks postinjury show satisfactory alignment of the fracture with the metaphyseal fragment healed to the proximal humerus. *D*, Films taken 9 months postinjury show that the metaphyseal fragment is almost completely resolved and range of motion is normal. (Courtesy Donald Plowman, M.D.)

there is interposed tendon or other tissue one would have to weigh the risks of surgical damage to the shoulder muscles against the benefit of achieving an anatomic reduction. In most cases, if an open reduction is required, the athlete's ability to recover fully, especially if he needs full shoulder motion and strength, would probably be severely compromised.

COMPLICATIONS

Nonskeletal complications are rarely reported with injuries in this area. Baxter and Wiley [337] described one patient with complete disruption of the brachial artery at the lateral border of the axilla. In some patients they also found severe tenting of the skin, which required operative intervention to prevent skin necrosis.

Dameron and Reibel [339] reported one case of brachial plexus paresis in a patient treated in a statue of liberty cast. Transient axillary nerve paralysis has also been described [349]. Usually, however, these problems resolve by the time the athlete is ready to start the recovery or rehabilitation phase.

Residual varus angulation and shortening, although they do occur, are rarely a problem in nonathletic individuals [337].

S E C T I O N   E

Fractures of the Humeral Shaft

Kaye E. Wilkins, M.D.

INCIDENCE

Fractures of the humeral shaft in skeletally immature patients are quite rare. They account for less than 2% of all pediatric fractures. In the pediatric age group, only 10% of all humeral fractures are isolated to the shaft [361]. The largest percentage of fractures of the humeral shaft occurring in patients older than 10 years is associated with athletic or recreational activities. Complete humeral shaft fractures usually are the result of severe indirect or direct trauma. In indirect trauma the force is rotational and produces a longitudinal or spiral pattern. In fractures due to direct blows there is usually a transverse fracture pattern. In both types, shortening occurs because of unopposed muscle contractures.

PHYSICAL EXAMINATION

The diagnosis is usually obvious. The arm is shortened, swollen, and very tender. Crepitus and angular motion may be palpable at the fracture site. Although vascular injuries are quite rare with closed humeral shaft fractures, a thorough examination of the function of the vascular system distally is essential. In open injuries it is crucial to examine the integrity of the vascular system to rule out a forearm compartment syndrome. It is important to check for ipsilateral injuries, especially in the distal forearm. Some of these may be minor, and their symptoms may be greatly overshadowed by the magnitude of the humeral shaft fracture.

DIAGNOSTIC STUDIES

The fracture is usually quite obvious on plain roentgenograms. One word of caution is necessary, however. Two views of the humerus are essential. These views should be obtained by rotating the patient, not the ex-tremity. Techniques requiring internal and external rotation of the arm are avoided. The anteroposterior view is usually easy. To obtain a lateral view it may be necessary to take a transthoracic lateral film. It is important to be sure that both the glenohumeral and elbow joints are visualized.

The prefracture integrity of the bone needs to be determined as well. The fracture site must be carefully evaluated to determine whether some defect such as a bone cyst or nonossifying fibroma may have made the bone more susceptible to fracture (see Fig. 14–7).

TREATMENT

Almost all humeral shaft fractures can be treated nonoperatively. There are very few instances in which operative methods are necessary in the pediatric athlete.

Nonoperative Techniques

In nondisplaced fractures a simple posterior splint or so-called Jacksonville sling [358] is usually all that is necessary (Fig. 14–53). When there is complete displacement, treatment must be directed toward controlling angulation. Shortening usually does not produce any significant clinical or functional effect [359]. In completely displaced fractures, angulation can be controlled by a number of simple noninvasive external mobilization techniques.

Hanging Arm Cast. The hanging arm cast was once a popular method of treating humeral shaft fractures. Its major advantage is that it can be wedged to the correct angulation (Fig. 14–54). Pollen [364] changed the position of the attachment to the suspension strap of the cast to correct angulation. The hanging arm cast has disadvantages such as discomfort and the need to sit up to sleep. The weight of the cast may overdistract the frac-

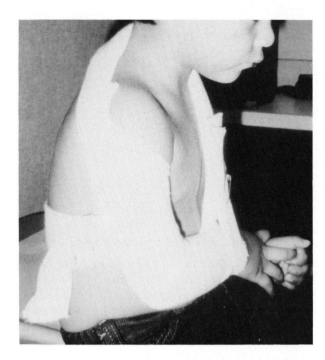

FIGURE 14–53
This Little League pitcher sustained an undisplaced fracture of the humeral shaft, which was treated with a Jacksonville sling [358] (modified stockinette Velpeau dressing). This type of sling both supports the extremity and prevents rotation.

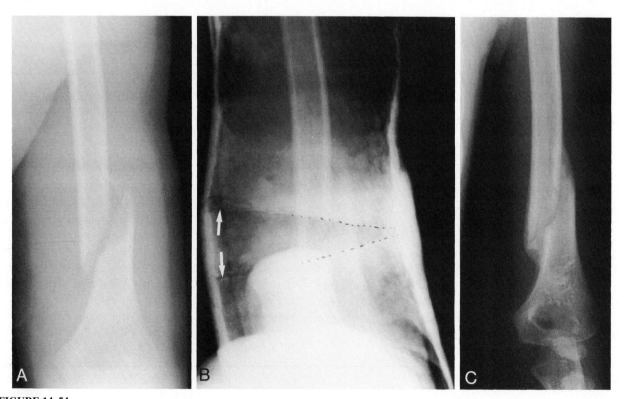

FIGURE 14–54
A, Injury films of a spiral distal shaft fracture in an 8-year-old gymnast. The fracture was placed in a hanging-arm cast but drifted into varus. *B*, Varus was corrected by performing a medial opening wedge of the distal portion of the cast (arrows). *C*, Six weeks postinjury there is good solid callus, and the linear alignment is maintained.

ture, which can lead to delayed or even nonunion [369].

Coaptation Splint. A coaptation (sugar tong) splint is easy to apply. It consists of a U-shaped slab of plaster that encases the arm from the axilla medially to the elbow and laterally to the deltoid. The splint is molded to control angulation in the coronal plane. It is usually secured with an elastic bandage wrapped around the arm. The forearm requires some type of sling suspension. If the forearm needs more support, such as in fractures in which there is an associated radial nerve paralysis, a second coaptation splint can be placed 90 degrees to the splint around the arm (Fig. 14–55). The advantages of the coaptation splint are the ease of application and the early return of elbow motion. Angulation in the coronal plane (varus-valgus) is easy to control. Angulation in the sagittal plane (flexion-extension) may be more difficult to manage.

Braces. These orthotic devices are usually reserved for the later stages in healing after some intrinsic stability has been obtained. They are more effective in the adolescent athlete. Their major advantages are their light weight and their ability to allow early motion [354].

Operative Indications

There are very few indications for operative intervention for humeral shaft fractures in the pediatric athlete. These special indications usually include multiple fractures in an athlete who must be treated in a recumbent position for the other injuries. In the patient with a closed head injury and spastic extremities, internal fixation may be the only means of controlling both angulation and excessive shortening. Associated radial nerve injury is not an indication for primary open reduction. Open fractures per se also are not always indications for internal fixation. The three major methods of operative intervention include traction, internal fixation with plates, and intramedullary rod fixation.

Traction. Skeletal traction applied distally through the olecranon with either a pin or a special screw may be useful in fractures that are severely comminuted (Fig. 14–56). Traction can be applied in either the overhead or side arm mode. It is useful in those who must remain recumbent for treatment of other injuries, an uncommon situation in modern polytrauma management. It is con-

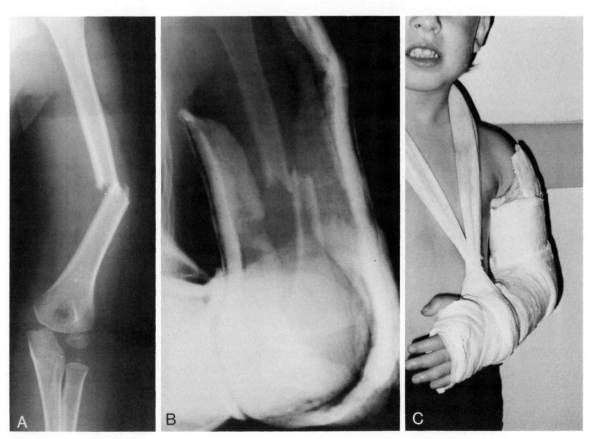

FIGURE 14–55

A, Injury films in a 6-year-old boy who was thrown from a horse, sustaining a midshaft fracture of the left humerus. There was also an associated paralysis of the radial nerve. *B*, Radiographs of the fracture fragments in the coaptation splint show satisfactory linear alignment but minimal bayonet apposition. *C*, Clinical photograph of the coaptation splint with molding around the midshaft. A forearm coaptation splint was added to support the wrist because of the radial nerve paralysis.

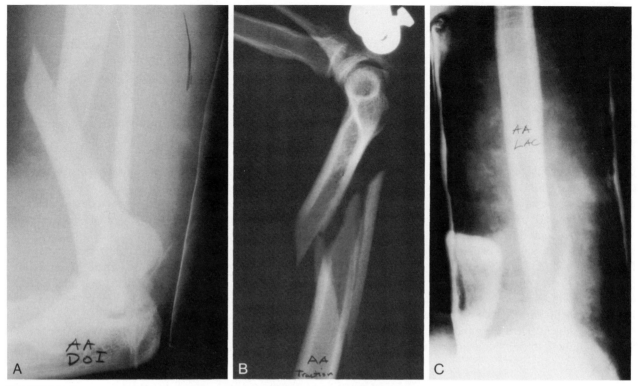

FIGURE 14–56
A, Injury film of a 15-year-old baseball player who sustained a comminuted fracture of the distal humeral shaft when he slid into home plate. Because of the marked comminution, he was treated with overhead olecranon pin traction for 10 days *(B)* until some early callus formed, and then he was placed in a long-arm cast *(C)*.

traindicated in the patient who is thrashing due to an associated head injury.

Open Reduction. Compressive plate fixation is an effective method of stabilizing shaft fractures. When applied properly this method has a low rate of complications and a high rate of union [370]. In patients with midshaft fractures the plate provides the best compressive force when applied to the posterior surface. In proximal and distal fractures the lateral surface of the shaft may need to be used. The major advantage is the security of fixation, which allows early motion and rehabilitation. A disadvantage is the need for a second operation to remove the plate.

Open reduction is usually mandatory in patients with vascular injuries. It may also be necessary if ipsilateral forearm fractures are present [362].

It is especially important to remove the plate in athletes, particularly those participating in collision sports. Thus with this type of treatment two recovery periods are needed. The first occurs after the initial fracture. The second occurs after plate removal because the bone must be protected until it is intrinsically stable—that is, until the defects produced by the screws and plate are completely filled with new bone, a time not exactly predictable. An ideal indication for the use of the lightweight coaptation brace may be during this second recovery period.

AUTHOR'S PREFERRED METHOD OF TREATMENT

In simple displaced closed fractures the use of the coaptation splint is ideal for both comfort and adequate stability. As the swelling subsides, the circular wrapping can be tightened. Early in the course of treatment the patient is started on isometric simultaneous biceps and triceps contractures to preserve muscle function and provide compressive forces across the fracture callus. In the pediatric athlete there is usually enough internal stability by 4 to 5 weeks to remove the splint. At this point shoulder motion can be initiated.

Postoperative Care

Once the fracture is stable the athlete progresses to a vigorous rehabilitation program emphasizing muscle strengthening not only of the biceps and triceps but also of the muscles about the shoulder girdle and forearm. The athlete can safely return to full activity depending on the nature of the sport. Athletes participating in swimming and tennis can return earlier than those in collision sports. Return to such sports may be best delayed until the callus has developed a distinct cortex. Added protection may be provided by a lightweight coaptation brace in the early stages.

SPECIAL FRACTURES

Pathologic Fractures

In fractures occurring through benign bone lesions the fracture should be allowed to heal. In the nonathlete unicameral bone cysts may heal in many cases with saline irrigation and steroid injection techniques. This usually is a prolonged process but does stabilize the bone for the stresses of normal activity. In the athlete, however, because rapid and complete reconstitution is desired, curettage and bone grafting are the best methods of restoring the bone to a stable condition to allow a return to activity as soon as possible.

Ipsilateral Fractures

If the forearm fracture is complex, it may need to be stabilized internally. The humeral shaft fracture can then often be treated nonoperatively. If a complex humeral fracture or other systemic problem is present, internal fixation of the humerus may be necessary [362].

COMPLICATIONS

Angular and Rotational Deformities

In the adolescent athlete angulation of up to 10 degrees usually has an insignificant effect on function or cosmetic appearance. Angulation greater than 10 degrees usually poses a cosmetic problem, especially if the distal fragment is in varus. Any angulation greater than 10 degrees needs to be corrected. Often this can be done with a delayed manipulation 3 to 4 weeks after the fracture when the callus is reasonably stable. In some cases, especially if angulation is in the sagittal plane, a manipulating cast can be applied with the elbow in extension. The athlete can usually tolerate this for the 2 to 3 weeks that are necessary until the fracture becomes stable enough to remove all immobilization devices.

In complete fractures treated with coaptation splints or hanging arm casts, the forearm rests against the anterior trunk. This can result in some internal rotation of the distal fragment. Usually this is no greater than 10 degrees and is not evident clinically [357]. If the extremity is used for throwing, this degree of rotation may be critical. In such patients, the upper extremity may have to be immobilized with the forearm directed anteriorly. This may require incorporating the arm cast into a thoracobrachial type of body cast.

Vascular Injuries

Vascular injuries usually result from severe violence and fortunately are rarely seen in the athletic setting. They most often occur with open injuries. When they do occur, they are surgical emergencies. A temporary vascular shunt may have to be placed to perfuse the extremity while bony repair is undertaken. These injuries require internal fixation to protect the vascular repair.

Nerve Injuries

Only one isolated median nerve injury has been reported in the pediatric age group [363]. This occurred in a patient with an incomplete greenstick midshaft fracture in which the artery was entrapped in the fracture site. Injuries to the ulnar nerve with humeral shaft fractures have not been reported.

The radial nerve is commonly injured in humeral shaft fractures. Twenty-five per cent of reported radial nerve injuries have occurred in patients under the age of 20 [365]. This injury is more common in shaft fractures of the middle third. Whitson [371] demonstrated anatomically that the radial nerve is separated posteriorly from the humeral shaft by a layer of deep triceps muscle and thus is relatively protected in this area.

The radial nerve is juxtaposed to the lateral cortex at the junction of the distal third and the middle third of the shaft where it passes from posterior to anterior through the lateral intermuscular septum. Because of this, Holstein and Lewis [360] suggested that all fractures in this area had a potential for acute or delayed radial nerve injury and thus should be fixed internally.

Subsequent follow-up studies have shown that from 73% to 93% of radial nerve injuries associated with fractures of the humeral shaft recover spontaneously, and there is no advantage to early exploration [356, 366, 367]. Szalay and Rockwood [368] outlined the method for estimating waiting time. They measure the distance from the tip of the most proximal spike to the medial epicondyle and then calculate 1 to 2 mm/day for regeneration plus 30 to 60 days for good measure. If there is no return of either gross muscle activity or EMG activity after this period of time, the nerve needs to be explored. They also noted that even if the nerve has been lacerated, the results with delayed repair are better than those with primary repair.

The major indications for primary open exploration are an open fracture or poor nerve function in a patient who needs open exploration for vascular repair.

Nerve Injuries

Kaye E. Wilkins, M.D.

Nerve injuries can be classified as *acute*, due to tension or blows directly to the nerve, or *chronic*, due to repeated pressure by the adjacent muscles, tendons, or ligaments. Acute injuries are usually manifest by the sudden onset of pain associated with development of a sensory or motor dysfunction in the distribution of the nerve involved. Chronic injuries are often manifest as pain syndromes with rather occult sensory and motor findings.

ACUTE NERVE INJURIES

These are usually the result of acute stretching of the nerve or a direct blow. Bateman [372] described the mechanism of acute nerve injuries in great detail. Initially, the symptoms of an acute traumatic nerve syndrome are complaints by the athlete of "burning numbness" in the shoulder or distally in the extremity. There may be other sensations such as radiating shocklike pain as well. Often the athlete is reluctant to move the extremity because of severe pain. One of the most important differentiations is whether the pain arises from compression in the area of the cervical spine and brachial plexus or distally in the shoulder region.

The initial assessment of motor function is often more helpful than looking for sensory deficits. All of the major muscle groups about the shoulder, elbow, and wrist need to be carefully evaluated. Two muscles that are often overlooked clinically are the trapezius and the serratus anterior. Nerve conduction velocities and electromyographic studies are helpful at appropriate times.

Bateman grouped the mechanisms causing acute traumatic shoulder neuropathies into five categories, usually based on the mechanism of the injury. He emphasized trying to reconstruct as much as possible the position of the player or players at the time of body contact or fall. His five categories are as follows: (1) projectile falls, (2) shoulder angle blows, (3) frontal force, (4) axillary injuries, and (5) twisting trauma.

Projectile Falls. A projectile fall is one in which the athlete falls directly on the point of the shoulder. Usually the head and neck are abducted in the opposite direction. The major nerve damage that occurs with this type of fall is to the supraclavicular portion of the brachial plexus. This usually places most of the stretch on the upper roots and spares the lower roots. Bateman believed that this was the most common traumatic nerve injury in the shoulder.

Shoulder Angle Blows. This type of injury involves a direct blow between the shoulder and the neck. This usually occurs in such stick handling sports as hockey and lacrosse and in certain riding and vehicular riding events. Usually most of the force is applied to the edge of the trapezius and the cephalad margin of the scapula. With this type of blow the accessory nerve can be injured at the cephaled margin of the trapezius. The major result here is paralysis of the middle and lower portions of the trapezius muscle. If the blow or stretch is more distal, the suprascapular nerve can be injured from either a direct contusion or an acute stretch. Again, the symptoms of weakness of the supraspinatus and infraspinatus muscles may be vague and difficult to elicit in the acute evaluation. The final nerve that can be injured is the axillary nerve as it courses posteriorly around the proximal humerus. This injury occurs very rarely because the bulk of the deltoid muscle provides protection against direct blows.

Frontal Force. This injury occurs when the player crouches forward and spreads his arms at the shoulder in an abducted and externally rotated position, as in blocking or tackling positions. In this position the infraclavicular branches of the brachial plexus can be crushed against the head of the humerus by a direct blow from an object such as a player's helmet or knee. The nerves most vulnerable to injury by this mechanism are the axillary and musculocutaneous nerves.

Axillary Injuries. Direct blows into the axilla from an inferior direction can crush the posterior cord of the brachial plexus against the upper aspect of the humerus and glenoid labium. This type of injury occurs in football, hockey, and ice vehicle racing sports. Because the posterior cord is accompanied by large venae comites, there may be significant hematoma formation with this injury. The deltoid and triceps muscles are often weakened because of injury to the posterior cord. The lower portion of the radial nerve often remains functional.

Twisting Trauma. This injury usually occurs in football when a twisting motion is applied to the shoulder. It also can occur with discus throwing. The most common associated injury complex is the injury to the axillary nerve that occurs in conjunction with dislocation of the glenohumeral joint.

Most of these acute neuropathies represent simple stretching (neurapraxia) of the nerve, and the dysfunction is temporary. In these instances the extremity needs to be rested and supported until the nerve has recovered. On rare occasions the nerve may be completely torn (axonotmesis), and surgical exploration and repair may be necessary.

CHRONIC NERVE INJURIES

The three major nerves affected by overuse or impingement syndromes of the shoulder are the axillary nerve in the quadrilateral space, the suprascapular nerve, and the long thoracic nerve. Priest and Nagel [381] reported a rare thoracic outlet syndrome in the depressed shoulder associated with the ''tennis shoulder'' syndrome.

Very little has been written about these syndromes in the pediatric athlete. The orthopedist who deals with adolescent athletes must be aware of the clinical manifestations of these syndromes in these often rather physically mature youngsters.

Suprascapular Nerve Syndrome. The suprascapular nerve is vulnerable to injury because of its anatomic characteristics. It is accompanied by a branch of the suprascapular artery, which originates from the thyrocervical trunk. When these structures reach the superior border of the scapula, they separate briefly. The nerve passes under the suprascapular ligament while the artery passes over it (Fig. 14–57). At this point the nerve is restricted in its motion and is thus vulnerable to traction or compression injury with extremes of shoulder motion. In the suprascapular fossa the artery and nerve are joined where the nerve supplies the supraspinatus muscle. The nerve then courses distally to the root of the acromion, where it gives off articular branches to the glenohumeral and acromioclavicular joints. At the root of the acromion it curves caudad around the spine of the scapula to supply the infraspinatus muscle. Although it supplies most of the sensory and sympathetic innervation to the

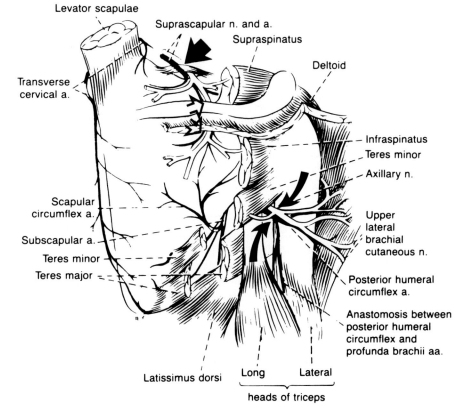

FIGURE 14–57
Neurologic injuries about the shoulder. The suprascapular nerve is bound down in the suprascapular notch by the transverse scapular ligament (large black arrow). Compression of the suprascapular nerve can also occur as it curves around the base of the acromion process to supply the infraspinatous muscle (double open arrows). The third area of compression is the axillary nerve as it emerges from the quadrangle space (double curved black arrows). (From Anderson, T. E., and Bergfield, J. A. Common throwing injuries of the shoulder. *Mediguide to Orthopedics* 4[1], 1982.)

Levator scapulae

Suprascapular n. and a.

Supraspinatus

Deltoid

Transverse cervical a.

Infraspinatus

Teres minor

Axillary n.

Scapular circumflex a.

Subscapular a.

Teres minor

Teres major

Upper lateral brachial cutaneous n.

Posterior humeral circumflex a.

Anastomosis between posterior humeral circumflex and profunda brachii aa.

Latissimus dorsi

Long   Lateral

heads of triceps

glenohumeral capsule, it has no cutaneous branches [376].

The symptoms of this nerve compression syndrome produce chronic posterior shoulder pain and weakness that often mimic the symptoms of a torn rotator cuff [377]. Drez [377] described a 16-year-old basketball player who developed weakness and pain after falling directly on his shoulder. Atrophy of the supraspinatus and infraspinatus muscles developed. An electromyogram showed denervation in both muscles. This athlete recovered with only supportive therapy. Drez felt that in this case (and in most other cases) the cause was a neurapraxia of the suprascapular nerve where it is stretched over the superior margin of the suprascapular notch (see Fig. 14–57). This injury can occur when the shoulder is acutely depressed. It has also been noted when the shoulder is repeatedly depressed, causing repeated microtrauma to the nerve. Bennett [373] suggested that traction on this nerve occurs in the follow-through phase of baseball throwing.

In cases that fail to respond to rest and rehabilitation, surgical release of the suprascapular ligament is felt to help by eliminating the point of nerve fixation. Jobe and his co-workers [379], however, believed that the point of injury in this syndrome is where the nerve crosses the base of the acromion (see Fig. 14–57). In their cases, which were more chronic, only the infraspinatus muscle was involved, and the supraspinatus was spared. This syndrome is often manifest as chronic pain that is misdiagnosed as ''tendinitis'' in high-level baseball pitchers. In their experience the residual infraspinatus muscle could be strengthened with exercises so that the pitcher could return to a competitive level. They did not believe that this type of suprascapular nerve syndrome would respond to surgical decompression. Electrical diagnostic studies may aid in differentiation of involved structures.

Quadrilateral Space Syndrome. This injury was originally described in baseball pitchers by Bennett [373] as an injury caused by a traction exostosis that occurred on the inferior border of the glenoid fossa due to the pull of the long head of the triceps and posterior glenohumeral capsule. He surmised that this exostosis irritated the axillary nerve as it coursed through the quadrilateral space. Cahill [374, 375] more recently suggested that the nerve may be injured when it is chronically compressed by fibrous bands in the quadrilateral space (see Fig. 14–57). This compressive force usually is greatest in the cocking phase of throwing. As a result of this compression, posterior shoulder pain occurs and increases when the shoulder is abducted and externally rotated. An arteriogram may be helpful by demonstrating compression of the posterior humeral circumflex artery when the shoulder is abducted and externally rotated. Treatment consists of rest and local steroid injections to decrease the inflamation. If this fails, surgical de-

compression of the quadrilateral space may be necessary.

The important aspect of these two chronic nerve syndromes is that their presence should always be kept in mind when evaluating the athlete who complains of chronic posterior shoulder pain. In athletes with this complaint the strength of the supraspinatus, infraspinatus, and deltoid muscles must be carefully evaluated. If there is any question about the diagnosis, electromyographic evaluation of these muscles may be helpful.

Long Thoracic Nerve Injury. This can occur as an idiopathic entity or following a traction injury to the shoulder such as occurs with bench press or shoulder resistance exercises. It has also been reported in young throwers with no major injury [378, 381].

The usual diagnostic test is to have the athlete push forward against a fixed object such as a wall while looking for winging of the scapula. This injury usually recovers with rest and prevention of reinjury. It must be remembered, however, that winging of the scapula can also be a manifestation of a C7 root neuropathy [380].

References

Epidemiology

1. Adams, J. E. Little League shoulder—Osteochondrosis of the proximal humeral epiphysis in boy baseball pitchers. *Calif Med* 105:22–25, 1966.
2. Albright, J. A., et al. Clinical study of baseball pitchers: Correlation of injury to the throwing arm with method of delivery. *Am J Sports Med* 6:15–21, 1978.
3. Atwater, A. E. Biomechanics of overarm throwing movements and of throwing injuries. *Exerc Sport Sci Rev* 7:43–85, 1979.
4. Barnett, L. S. Little League shoulder syndrome: Proximal humeral epiphysis in adolescent baseball pitchers. *J Bone Joint Surg* 67A:495–496, 1985.
5. Barone, G. W., and Rodgers, B. M. Pediatric equestrian injuries: A 14-year review. *J Trauma* 29:245–247, 1989.
6. Blyth, C. S., and Mueller, F. O. An epidemiologic study of high school football injuries in North Carolina 1968–1972. Consumer Product Safety Commission, final report. Washington D.C., U.S. Government Printing Office, 1973.
7. Blyth, C. S., and Mueller, F. O. When and where players get hurt. *Physician Sportsmed* 2:45–52, 1974.
8. Bixby-Hammett, D. M. Head injuries in the equestrian sports. *Physician Sportsmed* 11(8):86–87, 1983.
9. Cahill, B. R., and Tullos, H. S. Little League shoulder. *Sports Med* 2:150–153, 1974.
10. Carr, D., Johnson, R. J., and Pope, M. H. Upper extremity injuries in skiing. *Am J Sports Med* 9:378–383, 1981.
11. Chung, S. M. K., Batterman, S. C., and Brighton, C. T. Sheer strength of the human femoral capital epiphyseal plate. *J Bone Joint Surg* 58A:94–103, 1976.
12. Clarke, H. H. Physical fitness today: A status report. *Physical Fitness News Letter.* Series 27(5), 1981.
13. Committee on School Health. Competitive athletics. *Pediatrics* 18:672–675, 1956.
14. Consumer Product Safety Commission. Bicycle related injuries: Data from the National Electronic Injury Surveillance System. *JAMA* 257:3334–3337, 1987.
15. Cox, J. S. The fate of the acromioclavicular joint in athletic injuries. *Am J Sports Med* 9:50–53, 1981.
16. Collins, H. R. Contact sports in junior high school. *Tex Med* 63:67–69, 1967.

17. Culpepper, M. I., and Niemann, K. M. W. High school football injuries in Birmingham, Alabama. *S Med J* 76:873–878, 1983.

18. Dominquez, R. H. Shoulder pain in age group swimmers. *In* Eriksson, B., and Furberg, B. (Eds.), *Swimming Medicine IV.* Baltimore, University Park Press, 1978, pp. 105–109.

19. Dotter, W. E. Little Leaguer's shoulder—A fracture of the proximal epiphyseal cartilage of the humerus due to baseball pitching. *Guthrie Clinic Bull* 23:68–72, 1953.

20. Fulton, N. N., Albright, J. P., and El-Khoury, G. Y. Cortical desmoid-like lesion of the proximal humerus and its occurrence in gymnasts (ringman's shoulder lesion). *Am J Sports Med* 7:57–61, 1979.

21. Gainor, B. M., et al. The throw: Biomechanics and acute injury. *Am J Sports Med* 8:114–118, 1980.

22. Garrick, J. G., and Requa, R. K. Injuries in high school sports. *Pediatrics* 61:465–469, 1978.

23. Goldman, S. H. Personal communication, 1977.

24. Goldberg, B., Rosenthal, P. P., and Nicholas, J. A. Injuries in youth football. *Physician Sportsmed* 12:122–132, 1984.

25. Goldberg, B., et al. Children's sports injuries: Are they avoidable? *Physician Sportsmed* 7:93–101, 1979.

26. Hafner, J. Problems in matching young athletes: Body fat, peach fuzz, muscle and moustache. *Physician Sportsmed* 3:96–98, 1975.

27. Henry, J. H., and Neigut, B. L.: The injury rate in professional basketball. *Am J Sports Med* 10:16–18, 1982.

28. Hill, J. A., Lombardo, S. J., Kerlan, R. K., et al. The modified Bristow-Helfet procedure for recurrent anterior shoulder subluxations and dislocations. *Am J Sports Med* 9:283–287, 1981.

29. Hill, J. A. Epidemiologic perspective on shoulder injuries. *Clin Sports Med* 2:241–246, 1983.

30. Ireland, M. L., and Andrews, J. R. Shoulder and elbow injuries in the young athlete. *Clin Sports Med* 7:473–494, 1988.

31. Kirburz, D., et al. Bicycle accidents and injuries among adult cyclists. *Am J Sports Med* 14:416–419, 1986.

32. Landin, L. A. Fracture patterns in children. *Acta Orthop Scand* (Suppl)202:1–109, 1983.

33. Larson, R. L., and McMahan, R. O. The epiphyses and the child athlete. *JAMA* 196:607–612, 1966.

34. Lipscomb, A. B. Baseball pitching injuries in growing athletes. *J Sports Med* 3:25–34, 1975.

35. Mueller, F., and Blyth, C. Epidemiology of sports injuries in children. *Clin Sports Med* 3:343–352, 1982.

36. National Federation of State High School Associations. Sports participation survey indicates overall increase. National Federation Press, Vol. 2, October, 1981.

37. National Electronic Injury Surveillance System. Data highlights. Vol. 5, October–December, 1981.

38. Olson, O. C. The Spokane study: High school football injuries. *Physician Sportsmed* 7(12):75–82, 1979.

39. Peterson, C. A., and Peterson, H. A. Analysis of the incidence of injuries to the epiphyseal growth plate. *J Trauma* 12:275–281, 1972.

40. Priest, J. D., and Nagel, D. A. Tennis shoulder. *Am J Sports Med* 4:28–42, 1976.

41. Requa, R., and Garrick, J. G. Injuries in interscholastic wrestling. *Physician Sportsmed* 9:44–51, 1981.

42. Richardson, A. B., Jobe, F. W., and Collins, H. R. The shoulder in competitive swimming. *Am J Sports Med* 8:159–163, 1980.

43. Richardson, A. B. Overuse syndromes in baseball, tennis, gymnastics, and swimming. *Clin Sportsmed* 2:379–390, 1983.

44. Rockwood, C. A., Jr. Fractures and dislocations of the ends of the clavicle, scapulae and glenohumeral joint. *In* Rockwood, C. A., Jr., Wilkins, K. E., and King, R. E. (Eds.), *Fractures in Children,* Vol. 3, Philadelphia, J. B. Lippincott, 1984.

45. Slager, R. F. From Little League to big league, the weak spot is the arm. *Am J Sports Med* 5:37–48, 1977.

46. Snook, G. A. Injuries in women's gymnastics. A five year study. *Am J Sports Med* 7:242–244, 1979.

47. Snook, G. A. Injuries in intercollegiate wrestling—A 5-year study. *Am J Sports Med* 10:142–144, 1982.

48. Tibone, J. E. Shoulder problems of adolescents: How they differ from those of adults. *Clin Sports Med* 2:423–427, 1983.

49. Torg, J. S. The Little League pitcher. *Am Fam Physician* 6:71–76, 1972.

50. Torg, J. S., Pollack, H., and Sweterlitsch, P. The effect of competitive pitching on the shoulders and elbow of preadolescent baseball players. *Pediatrics* 49:267–272, 1972.

51. Tullos, H. S., and King, J. W. Lesions of the pitching arm in adolescents. *JAMA* 220:264–271, 1972.

52. Tullos, H. S., and Fain, R. H. Little League shoulder: Rotational stress fracture of proximal humeral epiphysis. *J Sports Med* 2:152–153, 1974.

53. Weseley, J. S., and Barenfeld, P. A. Ball throwers' fracture of the humerus: Six case reports. *Clin Orthop* 64:153–156, 1969.

54. Zariczny, B., et al. Sports related injuries in school age children. *Am J Sportsmed* 8:318–324, 1980.

Anatomy, Biomechanics, and Physiology
Anatomy

55. Abbott, L. S., and Lucas, D. B. The function of the clavicle. Its surgical significance. *Ann Surg* 140:583–597, 1954.

56. Anderson, H. Histochemistry and development of the human shoulder and acromioclavicular joints with particular reference to the early development of the clavicle. *Acta Anat* 55:124–165, 1963.

57. Bearn, J. G. Direct observations on the function of the capsule of the sternoclavicular joint in clavicular support. *J Anat* 101:159–170, 1967.

58. Chung, M. K., and Nissenbaum, M. M. Congenital and developmental defects of the shoulder. *Orthop Clin North Am* 6:381, 1975.

59. Codman, E. A. *The Shoulder.* Brooklyn, G. Miller, 1934.

60. DePalma, A. F. *Surgery of the Shoulder* (3rd ed.). Philadelphia, J. B. Lippincott, 1983.

61. Denham, R. H., and Dingley, A. F. Epiphyseal separation of the medial end of the clavicle. *J Bone Joint Surg* 49A:1179–1183, 1967.

62. Detrisac, D. A., and Johnson, L. L. *Arthroscopic Shoulder Anatomy. Pathological and Surgical Implications.* Thorofare, NJ, Slack, 1986.

63. Deutsch, A. L., Resnick, D., and Mink, J. H. Computed tomography of the glenohumeral and sternoclavicular joints. *Orthop Clin North Am* 16(3):497–511, 1985.

64. Gardner, E. The embryology of the clavicle. *Clin Orthop* 58:9–16, 1968.

65. Gardner, E., and Gray, D. J. Prenatal development of the human shoulder and acromioclavicular joints. *Am J Anat* 92:219–276, 1953.

66. Hollinshead, W. H. *Anatomy for Surgeons* (3rd ed), Vol. 3. Philadelphia: Harper & Row, 1982.

67. Kent, B. E. Functional anatomy of the shoulder complex. *Phys Ther* 51:867–887, 1971.

68. Laing, P. G. The arterial supply of the adult humerus. *J Bone Joint Surg* 38A:1105–1116, 1956.

69. Liberson, F. Os acromiale—A contested anomaly. *J Bone Joint Surg* 19:683–689, 1937.

70. Reeves, B. Experiments on the tensile strength of the anterior capsular structures of the shoulder in man. *J Bone Joint Surg* 50B:858–865, 1968.

71. Todd, T. W., and D'Errico, J. The clavicular epiphyses. *Am J Anat* 41:25–50, 1928.

Biomechanics

72. Atwater, A. E. Biomechanics of overarm throwing movements and of throwing injuries. *Exerc Sport Sci Rev* 7:43–85, 1979.

73. Basmajian, J. V., and Bazant, F. J. Factors preventing downward dislocation of the adducted shoulder joint. *J Bone Joint Surg* 41A:1182–1186, 1959.

74. Bechtol, C. O. Biomechanics of the shoulder. *Clin Orthop* 146:37–41, 1959.

75. Colachis, S. C., Jr., Strohm, B. R., and Brecher, V. L. Effects of axillary nerve block on muscle force in the upper extremity. *Arch Phys Med Rehabil* 50:647–654, 1969.

76. Colachis, S. C., Jr., and Strohm, B. R. Effects of suprascapular and axillary nerve blocks on muscle force in the upper extremity. *Arch Phys Med Rehabil* 52:22–29, 1971.

77. deDuca, C. J., and Forrest, W. J. Force analysis of individual muscles acting simultaneously in the shoulder joint during isometric abduction. *J Biomech* 6:385–393, 1973.

78. DePalma, A. F., Coker, A. J., and Probhaker, M. The role of the subscapularis in recurrent anterior dislocation of the shoulder. *Clin Orthop* 54:35, 1969.

79. Ekholm, J., Arborelius, U. P., Hillered, L., et al. Shoulder muscle EMG and resisting moment during diagonal exercise movements resisted by weight-and-pulley circuit. *Scand J Rehabil Med* 10:179–185, 1978.

80. Frankel, V. H., and Burstein, A. H. *Orthopaedic Biomechanics.* Philadelphia, Lea & Febiger, 1971.

81. Freedman, L., and Munro, R. R. Abduction of the arm in the scapular plane: Scapular and glenohumeral movements. *J Bone Joint Surg* 48A:1503–1510, 1966.

82. Fukuda, K., Craig, E. V., An, K., et al. Biomechanic study of the ligamentous system of the acromioclavicular joint. *J Bone Joint Surg* 68(3):434–440, 1986.

83. Gainor, B. J., Piotrowski, G., Puhl, J., et al. The throw: Biomechanics and acute injury. *Am J Sports Med* 8:114–118, 1980.

84. Glousman, R., Jobe, F., Tibone, J., et al. Dynamic electromyographic analysis of the throwing shoulder with glenohumeral instability. *J Bone Joint Surg* 70(2):220–226, 1988.

85. Howell, S. M., Galinat, B. J., Renzi, A. J. et al. Normal and abnormal mechanics of the glenohumeral joint in the horizontal plane. *J Bone Joint Surg* 70(2):227–232, 1988.

86. Howell, S. M., Imobersteg, A. M., Seger, D. H., et al. Clarification of the role of the supraspinatus muscle in shoulder function. *J Bone Joint Surg* 68(3):398–404, 1986.

87. Inman, V. T., Saunders, J. B., and Abbott, L. C. Observations on the function of the shoulder joint. *J Bone Joint Surg* 26:1–30, 1944.

88. Ivey, F. M., Calhoun, J. H., Rusche, K., et al. Isokinetic testing of shoulder strength: Normal values. *Arch Phys Med Rehabil* 66:384–386, 1985.

89. Jobe, F. W., Tibone, J. E., Perry, J., et al. An EMG analysis of the shoulder in throwing and pitching. *Am J Sports Med* 11:3–5, 1983.

90. Lucas, D. B. Biomechanics of the shoulder joint. *Arch Surg* 107:425–432, 1973.

91. Matsen, F. A., III. Biomechanics of the shoulder. *In* Frankel, V. H., and Nordin, M. (Eds.), *Basic Biomechanics of the Skeletal System.* Philadelphia, Lea & Febiger, 1980, pp. 221–242.

92. Nuber, G. W., Jobe, F. W., Perry, J., et al. Fine wire electromyography analysis of muscles of the shoulder during swimming. *Am J Sports Med* 14(1):7–11, 1986.

93. Perry, J. Anatomy and biomechanics of the shoulder in throwing, swimming, gymnastics, and tennis. *Clin Sports Med* 2:247–270, 1983.

94. Poppen, N. K., and Walker, P. S. Normal and abnormal motion of the shoulder. *J Bone Joint Surg* 58A:195–201, 1976.

95. Poppen, N. K., and Walker, P. S. Forces at the glenohumeral joint in abduction. *Clin Orthop* 136:165–170, 1978.

96. Richardson, A. R. The biomechanics of swimming: The shoulder and knee. *Clin Sports Med* 5:103–113, 1986.

97. Richardson, A. B., Jobe, F. W., and Collins, H. R. The shoulder in competitive swimming. *Am J Sports Med* 81:159–163, 1980.

98. Saha, A. K. Mechanics of elevation of glenohumeral joint. Its application in rehabilitation of flail shoulder in upper brachial plexus injuries and poliomyelitis and in replacement of the upper humerus by prosthesis. *Acta Orthop Scand* 44:668–678, 1973.

99. Saha, A. K. Dynamic stability of the glenohumeral joint. *Acta Orthop Scand* 42:491, 1971.

100. Turkel, S. J., Panio, M. W., Marshall, J. L., et al. Stabilizing mechanisms preventing anterior dislocation of the glenohumeral joint. *J Bone Joint Surg* 63A:1208–1217, 1981.

Physiology

101. Akeson, W. H., Amiel, D. and LaViolette, D. The connective-tissue response to immobility: A study of the chondroitin-4 and 6-sulfate and dermatan sulfate changes in periarticular connective tissue of control and immobilized knees of dogs. *Clin Orthop* 51:183–197, 1967.

102. Amiel, D., Woo, S. L-Y, Harwood, F. L., et al. The effect of immobilization on collagen turnover in connective tissue: A biochemical-biomechanical correlation. *Acta Orthop Scand* 53:325–332, 1982.

103. Cooper, R. R., and Misol, S. Tendon and ligament insertion. *J Bone Joint Surg* 52A:1–20, 1970.

104. Hooley, C. J., and McCrum, N. G. The viscoelastic deformation of tendon. *J Biomech* 13:521–528, 1980.

105. Muckle, D. S. Comparative study of ibuprofen and aspirin in soft-tissue injuries. *Rheumatol Rehabil* 13:141–147, 1974.

106. Noyes, F. R. Functional properties of knee ligaments and alterations induced by immobilization. *Clin Orthop* 123:210–242, 1977.

107. Noyes, F. R., DeLucas, J. L., and Torvik, P. J. Biomechanics of anterior cruciate ligament failure: An analysis of strain-rate sensitivity and mechanisms of failure in primates. *J Bone Joint Surg* 56A:236–253, 1974.

108. Noyes, F. R., Torvik, P. J., Hyde, W. B., et al. Biomechanics of ligament failure. II. An analysis of immobilization, exercise and reconditioning effects of primates. *J Bone Joint Surg* 56A:1406–1418, 1974.

109. Popov, E. P. *Mechanics of Materials* (SI version, 2nd ed.). Englewood Cliffs, NJ, Prentice-Hall, 1978.

110. Schmidt, K. L., Ott, V. R., Rocher, D. S., and Schaller, H. Heat, cold and inflammation. *Z Rheumatol* 38:391–404, 1979.

111. Tipton, C. M., James, S. L., Mergner, W., et al. Influence of exercise on strength of medial collateral knee ligaments of dogs. *Am J Physiol* 218:894–902, 1970.

112. Vailas, A. C., Tipton, C. M., Matthes, R. D., et al. Physical activity and its influence on the repair process of medial collateral ligaments. *Connect Tissue Res* 9:25–31, 1981.

Skeletal Injuries

Clavicle Fractures

113. Abbott, L. D., and Lucas, D. G. The function of the clavicle. *Ann Surg* 140:583–599, 1954.

114. Allman, F. L. Fractures and ligamentous injuries of the clavicle and its articulation. *J Bone Joint Surg* 49A:774, 1967.

115. Billington, R. W. A new (plaster yoke) dressing for fracture of the clavicle. *South Med J* 24:667–670, 1931.

116. Blount, W. P. *Fractures in Children.* Baltimore, Williams & Wilkins, 1955.

117. Bowen, A. D. Plastic bowing of the clavicle in children. *J Bone Joint Surg* 65A:403, 1983.

118. Curtis, R. J., and Rockwood, C. A. Fractures and dislocations of the shoulder in children. *In* Rockwood, C. A., and Matsen, F. A. (Eds.), *The Shoulder.* Philadelphia, W. B. Saunders, 1990.

119. Curtis, R. J., Dameron, T. B., and Rockwood, C. A. Fractures and dislocations of the shoulder. *In* Rockwood, C. A., Wilkins, K. E., and King, R. E. (Eds.), *Fractures in Children.* Philadelphia, J. B. Lippincott, 1991.

120. Dugdale, T. W., and Fulkerson, J. P. Pneumothorax complicating closed fracture of the clavicle. *Clin Orthop* 221:212–214, 1987.

121. Fairbanks, H. A. T. *Atlas of General Affections of the Skeleton.* Edinburgh, E & S Livingstone, 1951.

122. Ghormley, R. K., Black, J. R., and Cherry, J. H. Ununited fractures of the clavicle. *Am J Surg* 51:343–349, 1941.

123. Gumley, G. J., and Jupiter, J. J. Clavicle non-union—A review of management and presentation of a stable bone graft. *Orthop Trans* 9:29, 1985.

124. Howard, F. M., and Shafer, S. J. Injuries to the clavicle with neurovascular complications: A study of fourteen cases. *J Bone Joint Surg* 47A:1335–1346, 1965.

125. Jablon, M., Sutker, A., and Post, M. Irreducible fractures of the middle-third of the clavicle. *J Bone Joint Surg* 61A:296–298, 1979.

126. Katznelson, A., Nerubay, J., and Oliver, S. Dynamic fixation of the avulsed clavicle. *J Trauma* 16:841, 1976.

127. Key, J. A., and Conwell, H. E. Fractures of the clavicle. *In The Management of Fractures, Dislocations and Sprains.* St. Louis, C. V. Mosby, 1946, pp. 495–512.

128. Lester, C. W. The treatment of fractures of the clavicle. *Ann Surg* 89:600–606, 1929.

129. Liechtl, R. Fracture of the clavicle and scapula. *In* Weber, B. G., Brunner, C., and Freuler, F. (Eds.), *Treatment of Fractures in Children and Adolescents.* New York, Springer-Verlag, 1980, pp. 88–95.

130. Ljunggren, A. E. Clavicular function. *Acta Orthop Scand* 50:261–268, 1979.

131. Manske, D. J., and Szabo, R. M. The operative treatment of mid-shaft clavicular non-unions. *J Bone Joint Surg* 67A:1367, 1985.

132. Miller, D. S., and Boswick, J. A. Lesions of the brachial plexus associated with fractures of the clavicle. *Clin Orthop* 64:144, 1969.

133. Mital, M. A., and Aufranc, O. E. Venous occlusion following greenstick fracture of the clavicle. *JAMA* 206:1301–1302, 1968.

134. Moseley, H. G. The clavicle: Its anatomy and function. *Clin Orthop* 58:17–27, 1968.

135. Neer, C. S. II Nonunion of the clavicle. *JAMA* 172:1006–1011, 1960.

136. Nogi, J., Heckman, J. D., Hakala, M., et al. Non-union of the clavicle in a child. A case report. *Clin Orthop* 110:19, 1975.

137. Ogden, J. A., Conologue, G. J., and Bronson, M. L. Radiology of postnatal skeletal development, III. The clavicle. *Skeletal Radiol* 4:196–203, 1979.

138. Penn, I. The vascular complications of fractures of the clavicle. *J Trauma* 4:819–831, 1964.

139. Pollen, A. G. *Fractures and Dislocations in Children.* Baltimore, Williams & Wilkins, 1973.

140. Rang, M. Clavicle. *In* Rang, M. (Ed.), *Children's Fractures* (2nd ed.). Philadelphia, J. B. Lippincott, 1983.

141. Rowe, C. R. An atlas of anatomy and treatment of midclavicular fractures. *Clin Orthop* 58:29–42, 1968.

142. Salter, R. B. *Textbook of Disorders and Injuries of the Musculoskeletal System.* Baltimore, Williams & Wilkins, 1970, pp. 439–440.

143. Sayr, L. A simple dressing for fracture of the clavicle. *Am Pract* 4:1, 1871.

144. Slocum, D. B. The mechanisms of common football injuries. *JAMA* 170:1640, 1959.

145. Snyder, L. Loss of accompanying soft tissue shadow of clavicle with occult fracture. *South Med J* 72:243, 1979.

146. Stanley, D., Trowbridge, E. A., and Norris, S. H. The mechanism of clavicular fractures: A clinical and biomechanical analysis. *J Bone Joint Surg* 70B(3):461–464, 1988.

147. Tse, D. H. W., Slabaugh, P. B., and Carlson, P. A. Injury to the axillary artery by a closed fracture of the clavicle. *J Bone Joint Surg* 62A:1372, 1980.

148. Watson-Jones, R. Fractures of the clavicle. *In Fractures and Joint Injuries.* Baltimore, Williams & Wilkins, 1955.

149. Wilkins, R., and Johnston, R. M. Ununited fractures of the clavicle. *J Bone Joint Surg* 65A:773, 1983.

150. Wilson, J. C. Fractures and dislocations in children. *Pediatr Clin North Am* 14:659–662, 1967.

151. Zenni, E. J., Krieg, J. K., and Rosen, M. J. Open reduction and internal fixation of clavicular fractures. *J Bone Joint Surg* 63A:147–151, 1981.

Lateral End of Clavicle

152. Allman, F. L. Fractures and ligamentous injuries of the clavicle. *J Bone Joint Surg* 42B:312–319, 1963.

153. Asher, M. A. Dislocations of the upper extremity in children. *Orthop Clin North Am* 7:583, 1976.

154. Barber, F. A. Complete posterior acromioclavicular dislocation. *Orthopaedics* 10(3):493–496, 1987.

155. Bernard, T. M., Brunet, M. E., and Haddad, R. J. Fractured coracoid process in acromioclavicular dislocations. *Clin Orthop* 175:227–232, 1983.

156. Bjerneld, H., Hovelius, L., and Thorling, J. Acromioclavicular separations treated conservatively. *Acta Orthop Scand* 54:743–745, 1983.

157. Black, G. B., McPherson, J. A., and Reed, M. H. Traumatic pseudodislocation of the acromioclavicular joint in children. *Am J Sports Med* 19(6):644–646, 1991.

158. Bosworth, B. M. Acromioclavicular separation—A new method of repair. *Surg Gynecol Obstet* 73:866–871, 1941.

159. Browne, J. E., et al. Acromioclavicular joint dislocations: Comparative results following operative treatment with and without primary distal clavicectomy. *Am J Sports Med* 5:258, 1977.

160. Buckfield, C. T., and Castle, M. E. Acute traumatic dislocation of the clavicle. *J Bone Joint Surg* 66A:379, 1984.

161. Curtis, R. J., Dameron, T. B., and Rockwood, C. A. Fractures and dislocations of the shoulder. *In* Rockwood, C. A., Wilkins, R. E., and King, K. E., (Eds.), *Fractures in Children.* Philadelphia, J. B. Lippincott, 1991.

162. Eidman, D. K., Siff, S. J., and Tullos, H. S. Acromioclavicular lesions in children. *Am J Sports Med* 9(3):150–154, 1981.

163. Falstie-Jensen, S., and Mikkelsen, P. Pseudodislocation of the acromioclavicular joint. *J Bone Joint Surg* 64B:368–369, 1982.

164. Galpin, R. D., Hawkins, R. J., and Grainger, R. W. A comparative analysis of operative versus nonoperative treatment of grade III acromioclavicular separations. *Clin Orthop* 193:150–155, 1985.

165. Gerber, C., and Rockwood, C. A. Subcoracoid dislocation of the lateral end of the clavicle. *J Bone Joint Surg* 69A(6):924–927, 1987.

166. Glick, J. M., Milburn, L. J., Haggerty, J. F., et al. Dislocated acromioclavicular joint: Follow-up study of 35 unreduced acromioclavicular dislocations. *Am J Sports Med* 5(6):264–270, 1977.

167. Gurd, F. B. The treatment of complete dislocation of the outer end of the clavicle: A hitherto undescribed operation. *Ann Surg* 113:1094–1097, 1941.

168. Hall, R. H., Isaac, F., and Booth, C. R. Dislocation of the shoulder with special references to accompanying small fractures. *J Bone Joint Surg* 41A:489–494, 1959.

169. Havranek, P. Injuries of distal clavicular physis in children. *J Pediatr Orthop* 9(2):213–215, 1989.

170. Kennedy, J. C., and Cameron, H. Complete dislocation of the acromioclavicular joint. *J Bone Joint Surg* 36B(2):202–208, 1954.

171. Kohler, A., and Zimmer, E. A. *Borderlands of Normal and Early Pathologic in Skeletal Roentgenology* (3rd Am. ed. Translated by S. P. Wilke). New York, Grune & Stratton, 1968, pp. 156–159.

172. Larsen, E., Bjerg-Nielsen, A., and Christensen, P. Conservative or surgical treatment of acromioclavicular dislocation. *J Bone Joint Surg* 68(4):552–555, 1986.

173. McPherson, J. Traumatic ''pseudodislocation'' of the acromioclavicular joint in children (Abstract). *J Bone Joint Surg* 68B(3):507, 1987.

174. Montgomery, S. P., and Lloyd, R. D. Avulsion fracture of the coracoid epiphysis with acromioclavicular separation: Report of two cases in adolescents and review of literature. *J Bone Joint Surg* 59A:963–965, 1977.

175. Neer, C. S., II. Fractures of the distal third of the clavicle. *Clin Orthop* 58:43–50, 1968.

176. Ogden, J. A. Distal clavicular physeal injury. *Clin Orthop* 188:68–73, 1984.

177. Park, J. P., Arnold, J. A., Coker, T. P., et al. Treatment of acromioclavicular separations. *Am J Sports Med* 8(4):251–256, 1980.

178. Rockwood, C. A. Fractures of outer clavicle in children and adults. *J Bone Joint Surg* 64B:642, 1982.

179. Roper, B. A., and Levack, B. The surgical treatment of acromioclavicular dislocations. *J Bone Joint Surg* 64B:597, 1982.

180. Rowe, C. R. An atlas of anatomy and treatment of midclavicular fractures. *Clin Orthop* 58:29–42, 1968.

181. Smith, M. J., and Stewart, M. J. Acute acromioclavicular separations: A 20-year study. *Am J Sports Med* 7(1):62–71, 1979.

182. Taft, T. N., Wilson, F. C., and Oglesby, J. W. Dislocation of the acromioclavicular joint. *J Bone Joint Surg* 69A(7):1045–1051, 1987.

183. Taga, I., Yoneda, M., and Ono, K. Epiphyseal separation of the coracoid process associated with acromioclavicular sprain: A

case report and review of the literature. *Clin Orthop* 207:138–141, 1986.

184. Tibone, J., Sellers, R., and Tonino, P. Strength testing after third-degree acromioclavicular dislocations. *Am J Sports Med* 20(3):328–331, 1992.

185. Tossy, J. D., Mead, N. C., and Sigmond, H. M. Acromioclavicular separations: Useful and practical classification for treatment. *Clin Orthop* 28:111–119, 1963.

186. Walsh, W. M., Peterson, D. A., Shelton, G., et al. Shoulder strength following acromioclavicular injury. *Am J Sports Med* 13(3):153–161, 1985.

187. Weber, B. G., Brunner, C., and Freuler, R. *Treatment of Fractures in Children and Adolescents.* New York, Springer-Verlag, 1980, p. 89.

Medial End of Clavicle

188. Borowiecki, B., Charow, A., Cook, W., et al. An unusual football injury. *Arch Otolaryngol* 95:185–187, 1972.

189. Brooks, A. L., and Henning, G. D. Injury to the proximal clavicular epiphysis. *J Bone Joint Surg* 54A:1347, 1972.

190. Brown, J. E. Anterior sternoclavicular dislocation—A method of repair. *Am J Orthop* 31:184–189, 1961.

191. Buckerfield, C. T., and Castle, M. E. Acute traumatic retrosternal dislocation of the clavicle. *J Bone Joint Surg* 66A(3):379–385, 1984.

192. Clark, R. L., Milgram, J. W., and Yawn, D. H. Fatal aortic perforation and cardiac tamponade due to a Kirschner wire migrating from the right sternoclavicular joint. *South Med J* 67:316, 1974.

193. Denham, R. H., and Dingley, A. F. Epiphyseal separation of the medial clavicle. *J Bone Joint Surg* 49A:1179, 1967.

194. Destouet, J. M., Gilula, L. A., Murphy, W. A., et al. Computed tomography of the sternoclavicular joint and sternum. *Radiology* 138(1):123–128, 1981.

195. Deutsch, A. L., Resnick, D., and Mink, J. H. Computed tomography of the glenohumeral and sternoclavicular joints. *Orthop Clin North Am* 16:497–498, 1985.

196. Elting, J. J. Retrosternal dislocations of the clavicle. *Arch Surg* 104:35, 1972.

197. Heinig, C. F. Retrosternal dislocation of the clavicle: Early recognition, x-ray diagnosis and management. *J Bone Joint Surg* 50A:830, 1968.

198. Jit, I., and Kulkarni, M. Times of appearance and fusion of epiphysis at the medial end of the clavicle. *Indian J Med Res* 64(5):773–782, 1976.

199. Kennedy, J. C. Retrosternal dislocation of the clavicle. *J Bone Joint Surg* 31B:74, 1949.

200. Lemire, L., and Rossman, M. Sternoclavicular epiphyseal separation with adjacent clavicular fracture. *J Pediatr Orthop* 4:118, 1984.

201. Levisohn, E. M., Bunnell, W. P., and Yuan, H. A. Computed tomography in the diagnosis of dislocations of the sternoclavicular joint. *Clin Orthop* 140:12, 1979.

202. Lewonowski, K., and Bassett, G. S. Complete posterior retrosternal epiphyseal separation: A case report and review of the literature. *Clin Orthop* 281:84–88, 1992.

203. Lourie, A. A. Tomography in the diagnosis of posterior dislocation of the sterno-clavicular joint. *Acta Orthop Scand* 51:579, 1980.

204. Mazet, R., Jr. Migration of a Kirschner wire from the shoulder region into the lung: A report of two cases. *J Bone Joint Surg* 25A(2):477–483, 1943.

205. McCaughan, J. S., Jr., and Miller, P. R. Migration of Steinmann pin from shoulder to lung (letter to the editor). *JAMA* 207(10):1917, 1969.

206. McKenzie, J. M. M. Retrosternal dislocations of the clavicle. A report of two cases. *J Bone Joint Surg* 45B:138, 1961.

207. Mehta, J. C., Sachdev, A., and Collins, J. J. Retrosternal dislocations of the clavicle. *Injury* 591:79–83, 1973.

208. Rockwood, C. A. Injuries to the sternoclavicular joint. *In* Rockwood, C. A., Green, D. P., and Bucholz, R. W. (Eds.), *Fractures in Adults.* Philadelphia, J. B. Lippincott, 1991.

209. Rockwood, C. A. Dislocations of the sternoclavicular joint. *Instr Course Lect* 24:144, 1975.

210. Salvatore, J. E. Sternoclavicular joint dislocation. *Clin Orthop* 58:51, 1968.

211. Selesnick, F. H., Jablon, M., Frank, C., et al. Retrosternal dislocation of the clavicle. *J Bone Joint Surg* 66A:297, 1984.

212. Simurda, M. A. Retrosternal dislocation of the clavicle: A report of four cases and a method of repair. *Can J Surg* 11:487, 1968.

213. Tyer, H. D. D., Sturrock, W. D. S., and Callow, F. M. C. Retrosternal dislocation of the clavicle. *J Bone Joint Surg* 45B:132, 1963.

214. Winter, J., Sterner, S., Maurer, D., et al. Retrosternal epiphyseal disruption of medial clavicle: Case and review in children. *J Emerg Med* 7(1):9–13, 1989.

215. Worman, L. W., and Leagus, C. Intrathoracic injury following retrosternal dislocation of the clavicle. *J Trauma* 7(3):416–423, 1967.

Fractures of the Scapula

216. Ada, J. R., and Miller, M. E. Scapular fractures: Analysis of 113 cases. *Clin Orthop* 269:174–180, 1991.

217. Armstrong, C. P., and Van der Spuye, J. The fractured scapula: Importance and management based on a series of 62 patients. *Injury* 15:324–329, 1984.

218. Asher, M. A. Dislocations of the upper extremity in children. *Orthop Clin North Am* 7(3):583–591, 1976.

219. Aulicino, P. L., Reinert, C., Kornberg, M., et al. Displaced intra-articular glenoid fractures treated by open reduction and internal fixation. *Trauma* 26:1137–1141, 1986.

220. Benton, J., and Nelson, C. Avulsion of the coracoid process in an athlete. *J Bone Joint Surg* 53A(2):356–358, 1971.

221. Cain, T. E., and Hamilton, W. P. Scapular fractures in professional football players. *Am J Sports Med* 20(3):363–365, 1992.

222. Chung, S. M. K., and Nissenbaum, M. M. Congenital and developmental defects of the shoulder. *Orthop Clin North Am* 6(2):381–391, 1975.

223. Curtis, R. J., Dameron, T. B., and Rockwood, C. A. Fractures and dislocations of the shoulder in children. *In* Rockwood, C. A., Wilkins, K. E., and King, R. E. (Eds.), *Fractures in Children.* Philadelphia, J. B. Lippincott, 1991, pp. 829–919.

224. DePalma, A. F. *Surgery of the Shoulder* (2nd ed.). Philadelphia, J. B. Lippincott, 1973, p. 28.

225. Froimson, A. I. Fracture of the coracoid process of the scapula. *J Bone Joint Surg* 60A(5):710–711, 1978.

226. Goss, T. P. Current concepts review: Fractures of the glenoid cavity. *J Bone Joint Surg* 74A(2):299–305, 1992.

227. Guttentag, I. J., and Rechtine, G. R. Fractures of the scapula. A review of the literature. *Orthop Rev* 17:147–158, 1988.

228. Hall, R. H., Isaac, F., and Booth, C. R. Dislocation of the shoulder with special reference to accompanying small fractures. *J Bone Joint Surg* 41A:489–494, 1959.

229. Hardegger, F. H., Simpson, L. A., and Weber, B. G. The operative treatment of scapular fractures. *J Bone Joint Surg* 66B:725–731, 1984.

230. Heyse-Moore, G. H., and Stoker, D. J. Avulsion fractures of the scapula. *Skel Radiol* 9:27, 1982.

231. Ideberg, R. Unusual glenoid fractures: A report on 92 cases. *Acta Orthop Scand* 58:191–192, 1987.

232. Imatani, R. J. Fractures of the scapula: A review of 53 fractures. *J Trauma* 15:473–478, 1975.

233. Kohler, A., and Zimmer, E. A. *Borderlands of Normal and Early Pathologic in Skeletal Roentgenology* (3rd Am. ed., Translated by S. P. Wilke). New York, Grune & Stratton, 1968, pp. 156–159.

234. Liberson, R. Os acromiale: A contested anomaly. *J Bone Joint Surg* 19:683–689, 1937.

235. Mariani, P. P. Isolated fracture of the coracoid process in an athlete. *Am J Sports Med* 8(2):129–130, 1980.

236. McClure, J. G., and Raney, B. Anomalies of the scapula and related research. *Clin Orthop* 110:22–31, 1975.

237. McGahan, J. P., Rab, G. T., and Dublin, A. Fractures of the scapula. *J Trauma* 20:880–883, 1980.

238. Montgomery, S. P., and Lloyd, D. Avulsion fracture of the coracoid epiphysis with acromioclavicular separation. *J Bone Joint Surg* 59A(7):963–965, 1977.

239. Ogden, J. A., and Phillips, S. B. Radiology of postnatal skeletal development. VII. The scapula. *Skel Radiol* 9:157–169, 1983.

240. Rowe, C. R. Fractures of the scapula. *Surg Clin North Am* 43:1565, 1963.

241. Samilson, R. L. Congenital and developmental anomalies of the shoulder girdle. *Orthop Clin North Am* 11:219–231, 1980.

242. Thompson, D. A., Flynn, T. C., Miller, P. W., et al. The significance of scapular fractures. *J Trauma* 25:974–977, 1985.

243. Warwick, R., and Williams, P. L. *Gray's Anatomy* (35th ed.). Philadelphia, W. B. Saunders, 1973, p. 322.

244. Wilber, M. C., and Evans, E. B. Fractures of the scapula. *J Bone Joint Surg* 59A:358–362, 1977.

245. Zdravkovic, D., and Damholt, V. V. Comminuted and severely displaced fractures of the scapula. *Acta Orthop Scand* 45:60–65, 1974.

Glenohumeral Joint Instability

246. Aamoth, G. M., and O'Phelan, E. H. Recurrent anterior dislocation of the shoulder: A review of 40 athletes treated by subscapularis transfer (modified Magnuson-Stack procedure). *Am J Sports Med* 5(5):188–190, 1977.

247. Aronen, J. G., and Regan, K. Decreasing the incidence of recurrence of first time anterior shoulder dislocation with rehabilitation. *Am J Sports Med* 12(4):283–291, 1984.

248. Artz, T., and Huffer, J. M. A major complication of the modified Bristow procedure for recurrent dislocation of the shoulder. *J Bone Joint Surg* 54A(6):1293–1296, 1972.

249. Asher, M. A. Dislocations of the upper extremity in children. *Orthop Clin North Am* 7:583–591, 1976.

250. Bach, F. R., O'Brien, S. J., Warren, R. F., et al. An unusual neurological complication of the Bristow procedure: A case report. *J Bone Joint Surg* 70A(3):458–460, 1988.

251. Barratta, J. B., Lim, V., Mastomonaco, E., et al.: Axillary artery disruption secondary to anterior dislocation of the shoulder. *J Trauma* 23:1009–1011, 1983.

252. Barry, T. P., Lombardo, S. J., Kerlan, R. K., et al. The coracoid transfer for recurrent anterior instability of the shoulder in adolescents. *J Bone Joint Surg* 67A(3):383–386, 1985.

253. Blazina, M. E., and Satzman, J. S. Recurrent anterior subluxation of the shoulder in athletics—A distinct entity. *J Bone Joint Surg* 51A(5):1037–1038, 1969.

254. Boyd, H. B., and Sisk, T. D. Recurrent posterior dislocation of the shoulder. *J Bone Joint Surg* 54A(4):779–786, 1972.

255. Burkhead, W. Z., and Rockwood, C. A. Treatment of instability of the shoulder with an exercise program. *J Bone Joint Surg* 74A(6):890–896, 1992.

256. Carter, C., and Sweetnam, R. Recurrent dislocation of the patella and of the shoulder: Their association with familial joint laxity. *J Bone Joint Surg* 42B:721–727, 1960.

257. Curr, J. F. Rupture of the axillary artery complicating dislocation of the shoulder: Report of a case. *J Bone Joint Surg* 52B(2):313–317, 1970.

258. Curtis, R. J., Dameron, T. B., and Rockwood, C. A. Fractures and dislocations of the shoulder in children. *In* Rockwood, C. A., Wilkins, K. E., and King, R. E. (Eds.), *Fractures in Children.* Philadelphia, J. B. Lippincott, 1991.

259. DePalma, A. F., Cooke, A. J., and Probhakar, M. The role of the subscapularis in recurrent anterior dislocations of the shoulder. *Clin Orthop* 54:35–49, 1967.

260. DePalma, A. F., and Silverstein, C. E. Results following a modified Magnuson procedure in recurrent dislocation of the shoulder. *Surg Clin North Am* 43:1651–1653, 1963.

261. Detenbeck, L. C. Posterior dislocations of the shoulder. *J Trauma* 12(3):183–192, 1972.

262. Dimon, J. H., III. Posterior dislocation and posterior fracture dislocation of the shoulder: A report of 25 cases. *South Med J* 60(1):661–666, 1967.

263. Foster, W. S., Ford, T. B., and Drez, D. Isolated posterior shoulder dislocation in a child. *Am J Sports Med* 13(3):198–200, 1985.

264. Freundlich, B. D. Luxatio erecta. *J Trauma* 23(5):434–436, 1983.

265. Gerber, C., and Ganz, R. Clinical assessment of instability of the shoulder with special reference to anterior and posterior drawer tests. *J Bone Joint Surg* 66B(4):551–556, 1984.

266. Hawkins, R. J., Koppert, G., and Johnston, G. Recurrent posterior instability (subluxation) of the shoulder. *J Bone Joint Surg* 66(2):169–174, 1984.

267. Hawkins, R. J., and Mohtadi, N. G. H. Clinical evaluation of shoulder instability. *Clin J Sports Med* 1(1):59–64, 1991.

268. Heck, C. C., Jr. Anterior dislocation of the glenohumeral joint in a child. *J Trauma* 21:174–175, 1981.

269. Hernandez, A., and Drez, D. Operative treatment of posterior shoulder dislocations by posterior glenoidplasty, capsulorrhaphy and infraspinatus advancement. *Am J Sports Med* 14(3):187–191, 1986.

270. Hovelius, L. Anterior dislocation of the shoulder in teenagers and young adults. *J Bone Joint Surg* 69A(3):393–399, 1987.

271. Hovelius, L., Erikson, G. K., Fredin, F. H., et al. Recurrences after initial dislocation of the shoulder. *J Bone Joint Surg* 65(3):343–349, 1983.

272. Hovelius, L., Korner, G. L., Lundberg, G. B., et al. The coracoid transfer for recurrent dislocation of the shoulder. *J Bone Joint Surg* 65A(7):926–934, 1983.

273. Hovelius, L., Thorling, G. J., and Fredin, H. Recurrent anterior dislocation of the shoulder: Results after the Bankart and Putti-Platt operations. *J Bone Joint Surg* 61A(4):566–569, 1979.

274. Iftikhar, T. B., Kaminski, R. S., and Silva, I. Neurovascular complications of the modified Bristow procedure. *J Bone Joint Surg* 66A(6):951–952, 1984.

275. Karadimas, J., Rentis, G., and Varouchas, G. Repair of anterior dislocation of the shoulder using transfer of the subscapularis tendon. *J Bone Joint Surg* 62A(7):1147–1149, 1980.

276. Keiser, R. P., and Wilson, C. L. Bilateral recurrent dislocation of the shoulder (atraumatic) in a thirteen year-old girl. *J Bone Joint Surg* 43A(4):553–554, 1961.

277. Lawhon, S. M., Peoples, A. B., and MacEwen, G. D. Voluntary dislocation of the shoulder. *J Pediatr Orthop* 2:590, 1982.

278. Leach, R. E., Corbett, M., Schepsis, A., et al. Results of a modified Putti-Platt operation for recurrent shoulder dislocations and subluxations. *Clin Orthop* 164:20–25, 1982.

279. Lombardo, S. J., Kerlan, R. K., Jobe, F. W., et al. The modified Bristow procedure for recurrent dislocation of the shoulder. *J Bone Joint Surg* 58A(2):256–261, 1976.

280. Lucas, G. L., and Peterson, M. D. Open anterior dislocation of the shoulder: Case report. *J Trauma* 17:883–884, 1977.

281. Magnuson, P. B., and Stack, J. K. Bilateral habitual dislocation of the shoulders in twins: A familial tendency. *JAMA* 114(21):2103, 1940.

282. Marans, H. J., Angel, K. R., Schemitsch, E. H., et al. The fate of traumatic anterior dislocation of the shoulder in children. *J Bone Joint Surg* 74A(8):1242–1244, 1992.

283. Matthews, L. S., Vetter, W. L., Oweida, S. J., et al. Arthroscopic staple capsulorraphy for recurrent anterior shoulder instability. *Arthroscopy* 4(2):106–111, 1988.

284. May, V. R., Jr. Posterior dislocation of the shoulder: Habitual, traumatic and obstetrical. *Orthop Clin North Am* 11:271, 1980.

285. McLaughlin, H. L., and Cavallaro, W. U. Primary anterior dislocation of the shoulder. *Am J Surg* 80:615–621, 1980.

286. Miller, L. S., Donahue, J. R., Good, R. P., et al. The Magnuson-Stack procedure for treatment of recurrent glenohumeral dislocation. *Am J Sports Med* 12(2):133–137, 1984.

287. Mirick, M. J., Clinton, J. E., and Ruiz, E. External rotation method of shoulder dislocation reduction. *J Am Coll Emerg Physicians* 9(12):528–531, 1979.

288. Morgan, C. D., and Bodenstab, A. B. Arthroscopic Bankart suture repair: Technique and early results. *Arthroscopy* 3(2):111–122, 1987.

289. Morrey, B. F., and Janes, J. M. Recurrent anterior dislocation of the shoulder. *J Bone Joint Surg* 58A(2):252–256, 1976.

290. Neer, C. S., II. Involuntary inferior and multidirectional instability of the shoulder: Etiology, recognition and treatment. *Instr Course Lect* 34:232–238, 1985.

291. Neer, C. S., II, and Foster, D. R. Inferior capsular shift for involuntary inferior and multidirectional instability of the shoulder. *J Bone Joint Surg* 62A:897–908, 1980.

292. Norwood, L., and Terry, G. C. Shoulder posterior subluxation. *Am J Sports Med* 12(1):25–30, 1984.

293. Ogden, J. A. *Skeletal Injury in the Child*. Philadelphia, Lea & Febiger, 1982, pp. 227–228.

294. Rang, M. *Children's Fractures* (2nd ed.). Philadelphia, J. B. Lippincott, 1983.

295. Rao, J. P., Francis, A. M., Hurley, J., et al. Treatment of recurrent anterior dislocation of the shoulder by duToit staple capsulorrhaphy. *Clin Orthop* 204:169–176, 1986.

296. Richards, R. R., Hudson, A. R., Bertoia, J. T., et al. Injury to the brachial plexus during Putti-Platt and Bristow procedures: A report of eight cases. *Am J Sports Med* 15(4):374–380, 1987.

297. Rowe, C. R. Anterior dislocation of the shoulder: Prognosis and treatment. *Surg Clin North Am* 43:1609–1614, 1963.

298. Rowe, C. R. Prognosis in dislocation of the shoulder. *J Bone Joint Surg* 38A:957–977, 1956.

299. Rowe, C. R., Patel, D., and Southmayd, W. W. The Bankart procedure: A long term end-result study. *J Bone Joint Surg* 60A(1):1–16, 1978.

300. Rowe, C. R., Pierce, D. S., and Clark, J. G. Voluntary dislocation of the shoulder. *J Bone Joint Surg* 55A:445–459, 1973.

301. Samilson, R. L., and Miller, E. Posterior dislocations of the shoulder. *Clin Orthop* 32:69–86, 1964.

302. Shvartzman, P., and Guy, N. Voluntary dislocation of the shoulder. *Postgrad Med* 85(5):265–271, 1988.

303. Simonet, W. T., and Cofield, R. H. Prognosis in anterior shoulder dislocation. *Am J Sports Med* 12(1):19–24, 1984.

304. Tachdjian, M. O. *Paediatric Orthopaedics*. Philadelphia, W. B. Saunders, 1972.

305. Uhthoff, H. K., and Piscopo, M. Anterior capsular redundancy of the shoulder: Congenital or traumatic? An embryological study. *J Bone Joint Surg* 67B(3):363–366, 1985.

306. Vastamaki, M., and Solonen, K. A. Posterior dislocation and fracture dislocation of the shoulder. *Acta Orthop Scand* 51:479–484, 1980.

307. Wagner, K. T., and Lyne, E. D. Adolescent traumatic dislocations of the shoulder with open epiphysis. *J Pediatr Orthop* 3:61–62, 1983.

308. Yoneda, B., Welsh, P., and MacIntosh, D. L. Conservative treatment of shoulder dislocations in young males. *In* Bayley, I., and Kessel, L. (Eds.), *Shoulder Surgery*. Berlin, Springer-Verlag, 1982.

309. Zuckerman, J. D., and Matsen, F. A. Complications about the glenohumeral joint related to the use of screws and staples. *J Bone Joint Surg* 66A(2):175–180, 1984.

Impingement Syndrome

310. Altchek, D. W., Warren, R. F., Wickiewicz, T. L., et al. Arthroscopic acromioplasty. *J Bone Joint Surg* 72A(8):1198–1207, 1990.

311. Bigliani, L. U., D'Alessandro, D. F., Duralde, X. A., et al. Anterior acromioplasty for subacromial impingement in patients younger than 40 years of age. *Clin Orthop* 246:111–116, 1989.

312. Bigliani, L. U., and Morrison, D. S. The morphology of the acromion and its relationship to rotator cuff tears. *Orthop Trans* 10:459, 1986.

313. Cofield, R. H. Rotator cuff disease of the shoulder: Current concepts review. *J Bone Joint Surg* 67A(6):974–979, 1985.

314. Ellman, H. Arthroscopic subacromial decompression: Analysis of one- to three-year results. *Arthroscopy* 3(3):173–181, 1987.

315. Ellman, H., and Kay, S. P. Arthroscopic subacromial decompression for chronic impingement: Two- to five-year results. *J Bone Joint Surg* 73B(3):395–398, 1991.

316. Gartsman, G. M. Arthroscopic acromioplasty for lesions of the rotator cuff. *J Bone Joint Surg* 72A(2):169–180, 1990.

317. Hawkins, R. J., and Kennedy, J. C. Impingement syndrome in athletes. *Am J Sports Med* 8(3):151–157, 1980.

318. Jackson, D. W. Chronic rotator cuff impingement in the throwing athlete. *Am J Sports Med* 4(6):231–239, 1976.

319. Jobe, F. W., Giancarra, C. E., Kvitne, R. S., et al. Anterior capsulolabral reconstruction of the shoulder in athletes in overhand sports. *Am J Sports Med* 19(5):428–434, 1991.

320. Jobe, F. W., and Jobe, C. M. Painful athletic injuries of the shoulder. *Clin Orthop* 173:117–124, 1983.

321. Jobe, F. W., and Moynes, D. R. Delineation of diagnostic criteria in a rehabilitation program for rotator cuff injuries. *Am J Sports Med* 10:336–339, 1982.

322. Kennedy, J. C., Hawkins, R., and Krissoff, W. B. Orthopaedic manifestations of swimming. *Am J Sports Med* 6:309–322, 1978.

323. Micheli, L. J. Overuse injuries in children's sports, the growth factor. *Orthop Clin North Am* 14:337–360, 1983.

324. Neer, C. S. Anterior acromioplasty for the chronic impingement syndrome in the shoulder: A preliminary report. *J Bone Joint Surg* 54A:41–50, 1972.

325. Neer, C. S. Impingement lesions. *Clin Orthop* 173:70–77, 1983.

326. Richardson, A. B., Jobe, F. W., and Collins, H. R. The shoulder in competitive swimming. *Am J Sports Med* 8:159–163, 1980.

327. Tibone, J. E. Shoulder problems of adolescence. *Clin Sports Med* 2:423–426, 1983.

328. Tibone, J. E., Elrod, B., Jobe, F. W., et al. Surgical treatment of tears of the rotator cuff in athletes. *J Bone Joint Surg* 68A(6):887–891, 1986.

329. Torg, J. S., Pollack, H., and Sweterlisch, P. The effect of competitive pitching on the shoulders and elbows of preadolescent baseball players. *Pediatrics* 49:267–272, 1972.

Fractures of the Proximal Humerus

330. Dameron, T. B., Jr., and Reibel, D. B. Fractures involving the proximal humeral epiphyseal plate. *J Bone Joint Surg* 51A:289–298, 1969.

331. Dameron, T. B., and Rockwood, C. A. Fractures and dislocations of the shoulder. *In* Rockwood, C. A., Wilkins, K. E., and King, R. E. (Eds.), *Fractures in Children*. Philadelphia, J. B. Lippincott, 1984, pp. 589–593.

332. Grant, J. C. B. *Atlas of Anatomy*. Baltimore, Williams & Wilkins, 1962, pp. 101–102.

333. Laing, P. G. The arterial supply of the adult humerus. *J Bone Joint Surg* 38A:1105–1116, 1956.

334. Ogden, J. A., Conlogue, G. J., and Jensen, P. Radiology of postnatal skeletal development: The proximal humerus. *Skel Radiol* 2:153–160, 1978.

335. Ogden, J. A. *Skeletal Injury in the Child* (2nd ed.). Philadelphia, W. B. Saunders, 1990.

336. Aitken, A. P. End results of fractures of the proximal humeral epiphysis. *J Bone Joint Surg* 18A:1036–1041, 1936.

337. Baxter, M. P., and Wiley, J. Fractures of the proximal humeral epiphysis: Their influence on humeral growth. *J Bone Joint Surg* 68B:570–573, 1986.

338. Bourdillon, J. G. Fracture-separation of the proximal epiphysis of the humerus. *J Bone Joint Surg* 32B:35–37, 1950.

339. Dameron, T. B., and Reibel, D. B. Fractures involving the proximal humeral epiphyseal plate. *J Bone Joint Surg* 51A:289–297, 1969.

340. Dameron, T. B., and Rockwood, C. A. Fractures and dislocations of the shoulder. *In* Rockwood, C. A., Wilkins, K. E., and King, R. E. (Eds.), *Fractures in Children*. Philadelphia, J. B. Lippincott, 1984, pp. 589–607.

341. Danielsson, L. G., and Westlin, N. E. Riding accidents. *Acta Orthop Scand* 44:597–603, 1973.

342. Digby, K. H. The measurement of diaphyseal growth in proximal and distal directions. *J Anat Physiol* 50:187–188, 1916.

343. Kohler, R., and Trillaud, J. M. Fracture and fracture separation of the proximal humerus in children: Report of 136 cases. *J Pediatr Orthop* 3:326–332, 1983.

344. Landin, L. A. Fracture patterns in children. *Acta Orthop Scand* (Suppl)202:1–109, 1983.

345. Mc Bride, E. O., and Sisler, J. Fractures of the proximal humeral epiphysis and juxta-epiphyseal humeral shaft. *Clin Orthop* 38:143–153, 1965.

346. Neer, C. S., and Horowitz, B. S. Fractures of the proximal humeral epiphyseal plate. *Clin Orthop* 41:24–31, 1965.

347. Nilsson, S., and Svartholm, F. Fracture of the upper end of the humerus in children. *Acta Chir Scand* 130:433–439, 1965.

348. Ogden, J. A., Conlogue, G. J., and Jensen, P. Radiology of postnatal skeletal development: The proximal humerus. *Skel Radiol* 2:153–160, 1978.

349. Ogden, J. A. Humerus. *In* Ogden, J. A. (Ed.), *Skeletal Injury in the Child*. Philadelphia, W. B. Saunders, 1990, pp. 345–367.

350. Peterson, C. A., and Peterson, H. A. Analysis of the incidence of injuries to the epiphyseal growth plate. *J Trauma* 12:275–281, 1972.

351. Rang, M. *Children's Fractures* (2nd ed.). Philadelphia, J. B. Lippincott, 1983, pp. 143–151.

352. Sherk, H., and Probst, C. Fractures of the proximal humeral epiphysis. *Orthop Clin North Am* 6:401–413, 1975.

353. Williams, D. J. The mechanisms producing fracture separation of the proximal humeral epiphysis. *J Bone Joint Surg* 63B:102–107, 1981.

Humeral Shaft Fractures

354. Balfour, G. W., Mooney, V., and Asby, M. E. Diaphyseal fractures of the humerus treated with a ready-made fracture brace. *J Bone Joint Surg* 64A:11–13, 1982.

355. Baxter, M. P., and Wiley, J. Fractures of the proximal humeral epiphysis: Their influence on humeral growth. *J Bone Joint Surg* 68B:570–573, 1986.

356. Bostman, O., et al. Radial palsy in shaft fracture of the humerus. *Acta Orthop Scand* 57:316–319, 1986.

357. Dameron, T. B., Jr., and Grubb, S. A. Humeral shaft fractures in adults. *South Med J* 74:1461–1467, 1981.

358. Gilchrist, D. K. A stockinette Velpeau for immobilization of the shoulder girdle. *J Bone Joint Surg* 49A:750–751, 1949.

359. Hedstrom, O. Growth stimulation of long bones after fracture or similar trauma: A clinical and experimental study. *Acta Orthop Scand* (Suppl)122:1–62, 1969.

360. Holstein, A., and Lewis, G. B. Fractures of the humerus with radial nerve paralysis. *J Bone Joint Surg* 45A:1382–1396, 1963.

361. Landin, L. A. Fracture patterns in children. *Acta Orthop Scand* (Suppl)202:1–109, 1983.

362. Lange, R. H., and Foster, R. J. Skeletal management of humeral shaft fractures associated with forearm fractures. *Clin Orthop* 195:173–177, 1985.

363. MacNicol, M. F. Roentgenographic evidence of median nerve entrapment in a greenstick humeral fracture. A case report. *J Bone Joint Surg* 60A:98–100, 1978.

364. Pollen, A. G. *Fractures and Dislocations in Children*. Baltimore, Williams & Wilkins, 1973, pp. 7–22.

365. Pollock, F. H., et al. Treatment of radial neuropathy associated with fractures of the humerus. *J Bone Joint Surg* 63A:239–243, 1981.

366. Shah, J., and Bhatti, N. A. Radial nerve paralysis associated with fracture of the humerus: A review of 62 cases. *Clin Orthop* 172:171–176, 1983.

367. Sonneveld, G. J., Patka, P., Van Mourick, J. C., et al. Treatment of fractures of the shaft of the humerus accompanied by paralysis of the radial nerve. *Injury* 18:404–406, 1987.

368. Szalay, E. A., and Rockwood, C. A., Jr. Fractures of the distal shaft of the humerus associated with radial nerve injury. The University of Texas Health Science Center of San Antonio, San Antonio, 1981.

369. Tachdjian, M. *Pediatric Orthopedics*, Vol. 4. (2nd ed.). Philadelphia, W. B. Saunders, 1990.

370. Vander Griend, R., Tomasin, J., and Ward, E. F. Open reduction and internal fixation of humeral shaft fractures. *J Bone Joint Surg* 68A:430–433, 1986.

371. Whitson, R. O. Relation of the radial nerve to the shaft of the humerus. *J Bone Joint Surg* 36A:85–88, 1954.

Nerve Injuries

372. Bateman, J. E. Nerve injuries about the shoulder in sports. *J Bone Joint Surg* 49A:785–792, 1967.

373. Bennett, G. E. Elbow and shoulder lesions of baseball players. *Am J Surg* 98:484–492, 1959.

374. Cahill, B. R. Quadrilateral space syndrome. *In* Omer, G. E., Spinner, O., and Spinner, M. (Eds.), *Management of Peripheral Nerve Problems*. Philadelphia, W. B. Saunders, 1980, pp. 599–606.

375. Cahill, B. R., and Palmer, R. E. Quadrilateral space syndrome. *J Hand Surg* 8:65–69, 1983.

376. De Palma, A. F. Nerve entrapment syndromes. In DePalma, A. F. (ed.). *Surgery of the Shoulder*. Philadelphia, J. B. Lippincott, 1983, pp. 593–594.

377. Drez, D., Jr. Suprascapular neuropathy in the differential diagnosis of rotator cuff injuries. *Am J Sports Med* 4:43–45, 1976.

378. Ireland, M. L., and Andrews, J. R. Shoulder and elbow injuries in the young athlete. *Clin Sports Med* 7:473–494, 1988.

379. Jobe, F. W., et al. The shoulder in sports. *In* Rockwood, C. A., and Matsen, F. A. (Eds.), *The Shoulder*. Philadelphia, W. B. Saunders, 1990, pp. 961–987.

380. Makin, J. G., Brown, W. F., and Ebers, G. C. C7 radiculopathy: Importance of scapular winging in clinical diagnosis. *J Neurol Neurosurg Psychiatry* 49:640–644, 1986.

381. Priest, J. D., and Nagel, D. A. Tennis shoulder. *Am J Sports Med* 4:28–42, 1976.

UPPER EXTREMITY: ELBOW INJURIES IN CHILDREN AND ADOLESCENTS

James P. Bradley, M.D.

Elbow injuries in immature athletes are unique compared to those in mature individuals. The biomechanical and anatomic properties inherent in the epiphyseal plate, musculotendinous units, articular cartilage, and specific sport determine the site and pathologic response in the immature elbow. Most immature elbow maladies can be predicted based on the age and sport of the patient [35]. In young athletes, knowledge of these unique injury patterns combined with early modification of activity and appropriate treatment can often obviate functional disability and permanent deformity.

EPIPHYSEAL DEVELOPMENT

Skeletal maturation of the elbow centers around the primary ossification centers of the humerus, radius, and ulna and six distinct secondary centers of ossification. The chronologic appearance and closure of these centers has been well studied and documented [9, 21, 25, 57]. Usually secondary ossification centers appear radiographically as single bony foci; however, variations do occur. Variations in size, density, position, or number of secondary ossification centers, compared to the uninvolved extremity, often signal potential injury. An erudite knowledge of the normal developmental sequence of primary and secondary ossification centers of the elbow is paramount in evaluation of the young athlete.

Ossification of the Distal Humerus, Radius, and Ulna

Ossification of the distal humerus has extended distally to the condyles by birth [25]. The ossification proc-

ess proceeds at a predictable rate throughout childhood. The ossification rate in girls exceeds that in boys in most instances [21]. Throughout the first 6 months of life the distal humeral metaphyseal ossification line is symmetrical, and differentiation of the medial from the lateral side is difficult [9]. Beginning late in the first year or early in the second year, the ossific nucleus of the lateral condyle (capitellum) appears, and the distal humeral metaphysis becomes asymmetrical. Initially, the lateral humeral metaphysis slants laterally and then straightens; it then becomes well defined and sometimes concave to conform to the ossific nucleus of the lateral condyle [81].

The lateral condyle (capitellum) has the most variable pattern of ossification and time of appearance. Initially, it ossifies as a sphere and later flattens with maturation into its normal mature shape. Until about 8 years of age, the posterior portion of the physis is broader than the anterior portion [65]. In the absence of dislocation on a true lateral projection, the anterior humeral line (AHL) normally intersects the anterior third of the ossific nucleus of the lateral condyle (Fig. 15–1).

Radiographic changes in the elbow remain quiescent until late in the third year, when the ossific nucleus of the proximal radius begins to ossify. Elgenmark [21] noted the appearance of the proximal radius in 50% of girls at 3.8 years, whereas it was absent in the same percentage of boys until 4.5 years.

Commonly, the radial epiphysis begins as a sphere but often develops one or more flat sclerotic centers. Notches or clefts are sometimes noted in the proximal radial metaphysis; these are normal variations of maturation [41, 45].

Ossification of the medial epicondylar ossific nucleus

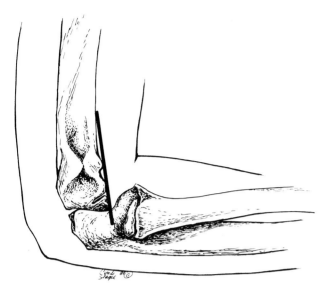

FIGURE 15–1
A line drawn along the anterior shaft of the distal humerus, the anterior humeral line (AHL), normally intersects the anterior third of the ossific nucleus of the capitellum.

begins between the fifth and sixth years with the semblance of a small concavity on the medial aspect of the humeral metaphyseal ossification border. Ossification of the medial epicondyle will become apparent in this area.

The medial epicondyle may arise from more than one ossific nucleus and is commonly the last epiphyseal center to fuse with the humeral shaft in the normal child, sometimes as late as 15 or 16 years [31]. During evaluation it is important to identify the presence and position of the medial epicondyle in each case [64]. Avulsion fractures of the medial epicondyle are commonly displaced into the normal position of the trochlear ossification center. Since the medial epicondylar nucleus appears chronologically before the trochlear center, any radiograph showing the presence of a trochlear center with no visualization of a medial epicondylar center should suggest that, in fact, a fracture or dislocation of the medial epicondylar center is present [31].

At birth the ulnar metaphyseal ossification margin lies halfway between the coronoid process and the tip of the olecranon. This margin usually progresses to enclose about two-thirds to three-fourths of the capitellar surface by 6 to 7 years of age [81]. The secondary ossification nucleus appears between 7 and 9 years of age. Sometimes two secondary ossification centers are visible, one being articular, the other a traction type [62]. The anterior center is almost always smaller than the posterior one [31]. The secondary ossification center of the olecranon may occasionally remain conspicuous into late adulthood [57].

The trochlea ossification center usually emerges between 9 and 10 years of age. The appearance of multiple irregular secondary trochlear ossification centers is not uncommon. The trochlear center often has an irregular outline, and this appearance should not be confused with an aberrant process [31].

The last secondary center to ossify is that of the lateral epicondyle, which appears initially after 10 years of age. It may be small and may rapidly fuse to the lateral condyle. The lateral epicondyle is not always apparent. The lateral epicondylar center first appears as a thin sliver rather than as the typical round or spherical ossific nucleus. Considering the relatively short time between the appearance and fusion of the center, it is sometimes uncertain whether ossification is delayed or fusion to the humerus has already occurred.

Subsequent to cessation of growth, the capitellum, trochlea, and lateral epicondyle fuse to produce one epiphyseal center, while the metaphyseal bone divides the extra-articular medial epicondyle from the new humeral epiphyseal center. The humeral epiphyseal center then fuses with the distal humeral metaphysis between 14 and 16 years of age [17]. At about this time, fusion of the proximal radial and ulnar epiphyseal centers with their appropriate metaphyses takes place. Last to fuse to the humeral metaphysis is the medial epicondylar center, which fuses between 14 + years in girls and 17 + years in boys [81] (Fig. 15–2).

An easy mnemonic with which to remember the sequence of progression of ossification of the distal humeral secondary centers of ossification is the word CRITOE. Each letter in the word stands for a separate secondary ossification center. The letter C represents capitellum (1 to 2 years), R represents radial epiphysis (3 to 4 years), I represents inner epicondyle (medial epicondyle, 5 to 6 years), T represents trochlea (9 to 10 years), O represents outer epicondyle (lateral epicondyle, more than 10 years), and E represents common epiphysis (14 to 16 years) (Fig. 15–3).

Fastidious examination of the radiographs is very helpful when evaluating young athletic elbow injuries. Usually a single bony focus is the mode of radiographic appearance of the secondary epiphyseal centers [59]. Sometimes two or more foci of ossification are apparent early, only to fuse later into a single bony focus. The ossific nucleus is typically homogeneous; variations in size, density, or position on comparative radiographs are harbingers of abnormal development. Irregular islets of ossification and fragmentation are considered abnormal. These anomalies usually represent alterations of the normal vascular genesis and ossification patterns of the secondary ossific centers. Repetitive throwing in young athletes may account for many of these aberrant ossific patterns [59].

Obviously, an intimate knowledge of the normal sequential pattern of appearance of the secondary ossification centers and temporal fusion rates is needed to eval-

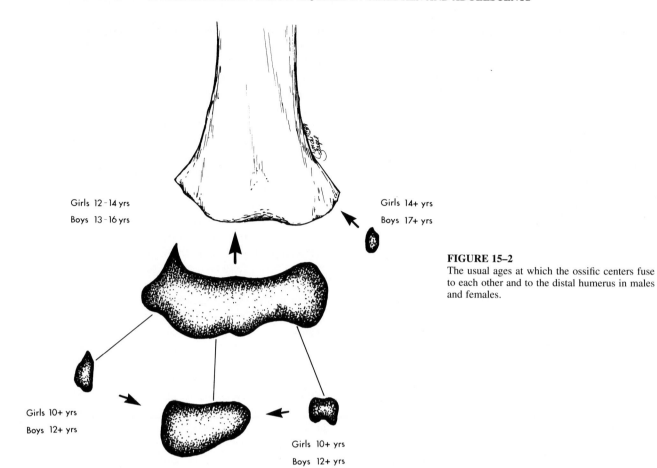

Girls 12 - 14 yrs
Boys 13 - 16 yrs

Girls 14+ yrs
Boys 17+ yrs

Girls 10+ yrs
Boys 12+ yrs

Girls 10+ yrs
Boys 12+ yrs

FIGURE 15–2
The usual ages at which the ossific centers fuse to each other and to the distal humerus in males and females.

FIGURE 15–3
The average ages of the appearance of the secondary ossification centers of the humerus for males and females.

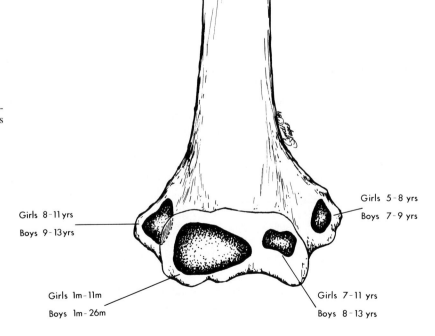

Girls 8 - 11 yrs
Boys 9 - 13 yrs

Girls 5 - 8 yrs
Boys 7 - 9 yrs

Girls 1m - 11m
Boys 1m - 26m

Girls 7 - 11 yrs
Boys 8 - 13 yrs

uate elbow injuries in young athletes thoughtfully. Failure to appreciate these subtle ossific differences may lead to delayed treatment.

Normal Bony Variants

Although normal ossific patterns of the developing elbow can be confusing, there are a few normal variations or unusual appearances that should be noted. The developing radial tuberosity, which is the site of insertion of the biceps brachii, may appear as an undermineralized focus. This appearance should not be misinterpreted as a destructive lesion of the bone [31]. The thin humeral olecranon fossa occasionally may appear to be totally lucent, the so-called perforated olecranon fossa [31]. Occasionally, a separate bony ossicle may be found within the perforated olecranon fossa. An anatomic anomaly that appears sporadically on the anterior medial distal humerus is a bony projection called the supracondylar process. This is an atavistic trait and is rarely significant.

THE BIOMECHANICS OF THE THROWING ELBOW

The throwing motion of the elbow is common to many sports, most notably the tennis serve, javelin throw, and football pass; however, the prototype in terms of abundance of biomechanical information is the baseball pitch. Many recent investigations have studied the elaborate pattern and synchrony of bony, ligamentous, and muscular interactions that occur in pitching [38, 39]. Recent electromyographic (EMG) observations have shed new light on the biomechanics and mechanisms of injury sustained by the throwing athlete [61].

The elbow articulation is one of the most congruous joints in the body and therefore is one of the most stable. This characteristic is the result of an almost equal contribution from the soft tissue constraints and the articular surfaces [7]. Static stability is provided by the articular surfaces and the ligamentous and capsular structures while dynamic stability is provided by the musculotendinous units crossing the elbow.

The Collateral Ligaments—Elbow Stability

The medial (or ulnar) collateral ligamentous complex of the elbow is broad and fan-shaped and is composed of three essential parts: an anterior oblique bundle, a posterior oblique bundle, and a transverse ligament (Fig. 15–4). The anterior oblique component of the medial collateral ligament is a thick substantial structure originating on the medial epicondyle and inserting into the coronoid process. Basically, in flexion the posterior fi-

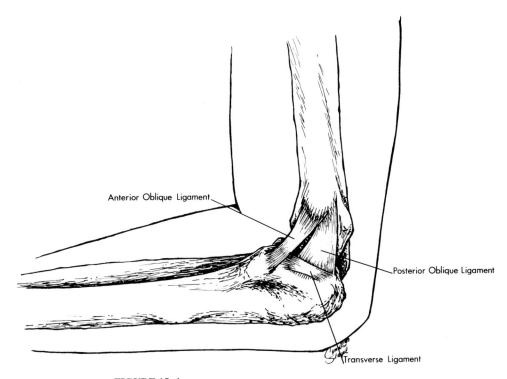

FIGURE 15–4
The medial (ulnar) collateral ligamentous complex of the elbow.

bers become tight while the anterior fibers become less tense [13]. Biomechanically and anatomically, the anterior oblique component of the medial collateral ligament is the major ligamentous support of the medial aspect of the elbow; this is especially true during throwing, when tremendous valgus tension is generated along the medial aspect of the elbow. The lateral (or radial) collateral ligamentous complex offers varus stability but is not well understood and shows more individual variation [7]. Basically, the complex is composed of three individual parts. (1) The radial collateral ligament originates from the lateral epicondyle and inserts onto the annular ligament. (2) The lateral ulnar collateral ligament originates from the posterior aspect of the lateral epicondyle, traverses the annular ligament, and attaches to the ulna at the crista supinatoris [56]. This division of the radial collateral complex accounts for the stability of the elbow after the radial head has been excised. (3) The accessory lateral collateral ligament originates from the inferior margin of the annular ligament and inserts onto the tubercle of the supinator (Fig. 15–5). Although not always present, the function of this ligament is to further stabilize the annular ligament during varus stress. The anconeus muscle and the lateral collateral ligaments form a complex that functions as both a static and dynamic stabilizer to the lateral elbow [13]. Interestingly, throwing athletes are not prone to varus stress injuries of the elbow.

The Bony Articulation—Elbow Stability

Theoretically, elbow stability can be considered to be approximately 50% a function of the collateral ligaments and anterior capsule and 50% a function of the bony articulation, primarily from the ulnohumeral joint [55]. An and Morrey [7] showed that with serial excision of the olecranon (25%, 50%, 75%, and 100%) there were near linear decreases in elbow stability provided by the ulnohumeral joint in both 0 degrees and 90 degrees of flexion. The stabilizing effect of the radial head on the elbow has been examined as well. The radial head does furnish some resistance to valgus stress varying from 15% to 30% depending on the load conformation and orientation of the elbow joint [7].

The resistance of the radial head to valgus stress may be greater during throwing, but additional information is required to better understand the role of the radial head in elbow stability. The amount of force transmitted across the elbow joint varies with the loading configuration and angular orientation of the joint, and a magnitude of nearly three times body weight has been surmised in certain functions [28, 32]. Surprisingly, activities of daily living necessitate a force of approximately half of body weight transmitted across the joint, with maximal loads noted at about 90 degrees of flexion [20, 46]. Halls and Travill [28] noted that 60% of the

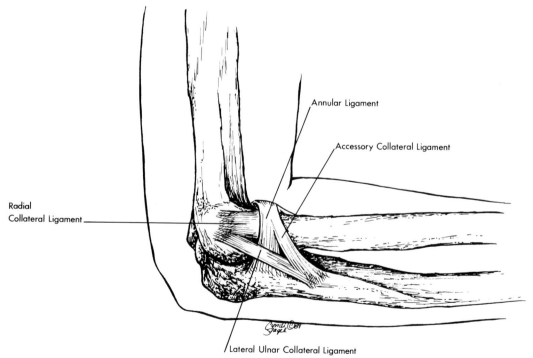

FIGURE 15–5
The lateral collateral ligamentous complex of the elbow.

axial load is transmitted across the joint at the radiohumeral joint and 40% at the ulnohumeral joint. These investigations primarily examined the elbow during activities of daily living and isometric lifting, and the results cannot be extrapolated to the tremendous demands imposed on the elbow during throwing. Considering this, it is not surprising that a small deficiency in the elaborate stability-controlling mechanisms of the elbow may have a significant and cumulative effect on elbow function.

Pitching

The throwing motion is common to many sports; however, the baseball pitch is the most studied and best understood example. The pitch is divided into five stages: Phase 1 is the wind-up or preparation phase, ending when the ball leaves the glove hand (Fig. 15–6); phase 2, termed early cocking, is a period of shoulder abduction and external rotation that begins as the ball is released from the nondominant hand and terminates with contact of the forward foot on the ground (Fig. 15–7); phase 3, the late cocking phase, continues until maximum external rotation at the shoulder is obtained (Fig. 15–8); phase 4 is the short propulsive phase of acceleration that starts with internal rotation of the humerus and ends with ball release (Fig. 15–9); and phase 5 is the follow-through phase, which starts with ball release and ends when all motion is complete (Fig. 15–10) [38, 39].

During the baseball pitch, the actions of the extensor

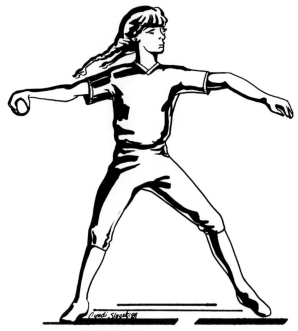

FIGURE 15–7
Throwing, phase II: Early cocking.

digitorum communis (EDC), brachioradialis (BR), flexor carpi radialis (FCR), flexor digitorum superficialis (FDS), extensor carpi radialis longus (ECRL), extensor carpi radialis brevis (ECRB), pronator teres (PT), and supinator (S) exemplify a complex concert of interdependence [66].

Dynamic EMG and high-speed film analysis of these muscles have expanded our understanding of the major

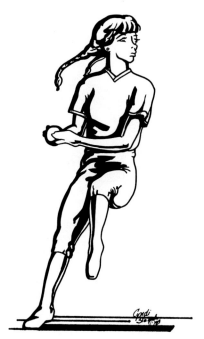

FIGURE 15–6
Throwing, phase I: Wind-up.

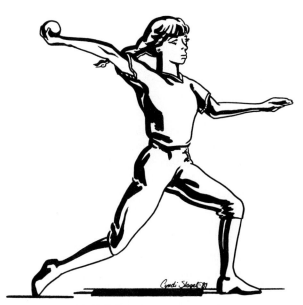

FIGURE 15–8
Throwing, phase III: Late cocking.

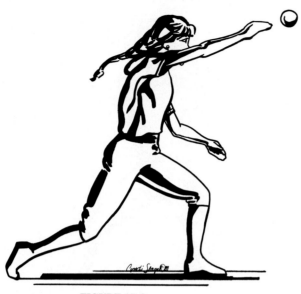

FIGURE 15–9
Throwing, phase IV: Acceleration.

muscles controlling the elbow. Basically, the EMG signal is recorded using the Basmajian single-needle technique [12]. Motion analysis using 16-mm cameras at speeds varying from 400 to 450 frames/second are synchronized to the EMG data recorded during throwing. A peak 1-second EMG signal obtained during a manual muscle strength test (MMT) is selected as a normalizing value (100%). During throwing, muscle activity patterns are assessed every 2 msec and expressed as a percentage of the normalized base. Assimilation of this type of EMG data combined with motion analysis has enhanced our understanding of the biomechanics of the elbow during throwing.

The wind-up phase demonstrates low activity in all muscle groups as the forearm is slightly pronated and flexed and the wrist extended. The ECRB, EDC, and PT show the highest activity. No significant differences in muscle activity have been noted in the fast ball versus the curve [61, 66].

During the early cocking phase the elbow is flexed, the wrist and metacarpophalangeal joints extended, and the forearm slightly pronated. The ECRB, ECRL, EDC (metacarpophalangeal extensors), BR, and PT all show moderate muscle activity during throwing of a fast ball. Muscle activity is noticeably lower in the BR when a curve ball is thrown, implying that less elbow flexion is required for its delivery [61, 66]. Throughout the late cocking phase, the wrist is extended, the elbow flexed, and the forearm pronated to 90 degrees; increased pronation is noted during the fast ball throw. Interestingly, there is increased activity in the wrist extensors and supinator when the curve ball is thrown, implying that

the ball position in the hand is different and the forearm is slightly more supinated during the curve ball throw [61, 66].

During acceleration the elbow is extended and the wrist and metacarpophalangeal joints are flexed to thrust the ball forward. A major difference between the fast ball and the curve is the increased activity of the ECRL and ECRB during the curve ball. The contrast probably represents the different posture needed at the release point of the curve [61, 66].

The follow-through phase is concluded with maximal pronation of the forearm, associated with internal rotation of the humerus, adducted across the chest. During the curve ball the wrist extensors again show more activity [61, 66].

EMG and high-speed film analysis demonstrate low to moderate activity of all elbow muscles during all phases of the pitch. This is in direct contrast to the data obtained of the shoulder musculature during the same evaluation. The shoulder muscles show higher EMG values and much more selectivity of muscles during throwing [38, 61].

The purpose of the elbow musculature during throwing is probably related to positioning necessary to accept the transfer of energy from the larger trunk and girdle structures. The most prominent difference between the fast ball and the curve ball is an increase in ECRL and ECRB activity during the late cocking, acceleration, and follow-through phases of the curve ball. This difference most likely represents the different posture needed at the release point of a curve.

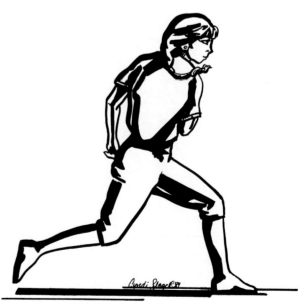

FIGURE 15–10
Throwing, phase V: Follow-through.

THROWING STRESSES ON THE ELBOW

In both the young throwing athlete and the mature thrower four distinct areas are vulnerable to throwing stress: (1) tension overload of the medial elbow restraints, (2) compression overload on the lateral articular surface, (3) posterior medial shear forces on the posterior articular surface, and (4) extension overload on the lateral restraints [33, 50, 59]. Specific injury patterns can be discerned during each phase of pitching.

During early cocking and especially during late cocking, a significant distraction force is applied to the medial aspect of the elbow [33, 59]. The resultant force presents as tension on the medial epicondylar attachments including the flexor muscle origin and the ulnar collateral ligaments. Commonly, with overuse or altered mechanics, the weakest link in the medial complex can be injured. In young athletes subsequent injury or avulsion of the medial epicondylar ossification center is often encountered (Fig. 15–11). The ulnar collateral ligaments may become overstretched, resulting in traction spurs on the coronoid process. Traction injuries to the ulnar nerve and flexor muscle strains may also ensue [30, 32, 33, 78].

Compression of the lateral articulation, in which the radial head abuts the capitellum, occurs mainly during early and late cocking. Sequelae include growth disturbances, chondral or osteochondral fractures of the capitellum (with resultant loose bodies), and growth disturbances and deformation of the radial head (Fig. 15–12) [33, 59].

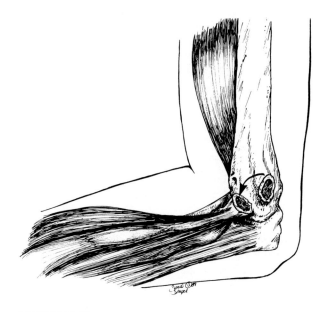

FIGURE 15–11
Avulsion fracture through the physis of the medial epicondyle with an attached anterior oblique ligament and flexor muscle mass.

Posterior articular surface damage develops in two phases of throwing. During late cocking, a posterior medial shear force develops about the olecranon fossa. Throughout follow-through, hyperextension of the elbow is prominent, placing stress on the olecranon and anterior capsule. These stresses commonly produce pathology at three sites: (1) posterior medial spurs, (2) true posterior olecranon spurs (triceps strain), and (3) traction spurs of the coronoid process [33, 59] (Fig. 15–13).

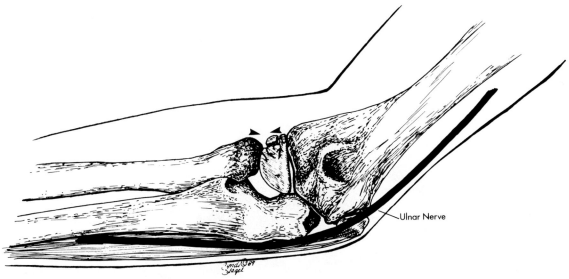

Ulnar Nerve

FIGURE 15–12
During early and late cocking, compression of the capitellum against the radial head and tension on the medial collateral ligament, flexor muscles and ulnar nerve medially usually are the forces that cause injury during throwing.

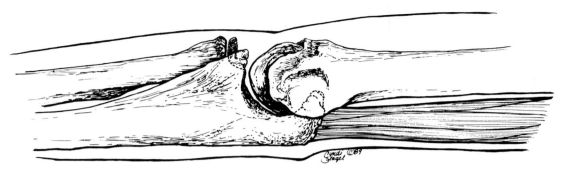

FIGURE 15–13
The sites of injury during the follow-through phase of throwing (coronoid and olecranon sprues).

Lateral extension overload occurs during acceleration when extreme pronation of the forearm results in a tension force applied to the lateral ligaments and lateral epicondyle. Consequently, lateral epicondylitis may develop [33, 59] (Fig. 15–14).

GYMNASTIC STRESSES OF THE ELBOW

The frequency of participation of young athletes in gymnastics during the past decade has increased significantly. Nearly one-third of injuries reported in gymnastics occur in the upper extremity with 7 percent involving the elbow [23]. In essence, the elbow, which normally is a nonweight-bearing joint, becomes a weight-bearing joint during routines such as one-arm balancing, handstands, tumbling, and trunk stabilization on the bars [24]. Goldberg [24] noted the presence of elbow compression and traction injuries very similar to those seen in Little League elbow, the most common of which presented as traction injuries of the medial aspect of the elbow. These injuries included partial tears of the flexor muscle mass, collateral ligament strains, and medial epicondylar traction injuries. The most significant injury noted by both Goldberg [24] and Snook [70] was a subluxation-dislocation of the elbow, often associated with an avulsion fracture of the medial epicondyle. Although infrequent, chondral or osteochondral fractures of the capitellum may occur as well [64].

The most prevalent problem afflicting the elbow in gymnasts is a posterior elbow injury [8]. Biomechanically, to support the body weight, the gymnast must repetitively "lock out" the elbow, thereby forcing the olecranon into the olecranon fossa, which results in posterior fossa inflammation [8].

LITTLE LEAGUE ELBOW

The term Little League elbow is used to depict a group of pathologic entities in and about the elbow joint in young developing throwers. It is important to realize that the throwing motion is common to the tennis serve, javelin throw, and football pass. The injury includes (1) medial epicondylar fragmentation and avulsion, (2) delayed or accelerated apophyseal growth of the medial epicondyle, (3) delayed closure of the medial epicondylar growth plate, (4) osteochondrosis and osteochondritis of the capitellum, (5) deformation and osteochondritis of the radial head, (6) hypertrophy of the ulna, and (7)

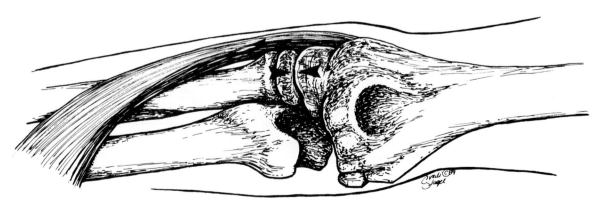

FIGURE 15–14
The sites of injury during the acceleration phase of throwing.

olecranon apophysitis with or without delayed closure of the olecranon apophysis [2, 27, 29, 48, 76, 77]. Many authors have emphasized that these abnormalities are secondary to the biomechanical throwing stresses placed on the young developing elbow [1, 2, 4, 11, 18, 19, 44, 48, 50, 54, 67, 68, 69, 71, 72, 75, 78, 79]. The physical stresses associated with throwing produce exceptional forces in and about the elbow [59]. These include traction, compression, and shear, which are localized to the medial, lateral, and posterior aspects of the elbow [33, 59]. Any or all of these forces may contribute to the alteration of normal osteochondral development of the elbow [59].

DIAGNOSIS

A timely and accurate diagnosis is the keystone to successful treatment of the many conditions associated with Little League elbow. A meticulous history and physical examination are the primary tools in the orthopedist's arsenal in achieving this goal. Special tests such as arthrography, computed tomography (CT) scan, magnetic resonance imaging (MRI), and bone scans are often necessary but play a confirmatory role rather than a diagnostic one.

History

Age, position, handedness, activity level, location of pain, duration of pain, radiation, trauma, mechanism of injury, nature of onset, and past medical history are all salient factors in the history.

The age of young throwers can be divided into three groups: (1) childhood, which terminates with the appearance of all secondary centers of ossification, (2) adolescence, which terminates with the fusion of all secondary centers of ossification to their respective long bones, and (3) young adulthood, which terminates with completion of all bone growth and the achievement of final muscular form [59]. During childhood, the most frequent complaints are sensitivity about the medial epicondyle, which is usually secondary to microinjuries at the apophysis and ossification center. Throwing stresses impede the normal chondro-osseous transformation and result in an irregular ossification pattern of the secondary ossification center [59]. When the athlete enters adolescence, muscle strength, muscle mass, and throwing force are increasing. The athlete increases the valgus stresses on the elbow, and the result can be an avulsion fracture of the entire medial epicondyle. Partial avulsion of the medial epicondyle becomes apparent as the thrower approaches the end of adolescence because the medial epicondyle begins to fuse. Some adolescents develop enough chronic stresses to cause delayed union or possibly nonunion of the medial epicondyle [59]. By young adulthood, the medial epicondyle is fused, and injuries of the muscular attachments and ligaments of the epicondyle become more prevalent. During this time the flexor muscles and ulnar collateral ligaments are at increased risk of injury [59]. Therefore, the age of the thrower can provide the examiner with useful information about the possible cause of the elbow problem.

The position played by the thrower provides insight into the magnitude of stresses placed on the elbow and the relative incidence of elbow complaints. Pitching inherently places more stress on the elbow during play, and pitchers most commonly complain of elbow injuries [33, 59]. The usual order of prevalence of elbow complaints among players is pitchers, infielders, catchers, and outfielders [59]. Although the magnitude of injury has not been proved to depend on position, intuitively it seems that pitchers have the greatest risk of elbow injury.

Handedness is very germane in the initial history. Most throwers present with elbow problems in the dominant extremity unless direct trauma is the cause of the problem.

Pain is the most common complaint. Localization, duration, character, temporal sequence (night, day, during or after activity), activity level, and nature of onset are all clues to the underlying pathology. Although pain is the most frequent complaint, related but less frequent problems include decreased elbow motion, mild flexion contracture, swelling, decreased performance, and local sensitivity of the elbow [59]. The pain is most often localized to the medial epicondyle; however, lateral and posterior pain may accompany or be the presenting complaint. The duration of pain is usually an indirect measure of the severity of the problem. Pain before, during, and after throwing is usually an ominous finding. The relationship of the pain to the specific activity must be delineated. Medial pain in a young adult that occurs with a specific phase of throwing (such as late cocking or acceleration) may be a harbinger of early instability, although medial pain in the same phases of throwing in childhood most commonly represents medial epicondylar injury.

Nocturnal pain is very uncommon, and the possible presence of a neoplastic process must be addressed. Burning or a vague ache centered around the medial aspect of the elbow and associated with dysesthesias or paresthesias of the ulnar two digits signifies ulnar nerve involvement and is a significant finding.

The duration of pain (acute versus chronic) is a very helpful sign. If a child presents with a single episode of injury, an acute traumatic condition such as avulsion of the medial epicondyle must be considered. If a young adult complains of similar symptoms, ulnar collateral ligament injury is possible. In other instances, the history may reveal an insidious onset of chronic pain connoting a form of overuse syndrome or possibly an osteochondrosis type of injury.

Ancillary information such as activities that aggravate or relieve the pain, types of pitches thrown, innings pitched, typical pitching rotation, and changes in the training schedule should be elucidated. Attention to detail is paramount because a neglected sprain or strain or the slightest change in the training schedule can sometimes lead to the correct diagnosis and treatment.

It is extremely helpful to remember that the elbow may be the site of referred pain, although this is uncommon in young throwers. Therefore, associated neck, shoulder, and wrist pain or restricted motion must be appraised.

A prior surgical history is essential when sorting through possible causes of the present pain. Surgical restoration of a displaced supracondylar fracture may sometimes change the intricate biomechanical relationships necessary for effective throwing. Prior shoulder surgery may place the elbow at risk for overuse syndromes secondary to altered shoulder throwing mechanics.

The past medical history and any recent medical work-ups should be evaluated. Inquiries are made about a history of family history of osteochondrosis including osteochondritis dissecans, Kohler's disease, Legg-Calvé-Perthes disease, and Osgood-Schlatter's disease. When such patients participate in activity that involves a high articular demand about the elbow, the likelihood of variations in epiphyseal osteochondral development is increased [59]. A history of delayed skeletal maturation combined with participation on an age-determined team commonly requires the child to throw beyond his physiologic tolerance and often leads to elbow problems [59].

A plethora of symptom complexes, some with subtle variations, may be evident on evaluation of young athletes with elbow pain, and only with a careful history can the orthopedist begin to localize the underlying pathology.

Normal Variations

An understanding of the normal geometry of the throwing elbow is needed to evaluate elbow injuries. At 90 degrees of flexion the medial and lateral epicondyles form an equilateral triangle with the tip of the olecranon. As the elbow is extended, these landmarks fall into a straight line. By understanding the relationship of these landmarks, the examiner can appraise the elbow for anatomic alignment and rotation, especially when evaluating the young athlete. Young throwers often have unilateral hypertrophy of the muscles and bone of the dominant extremity [27]. Twelve percent of male Little League pitchers in the Houston study (595 pitchers) had a flexion contracture of the elbow, and 37 percent of these young pitchers had a valgus deformity of the elbow [27]. The presence of hypertrophy, valgus deformity, and flexion contracture should not be considered uncommon in young throwers.

PHYSICAL EXAMINATION

Examination ideally begins with inspection of both elbows. Loss of motion, muscle atrophy or hypertrophy, bony deformity, and elbow asymmetry are ascertained. There may be some degree of hypertrophy or flexion contracture, or an alteration in the carrying angle of the dominant extremity. At this time, concomitant examination of the neck, wrist, shoulders, and hand is completed. The range of motion including flexion, extension, pronation, and supination is performed in comparing both extremities.

In assessing tenderness the medial and lateral epicondyles, olecranon process, radial head, and collateral ligaments are palpated. Palpation of the ulnar nerve in both flexion and extension is done to evaluate ulnar nerve subluxation. Slight flexion of the elbows is needed to examine the olecranon fossa; with gentle pressure, the examiner should be able to differentiate posteromedial from posterolateral pathology. The olecranon is unlocked with slight flexion (15 to 25 degrees), which will permit evaluation of the ligamentous stability of the elbow. The lateral ligaments are ideally tested with a varus stress and internal rotation of the arm, and the ulnar collateral ligaments are tested with a valgus stress and external rotation of the arm [83]. Stability testing requires ''sensitive fingers'' to detect the subtle differences indicative of elbow instability.

A complete neurologic and vascular examination of the extremity is performed routinely. Special attention is given to the ulnar nerve.

Radiography

Routine radiographs are essential in the diagnosis of elbow pathology. Standard anteroposterior, lateral, reverse axial [10], and comparison radiographs are needed. Stress films, when positive, are helpful in evaluating ligamentous compromise, but a negative stress film, even under anesthesia, does not exclude ligamentous disruption (Fig. 15–15). Common medial findings in the immature elbow include elbow enlargement, fragmenta-

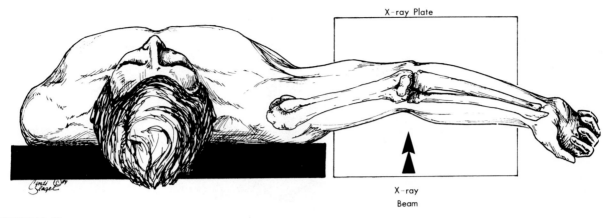

FIGURE 15–15
The gravity stress test of the medial elbow ligamentous complex. The arm is placed in full external rotation, permitting the weight of the forearm to deliver a valgus stress to the elbow.

tion, beaking of the epicondyle, and occasionally avulsion of the medial epicondyle. Lateral lesions usually involve the subchondral bone and manifest as osteochondrosis or osteochondritis dissecans of the capitellum or radial head and may eventually result in loose bodies and terminally degenerative arthritis. The initial finding is a lucent area in the capitellum best seen on the oblique film. A loose body that usually resides in the lateral compartment or anteriorly may develop. Posterior lesions commonly present with hypertrophy of the ulna that causes chronic impingement of the olecranon tip into the olecranon. Frequent impingement of the olecranon results in osteophytic enlargement with resultant loose bodies in the olecranon fossa. Rarely, stress fractures of the ulna, olecranon apophysitis, or delayed union of the olecranon apophysis transpires.

Tomograms are helpful in detailing the articular changes, loose bodies, spur formation, and trabecular changes that are sometimes associated with elbow problems.

Three-phase bone scans may be helpful in evaluating subtle changes noted in overuse injuries of the elbow. These are usually followed by tomograms or CT scans of the area of increased activity. Currently, ultrasound has been less beneficial in the diagnosis of lesions about the elbow. MRI is becoming a very useful modality in the evaluation of pediatric elbow injuries. MRI potentially has specific advantages in defining nonossified structures such as developing epiphyses and apophyses, joint capsules, fractures through cartilaginous structures, early avascular changes, and many ligaments and soft tissues not identified on plain radiographs. A thorough understanding of skeletal maturation and epiphyseal development is necessary for adequate evaluation of pathology in pediatric elbow injuries. The importance of comparison elbow views cannot be overemphasized in this population.

SPECIFIC CONDITIONS AND TREATMENT

Medial Tension Injuries

Most cases of Little League elbow present with medial elbow complaints. The triad of symptoms includes progressive medial pain, diminished throwing effectiveness, and decreased throwing distance. Repetitive valgus stresses and flexor forearm pull usually produce a subtle apophysitis or stress fracture through the medial epicondylar epiphyses. Physical manifestations include point tenderness, swelling over the medial epicondyle, and an elbow flexion contracture that is often greater than 15 degrees [13, 33, 73]. Radiographs show fragmentation and widening of the epiphyseal lines compared to the contralateral elbow [2, 13, 27, 77] (Fig. 15–16).

In most cases, a 4- to 6-week course of abstinence from throwing results in cessation of symptoms. Initially, ice and nonsteroidal anti-inflammatory medications help to alleviate the symptoms [13, 33, 73]. After the symptoms resolve, a gradual return to throwing is advisable. Occasionally, disability may continue for an extended period of time, and elbow pain may continue when throwing is resumed [52]. In these cases, throwing should be disallowed until the next baseball season.

Medial Epicondylar Fractures

When more substantial acute valgus stress is applied through violent muscle contraction during throwing an avulsion fracture of the medial epicondyle may ensue. The consequence is a painful elbow with point tenderness over the medial epicondyle and an elbow flexion contracture that may exceed 15 degrees. Radiographs

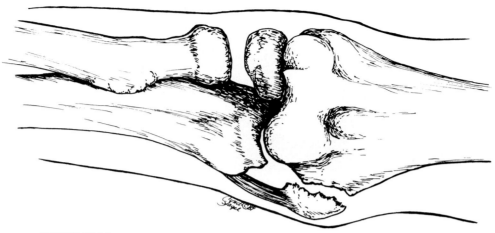

FIGURE 15–16
Medial tension injury with widening and fragmentation of the medial epicondylar ossification center.

most often show only a minimally displaced epicondylar fragment or significant displacement with or without displacement into the joint [13]. The extent of displacement is determined by the flexor-pronator muscles and the ulnar collateral ligaments, which originate on the medial epicondyle. The site of separation is usually the cartilaginous epiphyseal growth plate, which is the weakest area of the medial epicondyle during this period of growth [13]. Woods and Tullos [82] have divided these lesions into two types. Type 1 occurs in younger children and produces a large fragment that involves the entire medial epicondyle and often displaces and rotates (see Fig. 15–11). Type 2 occurs in adolescents and produces a small fracture fragment. This may be due to avulsion of the flexor tendon; the anterior oblique ligament is usually but not always intact.

Most treatment protocols center on how many millimeters the fracture fragment has been displaced. Hunter [33] noted that most avulsion fractures are best treated by splinting and rest; however, complete separation may require surgical repair if conservative treatment fails [33]. Bennett and Tullos [13] recommend that if displacement is in excess of 3 to 8 mm, a gravity stress radiograph should be performed to determine elbow stability. If elbow instability is found, surgical reattachment should be considered [13]. Irelano and Andrews [35] advocate anatomic surgical reduction and refuse to accept any degree of medial epicondylar displacement, noting that late sequelae of old medial avulsion epicondylar fractures and associated radiocapitellar degenerative changes can be seen in AP and lateral radiographs.

Medial Ligament Ruptures

Injuries to the ulnar collateral ligaments (UCL) are not common in young throwing athletes [35]. Most UCL injuries occur in adults and occasionally in young adults. Most patients have tenderness about the medial aspect of the elbow for months to years before the ligament is injured. Commonly, a rupture occurs as a sudden catastrophic event, after which the elbow is so painful that further throwing is not possible [40]. Clinically, with these injuries subtle findings of medial elbow instability are present, demonstrated by flexing the elbow to 25 degrees to unlock the olecranon from its fossa and gently stressing the medial side of the elbow [40]. Woods and Tullos [82] noted that a radiographic gravity medial stress test of the elbow is sometimes useful in diagnosing UCL injuries.

Treatment of complete tears of the UCL (with resulting instability) in young throwers who wish to return to repetitive throwing should consist of a surgical repair [13, 35, 40]. Irelano and Andrews [35] recommend direct surgical repair of the UCL. Bennett and Tullos [13] state that UCL ligament injuries associated with elbow instability may necessitate surgical reattachment. Jobe thinks that if elbow stability can be reconstituted, direct repair is indicated [36]; however, if a tenuous repair is imminent, reconstruction of the UCL using a palmaris longus tendon graft should be performed in association with an anterior submuscular transposition of the ulnar nerve [36] (Fig. 15–17).

Lateral Compression Injuries

Panner's Disease (Osteochondrosis)

Panner's disease is a malady of the growth or ossification centers in children that begins as a degeneration or necrosis of the capitellum and is followed by regeneration and recalcification [16]. The child (aged 7 to 12) presents with dull, aching elbow pain that is aggravated

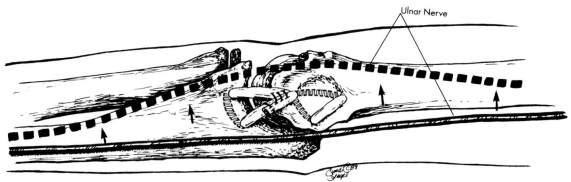

FIGURE 15–17
Medial collateral ligament reconstruction utilizing a tendon graft with an anterior submuscular transposition of the ulnar nerve.

by activity, especially throwing a ball. The elbow is usually swollen; however, lack of ability to extend it is not common. An important distinction must be made between Panner's disease (osteochondrosis) and osteochondritis dissecans. The difference focuses on age and degree of involvement of the capitellar secondary ossification center [16]. In the child, the most common cause of chronic lateral elbow pain is Panner's disease, but in the adolescent (aged 13 to 16), the most common cause of recurrent lateral elbow pain and limited motion is osteochondritis dissecans of the capitellum.

Panner's disease is a focal, localized lesion of the subchondral bone of the capitellum and its overlying articular cartilage [58]. The lesion is usually noted in the anterior central capitellum where it is in maximal contact with the articulation of the head of the radius [16]. Radiographs show that the capitellar ossification center is fragmented owing to irregular patches of relative sclerosis alternating with areas of rarefaction. The epiphysis may be irregular and smaller than that of the opposite side, and sometimes the entire epiphysis is involved. The natural history of Panner's disease is that as growth progresses, the capitellar epiphysis eventually assumes a normal appearance in size, contour, and subchondral architecture; the disease is a self-limited condition [13, 16].

Initial treatment should consist of rest, avoidance of throwing, and sometimes splinting until the pain and tenderness subsides [13, 16]. Radiographic follow-up is recommended to evaluate the healing response. Late deformity and collapse of the articular surface of the capitellum is uncommon [13, 16].

Osteochondritis Dissecans

Osteochondritis dissecans (OCD) is presently looked upon as a singular entity within the multiple entities encompassed by the term Little League elbow [14, 15, 51, 72]. Tullos and King [79] scrutinized the throwing motion and concluded that osteochondritis dissecans of the capitellum was secondary to compressive forces occurring between the radial head and the capitellum during throwing. Many other authors have noted the relationship between throwing and OCD [1, 2, 4, 11]. Osteochondritis is a focal lesion of the capitellum occurring in the 13- to 16-year-old age group, usually characterized by elbow pain and a flexion contracture of 15 degrees or more [13, 16]. The onset is insidious, with a focal island of subchondral bone demarcated by a rarefied zone on radiographs. Infrequently, the radial head appears larger than that on the uninvolved side [16]. Sequelae include loose bodies, residual deformity of the capitellum, and often residual elbow disability [13, 51]. Osteochondritis dissecans must be differentiated from Panner's disease, which is a distinct entity [13, 16, 51, 58]. Age, onset, loose body formation, radiographic findings, and deformity of the capitellum all aid in the differentiation. Panner's disease usually affects a younger population (less than 10 years), and the onset is acute with fragmentation of the entire capitellar ossific nucleus. The absence of loose bodies, minimal residual deformity of the capitellum, and no late sequelae are also unlike the findings in OCD.

The etiology of osteochondritis dissecans of the elbow has not yet been determined. Three popular theories include ischemia, trauma, and genetic factors [22, 49, 80]. One or all three may play a role in the development of OCD of the capitellum.

Typically, the patient with OCD presents with a dull, poorly localized pain that is aggravated by use, especially throwing, and relieved by rest. Unlike patients with Panner's disease, these patients commonly complain of limitation of motion, particularly extension. Later in the course of the disease, locking and catching with severe pain may supervene [16, 83]. Initial radiographs may be negative but usually show the typical rarefaction, irregular ossification, and a rarefied crater adjacent to the articular surface of the capitellum. Tomograms with contrast may be the most accurate method of establishing the diagnosis and determining whether the articular surface and subchondral bone are dissected from the capitellum [16, 51, 83]. Arthroscopy is an excellent method of determining the size of the lesion, its fixation, and the condition of the articular cartilage of the capitellum and radial head. Essentially, OCD lesions can be divided into three types [16]. Type I lesions are intact and show no evidence of displacement and no evidence of fracture of the articular cartilage. Treatment involves rest and avoidance of all vigorous activities. Splinting for 3 to 4 weeks may be employed if pain is a predominant complaint; this is followed by active range of motion exercises. Protection of the elbow should be continued until there is radiographic evidence of revascularization and healing [5, 16, 33, 51, 59, 83].

Type II lesions show evidence of fracture or fissure of the articular cartilage, or partial detachment of the lesion [16]. Controversy exists about which of three possible methods of treatment should be instituted. In 1981, Andrews [5] reported that an overly aggressive approach could lead to progressive loss of motion, although patients may experience some pain relief. He recommended conservative treatment until the patient is skeletally mature except in very unusual cases in which an obvious loose body mechanically interferes with motion [5]. In 1988 Irelano and Andrews [35] simply stated that surgical treatment of OCD includes removal of loose bodies, drilling, and debridement by arthrotomy or newer arthroscopic techniques. Yocum [83] believed that loosening of the fragment or frank displacement is a surgical situation. Pappas [59] stated that if the x-ray changes advance to potential compromise of the architectural support of the capitellum, surgical intervention (i.e., drilling to stimulate active repair or a subchondral bone graft) may be considered. He believes that osteocartilaginous fragments should be removed [59]. Hunter [33] reported that degenerative changes in the lateral compartment are associated with a poor prognosis, and osteophytes and loose bodies can be removed; however, ankylosis may remain, and the young athlete may be unable to throw. Bianco [16] concluded that two choices are apparent: (1) try to reattach the area of avascular bone surgically with Kirschner wires if possible, or (2) excise the loose area to prevent eventual loose body formation. He preferred to pin the lesion in situ with K-wires, noting that even with successful reattachment, subsequent collapse and deformation of the capitellar cartilage could occur [16].

Type III lesions are completely detached and lie free in the joint. Usually the loose body or bodies is hypertrophied and rounded, and the crater is obscured by fibrous tissue and is much smaller in diameter than the loose body [16]. Treatment usually consists of removal of the loose body by arthrotomy or arthroscopy with or without drilling or curettage [5, 16, 35, 83]. Bianco [16] stressed

that there is no evidence (in series of patients) that demonstrates that fragment reattachment is uniformly successful. Jobe [34], however, attempted reattachment of large loose bodies by means of arthrotomy and K-wire fixation. The results were good in these cases, and this method may prove to be useful. McManama and colleagues [51] reported that patients with large capitellar chondral defects associated with a locked elbow, evidence of loose bodies, or a failed course of conservative therapy require surgical intervention. They recommended removal of loose bodies, excision of capitellar lesions, and curettage to bleeding bone. Excellent or good results were demonstrated in 13 of 14 patients. They stated that complex surgical procedures such as lateral condylar excision, local bone grafting, or internal fixation of loose fragments are inappropriate [51].

Excision of loose bodies usually relieves the pain; however, there may be no improvement in range of motion, and late degenerative changes may still be the eventual outcome [16].

Posterior Extension and Shear Injuries

Injuries involving the posterior elbow are uncommon in young throwers. Pappas [59] reported only 18 instances in 111 elbows that involved the posterior joint structures, 11 of which were young adults. The causes of the various injuries are associated with the final stages of follow-through. During this throwing phase, extension overload at the olecranon tip and valgus stress that results in abutment of the medial aspect of the olecranon process against the olecranon fossa play roles in the pathology [5]. Injury during childhood usually centers on the secondary ossification center of the olecranon, which produces irregular patterns of ossification and secondary pain due to stress [59]. Pappas notes that the complaints, pathophysiology, and treatment are very representative of osteochondrosis [59]. During adolescence the injury pattern progresses to avulsion fragments or lack of fusion between the ossified secondary center and the olecranon [59]. This causes pain due to either loose bodies or nonunion of the olecranon [74]. Young adults may present with two additional problems: partial avulsion of the olecranon and secondary osteophyte formation at the tip and medial border of the olecranon (Fig. 15–18), limiting extension [5, 59, 83].

Treatment is tailored to the individual according to the age of the patient and the specific condition affecting the posterior elbow. Children with osteochondrosis usually respond to rest from pitching along with gentle range of motion exercises and a flexibility and strengthening program [5, 59, 83]. Adolescents with persistent pain associated with loose body formation or lack of

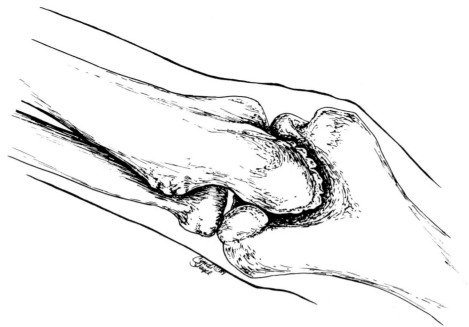

FIGURE 15–18
Typical location of posterior and posteromedial osteophytes of the olecranon associated with extension overload.

fusion may require surgical removal of the loose body and possibly a bone graft to induce union to the underlying physis [59]. Bone grafting is controversial, and rest and immobilization should precede any attempt at grafting. Yocum [83], Andrews [5], and Pappas [59] all recommend removal of symptomatic loose bodies employing arthrotomy or arthroscopic techniques.

In young adults, partial avulsion of the olecranon requires surgical reattachment [59]. Posterior and posteromedial osteophytes as well as loose bodies should be removed in symptomatic patients [5, 35, 59, 83] (see Fig. 15–18). Newer arthroscopic techniques have aided in treating these maladies [5, 35].

AUTHOR'S PREFERRED METHOD OF TREATMENT

Medial Tension Injuries

Medial Apophysitis

I find that a 4- to 6-week course of rest, specifically abstinence from throwing, results in cessation of symptoms. Initially, ice and nonsteroidal anti-inflammatory medications help to ease the symptoms. The use of steroid injections is neither necessary nor helpful. Rarely when the symptoms are advanced, the use of a removable posterior splint may be helpful. After 6 weeks, when the patient has no symptoms and a pain-free range of motion, strengthening exercises are begun. A progres-

sive throwing program is initiated at about 8 weeks. Medial apophysitis is usually a benign entity, and a good outcome is expected. Occasionally, symptoms may reappear when throwing is resumed; in these cases, throwing should be delayed until the next season.

Medial Epicondylar Fractures

Classification of these fractures according to size and amount of displacement is used as a guide in my treatment plan. In minimally displaced (less than 2 mm) or nondisplaced fractures, simple posterior splint immobilization is initiated. After the acute symptoms have subsided (1 to 2 weeks), the patient's arm may be removed from the splint periodically to begin active motion exercises. Radiographic evidence of healing should be apparent by 6 weeks, and immobilization is then discontinued. Aggressive active range of motion exercises as well as a progressive strengthening program are started. When radiographic evidence of union is obvious, the patient is allowed to begin a specific progressive throwing program. Competitive throwing is permitted when the patient demonstrates normal painless range of motion, strength, and endurance while on the throwing program.

In moderately displaced (more than 2 mm) fractures with a large fragment, open reduction with internal fixation is appropriate. Two small cancellous screws are required to prevent rotation of the fragment and to fix it securely. Early motion after open reduction is extremely advantageous in the adolescent, and I recommend it highly to regain flexion and extension. Depending on the quality of fixation, range of motion exercises begin between 1 and 2 weeks after surgery while the patient is wearing a functional orthosis. If radiographic evidence shows no displacement of the fragment at 6 weeks, the orthosis is removed, and more aggressive range-of-motion exercises are begun. Occasionally the medial collateral ligament avulses only a small fragment of bone (2-3 mm), or the small fragment is comminuted. In these cases, a radiographic valgus stress test is done. If no evidence of instability is noted, the arm is treated conservatively as described for minimally displaced fractures. However, if instability is noted, the fragment is excised, and the ligament and muscle origins are carefully reattached to the medial epicondyle. It is important that the anterior oblique portion of the medial collateral ligament is reattached or sutured; otherwise, latent valgus instability may develop. Occasionally, the retained small fragment in conservatively treated cases creates late symptoms of pain in adult throwers. In these cases, one can excise the fragment by performing a fiber-splitting flexor muscle incision. Care must be taken not to endanger the integrity of the medial collateral ligament.

If the medial epicondylar fragment is within the joint and there is no ulnar nerve dysfunction, open reduction and internal fixation with two small cancellous screws is undertaken. Care is taken to assess the integrity of the medial collateral ligament. If valgus instability is apparent with clinical stress testing after fixation, a primary repair of the medial collateral ligament should be done.

Ulnar nerve dysfunction can occur in as many as 50% of patients when the fragment is entrapped in the joint [3]. In the event of ulnar nerve impairment, decompression of the cubital tunnel with open reduction and internal fixation of the fragment is performed. I do not believe that anterior transposition of the ulnar nerve is necessary. After open reduction and internal fixation with or without cubital tunnel decompression, the patient is placed in a posterior splint initially, progressing to an elbow orthosis in from 1 to 2 weeks, depending on the quality of fixation. If at 2 weeks, no evidence of fixation failure is present, active range of motion exercises are encouraged. As the acute symptoms decrease, a progressive program of range of motion exercises is begun. At 6 weeks, the functional orthosis is removed if no evidence of fixation failure is apparent, and an aggressive program of range of motion exercises is begun. When the patient has no symptoms and a pain-free range of motion, strengthening exercises are started. A progressive throwing program is instituted when muscle strength and endurance have improved to 80% percent of that of the contralateral elbow as confirmed by isokinetic testing. Competitive throwing should not resume until the next season.

Medial Ligament Ruptures

True medial ligament ruptures are very uncommon in children and adolescent throwers, the majority occurring in young adults when muscle mass and force during throwing have increased. If the injury is detected in the early stages, conservative treatment is appropriate. Rest, for a longer time than may ordinarily be recommended, is crucial. Heat and ice should be applied alternately, and injections of lidocaine (Xylocaine) and steroids may be helpful in young adults. Injections should not be made into the ligament but on top of it to bathe it. It is preferable to give no more than three injections, and not more than once a month. If scarring and calcification are present and are accompanied by pain that does not respond to rest, the calcifications should be removed and the ligament repaired primarily if possible. If stability of the joint is all that is required, surgery is not necessary; however, if the patient desires to continue participation in a throwing sport, surgery is necessary.

Rarely, patients give a history of multiple episodes of pain over the medial elbow during throwing that initially restricts the throwing motion. However, after a few days to weeks of self-instituted conservative care, the pain resolves, only to become symptomatic with resumption of throwing. Valgus stress elicits pain and snapping at the medial elbow. Instability testing and stress x-rays are negative. If these patients do not respond to 6 months of supervised conservative treatment, open exploration of the medial ligaments is indicated.

Primary direct ligamentous repair is indicated when it is believed that a stable repair is attainable. Surgical reconstruction of the medial collateral ligament with a tendon graft is indicated in the following circumstances: (1) acute rupture in throwers who lack enough remaining ligament for a primary repair, (2) reestablishment of valgus stability in the presence of symptomatic chronic laxity, (3) following debridement for calcific tendinitis in athletes if there is not sufficient viable tissue left to effect a primary repair, and (4) multiple episodes of recurring pain with throwing after periods of conservative care. When surgical reconstruction of the medial collateral ligament is necessary, I prefer to use the technique described by Jobe and colleagues [36, 40].

Lateral Compression Injuries

Panner's Disease

It is salient to remember that Panner's disease and osteochondritis dissecans are two distinct entities with two separate processes. Initial treatment involves rest and avoidance of throwing. Sometimes pain and tenderness dictate splinting the extremity with a posterior splint until the acute symptoms resolve. Radiographic follow-up is necessary to ensure that an adequate healing response is present. Conservative treatment in most cases is satisfactory. Late deformity and collapse of the articular surface of the capitellum are uncommon.

Osteochondritis Dissecans

I find it very helpful to classify the lesion with regard to its size and fixation and the condition of the articular cartilage of the capitellum and radial head. Basically, OCD can be divided into three types using the above criteria as discussed earlier in this chapter.

Type I lesions are intact with no evidence of displacement and no fracture of the articular cartilage. Initial treatment usually consists of avoidance of all vigorous activity. If pain is a predominant complaint, splinting may be used until the acute symptoms subside. After the initial symptoms abate, active range of motion exercises are encouraged. The elbow should be protected until there is adequate radiographic confirmation of revascularization and healing.

Type II lesions on either radiographic or arthroscopic evaluation show fracture or fissuring of the articular cartilage or partial detachment of the lesion. It is important to determine the size of the lesion and the stability of the fragment. Generally, if the lesion is large enough to fix the fragment adequately, the lesion should be pinned in situ. Many methods have proved to be effective; however, arthroscopically aided pinning with either fine Kirschner wires or the newer absorbable fixation devices has proved useful. Under direct vision, the fragment is pinned in situ, bringing the K-wires out just under the skin in the lateral epicondylar area to aid in their removal. The ends of the pins are embedded deep into the articular cartilage so that they do not project into the joint. Generally, the pins are removed after 6 to 8 weeks. New absorbable fixation devices may alleviate the need for pin removal, but they are technically demanding, and meticulous attention to arthroscopic technique is paramount. If the fragment is small and pin purchase is tenuous, single excision to prevent future loose body formation and burring of the base of the lesion is undertaken. Sometimes even with successful reattachment of the detached area, subsequent collapse and deformation of the capitellum is the final outcome.

Type III lesions are completely detached, and the fragment is lying free in the joint. In most instances, the loose body or bodies have hypertrophied, and the edges have become rounded. The crater is usually smaller than the loose body and is filled with fibrous tissue. I prefer to remove the loose body or bodies and curette the base of the crater if loose fibrous tissue is present. In type III lesions, reattachment of the loose fragment is still experimental; however, newer techniques may make this option feasible. Although removal of the loose body is effective in relieving pain, there is usually no improvement in range of motion. The patient with a type III lesion should be seriously counseled about the effects of continued throwing, and in most instances abstinence from throwing should be recommended.

Posterior Extension and Shear Injuries

Posterior injuries are uncommon in young throwers, but as the thrower matures, the incidence of posterior problems increases. Basically, posterior injuries can be divided by age: (1) osteochondrosis of the olecranon in childhood, (2) avulsion fragments and lack of apophyseal fusion in adolescents, and (3) partial avulsion of the olecranon and osteophyte formation at the tip and medial border of the olecranon in young adults.

Osteochondrosis in childhood is best treated by rest from pitching and gentle range of motion exercises. When the acute symptoms abate, flexibility and strengthening programs are initiated. When normal strength and range of motion return, throwing is allowed.

Avulsion fragments in adolescence may become a chronic problem and usually require arthroscopic removal. Lack of apophyseal fusion is usually responsive to conservative measures including rest and sometimes immobilization. I have no experience in bone grafting procedures to induce bony union of the apophysis.

Partial avulsion of the olecranon in young adults requires open surgical reattachment of the olecranon and triceps. Symptomatic posterior and medial olecranon osteophytes should be removed to decrease pain and improve range of motion. I prefer arthroscopic removal of osteophytes utilizing a posterior and posterior lateral portal with the aid of an arthroscopic burring system.

SUMMARY

The specific emphasis in this chapter has been on sports-related elbow injuries in an immature population. Recent investigations have expanded our knowledge of the unique anatomic, biomechanical, and biochemical differences between immature and mature elbows. Extrapolation of these differences has enabled the orthopedist to understand the unique patterns of elbow injury sustained by immature athletes. A few basic principles are paramount in evaluating and understanding immature elbow injuries: (1) the anatomic and biomechanical properties inherent in the epiphyseal plate, musculotendinous units, and secondary centers of ossification predispose the immature elbow to specific injuries, (2) the term Little League elbow encompasses many entities about the elbow, (3) an astute understanding of the chronological radiographic appearance of the developing elbow is obligatory, (4) most immature elbow maladies can be predicted based on the age and sport of the patient, and (5) a knowledge of these unique injury patterns associated with early appropriate treatment can obviate functional disability and permanent deformity.

References

1. Adams, I. E. Bone injuries in very young athletes. *Clin Orthop* 58:129–140, 1968.
2. Adams, I. E. Injury to the throwing arm: A study of traumatic changes in the elbow joints of boy baseball players. *Calif Med* 102:127–132, 1965.
3. Aitken, A. P., and Childress, H. M. Intra-articular displacement of the internal epicondyle following elbow dislocation. *J Bone Joint Surg* 20:161–166, 1938.
4. Albright, J. A., Torl, P., Shaw, R., et al. Clinical study of baseball pitchers: Correlation of injury to the throwing arm with method of delivery. *Am J Sports Med* 6:15–21, 1978.
5. Andrews, J. R. Bony injuries about the elbow in the young throwing athlete. *Instr Course Lect* 34:323–331, 1985.
6. An, K. N., Jui, F. C., Morrey, B. F., et al. Muscles across the elbow joint: A biomechanical analysis. *J Biomech* 14:659–669, 1981.
7. An, K. N., and Morrey, B. F. Biomechanics of the elbow. *In* Morrey, B. F. (Ed.), *The Elbow and Its Disorders.* Philadelphia, W. B. Saunders, 1985.
8. Aronem, J. G. Problems of the upper extremity in gymnasts. *Clin Sports Med* 4:61–70, 1985.
9. Ashhurst, A. P. C. *An Anatomical and Surgical Study of Fractures of the Lower End of the Humerus.* Philadelphia, Lea & Febiger, 1910.
10. Ballinger, P. W. *Merrills Atlas of Radiological Positions and Radiographic Procedures.* St. Louis, C. V. Mosby, 1982.
11. Barnes, D. A., and Tullos, H. S. An analysis of 100 symptomatic baseball players. *AMJ Sports Med* 6:62–67, 1978.
12. Basmajian, J. B., and DeLuca, C. J. *Muscles Alive: Their Functions Revealed by Electromyography.* Baltimore, William & Wilkins, 1985, p. 285.
13. Bennett, J. B., and Tullos, H. S. Ligamentous and articular injuries in the athlete. *In* Morrey, B. F. (Ed.), *The Elbow and Its Disorders.* Philadelphia, W. B. Saunders, 1985.
14. Bennett, G. E. Shoulder and elbow lesions distinctive of baseball players. *Ann Surg* 126:107–110, 1947.
15. Bennett, G. E. Elbow and shoulder lesions of baseball players. *Am J Surg* 98:484–492, 1959.
16. Bianco, A. J. Osteochondritis dissecans. *In* Morrey, B. F. (Ed.), *The Elbow and Its Disorders.* Philadelphia, W. B. Saunders, 1985.
17. Brodeur, A. E., Silberstein, M. J., and Graviss, E. R. *Radiology of the Pediatric Elbow.* Boston, G. K. Hall, 1981.
18. Brogdon, B. G., and Crow, N. E. Little Leaguer's elbow. *Am J Roentgenol* 83:671–675, 1960.
19. Brown, R., Blazina, M. E., Kerlan, R. K., et al. Osteochondritis of the capitellium. *J Sports Med* 2:27–46, 1974.
20. Elkins, E. C., Leden, U. M., and Wakim, K. G. Objective recording of the strength of normal muscles, *Arch Phys Med* 32:639–647, 1951.
21. Elgenmark, O. The normal development of the ossific centers during infancy and childhood. *Acta Paediatr* (Suppl.) 33, 1946.
22. Gardiner, J. B. Osteochondritis dissecans in three members of one family. *J Bone Joint Surg* 37B:139, 1955.
23. Garrick, J. G., and Requa, R. K. Epidemiology of womens gymnastics injuries. *Am J Sports Med* 8:261–264, 1980.
24. Goldberg, M. J. Gymnastic injuries. *Orthop Clin North Am* 11:717–732, 1980.
25. Gray, D. J., and Gardner, E. Prenatal development of the human elbow joint. *Am J Anat* 88:429–469, 1951.
26. Green, W. R., and Banks, H. H. Osteochondritis dissecans in children. *J Bone Joint Surg* 35A:26–47, 1953.
27. Gugenheim, J. J., Stanley, R. F., Wood, G. W., et al. Little League survey: The Houston Study. *Am J Sports Med* 4:189–199, 1976.
28. Halls, A. A., and Travill, R. Transmission of pressures across the elbow joint. *Anat Rec* 150:243, 1964.
29. Hang, Y. S. Little League elbow: A clinical and biomechanical study. *Int Orthop* 3:70, 1982.
30. Hang, Y. S. Tardy ulnar neuritis in a Little League baseball player. *Am J Sports Med* 8:333, 1980.
31. Hoffmann, A. D. Radiography of the pediatric elbow. *In* Morrey, B. F. (Ed.), *The Elbow and Its Disorders.* Philadelphia, W. B. Saunders, 1985.
32. Hui, F. C., Chao, E. Y., and An, K. N. Muscle and joint forces at the elbow during isometric lifting (Abstract). *Orthop Trans* Z2:169, 1978.
33. Hunter, S. C. Little League elbow. *In* Zarins, B., Andrews, J. R., and Carson, W. G. (Eds.), *Injuries to the Throwing Arm.* Philadelphia, W. B. Saunders, 1985.
34. Indelicato, P. A., Jobe, F. W., Kerlin, R. K., et al. Correctable elbow lesions in professional baseball players. *Am J Sports Med* 7:72–79, 1979.
35. Irelano, M. L., and Andrews, J. R. Shoulder and elbow injuries in the young athlete. *Clin Sports Med* 7:473–494, 1988.
36. Jobe, F. W. Personal communication, 1988.
37. Jobe, F. W., and Bradley, J. P. Ulnar neuritis and ulnar collateral ligament instabilities in overarm throwers. *In* Torg, J. (Ed.), *Current Therapy in Sports Medicine,* Vol. 2. Toronto, B. C. Decker, 1990, pp. 419–424.
38. Jobe, F. W., and Bradley, J. P. The diagnosis and nonoperative treatment of shoulder injuries in athletes. *Clin Sports Med* 8:419–437, 1989.
39. Jobe, F. W., and Bradley, J. P. Rotator cuff injuries in baseball: Prevention and rehabilitation. *Sports Med* 6:337–386, 1988.
40. Jobe, F. W., Stark, H., and Lombardo, S. L. Reconstruction of the ulnar collateral ligament in athletes. *J Bone Joint Surg* 68A:1158–1163, 1986.
41. Keats, T. E. *An Atlas of Normal Roentgen Variants That May Simulate Disease* (2nd ed.). Chicago, Yearbook, 1979, pp. 241–268.
42. King, D. Osteochondritis dissecans: A clinical study of twenty-four cases. *J Bone Joint Surg* 14:535, 1932.
43. King, I. W., Brelsford, A. J., and Tullos, H. S. Analysis of the pitching arm of the professional baseball pitcher. *Clin Orthop* 67:116–123, 1969.
44. King, I. W., Brelsford, A. J., and Tullos, H. S. Epicondylitis and osteochondritis of the professional baseball pitchers elbow. American Association of Orthopaedic Surgeons, Symposium on Sports Medicine, 1987, pp. 75–78.
45. Kohler, A., and Zimmer, E. A. *Borderlands of the Normal and Early Pathologic in Skeletal Roentgenology* (3rd ed.). New York, Grune & Stratton, 1968.
46. Larson, R. F. Forearm positioning on maximal elbow flexor force. *Phys Ther* 49:748–756, 1969.
47. Larson, R. L., and McMahan, R. O. The epiphyses and the childhood athlete. *JAMA* 196:99–104, 1966.
48. Larson, R. L., Singer, K. M., Bergstrom, R., et al. Little League Survey: The Eugene Study. *Am J Sports Med* 4:201–209, 1976.
49. Lindholm, T. S., Osterman, K., and VanKkae, E. Osteochondritis dissecans of the elbow, ankle, and hip. *Clin Orthop* 148:245, 1980.
50. Lipscomb, A. B. Baseball pitching injuries in growing athletes. *Am J Sports* 3:25–34, 1975.

51. McManama, G. B., Micheli, L. J., Berry, M. V., et al. The surgical treatment of osteochondritis of the capitellum. *Am J Sports Med* 13(1):11–21, 1985.

52. Micheli, L. J. The traction apophysitises, *Clin Sports Med* 6:389–404, 1987.

53. Micheli, L. J. Sports injuries in children and adolescents. *In* Strauss, R. H. (Ed.), *Sports Medicine and Physiology*. Philadelphia, W. B. Saunders, 1979, pp. 288–303.

54. Middlman, I. C. Shoulder and elbow lesions of baseball players. *Am J Surg* 102:627–632, 1961.

55. Morrey, B. F., and An, K. N. Articular and ligamentous contributions to the stability of the elbow joint. *Am J Sports Med* 11:315, 1983.

56. Morrey, B. F., and An, K. N. Functional anatomy of the collateral ligaments of the elbow joint. *Clin Orthop* 201:84–90, 1986.

57. O'Donoghue, D. H., and Stanley, L. Persistent olecranon epiphyses in adults. *J Bone Joint Surg* 24:677–680, 1942.

58. Panner, H. I. A peculiar affection of the capitellum humeri, resembling Calvé-Perthes disease of the hip. *Acta Radiol* 10:234, 1928.

59. Pappas, A. M. Elbow problems associated with baseball during childhood and adolescence. *Clin Orthop* 164:30–41, 1982.

60. Pappas, A. M. Elbow problems associated with baseball during childhood and adolescence. *Clin Orthop* 164:30, 1982.

61. Perry, J., and Glousman, R. Biomechanics of throwing. *In* Nicholas, J. A., and Hershman, E. B. (Eds.), *The Upper Extremity in Sports Medicine*. St. Louis, C. V. Mosby, 1990, pp. 727–750.

62. Porteous, C. J. The olecranon epiphyses. *J Anat* 94:286, 1960.

63. Priest, J. D., and Weise, D. J. Elbow injury in women's gymnastics. *Am J Sports Med* 9:288–295, 1981.

64. Rogers, L. F. *Radiology of Skeletal Trauma*. New York, Churchill Livingstone, 1982, pp. 435–501.

65. Silberstein, M. J., Brodeur, A. E., and Graviss, E. R. Some vagaries of the capitellum. *J Bone Joint Surg* 61A:244, 1979.

66. Sisto, D., Jobe, F. W., and Moynes, D. R. An electromyographic analysis of the elbow in pitching. *Am J Sports Med* 15:260–263, 1987.

67. Slager, R. F. From Little League to big league, the weak spot is the arm. *Am J Sports Med* 5:37–48, 1977.

68. Slocum, D. B. Classification of elbow injuries from baseball pitching. *Tex Med* 64:48–53, 1968.

69. Smith, M. G. H. Osteochondritis of the humeral capitellum. *J Bone Joint Surg* 468:50–54, 1964.

70. Snook, G. A. Injuries in women's gymnastics, *Am J Sports Med* 7:242–244, 1979.

71. Tiynon, M. C., Anzel, S. H., and Waugh, T. R. Surgical management of osteochondritis dissecans of the capitellum. *Am J Sports Med* 4:121–128, 1976.

72. Torg, J. S. Little League: "The theft of a carefree youth." *Physician Sportsmed* 1:72–78, 1973.

73. Torg, J. S. The Little League pitcher. *Am Fam Physician* 6:71–76, 1972.

74. Torg, J. S., and Moyer, R. A. Non-union of a stress fracture through the olecranon epiphyseal plate observed in an adolescent baseball pitcher. *J Bone Joint Surg* 59A:264–268, 1977.

75. Torg, J. S., Pollack, H., and Sweterlitsch, P. The effect of competitive pitching on the shoulders and elbows of pre-adolescent baseball players. *Pediatrics* 49:267–272, 1972.

76. Trias, A., and Ray, R. D. Juvenile osteochondritis of the radial head-report of a bilateral case. *J Bone Joint Surg* 45A:576–582, 1963.

77. Tullos, H. S., Erwin, W. D., Woods, G. W., et al. Unusual lesions of the pitching arm. *Clin Orthop* 88:169–182, 1972.

78. Tullos, H. S., and King, J. W. Lesions of the pitching arm in adolescents. *JAMA* 220:264–271, 1972.

79. Tullos, H. S., and King, J. W. Throwing mechanisms in sports. *Orthop Clin North Am* 4:709–720, 1973.

80. Woodward, A. H., and Bianco, A. J. Osteochondritis dissecans of the elbow. *Clin Orthop* 110:35, 1975.

81. Wilkens, K. E. Fractures and dislocations of the elbow region. *In* Rockwood, C. A., Wilkens, K. E., and King, R. E. (Eds.), *Fractures in Children*. Philadelphia, J. B. Lippincott, 1984, pp. 363–501.

82. Woods, G. W., and Tullos, H. S. Elbow instability and medial epicondyle fractures. *Am J Sports Med* 5:23–30, 1977.

83. Yocum, L. A. The diagnosis and non-operative treatment of elbow problems in the athlete. *Clin Sports Med* 8:439–451, 1989.

HAND AND WRIST INJURIES

Jeffrey L. Lovallo, M.D.
Barry P. Simmons, M.D.

As the entire country becomes more sports oriented with multimillion dollar athletic contracts adorning sports pages daily, there has been a concomitant increase in athletic participation by both boys and girls. Women's athletics have especially seen an increase in participation with the highest injury rate at the 1985 Junior Olympics being in field hockey [36]. The increasing participation by younger athletes in competitive sports is accompanied by pressure on the medical community from both parents and coaches to return players to competition as soon as possible after an injury. It is therefore imperative that physicians and paramedical personnel be fully trained in the prevention and treatment of athletic injuries.

In most sports the hand and wrist are exposed, causing them to have a very high incidence of injury. Zariczny and colleagues found that 30% of all injuries in children were to the hand and wrist, with boys having twice the number of injuries as girls [73]. Backx in the Netherlands found a 15% injury rate to the wrist and hand [3]. Chambers, studying a group of military children, found that 65% of all injuries were to the hand and wrist with basketball and football having the highest incidence [9]. There is a very high incidence of hand and wrist injuries in boxing and 16-inch softball [12, 45]. The thumb is most commonly injured in the adolescent downhill skier, and 50% of all skateboarding fractures occur in the hand [14]. Overall, the incidence of injuries to the hand and wrist depend on the amount of contact and stress loading applied to the limb. Injury rates range from 3% to 65%, with swimming and soccer having the lowest incidence and football and basketball having the highest [6, 8, 15, 16, 61, 65, 68].

This chapter emphasizes the preventive, diagnostic, conservative, and surgical management of injuries in the pediatric wrist and hand. Emphasis is placed on common

pitfalls and errors occurring during diagnosis and treatment. Diagnostic and therapeutic treatment protocols are outlined, but this outline should never substitute for good clinical judgment. The spectrum of bony, tendinous, and ligamentous injuries is covered as well as the increasing incidence of stress-related injuries in the upper extremity. Before any athletic injury can be adequately treated, a thorough understanding of the anatomy and biomechanics of the injured limb is mandatory.

DISTAL FRACTURES OF THE RADIUS AND ULNA

Distal radial and ulnar fractures are quite common and usually result from a fall on the outstretched hand. Forty-five percent of all long bone fractures in children occur in the radius, and 75% of these occur in the distal third of the radius. These fractures, if treated properly, almost always heal without residual disability. Compared with adult fractures, radial collapse, loss of motion, and distal radial ulnar joint impingement problems are rare.

There are four types of distal radial or ulnar fractures: torus, greenstick, physeal, and complete fractures [54]. Initial treatment of these injuries on the field should include splinting, elevation, and application of a cooling agent to decrease edema. A thorough neurologic and vascular examination must be performed, although neurovascular injuries in these fractures are rare. After radiographic assessment, most of these fractures can be treated with cast immobilization with or without closed reduction. Salter type I or II physeal fractures can be treated by closed reduction (Fig. 16–1) [58]. Following closed reduction of a type III or IV distal radial fracture, if there is articular displacement of more than 2 mm, open reduction with Kirschner wire pin fixation is indi-

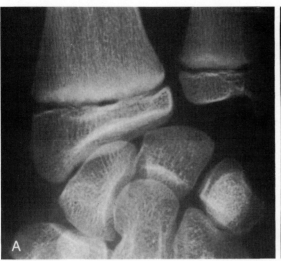 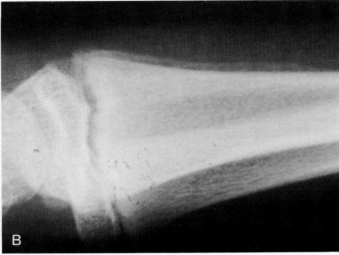

FIGURE 16–1
A, This patient was a 14-year-old white boy who fell on his outstretched hand while playing soccer. Initial radiographs were negative. Physical examination demonstrated tenderness over the distal radius, and he was placed in a short-arm cast. *B,* Four weeks later, volar callus formation is consistent with a nondisplaced Salter I fracture.

cated. Four to six weeks of cast immobilization are required with pin removal at 4 to 6 weeks. Torus fractures can be treated by simple short-arm cast immobilization for 4 to 6 weeks depending on the child's age. Greenstick fractures and complete fractures of the distal radius need to be treated with a long-arm cast for 4 weeks followed by a short-arm cast for 2 weeks. Depending on the child's age, up to 20 to 30 degrees of volar or dorsal angulation can be tolerated without permanent residual deformity. A major complication of distal radial and ulnar fractures in the immature skeleton is fracture redisplacement. This necessitates careful observation of the fracture with weekly x-rays during the first 2 weeks following injury. Residual deformity after treatment is best observed until growth ceases because many deformities will correct themselves with time. If after plate closure a deformity remains in either the radius or the ulna, an osteotomy can be performed.

STRESS INJURIES TO THE DISTAL RADIAL AND ULNAR PHYSES

In 1985, Roy and colleagues [55] reported on 21 young gymnasts who suffered stress changes to the distal radial epiphysis. These gymnasts were of Class II or better and practiced for approximately 36 hours/week. Stiffness and pain with dorsiflexion were the presenting symptoms. Roentgenograms demonstrated widened epiphyses, cystic changes, and beaking of the distal metaphysis. Treatment consisted of rest with or without cast immobilization. All patients but one returned to competitive gymnastics with no evidence of growth arrest. Ven-

der and Watson [67] reported a case of acquired Madelung's deformity in a 17-year-old gymnast. This resulted in distal radioulnar joint incongruity and was treated with a matched ulnar arthroplasty with relief of symptoms. Mandlebaum and associates [34], in evaluating pain in collegiate gymnasts, found a significant increase in ulnar variance compared with controls. They also found that the ulnar variance increased in proportion to the time spent in gymnastics. Although Roy and colleagues [55] concluded that there was no evidence of distal radial growth arrest, there is compelling evidence that repeated dorsiflexion stress loading of the wrist leads to partial distal radial growth arrest creating a positive ulnar variance. Gerber and co-workers [19] reported a similar case involving the distal ulnar epiphysis with a widened physis and metaphyseal irregularity. Complete resolution of symptoms occurred after 6 weeks of cast immobilization. An ulnar diaphyseal stress fracture treated successfully with cast immobilization has been reported in a weight lifter [48]. Although no cases of severe distal radial or ulnar epiphyseal growth arrest have been reported, if a child develops changes of the distal radius or ulna, the family should be informed that growth arrest may be significant enough to require future surgical intervention.

DISTAL RADIOULNAR JOINT INJURIES

Distal radial ulnar joint injuries in the child and adolescent athlete are rare. The two major types of injuries are acute dislocations of the distal radioulnar joint and triangular fibrocartilage complex (TFCC) lesions. Acute dislocations of the distal radionulnar joint should be treated with 6 weeks of long-arm cast immobilization. In acute dorsal dislocations, the forearm should be immobilized in full supination, and in volar dislocations the forearm should be placed in pronation. The athlete can anticipate a return to competition after 6 to 8 weeks of adequate rehabilitation. Triangular fibrocartilage complex tears are increasingly recognized in patients with repeated dorsiflexion stress impact loading on the wrist, which is common in gymnasts. Mandlebaum and associates [34] reported a 75% incidence of ulnar wrist pain in gymnasts with wrist pain syndrome. Palmer and Linscheid [47] recently outlined a classification of TFCC tears. In most TFCC tears a positive ulnar variance causes ulnar carpal impingement, leading to wear and possible perforation of the central disc of the TFCC. Treatment of TFCC injuries is in its infancy, with Darrach's procedure, ulnar shortening, hemiresection interposition arthroplasty, matched ulnar resection, and arthroscopic debridement of the TFCC being recommended [11, 42]. Currently, if conservative treatment fails, patients with neutral or negative ulnar variance with TFCC central tears are best treated by arthroscopic debridement. Patients with TFCC tears and ulnar positive or neutral variance should be treated with ulnar shortening and/or debridement of the tear (Table 16–1). In a child or adolescent bony resection procedures on the ulnar side of the wrist should be delayed until growth ceases. At this time, there are limited data on whether a competitive gymnast or other athlete undergoing these ulnar-sided wrist procedures can return to his or her preinjury status. Ishibe and colleagues [26] reported one case of osteochondritis dissecans of the distal radioulnar joint that became asymptomatic after open debridement of the joint.

TABLE 16–1
Distal Radioulnar Joint Injuries

Injury	Treatment
Acute	
Volar dislocation	Long-arm cast 6 weeks (pronation)
Dorsal dislocation	Long-arm cast 6 weeks (supination)
Chronic	
Ulnocarpal impingement (no TFCC tear)	Ulnar shortening
TFCC perforation (ulnar variance negative)	Arthroscopic debridement
TFCC perforation (ulnar variance neutral)	Arthroscopic debridement and/or ulnar shortening
TFCC perforation (ulnar variance positive)	Ulnar shortening and TFCC debridement

TFCC, triangular fibrocartilage complex.

WRIST INJURIES

Scaphoid Fractures

The scaphoid fracture is the most common carpal fracture in children and has a peak incidence between 12 and 15 years of age [54]. Only six cases have been reported in children under 10 years of age [20,62]. It has been estimated that 1 in 10,000 children will suffer a scaphoid fracture with approximately 75% being distal pole fractures, 20% waist fractures, and 5% proximal pole fractures. This distribution differs from that seen in adults. These fractures usually occur following a fall on the outstretched hand. Early recognition is the key to proper treatment of scaphoid fractures. Most pediatric scaphoid fractures heal with cast immobilization [20, 33, 39, 63]. A child typically complains of pain in the periscaphoid area. Physical examination demonstrates a decreased range of motion and tenderness in the anatomic "snuff box." Initial evaluation should include a standard radiographic scaphoid series. If initial radiographs are negative and there is a high index of suspicion for fracture, the limb should be immobilized in a short-arm thumb Spica cast. Repeat radiographs should be taken in 2 weeks. If these radiographs are negative and there is still a high clinical suspicion of fracture, a bone scan should be obtained. If the bone scan is positive, the child should be immobilized in a short-arm thumb Spica cast for 6 weeks. If all imaging examinations are negative, one should suspect acute scapholunate disassociation [28]. Fractures of the distal pole and tubercle can be treated with 6 weeks of short-arm thumb Spica cast immobilization. The child can participate in athletic competition with padding on the cast. Waist fractures and proximal pole fractures should be treated with 4 weeks of a long-arm cast followed by a short-arm cast until union occurs or for 5 months [17]. If nonunion with cystic changes is diagnosed in a child, immobilization for 3 to 6 months is recommended. If union is not achieved, autogenous bone grafting should be performed. Southcott and Rosman [62] reported union in eight cases of scaphoid nonunion treated by autogenous bone grafting in patients ranging from 9 to 14 years old. Huene [25] recommended primary internal fixation of carpal waist fractures followed by return to competitive athletics including football in approximately 6 to 8 weeks without external support. Riester and colleagues [53] treated 12 fractured scaphoids in football players with short-arm cast immobilization and allowed immediate athletic participation with padded short-arm casts. Ten of twelve healed in 6 months, but two proximal pole fractures progressed to nonunion requiring bone grafting.

Manzione and Pizzutillo [35] and more recently Hanks and colleagues [21] reported stress fractures of

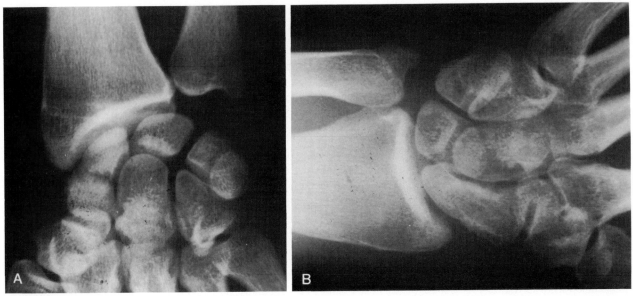

FIGURE 16–2
A, This patient was a 17-year-old elite gymnast who had complained of chronic wrist pain for approximately 3 months. Two previous radiographs were normal. This x-ray demonstrates a transverse wrist fracture of the scaphoid consistent with a stress fracture. *B,* Five months later following volar autogenous bone grafting without internal fixation, there is complete healing of the scaphoid fracture, and the patient has returned to competitive gymnastics.

the scaphoid waist. Of the five reported cases, four were gymnasts, and all healed with cast immobilization. A 17-year-old elite class gymnast complained of insidious onset of right wrist pain. Initial radiographs were negative, but follow-up radiographs revealed a stress fracture of the scaphoid. Despite cast immobilization for 4 months, nonunion occurred. Six months after volar autogenous bone grafting, the athlete returned to unrestricted gymnastic participation (Fig. 16–2) [57].

Our current treatment protocol is to immobilize distal third and tubercle fractures with a short-arm thumb Spica cast while allowing athletic participation. Scaphoid waist, proximal pole, and nonunions are treated for 4 weeks with a long-arm thumb Spica cast followed by a short-arm thumb Spica cast until union occurs. Contact sports are not allowed during this time. Established scaphoid nonunions and acute displaced fractures require surgical intervention. We prefer to treat nonunions with volar autogenous bone grafting placed through a volar approach [57]. There is no contraindication to use of the Herbert screw in the pediatric age group, and it may shorten the period of immobilization. Acute displaced fractures should be treated with Kirschner wires or a Herbert screw following open reduction.

Other Carpal Bone Fractures

Fractures of the other carpal bones are extremely rare. Capitate fractures can be treated by cast immobilization for 4 to 6 weeks [2]. Dorsal triquetral fractures secon-

dary to either acute dorsiflexion or a direct blow can be treated for 3 to 4 weeks with short-arm cast immobilization while allowing athletic participation [54]. Hook of hamate fractures are rare in children. The fractures usually occur secondary to torquing of the hand around a shafted object such as a golf club, tennis racket, or baseball bat. This injury should be suspected if a patient complains of pain on the ulnar palm. A carpal tunnel and oblique roentgenogram of the wrist should be ordered. If these are negative, a CT scan of the hamate should be obtained. This injury requires 6 weeks of short-arm cast immobilization. If there is persistent pain and nonunion, the hamate hook should be excised, taking care not to injure the ulnar nerve (Fig. 16–3) [5].

Ligamentous Injuries of the Wrist

Ligamentous injuries in children are rare with only two reported cases in the literature. A common ligamentous injury is scapholunate dissociation with a scapholunate ligament tear that may be either chronic or acute. Patients present with limited range of motion, dorsal wrist pain, pain with extension of the wrist, and pain with grasping. Roentgenograms may demonstrate a Terry Thomas sign or cortical ring sign, or the scapholunate angle may be increased on the lateral plain film. If plain films are negative and clinical suspicion persists, a radial carpal arthrogram can be performed. With a tear of the scapholunate ligament there will be leakage of dye into the midcarpal joint. In the acute injury, if the

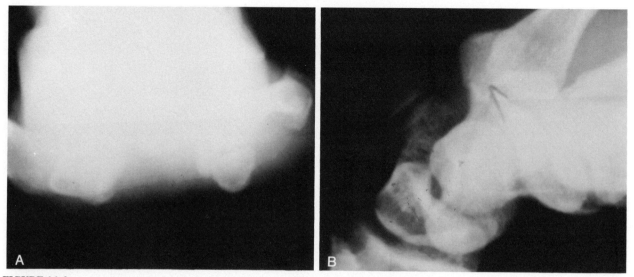

FIGURE 16–3

A, The patient was a 19-year-old youth who complained of pain in his ulnar palm (for approximately 3 months) following batting practice. An initial carpal tunnel view was negative for a fracture. *B,* An oblique roentgenogram demonstrated a hook of hamate fracture. Despite cast immobilization, the fracture remained painful and nonunited. Subsequent excision was required.

scapholunate alignment is normal, the arm should be immobilized for 6 weeks in a long-arm cast. If the scapholunate alignment is abnormal, then either percutaneous or open reduction of the scapholunate joint with pinning should be performed, followed by 6 to 8 weeks of cast immobilization. The treatment of chronic scapholunate dissociation is controversial. Current treatment options include scapholunate ligament reconstruction, dorsal capsulodesis, volar capsulodesis, and intercarpal arthrodesis. Gerard [18] reported an excellent result following ligamentous reconstruction of the scapholunate ligament utilizing a portion of the extensor carpi radialis longus tendon. We recommend deferment of treatment for scapholunate dissociation until adulthood. If treatment is necessary during childhood, the surgeon should use the procedure with which he is most comfortable.

AVASCULAR NECROSIS OF CARPAL BONES

Kienböck's Disease

Kienböck's disease, or avascular necrosis of the lunate, is rare in the immature carpus but does occur in the adolescent. The goals of treatment for Kienböck's disease are to reduce pain, maintain wrist motion, promote revascularization of the lunate, prevent carpal collapse, and prevent secondary arthritis. The most widely used classification of Kienböck's disease has been proposed by Lichtman; we have modified this to include carpal collapse (Table 16–2). Current treatments suggested for Kienböck's disease, depending on the stage,

include lunate resection with either silicone or tendon interposition arthroplasty, intercarpal arthrodesis, ulnar lengthening, radial shortening, wrist arthrodesis, proximal row carpectomy, fibrous arthroplasty, radial carpal arthrodesis, and cast immobilization (Fig. 16–4) [1, 4, 69]. No treatment mode has been universally successful. Our current treatment protocol includes radial shortening, a scaphoid-trapezial-trapezoid arthrodesis, fibrous arthroplasty, or radiocarpal arthrodesis (Table 16–3). We no longer use the lunate silicone prosthesis, with or without intercarpal arthrodesis, because silicone synovitis may occur secondary to wear debris of the silicone lunate. In patients with this disease, a return to preinjury status is unpredictable.

Avascular Necrosis of Other Carpal Bones

Larson and colleagues [29] reported a 6-year-old child with avascular necrosis of the proximal pole of the scaphoid following a fracture. The proximal pole revascularized, but the scaphoid remained nonunited. At 12 years of age the patient remained asymptomatic. Murakami and Nahajima [42] reported two cases of avascular necrosis of the capitate in two competitive gymnasts. The avascular necrosis was thought to be secondary to repetitive dorsiflexion with formation of microfractures. At surgery, avascular necrosis was detected in the head of the capitate. This area was resected without bone grafting. Both patients returned to competitive gymnastics.

TABLE 16–2
Classification of Kienbock's Disease

Stage	Pain	Plain Radiographs	Lunate Collapse	Carpal Collapse	Arthritis
1	+	−	−	−	−
2	+	+	−	−	−
3	+	+	+	+/−	−
4	+	+	+	+	+

Kienbock's disease can be classified according to radiographic finding. Stages 1, 2, and 3 are most likely in the adolescent age group.

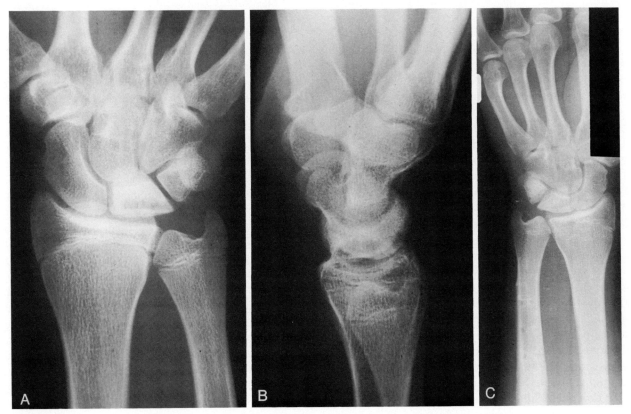

FIGURE 16–4
A, Kienbock's disease in a 15-year-old boy who presented with pain following a fall playing basketball. Note that the distal ulna is shorter than the distal radius (negative ulna variance). *B,* Lateral radiograph shows maintenance of carpal height. *C,* Ulnar lengthening in the mid-shaft resulted in healing of the lunate without collapse.

TABLE 16–3
Treatment of Kienbock's Disease

Stage	Procedure	Lunate Collapse	Carpal Collapse	Ulnar Variance	Radiolunate Arthritis	Radioscaphoid Arthritis
1 and 2	Radial shortening ⎤	N	N	− or neutral	N	N
	Ulnar lengthening ⎦	N	N	+	N	N
3	Radial shortening	Y	None or moderate	− or neutral	N	N
	Ulnar lengthening	Y	Y-Severe	− or +	N	N
4	STT arthrodesis; excision of lunate, no silicone	Y	Y	− or +	Y	N
	Fibrous arthroplasty or Radiocarpal fusion	Y	Y	− or +	Y	Y

STT, Scaphoid-trapezial-trapezoid; N, no; Y, yes; −, negative; +, positive.

CARPOMETACARPAL JOINT INJURIES

Carpometacarpal dislocations with or without associated fractures are rare in children. These injuries are the result of significant trauma. Most dislocations are associated with a fracture except in the case of the thumb. The most common carpometacarpal joint to be injured is the thumb, and injury results from an axial compressive force on the thumb tip during contact sports. A bony fragment may stay with the deep volar ligament producing a Salter-Harris type III fracture. These fractures are usually easily reduced, but resubluxation may occur.

Reduction is accomplished by applying distal traction on the thumb with direct pressure over the base of the metacarpal. The thumb should then be placed in a well-molded short-arm thumb Spica cast in maximum abduction with pressure applied over the ulnar aspect of the first metacarpal distally and the radial aspect proximally. If there is an inadequate reduction, K-wire fixation or open reduction may be required. A cast should be worn for 6 weeks, and contact sports should be avoided. After 3 weeks sports participation is allowed with the cast brought over the tip of the thumb. If percutaneous wire fixation is used, sports participation is not allowed. After removal of the cast, a short oppenons splint should be worn for an additional 6 weeks during participation in contact sports. An unstable joint after treatment can be stabilized with a flexor carpi radialis tenodesis (Fig. 16–5) [14]. If the patient still has open epiphyses the drill hole in the first metacarpal should be made distal to the metacarpal physis.

Carpometacarpal dislocations of the digits are even less common in children [71]. These occur secondary to an axial compressive force, usually from a fight. Treatment for these is similar to that used for first carpometacarpal dislocations with closed reduction followed by 4 to 6 weeks of cast immobilization. If the reduction is unstable, closed or open reduction with K-wire fixation is required.

METACARPOPHALANGEAL JOINT INJURIES

Dorsal dislocation of the thumb metacarpophalangeal (MP) joint is the most common dislocation in the child's hand [54]. The joint dislocates following forced hyperextension either from a fall or jamming injury against a helmet. The proximal phalanx may be partially or fully displaced dorsally, lying parallel to the first metacarpal. If the proximal phalanx is colinear with the metacarpal, the volar plate is usually interposed in the joint (Fig. 16–6). When the proximal phalanx is noncolinear, volar plate interposition is rare. An initial attempt at closed reduction should always be attempted. Following an adequate anesthetic, either local or general, the proximal phalanx is hyperextended at the MP joint with pressure applied over the base of the proximal phalanx to relocate it over the metacarpal head. Distal traction is to be avoided because reduction with this manuever is impossible. One manuever that may aid in reduction is to float the volar plate out of the joint by distending it with 1% lidocaine (Xylocaine). Following reduction, the joint is usually stable and is not prone to redislocation. Cast immobilization for 3 weeks is adequate, and athletic participation is allowed. If required, open reduction is performed using either a volar or dorsal approach. This allows easy extraction of the volar plate without having to divide it longitudinally. The thumb should be immobilized for 3 weeks, although early flexion may help avoid stiffness [7, 13, 49, 56].

MP dislocations of the fingers are rare, the most common occurring in the index finger. This dislocation occurs after a hyperextension injury to the digit. Initial assessment shows a digit with a prominent metacarpal head and a finger that is slightly supinated and ulnarly deviated. Radiographic examination should include anteroposterior, lateral, and obique views. These demonstrate a proximal phalanx that is dorsal to the metacarpal head. Volar plate entrapment usually precludes closed reduction [67]. Open reduction is performed through a

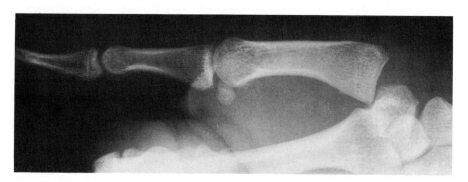

FIGURE 16–5
This thumb trapeziometacarpal joint was initially dislocated at age 15 while the patient was playing football. It was easily reduced on the sidelines and never immobilized. Two years later painful chronic subluxation was noted, requiring a flexor carpi radialis tenodesis to stabilize the joint.

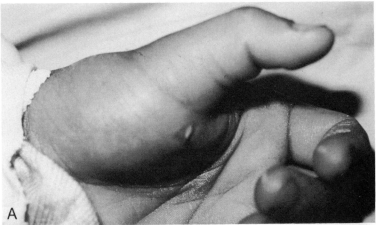

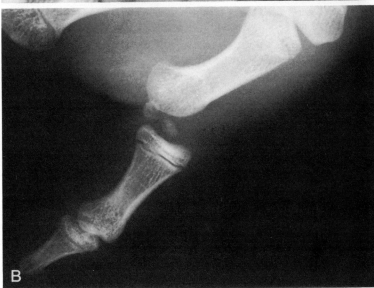

FIGURE 16–6
A and *B*, Hyperextension of the thumb metacarpopha-langeal joint resulted in this complex dislocation. In-terposition of the volar plate often prevents closed reduction.

volar or dorsal approach, with care being taken to avoid injury to the radial digital nerve, which is tented over the metacarpal head and lies just beneath the skin meta-carpal head and lies just beneath the skin [7, 49, 56, 67]. The lumbrical tendon is radial to the metacarpal head, and the flexor tendon is ulnar. After visualization of the metacarpal head, an attempt at volar plate extraction can be made with a hook. Often a longitudinal split in the volar plate is required to obtain reduction. After reduc-tion the finger is splinted for 10 days followed by im-mediate mobilization.

Gamekeeper's Thumb

The thumb MP joint is the most commonly injured joint in downhill skiers from ages 11 to 16 (Fig. 16–7) [6, 8, 16, 54]. These injuries result from an excessive radial deviation force on the thumb after falling on the outstretched hand with the thumb in the abducted posi-tion. In the immature skeleton, this results in either a Salter-Harris fracture or ligamentous injury (which is much less common). Salter-Harris type II fractures are common in children, whereas adolescents typically pre-sent with a Salter-Harris III fracture. When athletes give a history of a radial deviation force on the MP joint and tenderness is present along the ulnar collateral ligament, a radiograph must be obtained before the joint is stressed. Stressing the joint could theoretically displace a nondisplaced Salter-Harris fracture. Nondisplaced Sal-ter-Harris types I and II fractures are best treated with 4 weeks of a short-arm thumb Spica cast. Athletic partici-pation can be allowed. Displaced fractures should be treated by closed reduction and cast immobilization.

The ulnar collateral ligament inserts onto the epiphy-sis with no insertion onto the shaft of the proximal phalanx. This anatomic alignment predisposes adoles-cents to Salter-Harris type III fractures, while type IV fractures are rare. On radiographs the Salter-Harris III or IV fracture serves as a marker for the location of the ulnar collateral ligament. Nondisplaced or minimally displaced Salter-Harris III or IV fractures can be treated

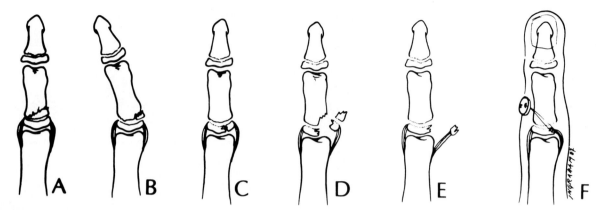

FIGURE 16–7

The spectrum of thumb fractures of the proximal phalanx at the metacarpophalangeal joint level as a result of a radial directed force. The Salter II fractures (*A,B*) are usually seen in the 5- to 11-year-old age group. The remainder occur mainly in adolescents, often in skiing accidents. *A,* Undisplaced Salter II fracture requiring no reduction. *B,* Displaced Salter II fracture requiring reduction. *C,* Minimally displaced Salter III fracture requiring no reduction. *D,* Salter IV fracture in which healing may or may not provide adequate ligamentous stability but would result in a significantly abnormal joint surface. This needs open reduction and K-wire fixation. *E,* Small, significantly displaced Salter III fracture now proximal to the dorsal apparatus (Stener lesion). Left displaced, there would be no significant articular surface abnormally, but severe ligamentous laxity would result. This requires open reduction. If the fragment is sufficiently large, it can be held with a K-wire. *F,* If the fragment is small it can be removed and the ulnar collateral ligament repaired directly with a pull-out suture. The same procedure is used when the ligament tear occurs without a fracture.

by a short-arm thumb Spica cast for 4 weeks [3, 9, 70]. Athletic participation can be allowed while wearing the cast. In skiers the cast can be molded to the ski pole grip by allowing the athlete to grasp the pole while the cast material is soft. The cast can then be covered with either a mitten or sock during skiing. If the fracture fragment is displaced, open reduction and internal fixation are required. Fixation is best achieved with two retrograde K-wires. Athletic participation is not allowed. If the radiograph discloses a large displaced fragment, open reduction is indicated to restore a normal joint surface regardless of the status of the collateral ligament. Articular incongruities do not remodel any better in children than in adults. Simmons and Hastings [59] demonstrated that untreated displaced intra-articular fractures are the leading cause of long-term disability following fracture treatment in the pediatric age group.

If x-rays are negative, the integrity of the ulnar collateral ligament must be assessed. This is accomplished by performing radial deviation of the MP joint in both full extension and 30 degrees of flexion. Radial deviation of greater than 30 degrees indicates at least a partial tear of the ulnar collateral ligament. The opposite side can be used for comparison (assuming it has not previously been injured). The examiner needs to develop a sense of the instability of the MP joint. If there is no firm end point, especially in full extension, there is a complete tear of the ulnar collateral ligament and a partial tear of the volar plate. If there is no firm end point, surgical repair is required. If there is more than 30 degrees of radial deviation and no firm end point while testing MP flexion, a complete tear is suggested. The unique anat-

omy on the ulnar side of the thumb MP joint allows the avulsed ulnar collateral ligament to migrate proximal to the adductor aponeurosis and does not allow healing to take place. Therefore, an ulnar collateral ligament with evidence of instability or no firm end point needs to be treated surgically. Surgery is best accomplished by securing the ulnar collateral ligament with a pull-out wire over a button followed by cast immobilization for 4 weeks. After 4 weeks, the button can be removed and a new cast applied; athletic participation is then allowed. The decision to operate can be made routinely by plane radiographs and clinical examination. Radiographic stress views, MP arthrograms, MRI, and anesthesia are usually not required.

Digital MP Joint Injuries

Ligamentous injuries to the MP joints of a digit are rare. They are almost always associated with a fracture. Unlike the thumb, the fracture may involve either the proximal phalanx or the metacarpal head. If the fracture fragments are displaced, open reduction and internal fixation with K-wires are required to restore articular congruity (Fig. 16–8). Postoperatively the joint should be immobilized in 30 to 40 degrees of flexion to avoid contracture of the collateral ligament. Commencement of therapy must be individualized according to stability after fracture reduction. Athletic partipation is allowed at 4 to 6 weeks with buddy taping to a border digit for an additional 4 weeks. Purely ligamentous injuries are best treated with cast immobilization for 2 weeks fol-

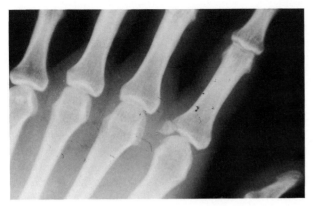

FIGURE 16–8
Displaced intra-articular proximal phalanx avulsion fracture requiring open reduction and internal fixation.

lowed by buddy taping to an adjacent digit for 4 weeks. Collateral ligament stability of the MP joint is tested by applying a radial or ulnar deviation force with the MP joints in 90 degrees of flexion.

Dorsal Capsular Rupture of the Digital MP Joints

Dorsal capsular rupture is a recently described entity that usually occurs after striking an object with a closed fist [50]. In a recent report, four of six people with this injury were boxers. This injury is most common in the index and long finger MP joints. Presenting symptoms are recurrent pain and swelling over the dorsal aspect of the MP joints. Physical examination reveals tenderness over the dorsum of the MP joint with a palpable defect representing a rent in the dorsal capsule. Initial treatment should consist of rest and conservative therapeutic measures. If pain persists, surgical intervention is indicated. At surgery a tear of the dorsal capsule is identified and repaired with nonabsorbable sutures. The repair should not be so tight that full flexion of the MP joint in the operating room suite cannot be obtained. Splinting is required in the postoperative period, followed by range of motion and strengthening exercises. Six months may be required before a full return to boxing is allowed.

INTERPHALANGEAL JOINT INJURY

The "jammed finger" is the most common joint injury in the child and adolescent athlete's hand. This injury results from an axial compressive force being applied to the end of the digit and can result in proximal interphalangeal (PIP) joint hyperextension with or without dislocation. This is a common injury in any ball-catching sport. Unlike metacarpophalangeal joint dislocations, reduction is easily accomplished by traction followed by joint flexion. This is often done by the athlete or coach, hence the term "coach's finger." The digit can be taped to the adjacent finger, and if the athlete is sufficiently comfortable, he or she can return to the game [7, 22, 38, 49]. It is imperative that medical attention be sought subsequently. Significant complications such as stiffness or chronic dislocation can occur. There is also the possibility of a fracture [37, 40].

Frequently, this injury is associated with a volar Salter-Harris type III fracture at the base of the middle phalanx (Fig. 16–9). Unless the fracture is so large that the joint is subluxed, this should be treated as a soft tissue injury. Control of edema will allow the earliest return of full function. This can be accomplished by

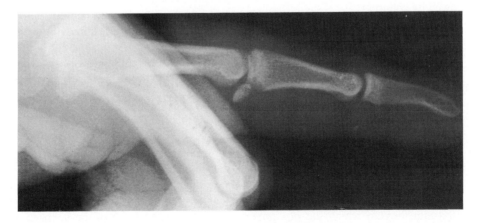

FIGURE 16–9
Axial compression as a result of the fingertip being struck by a ball results in distal interphalangeal joint flexion and proximal interphalangeal joint extension. The "jammed finger" may thus have either a mallet deformity or a PIP injury, usually the latter. This often results in a Salter III fracture from the base of the middle phalanx. Unless the fragment is sufficiently large to result in joint incongruity and subluxation, which is extremely rare in the child and adolescent age groups, this should be treated as a soft tissue injury. Although this radiograph shows a large fragment, there is no chronic subluxation, and the patient can be treated nonoperatively; this fragment usually does not block flexion.

application of a chronic pressure, self-adherent elastic wrap. A dorsal padded malleable aluminum splint can be applied with the PIP joint in 20 degrees of flexion. A dorsal splint is better tolerated than a volar splint because it allows metacarpophalangeal joint flexion and use of the fingertip [56]. Treatment following splinting must be individualized. Range of motion, especially flexion of the PIP joint, is encouraged. If symptoms persist, a formal hand therapy rehabilitation program may have to be instituted. Most patients can return to sports in 2 weeks. These injuries may produce persistent pain and swelling for up to 6 months. In many cases, the PIP joint never returns to its preinjury size. Chronic dorsal hyperextension instability is extremely uncommon in the pediatric age group. A fixed flexion (pseudoboutonniere) deformity is the most common sequela following this injury; it most commonly occurs when a knowledgeable physician is not consulted. Chronic hyperextension of the PIP joint is easily treated by repair of the volar plate through a Brunner incision. This can be done several years after the initial injury.

Boutonniere Deformity

A boutonniere deformity occurs secondary to rupture of the central slip or a dorsal displaced Salter-Harris III fracture at the base of the middle phalanx. This injury results from either direct trauma to the dorsum of the PIP joint or a volar dislocation of the PIP joint [7, 49, 56]. Central slip rupture with no fracture is treated by splinting the PIP joint in full extension for 5 weeks. PIP flexion is not allowed during the entire time of splinting. A dorsal Salter-Harris type III fracture, if nondisplaced, is treated by splinting for 3 to 4 weeks. A displaced fracture requires open reduction and internal fixation with K-wires, followed by splinting.

Collateral Ligament Injuries

A pure lateral force will result in either a sprain or a complete tear of a collateral ligament, with or without a dislocation. These injuries are most common in the border digits, especially the little finger. Treatment consists of buddy taping to an adjacent digit for 4 weeks. Again, therapy is critical to maintaining a full range of motion. Occasionally, one may encounter an irreducible lateral dislocation. This results from a tear between the lateral band and the central slip through which the proximal phalangeal condyle herniates. Reduction can be achieved by making a dorsal incision and repairing the central tendon, lateral slip tear. Collateral ligament tears never need to be repaired.

DISTAL INTERPHALANGEAL JOINT

The most common injury occurring at the distal interphalangeal (DIP) joint is either a bony or tendinous mallet finger. This fracture is similar to that of a bony boutonniere deformity with a dorsal Salter-Harris III fracture of the distal phalangeal physis. Mallet fingers result from forced hyperflexion of the DIP joint secondary to a jamming injury. The patient is unable to actively extend the DIP joint but has full passive extension [54]. Unless there is significant displacement of the Salter-Harris III fracture, all of these injuries can be treated with dorsal splinting of the DIP joint for 6 weeks. If the patient has full active extension at 6 weeks, flexion exercises are started, and a splint is worn during athletic activities for another month. If an extensor lag continues after 6 weeks, full-time splinting is continued for another 4 weeks. During splinting, the patient must be emphatically informed that he or she is not to allow flexion at the DIP joint. If an extension lag is present at 10 weeks, terminal tendon repair can be considered. In the authors' experience, this has never been necessary in children or adolescents. Large displaced epiphyseal fractures should be treated with open reduction and internal fixation.

Following hyperextension injury, a distal dorsal interphalangeal dislocation can occur. This is often reduced by the trainer on the field. Following reduction, the patient should be able to extend and flex the DIP joint. True anteroposterior, lateral, and oblique roentgenograms of the digit should be obtained to rule out an associated fracture. There have been two reported cases of irreducible DIP dislocations secondary to interposition of the volar plate and an osteochondral fragment within the joint [47, 64]. If reduction cannot be obtained by closed manipulation, open reduction is required. Following reduction, the patient should be treated with control of edema and dorsal splint immobilization [7, 13]. Therapy is begun with an early return to athletics.

AVULSION OF THE FLEXOR DIGITORUM PROFUNDUS

Avulsion of the flexor digitorum profundus is the most common closed flexor tendon injury in the adolescent athlete. This injury occurs most commonly to the ring finger [30, 51]. The injury results when a hyperextension force is applied to the DIP joint with concomitant attempted flexion of the flexor digitorum profundus tendon. This occurs almost exclusively in football or rugby as the finger catches on the opposing player's shirt or jersey—thus the name ''jersey finger.'' If identified early, the injury can be treated successfully. The main complication of this injury is the inability to diagnose it promptly.

The patient often assumes that the injury is a slight sprain of the distal joint and does not seek medical treatment. At the initial examination it is imperative that the patient be able to flex the distal joint. If he is unable to flex the joint it should be assumed that avulsion has occurred. A missed diagnosis occurs when the physician believes that inability to flex the DIP joint is secondary to pain and swelling. In almost no case is a patient with an intact flexor digitorum profundus unable to flex the distal phalanx at least 10 degrees. The tendon can also be palpated if flexion is antagonized. Examination of the patient must include palpation of the entire volar aspect of the digit and palm.

The avulsed tendon classically retracts to one of three levels: (1) just distal to the A4 pulley, often with a chip of bone; (2) at the level of the PIP joint; or (3) within the palm. The treatment for all three of these is similar in the acute situation. Radiographic examination with true AP and lateral views of the digit should always be obtained. A small fleck of bone can be seen at the level of the A4 pulley or PIP joint and will aid the surgeon in identifying the level to which the tendon has retracted and the degree of vascular disruption that has occurred [30, 51]. Obviously, a tendon in the palm is associated with rupture of both the long and short vincula and will be relatively avascular, whereas a tendon that has retracted to the level of the PIP joint has an intact long vincula and a ruptured short vincula, and a tendon at the level of the A4 pulley has both long and short vincula intact. A tendon with less retraction has better vascularity and a more favorable prognosis. Treatment of the acute injury consists of making Brunner incisions on the volar aspect of the digit. The tendon is passed under both A2 and A4 pulleys causing as little damage as possible to the tendon sheath. The tendon is then brought out through the distal phalanx using a pull-out wire and button and taking care not to injure the distal phalangeal physis [7, 50, 56]. Postoperative rehabilitation is similar to that used for any lacerated flexor tendon within the digit (Fig. 16–10).

FIGURE 16–10
A, A 13-year-old boy presented 6 weeks after a slight sprain to the DIP joint of his ring finger while playing football. On examination, the patient was unable to flex the DIP joint of his right ring finger. *B,* Lateral radiograph of the involved digit demonstrated a defect in the volar base of the distal phalanx. No fragment was identified in the digit, indicating possible retraction of the tendon into the palm. At surgery, a necrotic tendon was found in the palm, necessitating a free tendon graft.

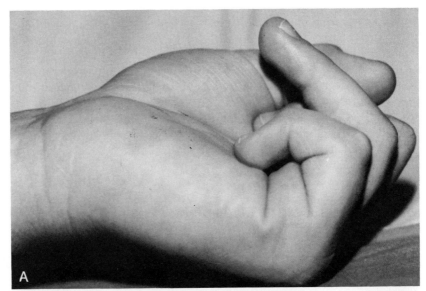
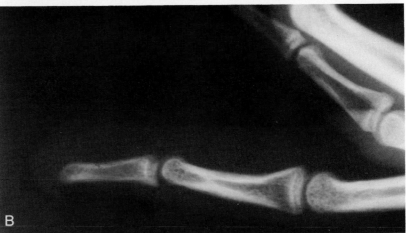

The difficulty with flexor digitorum profundus avulsion occurs when the initial diagnosis is delayed. If a diagnosis is made within 3 weeks, the tendon can usually be reattached, whether the tendon is retracted to the level of the digit or the palm. If the diagnosis is not made until 6 weeks it is virtually impossible to repair the tendon because it has usually retracted into the palm and has become fibrotic. In a late diagnosis, flexion at the PIP joint needs to be assessed. If the patient has full flexion of the PIP joint and is asymptomatic, reconstructive surgery may not be indicated [30, 51, 63]. However, free tendon grafts around an intact superficialis in the adolescent and young adult have had excellent results; in our experience patients are usually symptomatic, and we suggest tendon grafts.

DIGITAL FRACTURES

Fractures are the most common athletic injuries that require treatment. Epiphyseal fractures account for 41% of hand fractures compared with 10% to 15% for other long bone fractures [22, 59]. The specific ossific nuclei of the epiphyses appear in the metacarpals and phalanges by 3 years of age and fuse between 14 and 17 years of age [54]. The difference between adult and pediatric hand fractures is the presence of open physes in the child. Hand fractures in children have the capacity for remodeling, especially when the fracture is near the epiphysis and angulates in the plane of motion of the digit. Regardless of age, there is minimal or no remodeling of rotational displacement, and therefore a rotated displaced fracture should not be accepted. Lateral displacement is not in the plane of motion and also does not remodel. Most childrens' fractures can be treated conservatively, with only 10% requiring open reduction and internal fixation [31].

Distal Phalangeal Fractures

Crush injuries and hyperflexion injuries are the two major injuries that occur to the distal phalanx. These injuries are often open. Crush injuries during athletic activities usually occur when a finger is caught between two helmets. These injuries result in tuft fractures. They should be treated like any open injury with debridement and repair of the nailbed laceration using interrupted 6–0 chromic sutures under loop magnification [22, 31, 72]. Aluminum splint application with buddy taping for approximately 3 to 4 weeks will allow the patient to return to sports. Hyperflexion injuries of the distal phalanx result in either a bony mallet finger or an open Salter-Harris type I epiphyseal fracture at the base of the phalanx. Open epiphyseal fractures require irrigation and

replacement of the avulsed nail plate beneath the eponychium followed by splinting for 4 weeks. Kirschner wire fixation is not necessary. Hastings and Simmons [22] reported that this injury has a high complication rate.

Middle and Proximal Phalangeal Fractures

The proximal and middle phalanges of the border digits are most frequently fractured. There are four major fracture patterns in the immature skeleton: (1) condylar fractures of the head, either unicondylar or bicondylar, (2) subcondylar fractures, (3) shaft fractures, and (4) epiphyseal fractures [54]. In evaluating any phalangeal fracture, it is imperative that true AP, lateral, and oblique radiographs be obtained. Intra-articular fractures of the head of the proximal or middle phalanx can be either unicondylar or bicondylar. Nondisplaced fractures can be treated conservatively with plaster immobilization for 4 weeks. These fractures need to be monitored with weekly x-rays because they have a tendency to displace. Displaced fractures require gentle closed reduction. Unreducible fractures should be treated by open reduction [22, 31, 72]. A dorsolateral incision entering the joint volar to the lateral band is best. Unicondylar fractures are treated with two transverse K-wires. Bicondylar fractures are similarly treated and then pinned to the phalangeal shaft. If the reduction is sufficiently stable, gentle early motion is preferred; athletic participation is not allowed. Subcondylar phalangeal neck fractures are common in children between 5 and 10 years of age and occur following a direct blow to the digit. Phalangeal neck fractures are more common in the proximal phalanx but can occur in the middle phalanx. These fractures normally displace dorsally and can rotate up to 90 degrees [31, 72]. Again, a true lateral roentgenogram is mandatory for adequate assessment of this injury. Displaced fractures should be treated by closed manipulation. These fractures are notorious for redisplacement and should be followed weekly with serial AP and lateral roentgenograms. If the fracture cannot be reduced or if redisplacement occurs, open reduction with internal fixation is indicated. This is accomplished by crossed K-wire fixation. The pins are removed after 4 to 6 weeks, and physical therapy is started. Shaft fractures of the middle and proximal phalanges are far less common in children than in adults. Most of these fractures are nondisplaced and can be treated with plaster immobilization for 4 weeks. Twenty degrees of angulation may be acceptable in the plane of motion in children under 10 years of age, but no more than 10 to 15 degrees of deformity are acceptable in older children. Malrotation or deviation is not acceptable. Most fractures, owing to a thickened periostium, remain nondisplaced. A displaced midshaft fracture requires closed reduction. If unstable, it can be held with two parallel longitudinal K-wires inserted across the flexed MP joint. These fractures have the highest incidence of nonunion. Salter-Harris type II fractures at the base of the proximal phalanx are the most common fractures in the child's hand [22]. Following digital block anesthesia, this type of fracture can be reduced by flexing the MP joint to 90 degrees and adducting or abducting the proximal phalanx. The alternative of levering the fracture over a pen or pencil placed deep in the web space is discouraged. This fracture should be immobilized in plaster for 3 to 4 weeks. As these are epiphyseal fractures, they have a great potential for remodeling, and 30 degrees of volar or dorsal angulation are acceptable. Again, no rotational deformities should be accepted.

METACARPAL FRACTURES

Metacarpal fractures in children are less common than in adults. Neck fractures (boxer's fractures) of the little finger are the most common metacarpal fractures [43]. Neck fractures are treated by closed reduction and cast immobilization for 3 weeks (Fig. 16–11) [34]. Intra-articular fractures through the physes are rare [32]. If the fracture is displaced, it should be treated by open reduction and internal fixation [53]. Almost all shaft fractures can be treated by closed reduction and cast immobilization. It is imperative that finger rotation be checked following reduction. This can be done by either actively flexing or passively extending the wrist, using the tenodesis effect of the long flexor tendons, to flex the digit. Metacarpal base fractures are usually nondisplaced and can be treated by simple cast immobilization for 3 to 4 weeks. Should any metacarpal fracture have rotational malalignment, open reduction and crossed K-wire fixation are indicated.

Thumb Metacarpal Fractures

Thumb metacarpal fractures are quite common and occur frequently during skiing. A Salter-Harris II fracture through the base of the metacarpal is the most common injury. These fractures can be displaced either radially or ulnarly. Radially displaced fractures can be treated by closed reduction and cast immobilization for 4 weeks. Ulnarly displaced fractures are inherently un-

FIGURE 16–11
A, This 14-year-old white boy injured his right index finger while playing football. Radiographs were equivocal, but on physical examination the patient had a swollen tender distal index metacarpal. *B,* Four weeks following cast immobilization abundant callus is present, indicating a nonepiphyseal metacarpal neck fracture.

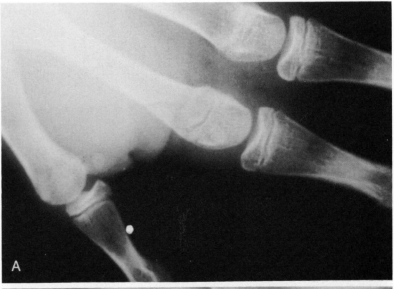
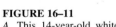
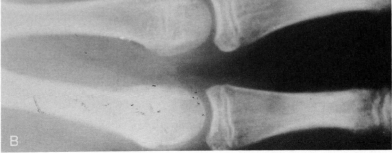

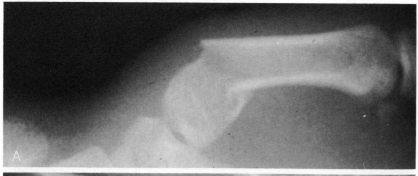

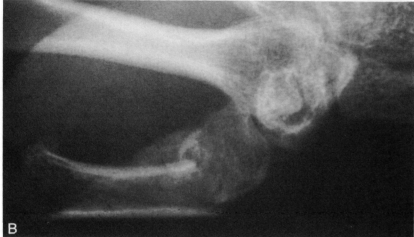

FIGURE 16–12
A, This patient was a 17-year-old high school quarterback who struck his right thumb on an opposing player's helmet. The fracture was treated with cast immobilization for 4 weeks. *B,* At 4 weeks there was abundant callus. Clinically, the patient had a slightly prominent metacarpal but no functional deficit.

stable and are difficult to reduce by closed methods [22, 31, 54, 72]. A reduced ulnarly displaced fracture must be followed by serial roentgenograms. Irreducible fractures require open reduction and internal fixation with K-wires. Thirty degrees of residual angulation are acceptable for this fracture (Fig. 16–12).

FROSTBITE

Mild frostbite injuries frequently occur following winter sports activities. In most cases, gentle rewarming of the hands in water at a temperature of 100°F will resolve the frostbite with no permanent tissue damage. Prolonged cold exposure can lead to deep freezing of the tissues. In these cases, premature fusion of the distal and often the middle phalangeal physes can occur. The thumb is usually spared because the child tends to clench the thumb in his palm. Premature fusion can lead to an acquired brachydactyly with mild flexion contractures of the digits. Partial premature fusions can result in angular deformities [44]. Obviously, the best way to prevent severe frostbite is to supply adequately insulated gloves or mittens to all children who are participating in winter sports. At the earliest sign of exposure, the child should be brought indoors, and immediate rewarming of the involved digits should be initiated.

SUMMARY

Sports injuries of the hand and wrist in children demand a thorough knowledge of the anatomy and biomechanics of the hand as well as the specific modalities of treatment. Children have a tremendous capacity for remodeling of fractures, and the treating physician needs to recognize the acceptable limits of fracture deformity. If there is any doubt about a treatment plan, a hand specialist should be consulted. Most children's injuries, if recognized promptly and treated by a knowledgeable physician, have a successful outcome. Permanent disabilities after injuries to the hand in children result from delayed diagnoses and improper treatment. If appropriately managed, most hand injuries in children should not prevent the child from continuing to be an active participant in sports.

References

1. Almquist, E. E., Burns, J. F., and Wash, S. Radial shortening for the treatment of Kienbock's disease—a 5 to 10 year followup. *J Hand Surg* 7:348–357, 1982.
2. Anderson, W. J. Simultaneous fracture of the scaphoid and capitate in a child. *J Hand Surg* 12A:271–273, 1987.
3. Backx, F. J., Erich, B. M., Kemper, A. B., et al. Sports injuries in school-aged children: An epidemiologic study. *Am J Sports Med* 17:234–240, 1989.

4. Bianco, R. H. Excision of the lunate in Kienbock's disease: Long-term results. *J Hand Surg* 10A:1008–1013, 1985.

5. Bishop A. T., and Beckerbaugh, R. D. Fracture of the hamate hook. *J Hand Surg* 13A:136–139, 1988.

6. Blitzer, C. M., Johnson, R. J., Ettlinger, C. F., et al. Downhill skiing injuries in children. *Am J Sports Med* 12:142–147, 1984.

7. Burton, R. I. and Eaton, R. G. Common hand injuries in the athlete. *Orthop Clin North Am* 4:809–838, 1973.

8. Carr, D., Johnson, R. J. and Pohlman, M. H. Upper extremity injuries in skiing. *Am J Sports Med* 9:378–383, 1981.

9. Chambers, R. B. Orthopedic injuries in athletes (ages 6 to 17). *Am J Sports Med* 7:195–197, 1979.

10. Coonrad, R. W., and Pohlman, M. H. Impacted fractures in the proximal portion of the proximal phalanx of the finger. *J Bone Joint Surg* 51A:1291–1296, 1969.

11. Darrow, J. C., Linscheid, R. L., Dobyns, J. H., et al. Distal ulnar recession for disorders of the distal radio-ulnar joint. *J Hand Surg* 10A:482–491, 1985.

12. Degroot, H., and Mass, D. P. Hand injury patterns in softball players using a 16 inch ball. *Am J Sports Med* 16:260–265, 1988.

13. Dobyns, J. H., Sim, F. H., and Linscheid, R. L. Sports stress syndromes of the hand and wrist. *Am J Sports Med* 6:236–254, 1978.

14. Eaton, R. G., and Littler, J. W. Ligament reconstruction for the painful thumb carpometacarpal joint. *J Bone Joint Surg* 55A:1655, 1973.

15. Garrick, J. F., and Regua, R. K. Epidemiology of women's gymnastics injuries. *Am J Sports Med* 8:261–264, 1980.

16. Garrick, J. F., and Regua, R. K. Injury patterns in children and adolescent skiers. *Am J Sports Med* 7:245–248, 1980.

17. Gellman, H. S., Caputo, R. J., Carter, V., et al. Comparison of short and long thumb-spica casts for non-displaced fractures of the carpal scaphoid. *J Bone Joint Surg* 71A:354–357, 1989.

18. Gerard, F. M. Post-traumatic carpal instability in a young child. *J Bone Joint Surg* 62A:131–133, 1980.

19. Gerber, S. D., Griffin, P. P., and Simmons, B. P. Breakdancer's wrist. *J Pediatr Orthop* 6:98–99, 1986.

20. Greene, M. H., Hadied, A. M., and LaMont, R. L. Scaphoid fractures in children. *J Hand Surg* 9A:536–541, 1984.

21. Hanks, G. A., Kalenak A., Bowman, L. S., et al. Stress fractures of the carpal scaphoid. *J Bone Joint Surg* 71A:938–941, 1989.

22. Hastings, H., and Simmons, B. P. Hand fractures in children. *Clin Orthop* 188:120–130, 1984.

23. Hawkins, R. W., and Lyne, E. D. Skateboarding fractures. *Am J Sports Med* 9:99–102, 1981.

24. Ho, P. K., Dellon, A. L., and Wilgis, E. F. True aneurysms of the hand resulting from athletic injury. *Am J Sports Med* 13:136–138, 1985.

25. Huene, D. R. Primary internal fixation of carpal navicular fractures in the athlete. *Am J Sports Med* 7:175–177, 1979.

26. Ishibe, M., Ogino, T., and Sato, Y. Osteochondritis dissecans of the distal radioulnar joint. *J Hand Surg* 14A:818–821, 1989.

27. Itoh, Y., Wakano, K., Takeda, T., et al. Circulatory disturbances in the throwing hand of baseball pitchers. *Am J Sports Med* 15:264–269, 1987.

28. Kuschner, S. H., Gellman, H., and Bindiger, A. Extensor digitorum brevis manus, and unusual cause of exercise-induced wrist pain. *Am J Sports Med* 17:440–441, 1989.

29. Larson, B., Light, T. R., and Ogden, J. A. Fracture and ischemic necrosis of the immature scaphoid. *J Hand Surg* 12A:122–127, 1987.

30. Leddy, J. P., and Packer, J. W. Avulsion of the profundus tendon insertion in athletes. *J Hand Surg* 2:66–69, 1977.

31. Leonard, M, H., and Dubravcik, P. Management of fractured fingers in the child. *Clin Orthop* 73:160–168, 1970.

32. Light, T. R., and Ogden, J. A. Metacarpal epiphyseal fractures. *J Hand Surg* 12A:460–464, 1987.

33. MacDonald, J. W. Delayed union of the distal scaphoid in a child. *J Hand Surg* 12A:520–522, 1987.

34. Mandelbaum, B. R., Bartolozzi, A. R., Davis, C. A., et al. Wrist pain syndrome in the gymnast. *Am J Sports Med* 17:305–317, 1989.

35. Manzione, M., and Pizzutillo, P. D. Stress fracture of the scaphoid waist. *Am J Sports Med* 9:268–269, 1981.

36. Martin, R. K., Yesalis, C. E., Foster, D., et al. Sports injuries at the 1985 Junior Olympics: An epidemiologic analysis. *Am J Sports Med* 15:603–608, 1987.

37. McCue, F. C., Andrews, J. R., Hakala, M., et al. The coach's finger. *Am J Sports Med* 2:270–275, 1974.

38. McCue, F. C., Baugher, W. H., Kulund, D. N., et al. Hand and wrist injuries in the athlete. *Am J Sports Med* 7:275–286, 1979.

39. McCue, F. C., Hakala, M. W., Andrews, J. R., et al. Ulnar collateral ligament injuries of the thumb in athletes. *Am J Sports Med* 2:70–79, 1974.

40. McCue, F. C., Honnor, R., Johnson, M. C., et al. Athletic injuries of the proximal interphalangeal joint requiring surgical treatment. *J Bone Joint Surg* 52A:937–956, 1970.

41. Minami, A., Ogino, R., and Minami, M. Treatment of distal radioulnar disorders. *J Hand Surg* 12A:189–195, 1987.

42. Murakami, S., and Nahajima, H. Aseptic necrosis of the capitate bone in two gymnasts. *Am J Sports Med* 12:170–173, 1984.

43. Murakami, Y. Stress fracture of the metacarpal in an adolescent tennis player. *Am J Sports Med* 16:419–420, 1988.

44. Nakazato, R., and Ogino, T. Epiphyseal destruction of children's hands after frostbite: A report of two cases. *J Hand Surg* 11A:289–292, 1986.

45. Noble, C. Hand injuries in boxing. *Am J Sports Med* 15:342–346, 1987.

46. Palmar, A. K. Triangular fibrocartilage complex lesions: A classification. *J Hand Surg* 14A:594–606, 1989.

47. Palmar, A. K., and Linscheid, L. R. Irreducible dorsal dislocation of the distal interphalangeal joint of the finger. *J Hand Surg* 2:406–408, 1977.

48. Patel, M. E., Iritarry, J., and Stricevic, M. Stress fracture of the ulnar diaphysis: Review of the literature and report of a case. *J Hand Surg* 11A:443–445, 1986.

49. Posner, M. A. Injuries to the hand and wrist in athletes. *Orthop Clin North Am* 8:593–617, 1977.

50. Posner, M. A., and Ambrose, L. Boxers knuckle-dorsal capsular rupture of the metacarpophalangeal joint of a finger. *J Hand Surg* 14A:229–236, 1989.

51. Reef, T. C. Avulsion of the flexor digitorum profundus: An athletic injury. *Am J Sports Med* 5:281–285, 1977.

52. Rettig, A. C., Ryan, R., Shelbourne, K. D., et al. Metacarpal fractures in the athlete. *Am J Sports Med* 17:567–572, 1989.

53. Riester, J. N., Baker, B. E., Mosher, J. F., et al. A review of scaphoid fracture healing in competitive athletes. *Am J Sports Med* 13:154–161, 1985.

54. Rockwood, C. A., and Green, D. P. *Fractures in Children.* Philadelphia, J.B. Lippincott, 1984.

55. Roy, S., Caine, D., and Singer, K. M. Stress changes of the distal radius epiphysis in young gymnasts. *Am J Sports Med* 13:301–308, 1985.

56. Ruby, L. K. Common hand injuries in the athlete. *Orthop Clin North Am* 11:820–834, 1980.

57. Russe, O. Fracture of the carpal navicular. *J Bone Joint Surg* 42A:759–768, 1960.

58. Ryan, J. R., and Salciccioli, G. G., Fractures of the distal radial epiphysis in adolescent weight lifters. *Am J Sports Med* 4:1, 1976.

59. Simmons, B. P. and Hastings, H. Hand fractures in children: A statistical analysis. *In* Tubiana, R. (Ed.), *The Hand,* Vol. 2. Philadelphia, W.B. Saunders, 1985.

60. Simmons, B. P., and Lovallo, J. L. Hand and wrist injuries in children. *Clin Orthop Sports Med* 7:495–512, 1988.

61. Snook, G. A. Injuries in women's gymnastics. *Am J Sports Med* 7:242–244, 1979.

62. Southcott, R., and Rosman, M. A. Non-union of carpal scaphoid fractures in children. *J Bone Joint Surg* 59B:20–23, 1977.

63. Stark, H. H., Zemel, N. P., Boyes, J. H., et al. Flexor tendon graft through intact superficialis tendon. *J Hand Surg* 2:456, 1977.

64. Stripling, W. D. Displaced intra-articular osteochondral fracture—cause for irreducible dislocation of the distal interphalangeal joint. *J Hand Surg* 7:77–78, 1982.

65. Sullivan, J. A., Gross, R. H., Grana W. A., et al. Evaluation of injuries in youth soccer. *Am J Sports Med* 8:325–327, 1980.

66. Sweterlitsch, P. R., Torg, J. S., and Pollack, H. Entrapment of a sesamoid in the index metacarpophalangeal joint. *J Bone Joint Surg* 51A:995–998, 1969.

67. Vender, M. I., and Watson, H. K. Acquired Madelung-like deformity in a gymnast. *J Hand Surg* 13A:19–21, 1988.

68. Watson, A. Sports injuries during one academic year in 6,799 Irish school children. *Am J Sports Med* 12:65–71, 1984.

69. Watson, H. K., Ryan, J., and Dibella, A. An approach to Kienbock's disease: Triscaphe arthrodesis. *J Hand Surg* 10A:179–187, 1985.

70. White, G. M. Ligamentous avulsion of the ulnar collateral ligament of the thumb of a child. *J Hand Surg* 11A:669–672, 1986.

71. Whitson, R. O. Carpometacarpal dislocation: A case report. *Clin Orthop* 6:189–195, 1955.

72. Wood, V. E. Fractures of the hand in children. *Orthop Clin North Am* 7:527–542, 1976.

73. Zariczny, B., Shattuck, L. J., Mast, T. A., et al. Sports-related injuries in school-aged children. *Am J Sports Med* 8:318–324, 1980.

HIP AND PELVIC INJURIES IN THE YOUNG ATHLETE

Peter M. Waters, M.D.
Michael B. Millis, M.D.

Hip and pelvic injuries in the young athlete comprise a broad spectrum of trauma to the pelvic skeleton and soft tissues (Table 17–1). The character of the injury depends on the skeletal age and physiologic conditioning of the athlete, the sport involved, and the nature of the trauma to the athlete. As with other sports-related injuries in this age group, the injuries may be classified as macrotrauma or repetitive microtrauma. Skeletal trauma may be epiphyseal, apophyseal, or diaphyseal, depending on the age of the patient and the velocity of the injury. Soft tissue injuries are predominantly acute strains or repetitive overuse syndromes. In the skeletally immature individual, growth plate injuries are more common than ligamentous or musculotendinous injuries. The conditioned state of the athlete, the training routine, and the equipment utilized are important factors in these injuries.

ASSESSMENT OF HIP AND PELVIC INJURIES

The child with a hip or pelvic injury may present to the sports practitioner either with an acute injury requiring immediate attention or a chronic condition that needs definitive diagnosis and treatment. An acute injury may present, after significant trauma on the field, with pain in the hip or pelvic region, inability to bear weight, tenderness at the specific site of injury, and deformity if the injury results in an acute fracture or dislocation. In assessing the child with a severe, acute injury in the field, the practitioner should stabilize the extremity and transport the patient as rapidly as possible to an emergency facility where definitive diagnosis and therapy can occur. A hip fracture or dislocation should be considered an operative emergency in order to preserve the blood supply to the femoral head and neck. Reduction should not be carried out on the field, unless there is serious neurovascular compromise of the distal extremity.

More commonly, the sports practitioner encounters an athlete with persistent restricting pain in the hip and pelvic region with sports activity. The injured athlete requires a thorough physical assessment including the following: specific areas of tenderness, limitation of hip range of motion in all planes, muscle strength, presence or absence of muscle atrophy, and distal neurologic examination. Diagnostic considerations include apophyseal injuries, stress fractures, slipped capital femoral epiphysis, Legg-Calvé-Perthes disease, and musculotendinous strains, among others. The physical examination frequently provides definitive information for diagnosis. Standard anteroposterior and lateral radiographs are often necessary for diagnosis. In cases of diagnostic dilemmas, a bone scan may elucidate an unrecognized stress fracture, apophysitis, or pathologic lesion.

ANATOMIC CONSIDERATIONS

As Ogden [44] emphasized, understanding the effects of traumatic injury on the skeletally immature hip and pelvis demands a knowledge of the progression of skeletal and vascular growth. The development of the femoral head and neck region into its three separate ossification centers (capital femoral epiphysis, greater trochanter, and lesser trochanter) progressively alters the biomechanics of the proximal femur and thus its injury patterns. The changing vascular pattern of the femoral head and neck greatly influences the risk of the many possible complications of trauma to the hip and pelvis such as avascular necrosis, nonunion, malunion, and possible eventual degenerative disease. On the pelvic side of the

279

TABLE 17–1
Classification of Hip and Pelvic Injuries

I. Skeletal Injuries
  A. Apophyseal Avulsion Fractures
    1. Iliac crest (abdominal musculature)
    2. Anterior superior iliac spine (sartorius)
    3. Anterior inferior iliac spine (rectus femoris)
    4. Lesser trochanter (iliopsoas)
    5. Ischium (hamstring)
  B. Growth Plate Injuries
    1. Slipped capital femoral epiphysis
    2. Salter-Harris physeal fractures
  C. Nonphyseal Fractures
    1. Pelvic Fractures
      a. Iliac wing fractures
      b. Acetabular fractures
      c. Stable pelvic ring fractures
      d. Unstable pelvic ring fractures
    2. Femoral Neck Fractures
      a. Transcervical fracture
      b. Cervicotrochanteric fracture
      c. Intertrochanteric fracture
    3. Subtrochanteric fracture
  D. Hip Dislocations
  E. Stress Fractures
    1. Femoral neck
    2. Pelvis
  F. Pathologic Fractures
II. Soft Tissue Injuries
  A. Musculotendinous Strains
    1. Snapping hip syndrome
    2. Iliac apophysitis
    3. Osteitis pubis
  B. Contusions

hip joint, undisturbed triradiate cartilage growth is crucial for normal acetabular development, and skeletal injuries in this region may have long-term sequelae for the patient in terms of acetabular dysplasia and degenerative hip disease.

There are several apophyses about the hip and pelvis with large muscle attachments, accounting for the frequency of apophyseal avulsion fractures seen in adolescent athletes. These secondary centers of ossification appear between the ages of 11 and 15 years and account for circumferential but not longitudinal growth of the bones [17, 37]. In general, the physis is the weakest structure of the growing skeleton and is most vulnerable to direct trauma and avulsion injuries. However, other than slipped capital femoral epiphyses, physeal injury in the proximal femur and acetabulum is a rare occurrence.

SPECIFIC INJURIES AND THEIR MANAGEMENT

Avulsion Fractures

The mechanism of injury is either a sudden violent muscular contraction or an excessive amount of muscle stretch across an open apophysis. There is often no external trauma [17, 37]. The injury occurs most often in adolescent athletes between the ages of 14 and 17 years. A similar overload in an adult would most likely result in a muscle strain. Avulsion fractures are more frequent in males than in females, but this pattern may be changing with the greater frequency of female athletic programs. The most common sites of avulsion fracture are the anterior superior iliac spine (at the origin of the sartorius), the ischium (hamstrings) (Fig. 17–1), the lesser trochanter (iliopsoas, Fig. 17–2), the anterior-inferior iliac spine (rectus), and the iliac crest (abdominal muscles). A greater trochanteric avulsion at the insertion of the abductors is extremely rare [44]. These injuries occur in a broad spectrum of individual and team sports, usually in competitive athletes (particularly sprinters, jumpers, soccer and football players) during the course of an extreme effort. The athlete generally presents with localized swelling, tenderness, and limitation of motion about the site of the avulsion fracture. Pain may be extreme. Radiographs should confirm the diagnosis. On occasion, pelvic inlet, outlet, or oblique views may be necessary to define the lesion and the extent of displacement.

Therapy with bed rest, ice application, and positioning of the limb to lessen the stretch on the affected muscle and apophysis frequently improves the patient's symptoms and decreases the risk of further displacement of the apophysis. Metzmaker and Pappas [37] outlined a five-stage progressive rehabilitation program that was successful in 27 athletes with acute avulsion fractures of the hip and pelvis. The stages are as follows: (1) *Rest* with positioning to relax the involved muscle group, ice application, and analgesia are initiated at the time of injury. (2) The patient is allowed to *gradually increase the excursion* of the injured musculotendinous unit when pain has subsided. (3) When he or she has obtained full, active range of motion, the athlete institutes a comprehensive *resistive exercise program.* (4) When 50% of anticipated strength has been achieved, the athlete *integrates* the use of the injured musculotendinous unit with the other muscles of the pelvis and lower extremity. This is the stage when the risk of reinjury is high if the patient returns to full participation before normal strength and function are achieved. (5) Only when the athlete has achieved full strength and integration of the injured muscle into his athletic activity is he allowed to *return to competitive sports.*

Isokinetic strength testing can be utilized as a more objective assessment of progress during strength rehabilitation. The great majority of athletes can be successfully treated nonoperatively with a guided rehabilitation program. Rarely, the degree of displacement may be significant enough to lead to either fibrous union or nonunion [21]. This may be associated with chronic pain and func-

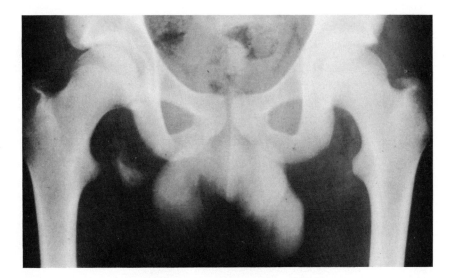

FIGURE 17–1
Ischial avulsion fracture by forceful hamstring contractures in a track athlete.

tional disability. In these cases, chronic pain may be an indication for excision of the separated apophysis. Early open reduction and internal fixation have been advocated when there is significant displacement of a fragment [5]. However, exact surgical indications are unclear. Functional disability in competitive athletes has been described rarely following this injury [50]. We treat our athletes conservatively utilizing a progressive program of isometric strengthening during the early postinjury phase, advancing to resistive isokinetic strengthening prior to return to competitive sports. Other than circumferential wraps for symptomatic relief, we do not utilize any special equipment during the athlete's return to sports.

EPIPHYSEAL INJURIES

Salter-Harris Physeal Fractures of Proximal Femur and Acetabulum

Although these injuries are rare in sports [34], their presence indicates either severe trauma or an associated disease process [3, 4, 8], and their morbidity demands attention. Transphyseal fractures of the femoral neck represent a type I Salter-Harris fracture. In a young child, severe violence is necessary to produce this separation. In the adolescent, this may represent one end of the spectrum of slipped capital femoral epiphysis. It may occur with an associated pathologic state such as renal osteodystrophy or hypothyroidism [8]. High-energy fractures may be associated with dislocation of the femoral head from the acetabulum. Emergent, careful open reduction and internal fixation are advocated, using smooth pins across the epiphysis. The risk of premature closure of the epiphysis is high. The results from treat-

ment of this fracture are frequently poor owing to avascular necrosis of the femoral head [56].

Slipped Capital Femoral Epiphysis

Slipped capital femoral epiphysis is the most common hip disorder in the adolescent [2]. This condition represents a mechanical shearing failure of the proximal femoral physis [5, 12], which results in variable degrees of posterior and medial slippage of the proximal femoral epiphysis and concomitant extension and external rotation of the femoral neck and shaft (Fig. 17–3). This rarely occurs as an acute fracture associated with a discrete injury. It is usually a chronic microfracturing process of the physis under physiologic loads during the preadolescent and adolescent growth spurt [24, 60].

Most children who suffer from slipped capital femoral epiphysis are either heavy or are rapidly growing [20, 29, 30]. Relative femoral retroversion is another risk factor [14]. Slipped capital femoral epiphysis is more common in males. It rarely occurs before age 9 in girls or age 11 in boys unless there is an underlying endocrinologic disorder. It almost always begins before puberty, but if untreated the condition can progress until skeletal maturity is attained. The condition is ultimately bilateral in nearly 50% of cases [28], although the presentation is often *not* simultaneous.

Classification

Slipped capital femoral epiphysis usually is classified in terms of either the acuity of the process or the severity of the anatomic abnormality. Chronologically, the condition is either acute or chronic. In an acute slipped

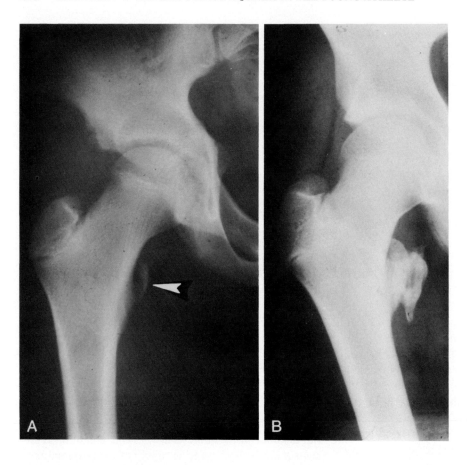

FIGURE 17–2
A, Avulsion fracture of lesser trochanter by iliopsoas in adolescent athlete. *B,* Healing of bony avulsion, which was treated with observation, rest, anti-inflammatory agents, and physical therapy.

epiphysis the symptoms are more severe and of shorter duration [9]. The patient is typically in great distress, which is greatly increased by any attempt to move the involved leg. The leg typically lies in significant external rotation. An acute slipped capital femoral epiphysis represents an acute physeal fracture with concomitant in-

creased instability, risk of avascular necrosis, and malunion.

The patient with a chronic slipped capital femoral epiphysis typically has prolonged symptoms that may never have been dramatic and indeed may be minimal. Physical examination reveals limitation of hip internal

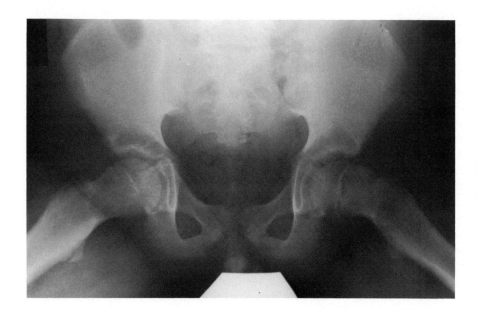

FIGURE 17–3
Left slipped capital femoral epiphysis (SCFE) in an athlete who had left groin pain for several weeks. The frog lateral position provides the most sensitive radiographic image for detecting an SCFE.

rotation, especially in flexion. Unlike most hip disorders, there is no hip flexion contracture. Distress during attempted range of motion is much less than that with an acute slipped capital femoral epiphysis. Radiographs typically show bony remodeling of the femoral neck with posteromedial displacement of the femoral head through the physis.

A third category of patients with slipped epiphysis is the patient with an acute on chronic slip. In this injury there is an element of acute physeal separation superimposed on a chronic slipped capital femoral epiphysis.

Characterizing the severity of deformity in slipped capital femoral epiphysis is important because the degree of deformity, barring complications [23], ultimately correlates best with long-term problems, specifically osteoarthritis of the hip [2, 5].

Slipped capital femoral epiphyses have been characterized by the degree or percentage of the slipped epiphysis (grade 1, 0–25%; grade 2, 25%–50%; grade 3, 50%–75%; grade 4, 75%–100%), but this system is notorious for underestimating the true amount of deformity. It is more accurate to characterize the malposition of the capital femoral epiphysis with regard to the femoral shaft as seen in the frog lateral view [51] (the physis-shaft angle). Another method of measuring the amount of slip is to use a computed tomography (CT) scan to define the slip angle [14].

Diagnosis

A young athlete with a chronic slipped capital femoral epiphysis will have difficulty with athletic activities. A limp or external rotation gait may be present. Symptoms are often vague, and pain may not be present at all. When there is a complaint of discomfort, it is usually an aching discomfort that may be located anywhere from the groin proximally to the medial knee region distally. Symptoms are typically worse with physical activity.

Slipped capital femoral epiphysis is among the most poorly diagnosed of all pediatric orthopedic conditions, and the diagnosis must be considered in any child between the ages of perhaps 8 and 15 who has any gait abnormality or any symptoms between the pelvis and tibia. In its early stages, this condition is easily treated and usually has minimal sequelae. If the slipped epiphysis is not diagnosed in a timely fashion [15] and the subsequent deformity becomes severe, the measures needed to treat it are more extreme, and both the surgical risks and the chances of long-term dysfunction are much greater.

Physical examination usually reveals limited internal rotation or at least a preponderance of external rotation over internal rotation. In more severe cases, when the hip is flexed, the leg tends to ride into external rotation

as the prominent anterior neck abuts against the anterior acetabulum. Laboratory tests other than plain radiographs are usually unrevealing.

Anteroposterior and particularly frog lateral radiographs of both hips are crucial to making this diagnosis (see Fig. 17–3). The diagnosis can be subtle in its earlier stages, but a widening and blurring of the proximal femoral physis is an early sign, even before the proximal femoral epiphysis starts to undergo its characteristic posterior tilting. At this stage, a high-resolution bone scan usually shows increased uptake at the top of the femoral neck, and a magnetic resonance imaging (MRI) scan reveals physeal changes.

In a patient with acute slipped capital femoral epiphysis, there is obvious discontinuity between the anterosuperior portion of the femoral neck and the anterolateral corner of the capital femoral epiphysis. In more chronic cases of slipped epiphysis, the superior neck may remodel rapidly enough to follow the epiphysis as it falls posteriorly and medially. There is characteristic deformation of the femoral neck, bone formation along the posterior neck, and malalignment of the epiphysis with relation to the femoral shaft.

Treatment

If the physis is still open, the first priority in treatment is to stabilize the epiphysis to prevent further slippage. This is most commonly done with a transphyseal screw or pin. Biplanar image intensification is mandatory for intraoperative control because the direction of the slippage of the epiphysis dictates the direction of the internal fixation devices. This is usually at some angle to the plane of the femoral neck (*not* in the same plane as the neck) if the device is to cross the physis into the epiphysis at a right angle to the growth plate, as is most desirable biomechanically [40].

Knowles pins or cannulated screws are the most frequently used internal fixation device for fixation of mild to moderate slipped capital femoral epiphyses. In a very chronic slip, a single screw may be strong enough to provide adequate fixation, provided that it is placed ideally through the middle of the physis into the center of the epiphysis. If there is any question about the acuity of the slippage, it is probably safer to use two screws with a lag effect if possible.

More severely slipped capital femoral epiphyses, in which the angle of the slippage is 45 degrees or more, are associated not only with present dysfunction in the form of a limitation of flexion and a severe external rotation deformity but also with a significant risk of osteoarthritis in the distant future. Patients with this much deformity must be considered not only for stabilization but also for some sort of realignment procedure in which the epiphysis is realigned in a more physiologic position in the acetabulum.

The problem with realigning procedures is that they are not only technically more demanding but also more dangerous in terms of the blood supply to the femoral head than are simple stabilization procedures. The choices among realignment procedures include acute manipulative reduction (only to be considered in an acute slip) [9], cuneiform osteotomy [6, 18], intertrochanteric osteotomy of the flexion-valgus-derotational type [25, 42], and base of neck osteotomy (anterolateral closing wedge osteotomy after the method of Warren Kramer) [32]. Of all the realigning procedures, intertrochanteric osteotomy is probably the most desirable in terms of being not only efficacious but also relatively safe [25, 42]. AO blade plates provide very rigid and reliable fixation. Some compensatory deformity is created because the realignment is done in the intertrochanteric region at a distance of a few centimeters from the true deformity at the top of the neck. Cuneiform osteotomy is an open reduction of the epiphysis with resection of reactive bone to allow gentle reduction of the epiphysis onto the femoral neck without tension. It should be reserved for severe slips and carries a high risk of avascular necrosis [6, 18].

Complications

Complications of slipped capital femoral epiphysis may be associated with the condition itself or with the treatment. In a patient with an acute slipped capital femoral epiphysis avascular necrosis of the femoral head can result from injury to the retinacular vessels at the moment of the acute slip or during reduction maneuvers. With this in mind, the treating physician should be as gentle as possible in dealing with a patient with a slipped capital femoral epiphysis. There is no uniform agreement about whether the patient with a severe slippage (greater than 60-degree slip angle) is best treated by general traction overnight, with pinning in whatever position results, or a ''gentle manipulation'' under general anesthesia to bring the knee to a straight-up position. We prefer to keep the patient with a severe acute slipped epiphysis in a comfortable position with the leg on a pillow until he can be brought to the operating room. We then open the joint through an anterior or anterolateral approach to reduce the deformity under direct vision to the point where the neck and head start to move as a unit. At this point, if the deformity seems to be reduced to an acceptable position, the epiphysis is pinned in situ. If the deformity is still judged to be so unacceptable that very poor function is likely to result, the epiphysis is pinned as it is, and an acute or late realignment through the intertrochanteric region is carried out.

The other major complication of slipped capital femoral epiphysis is chondrolysis. Destruction of the articular cartilage can occur, either by a poorly understood autoimmune process or by mechanical injury to acetabular cartilage from protruding pins [41, 57]. Chondrolysis rarely occurs in the absence of treatment. It is diagnosed by progressive pain and limitation of motion on physical examination with progressive narrowing of the cartilage space on radiography. It is to be suspected when, after in situ pinning, the patient becomes progressively more uncomfortable. It can be treated by removing the offending internal fixation devices, if they are the cause, and by administering nonsteroidal anti-inflammatory drugs, heavy traction, and physical therapy. Prognosis is guarded, and occasionally hip fusion or arthroplasty may be necessary.

In summary, slipped capital femoral epiphysis is a condition that is relatively easy to treat in its early stages, but the diagnosis must be considered and the appropriate radiographs taken if treatment is to be rendered in a timely fashion. If the diagnosis is made, the young athlete with this condition must cease athletic activities entirely until the slipping epiphysis is stabilized by internal fixation devices. It must be remembered that the contralateral hip will ultimately slip in almost 50% of cases, and follow-up radiographs must at least occasionally show both hips. Any contralateral symptoms must be investigated thoroughly.

Sports may be possible once the growth plate starts to fuse, although the stress-rising effect of internal fixation devices is associated with a risk of pathologic fracture. The safest course is to limit athletic activity until several months after the internal fixation devices have been removed. In the meantime, noncontact cardiovascular fitness training, lower extremity range of motion exercises, and progressive resistive exercises should be initiated. The pins always remain in place until the growth plate is completely fused on radiography. After removal of the hardware, activity should be restricted for 2 or 3 months to allow bony healing across the pin sites. At that point, full athletic activity may resume.

NONPHYSEAL FRACTURES

These injuries are infrequently caused by skeletal trauma in the athlete [3, 7, 55, 58]. However, violent trauma or a predisposing pathologic state may result in a pelvic or proximal femoral fracture.

Pelvic Fractures

In Torode and Zieg's [55] series of 141 children with pelvic fractures, five were secondary to sporting events.

These injuries are classified into avulsion fractures, iliac wing fractures, simple ring fractures, and unstable ring fractures. Avulsion fractures have already been discussed. Iliac wing and simple ring fractures can be treated nonoperatively. However, type IV injuries with pelvic disruption represent an unstable pelvis that often requires treatment either by open reduction and internal fixation or by external fixation. These injuries have a high rate of associated genitourinary, abdominal, neurologic, and other musculoskeletal injuries [7, 55, 58] that need to be addressed when the patient presents to the emergency room.

Return to sports participation by patients with stable pelvic injuries depends on the level of discomfort and the conditioned state of the athlete. Protected weight bearing as tolerated is allowed for 3 to 6 weeks until the fracture is clinically and radiographically healed. Return to sports is then determined by the time needed to attain full range of motion and lower extremity strength. Isokinetic analysis of strength is helpful in obtaining an objective measurement of strength to lessen the risk of recurrent injury by premature return to competitive sports.

Femoral Neck Fractures

These fractures are classified as transphyseal, transcervical, cervicotrochanteric, and intertrochanteric [4, 44, 56]. These injuries are the result of severe trauma, most frequently from motor vehicle accidents or falls from extreme heights. If any femoral fracture follows minimal trauma, the presence of an underlying pathologic lesion should be suspected. Displaced femoral neck fractures require immediate reduction to lessen the risk of avascular necrosis. Internal fixation is recommended to prevent malunion and nonunion. Intraoperative anatomic alignment of the femoral neck is a prerequisite for internal fixation. This may be achieved by gentle traction but may require open reduction of the femoral neck fracture (Fig. 17–4). Internal fixation with multiple threaded pins or screws that do not cross the physis are preferred in neck and intertrochanteric fractures. Care must be taken to minimize interference with the intraosseous and retinacular blood supply to the epiphysis because the risk of avascular necrosis is high. Bone scans or MRI scans are utilized to monitor the postinjury vascularity of the femoral head. Protected weight bearing and range of motion exercises are prescribed until healing of the fracture occurs radiographically. Sports are allowed after fracture healing and full rehabilitation, even with internal fixation. Hardware removal is performed approximately 1 year after fracture healing. Protected weight bearing and prohibition from sports are prescribed for 2 months after hardware removal to lessen the risk of refracture.

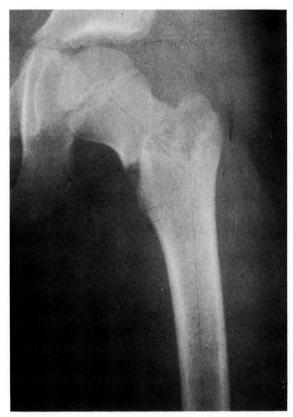

FIGURE 17–4
Acute femoral neck fracture that requires emergency reduction anatomically.

Subtrochanteric Femoral Fractures

These fractures are also a result of a violent injury. Ireland and Fisher [26] noted that 2 of their 20 patients with subtrochanteric fractures were football players. The proximal fragment usually lies in flexion, abduction, and external rotation because of the influence of the iliopsoas, hip abductors, and external rotators. In patients under the age of 10, closed reduction, femoral skeletal traction in the 90/90-degree position, and Spica casting comprise the standard therapy. In older children and adolescents, open reduction and internal fixation (with a plate or intermedullary rod) may be desirable, particularly if acceptable alignment cannot be achieved by closed means. Criteria for return to sports and removal of hardware are similar to those outlined for femoral neck fractures.

HIP DISLOCATIONS

Hip dislocations in children are usually posterior. Classically, the leg is flexed, adducted, and internally rotated on presentation [43]. Hip dislocations in skeletally mature individuals are caused by more severe trauma and are associated with femoral neck and acetabular fractures. A prereduction neurologic examination must be done to evaluate sciatic nerve function. Pretreatment radiographs to define the type of dislocation and associated injuries should be performed. In particular, it is imperative to rule out an associated femoral neck fracture prior to manipulation. A hip dislocation should be considered an emergency. Closed reduction, under anesthesia if possible, should be performed urgently to lessen the risk of avascular necrosis. If closed reduction is not possible, open reduction and release of an inverted limbus or removal of an osteochondral fragment is necessary. Postreduction radiographs and CT scans of the hip are necessary to be certain that no soft tissue or bony interposition is blocking complete concentric reduction of the hip.

In skeletally immature athletes, less severe trauma such as a fall (Fig. 17–5) can result in a posterior hip dislocation. In these situations there is usually no associated femoral neck or acetabular fracture. Closed or open reduction should be performed emergently as outlined above.

Postreduction treatment varies from skin or skeletal traction to Spica cast immobilization to protected weight

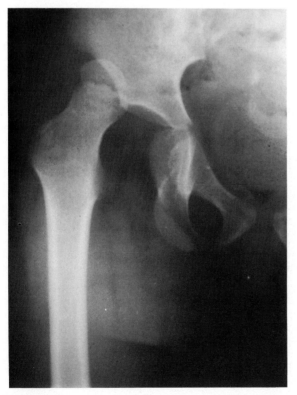

FIGURE 17–5
Hip dislocation without a fracture. This is an emergent situation requiring reduction under anesthesia to lessen the risk of avascular necrosis.

bearing with crutches. In the absence of associated femoral neck or acetabular fractures we have found these hips to be stable and do not immobilize them in a Spica cast. Protected weight bearing with crutches is used for 6 weeks. Rehabilitation with range of motion and strengthening exercises is performed for 6 more weeks. Radiographs, bone scans, and MRI scans are used to assess the potential complications of avascular necrosis or myositis ossificans. If these problems are absent, the athlete commences a gradual return to competition at 3 months.

STRESS FRACTURES

Stress fractures of the femoral neck are secondary to chronic repetitive microtrauma [22, 39]. This diagnosis should be considered in a competitive track or cross-country athlete with persistent discomfort in the groin. Local tenderness in the region of the femoral neck and limited range of hip motion, particularly flexion and internal rotation, may be seen (Fig. 17–6). Plain radiographs may initially be negative. When a stress fracture is suspected clinically, early diagnosis may be made by a technetium-99 bone scan. On diagnosis, immediate cessation of athletic activity is mandatory to prevent the disastrous progression of a stress fracture to a displaced femoral neck fracture (Fig. 17–7). Devas [16] has identified two types of femoral neck stress fractures. The first is a transverse stress fracture in the superior portion of the neck that may become displaced. This is more frequently seen in adults. Internal fixation with threaded pins is recommended before displacement, with its accompanying risks of avascular necrosis and nonunion, occurs. The second type is a compression stress fracture in the inferomedial neck that rarely becomes displaced. These fractures frequently can be treated with limited weight bearing until there is radiographic evidence of callus formation and healing. In younger athletes, these injuries are usually compression stress fractures and are not at risk for displacement. Protected weight bearing, range of motion exercises, and nonimpact-loading cardiovascular conditioning, such as bicycling and swimming, are recommended until healing occurs.

When range of motion is unrestricted the Trendelenburg test is negative, and activities of daily living are pain-free, then we consider a return to competitive sports. This must be a graduated, supervised process with care taken to avoid excessive stress in a relatively deconditioned state, which may cause recurrent injury. We work closely with our physical therapist, sports trainers, coaches, and athletes to outline an individual program of progressive return to sports. Recurrence of symptoms is a clear indication to reduce activity and slow the rehabilitative process.

Stress fractures of the pelvis at the junction of the

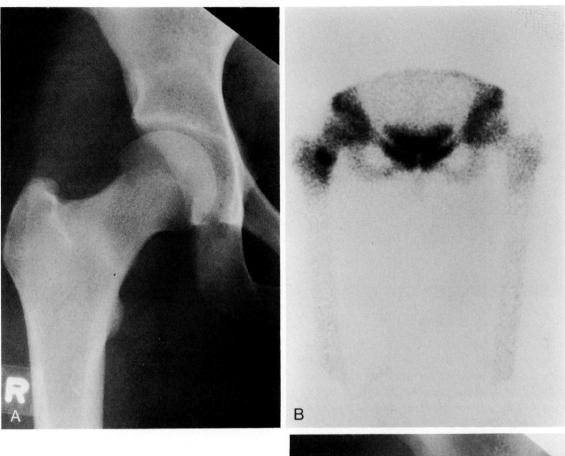

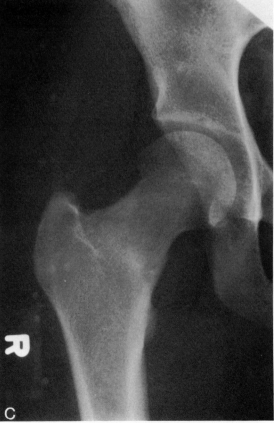

FIGURE 17–6
Stress fracture in a long distance runner. Initial radiograph *(A)* was normal, but bone scan *(B)* was positive, and subsequent radiographs *(C)* were diagnostic.

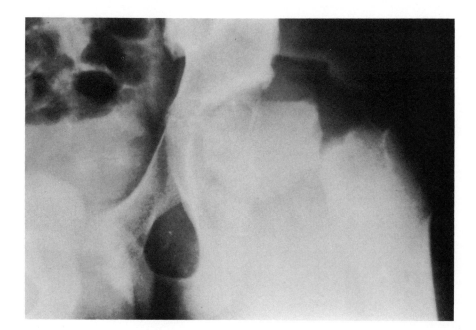

FIGURE 17–7
Long distance runner with a 1-month history of groin pain initially diagnosed as a "pulled muscle" presented emergently with this displaced femoral neck fracture through an area of chronic stress. Open reduction with internal fixation was performed emergently.

ischium and inferior pubic ramus have been described in runners. Bone scans are positive early, and radiographs taken 2 to 3 weeks after injury reveal periosteal new bone and sclerosis at the junction of the ischial-inferior pubic ramus. This radiographic appearance may raise extreme concern about a malignant tumor if a stress fracture is not considered in the differential diagnosis. Therapy is similar to that described for femoral neck stress fractures.

Osteitis pubis is an unusual injury that occurs more commonly in long distance runners but has been described in a variety of athletic activities [31]. The mechanism of injury appears to be strenuous conditioning of the rectus abdominis and adductor muscles. The individual is tender directly over the symphysis pubis. Bone scans are positive in the symphysis early, and radiographs at 2 to 3 weeks after injury reveal sclerosis on one or both sides of the symphysis pubis. The differential diagnosis includes ostitis secondary to chronic prostatism in males. Rest, heat, and conditioning exercises that do not cause pain are recommended.

PATHOLOGIC FRACTURES AND CONDITIONS

A pathologic fracture is a fracture through abnormal bone. When the severity of injury exceeds the trauma that caused the injury, a pathologic lesion or state should be suspected. Similarly, when a rare skeletal injury is present, screening should be done for pathologic conditions. Pathologic conditions present either with an acute fracture through a lesion or with complaints of persist-

ent, activity-related pain similar to symptoms of an overuse injury. Radiographs are necessary for definitive diagnosis. Unfortunately, many busy sports medicine centers have examples of neoplasias in athletes that have been misdiagnosed and incorrectly treated as sprains or strains. Conditions that may present as pathologic injuries include benign lesions (osteoid osteoma, unicameral bone cysts, fibrous dysplasia), malignant neoplasias (Ewing's sarcoma, osteogenic sarcoma), and endocrinopathies (hypothyroidism, renal osteodystrophy) and may be appreciated only on radiographs.

Our policy has been to screen our symptomatic athletes radiographically on presentation. We feel that this lessens our risk of inadvertently missing an underlying pathologic condition that is unrecognized clinically (Fig. 17–8).

Legg-Calvé-Perthes Disease

This is a condition of unknown etiology that affects the growth and development of the capital femoral epiphysis; it usually presents between the ages of 4 and 10 years (peak incidence 5 to 7 years). Although it was first described clinically about 1910 by many authors, its pathophysiology remains incompletely understood and its treatment imperfect. There is an associated circulatory disturbance in the capital femoral epiphysis and a generalized mild retardation of skeletal growth [11, 33]. There is a definite male preponderance (4:1), and both hips are involved in at least 20% of cases, though rarely simultaneously. The disease has an extremely variable clinical course but a very characteristic series of radiologic findings [10, 45].

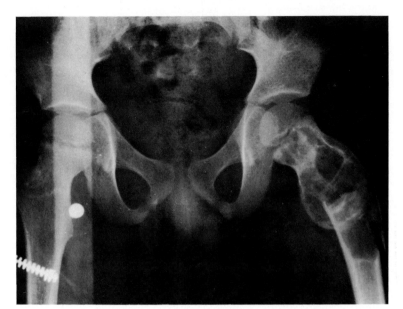

FIGURE 17–8
Eight-year-old boy presented with acute pain during a soccer game. In retrospect, it was noted that he had had recurring activity-related pain. Radiographs were diagnostic of a pathologic fracture through a cystic lesion of the femoral neck.

Diagnosis

The typical patient presents with a history of an intermittent, mildly symptomatic limp of a few weeks' duration. What follows thereafter may range from complete cessation of symptoms to recurring stiffness and pain culminating in early osteoarthritis and permanently disturbed hip function. This frustrating variability in the natural history of the disease seems to depend to a large extent on the age at which the disease begins and the amount of the femoral head that is involved. Younger patients and patients with less than 50% femoral head involvement have the best prognosis [9, 10, 48]. The nature of the primary pathology in Perthes disease is still

uncertain, but it seems not to be primarily inflammatory, neoplastic, or traumatic. The obvious component of hypovascularity during the early stages in the involved part of the epiphysis may be only a secondary finding [45].

Physical examination at presentation usually reveals a characteristic limitation of internal rotation, extension, and abduction, as noted with any hip condition associated with a synovitis. There may be some atrophy of the thigh. Tenderness and swelling are rare. Other joints are characteristically uninvolved (with the occasional exception of the other hip). Some degree of limp is usual.

Radiographs are usually diagnostic (Fig. 17–9). The sequential characteristic findings are temporary cessation in the growth of the bony epiphysis, a sclerotic appear-

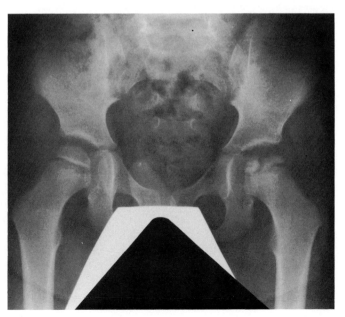

FIGURE 17–9
Radiograph of a 5-year-old boy who had chronic groin pain and a limp while playing soccer. Legg-Calvé-Perthes disease frequently presents with activity-related pain.

ance of the epiphysis, fragmentation and apparent collapse of the bony epiphysis, and finally, reossification of the epiphysis with new bone. These radiographic stages are thought to correlate with a circulatory disturbance to the bony epiphysis, with necrosis of the epiphyseal bone followed by reinstitution of the epiphysis by new living bone. The shape of the entire epiphyseal osteocartilaginous model may or may not be disturbed depending on whether the function of the proximal femoral growth plates is disturbed by the disease process. Perthes disease is primarily a disorder of the bony epiphysis, but it may have secondary effects on the proximal femoral physis and subarticular hemispherical microphysis.

Arthrography may be necessary to determine the shape of the femoral head during active disease in patients with major femoral head involvement. In the very early stages, before any plain radiographic findings are present, technetium bone scanning [35] or MRI may be helpful.

Catterall [10] and Salter [48, 49] both have found that certain radiographic findings are associated with a greater or lesser risk of femoral head deformation and have used these parameters as guides for instituting treatment. Both agree that patients in whom more than 50% of the femoral head is involved generally have worse prognoses and merit any treatment that can reduce the incidence of femoral head deformation. They both agree that preservation of the lateral column of the epiphysis on the anteroposterior radiograph is a good sign. Catterall classifies patients into four groups depending on whether the involvement of the epiphysis is 25%, 50%, 75%, or 100%. Salter classifies patients into groups A and B, with A having up to 50% of the femoral head involved, and B having more than 50% of the femoral head involved. Salter noted that careful anteroposterior and frog radiographs early in the disease often show the "crescent sign," which he believes is a subchondral fracture whose extent equals the subsequent extent of maximum resorption of the epiphysis due to Perthes disease [49]. These radiographic prognostic classifications are problematic in that patients in the earliest stages of disease are not classifiable as to prognosis, meaning that one must make a blind choice in the very early stages between not treating any patients, which means leaving untreated a few who might benefit from it, and treating all of them, which means that containment treatment is used on many who do not need it.

Treatment

The initial aim of treatment in Perthes disease is to control the symptoms and the disturbed function of the hip joint by instituting restriction of activity, crutches, and perhaps even bedrest with Buck's traction and balanced suspension until the pain and limitation of motion subside. The second goal of treatment is to prevent deformation of the affected femoral head, because deformation of the femoral head due to Perthes disease is a potential risk for osteoarthritis in adulthood [35, 53]. If at the time treatment is instituted the femoral head is already deformed, the goal of treatment is to at least prevent further deformation and at most restore the femoral head to a round configuration.

The difficulty with selecting and executing treatment programs for Perthes disease arises from the fact that there is no agreement on the primary pathophysiology or on the efficacy of different treatment programs. There is general agreement that younger patients and those in whom there is less involvement of the femoral head tend to do better than older patients and those in whom more femoral head is involved. Patients older than age 6 in whom more than 50% of the femoral head is involved seem to have the highest risk of osteoarthritis in adulthood; the female sex seems to be an additional risk factor [35, 53].

Virtually all orthopedists agree on treating the stage of synovitis with activity restriction. Further intervention is based on the concept that containment of the anterior and lateral portions of the femoral head in the acetabulum will reduce the tendency toward deformation [46, 48]. The assumption is that uncontrolled growth of the anterior and lateral growth centers in the femoral head is responsible for deformation and that pressure by the interior of the acetabulum on this portion of the femoral head will keep it growing in proportion to the rest of the head. Containment methods, past and present, include (1) ambulatory and nonambulatory abduction casts [46] and braces [47] of various designs, most with a flexion and internal rotation component added; (2) varus intertrochanteric osteotomy [48]; (3) innominate osteotomy [48, 52]; and (4) Chiari pelvic osteotomy [9] (usually reserved for already deformed and irreducibly subluxated femoral heads). All these containment methods presuppose an aggressive attempt to restore a normal or near normal range of motion by restricting activity and instituting physical therapy before applying the splints or operative methods themselves. Treatment is continued until radiographs suggest that the involved portion of the femoral head is being covered by at least a rim of new bone [54]. This may require as short a period of time as a few months in a 2- or 3-year-old patient, to as long as 2 or 3 years in a patient 10 to 12 years of age.

Most observers agree that noncontainment methods of treatment do not influence the natural course of Perthes disease. Noncontainment methods used have included a variety of unilateral braces, such as the Snider sling, and simple crutches. Even containment devices, such as the Scottish Rite orthosis or the Toronto brace, must be monitored by radiographs to be certain that the affected hip is abducted sufficiently to ''contain'' the lateral portion of the femoral head under the acetabular labrum.

Return to Athletics

Most orthopedists restrict high-impact athletic activity until Perthes disease is well into the healing phase on the assumption that loading trauma to the epiphysis negatively affects its growth during this sensitive period. Exceptions to this proscription of sports include patients with apparently mild Perthes disease involving less than 50% of the femoral head.

The treating physician must be attentive to the patient with healed Perthes disease because residual deformation of some degree follows in most patients. This deformation may range from mild coxa magna to significant femoral head collapse and joint incongruity. These patients are probably more at risk for an overuse syndrome around the hip than the normal patient depending on the amount of residual deformation that is present. Younger patients usually tend to do better during the posthealing years because the acetabulum and femoral head have had more time to remodel. The patient whose Perthes disease begins in the later years of childhood may be left with a worse situation. The femoral head may heal in an aspherical position, incongruent with an acetabulum that does not have time to remodel before skeletal growth ends. It is this last type of patient that is most prone to develop early osteoarthritis.

In summary, Perthes disease is often undiagnosed during its active phase. Hip radiographs taken anytime thereafter may show the characteristic femoral head deformities associated with severe Perthes disease. This radiographic appearance should lead the orthopedist to give advice about either restricting activity or instituting active treatment according to the type of deformity present.

SOFT TISSUE INJURIES

Contusions

Contusions, abrasions, and sprains constitute the most common form of injury suffered by young athletes [1, 19, 27]. These injuries are frequently minor and can be treated with a brief period of rest, ice, elevation, and return to athletic activity when pain is absent. On occasion, contusions cause significant muscular hemorrhage resulting in prolonged muscle spasm, disuse atrophy, and decreased range of motion. Formal rehabilitation with flexibility and strengthening exercises beginning after the acute inflammation has subsided may be necessary. Consideration should be given to the possibility

of myositis ossificans [8] if the hemorrhage is severe. The athlete should return to competitive activities only after he has regained full strength and coordination. Early, unguided return to sports participation may result in repetitive microtrauma that prolongs disability.

ILIAC APOPHYSITIS

Clancy and Foltz [13] described a syndrome of iliac crest tenderness on palpation and muscular contraction in the adolescent long distance runner. These athletes had no history of local trauma but were enrolled in intensive training programs. The radiographs were normal. The syndrome seems to be a traction apophysitis similar to Osgood-Schlatter's disease. Therapy consists of 4 to 6 weeks of rest with an adjunct of ice application and anti-inflammatory medications. Progressive return to sports is initiated with close monitoring of recurrent pain.

SNAPPING HIP SYNDROME

This entity is most commonly associated with iliotibial band irritation of the greater trochanteric bursa with hip flexion and extension, especially during internal rotation. Athletes frequently describe a sensation of hip dislocation. This entity usually responds to conservative therapy of rest and nonsteroidal anti-inflammatory medication followed by stretching exercises of the fascia lata [38]. Release of the iliotibial band has been performed in the rare athlete who does not respond to conservative therapy.

Athletes may also develop a tenosynovitis of the iliopsoas tendon near its insertion at the lesser trochanter. In this condition, the discomfort and snapping sensation are localized medially along the femoral neck. As with iliotibial band irritation, this entity usually responds to conservative therapy of anti-inflammatory medications, hip abduction and external rotation stretching exercises, and deep heat and ultrasound therapy. Rarely, release of the iliopsoas tendon sheath may be necessary [38].

SPRAINS

As an adolescent approaches skeletal maturity, the ligamentous and musculotendinous structures become more vulnerable to injury. With fusion of the epiphyses and apophyses, the growth plates no longer form the path of least resistance, and micro- and macrotrauma are transmitted through the soft tissue structures. These injuries result either from an acute event of excessive passive stretch or violent muscular contracture against resistance or from a chronic overuse syndrome. If the injury is acute, therapy consisting of rest, ice massage, and progressive flexibility and strengthening exercises when the patient is pain-free results in rehabilitation of the musculotendinous injury. If the injury is secondary to chronic overuse, the underlying factor of improper conditioning, inadequate equipment, or anatomic malalignment must be identified and alleviated to achieve successful therapy [39].

DIFFERENTIAL DIAGNOSIS

In addition to the pathologic conditions that may present as fractures, the clinician treating sports injuries in children should keep in mind a differential diagnosis of medical problems that may present with hip and pelvic pain during athletic activities. These include Perthes disease, congenital dislocation of a hip (in the young child), toxic synovitis or septic arthritis (with acute pain), or inflammatory synovitis (with chronic pain). Leukemia and neuroblastoma may present with limb pain. Not all ''sports injuries'' result from trauma, and the sports clinician needs to be ever conscious of the unexpected.

SUMMARY

Hip and pelvic injuries are relatively rare in the young athlete. Contusions and musculotendinous sprains are the most common injuries about the hip and pelvis. Apophyseal avulsion fractures and stress fractures are the most frequently encountered skeletal injuries. Each of these entities can be successfully treated with guided physical therapy following conservative management with rest, anti-inflammatory medications, and ice massage until the patient is pain-free. Rehabilitation requires restoration of full joint motion, flexibility, and isokinetic strengthening before return to competitive sports is allowed. Epiphyseal, diaphyseal, or pathologic fractures are rare entities that are secondary to violent trauma. These injuries are severe and often require operative intervention. Femoral neck fractures have a high rate of complications from avascular necrosis, nonunion, or malunion. Pelvic fractures are frequently associated with genitourinary, abdominal, neurologic, and musculoskeletal injuries. Pathologic fractures are most commonly secondary to benign lesions, such as unicameral bone cysts, and are less likely to be due to malignancy. All of these musculoskeletal injuries require skeletal healing before strenuous rehabilitation can begin. During this phase, we maintain range of motion, isometric strength, and nonweight-bearing cardiovascular fitness. After bony healing, isokinetic strengthening is initiated. Finally, in children with hip pain during athletic activities, even with antecedent trauma, the sports clinician must screen for slipped capital femoral epiphysis, Perthes disease, congenital subluxation of the hip, toxic synovitis, systemic neoplasia, or an infectious process.

References

1. Andrish, J.G. Overuse syndromes of the lower extremity in youth sports. *In* Boileau, R. (Ed.), *Advances in Pediatric Sports Sciences.* Champaign, IL, Human Kinetics Publishers, 1984.
2. Aronson, J. Osteoarthritis of the young adult hip: Etiology and treatment. *Instr Course Lect* 35:119–128, 1986.
3. Blatter, R. Fractures of the pelvis and acetabulum. *In* Weber, B.G., Brunner, C., and Frueler, F. (Eds.), *Treatment of Fractures in Children and Adolescents.* Berlin, Springer-Verlag, 1980.
4. Bortzy, A. Fractures of the proximal femur. *In* Weber, B.G., Brunner, C.H., and Frueler, F. (Eds.), *Treatment of Fractures in Children and Adolescents.* Berlin, Springer-Verlag, 1980.
5. Boyer, D.W., Mickelson, M.R., and Ponseti, I.V. Slipped capital femoral epiphysis. A long-term follow-up study of under 21 patients. *J Bone Joint Surg* 63A:85–95, 1981.
6. Broughton, N.S., Todd, R., Dunn, D., et al. Open reduction of the severely slipped upper femoral epiphysis. *J Bone Joint Surg* 70B:435–439, 1988.
7. Bryan, W.J., and Tullos, H.S. Pediatric pelvis fractures. *J Trauma* 19:799–805, 1979.
8. Canale, T.S., and King, R.E. Pelvic and hip fractures. *In* Rockwood, C.A., Wilkins, K.E., and King, R.E. (Eds.), *Fractures in Children.* Philadelphia, J.B. Lippincott, 1984.
9. Casey, B., Hamilton, H., and Bobechko, W. Reduction of acutely slipped upper femoral epiphysis. *J Bone Joint Surg* 54A:94, 1976.
10. Catterall, A. The natural history of Perthes disease. *J Bone Joint Surg* 53B:37, 1971.
11. Chung, S.M.K. Diseases of the developing hip joint. *Pediatr Clin North Am* 33:1457, 1986.
12. Chung, S., Batterman, S., and Brighton, C. Shear strength of the human femoral capital epiphyseal plate. *J Bone Joint Surg* 58A:94, 1976.
13. Clancy, W.G., and Foltz, A.S. Iliac apophysitis in stress fractures in adolescent runners. *Am J Sports Med* 4:214–218, 1976.
14. Cohen, M., Gelberman, R.H., Kasser, J., et al. Slipped capital femoral epiphysis: Assessment of epiphyseal displacement and angulation. *J Pediatr Orthop* 6:259–264, 1986.
15. Cowell, H.R. The significance of early diagnosis and treatment of slipping of the capital femoral epiphysis. *Clin Orthop* 48:89–94, 1966.
16. Devas, M.E. Stress fractures of the femoral neck. *J Bone Joint Surg* 47B:728–738, 1965.
17. Fernbach, S.K., and Wilkinson, R.H. Avulsion fractures of pelvis and proximal femur. *Am J Roentgenol* 137:581–584, 1981.
18. Fish, J.B. Cuneiform osteotomy of the femoral neck in the treatment of slipped capital femoral epiphysis. *J Bone Joint Surg* 66A:1153–1164, 1984.
19. Garrick, J.G. Sports medicine. *Pediatr Clin North Am* 33:1541, 1986.
20. Gelberman, R.H., et al. Association of femoral retroversion with slipped capital femoral epiphysis. *J Bone Joint Surg* 68A:1000–1006, 1986.
21. Godshall, R.W., and Hansen, C.A. Incomplete avulsion of a portion of the iliac epiphysis. *J Bone Joint Surg* 55A:1301–1302, 1973.
22. Halek, M., and Noble, B. Stress fractures of the femoral neck in joggers. *Am J Sports Med* 10:112, 1982.
23. Hall, J.E. The results of treatment of slipped femoral epiphysis. *J Bone Joint Surg* 39B:659, 1957.
24. Harris, W.R. The endocrine basis for the slipping of the femoral epiphysis. *J Bone Joint Surg* 32B:5, 1950.
25. Imhauser, G. Spatergednisse der sog. Imhauser-Osteotomie bei der Epiphysenlosung. *Z Orthop* 115:716–725, 1977.

26. Ireland, D.C., and Fisher, R.L. Subtrochanteric fractures of the femur in children. *Clin Orthop* 110:157–166, 1975.
27. Izant, R.J., and Hubay, C.A. The annual injury of fifteen million children. *J Trauma* 6:65–74, 1966.
28. Kasser, J., et al. Unpublished data, 1988.
29. Kelsey, J., Acheson, R., and Keggi, K. The body build of patients with slipped capital femoral epiphysis. *Am J Dis Child* 124:276, 1972.
30. Kelsey, J., Keggi, K., and Southwick, W. The incidence and distribution of slipped capital femoral epiphysis in Connecticut and the southwestern United States. *J Bone Joint Surg* 52B:1203, 1970.
31. Koch, R., and Jackson, D. Pubic symphysitis in runners. *Am J Sports Med* 9:62, 1981.
32. Kramer, W. Compensatory osteotomy of the base of the femoral neck after in situ pinning for slipped capital femoral epiphysis. *J Bone Joint Surg* 58A:796–800, 1976.
33. Kristmandsduttir, F., Burwell, R.G., and Harrison, M.H.M. Delayed skeletal maturation in Perthes disease. *Acta Orthop Scand* 58:277, 1987.
34. Larson, R.L. Epiphyseal injuries in the adolescent athlete. *Orthop Clin North Am* 4:839–851, 1973.
35. McAndrew, M., and Weinstein, S. A long term follow up of Legg-Calvé-Perthes disease. *J Bone Joint Surg* 66A, 860, 1984.
36. Melby, A., Hoyt, W., and Weiner, D. Treatment of chronic slipped capital femoral epiphysis by bone graft epiphyseodesis. *J Bone Joint Surg* 62A:119, 1980.
37. Metzmaker, J.N., and Pappas, A.M. Avulsion fractures of the pelvis. *Am J Sports Med* 13:349–358, 1985.
38. Micheli, L.J. Sites of overuse injury. *In* Lovell, W., and Winter, R. (Eds.), *Pediatric Orthopaedics.* Philadelphia, J.B. Lippincott, 1986.
39. Micheli, L.J. Overuse injuries in children's sports. *Orthop Clin North Am* 14:337–359, 1983.
40. Morrissy, R.T. Slipped capital femoral epiphysis—Natural history, etiology, and treatment. *Instr Course Lect* 29:81, 1980.
41. Morrissy, R.T., Kalderon, A.E., and Gurdes, M.H. Synovial immuno-fluorescence in patients with slipped capital femoral epiphysis. *J Pediatr Orthop* 1:55, 1981.
42. Muller, M. Intertrochanteric osteotomy: Indications, pre-operative planning, and technique. *In* Schatzker, J. (Ed.), *The Intertrochanteric Osteotomy.* Berlin, Springer-Verlag, 1984, pp. 25–66.
43. Offrieski, C. Traumatic dislocations of the hip in children. *J Bone Joint Surg* 63B:194, 1981.
44. Ogden, J.A. Trauma, hip development, and vascularity. *In* Tronzo,

R.G. (Ed.), *Surgery of the Hip Joint.* New York, Springer-Verlag, 1984.
45. Paterson, D., and Savage, J.P. The nuclide bone scan in the diagnosis of Perthes disease. *Clin Orthop* 206:23, 1986.
46. Petrie, J.G., and Bitenc, I. The abduction weight bearing treatment in Legg Perthes disease. *J Bone Joint Surg* 53B:54, 1971.
47. Purvis, J.M., Dimon, J.H., III, Meehan, P.L., et al. Preliminary experience with the Scottish Rite abduction orthosis for Legg Perthes disease. *Clin Orthop* 150:49, 1980.
48. Salter, R.D. Current concepts review. The present status of surgical treatment for Legg-Perthes disease. *J Bone Joint Surg* 66A:961, 1984.
49. Salter, R.D., and Thompson, G.H. Legg-Calvé-Perthes disease: The prognostic significance of the subchondral fracture and a two-group classification of the femoral head involvement. *J Bone Joint Surg* 66A:479, 1984.
50. Schlonsky, J., and Olix, M.L. Functional disability following avulsion fracture of the ischial epiphysis. *J Bone Joint Surg* 54A:641–644, 1972.
51. Southwick, W.O. Osteotomy through the lesser trochanter for slipped capital femoral epiphysis. *J Bone Joint Surg* 49A:807–835, 1967.
52. Sponseller, P.D., Desai, S., and Millis, M.B. A comparison of femoral and innominate osteotomies in the primary treatment of Perthes disease. *J Bone Joint Surg* 70A:1131–1139, 1989.
53. Stulberg, S.D., Cooperman, D.R., and Wallensten, S. The natural history of Legg Perthes disease. *J Bone Joint Surg* 63A:1095, 1981.
54. Thompson, G.H., and Westin G.W. Legg-Calve-Perthes disease: Results of discontinuing treatment early in the reossification state. *Clin Orthop* 139:70, 1979.
55. Torode, I., and Zieg, D. Pelvic fractures in children. *J Pediatr Orthop* 5:76–84, 1985.
56. Tronzo, R.G. Fractures in children. *In* Tronzo, R.G. (Ed.), *Surgery of the Hip Joint.* New York, Springer-Verlag, 1984.
57. Walters, R., and Simon, S. Joint destruction—A sequel of unrecognized pin penetration in patients with slipped capital femoral epiphysis. *In The Hip: Proceedings of the Eighth Open Scientific Meeting of the Hip Society.* St. Louis, C.V. Mosby, 1980, p. 145.
58. Watts, H.G. Fractures of the pelvis in children. *Orthop Clin North Am* 7:615–624, 1976.
59. Weinstein, S.L., Morrissy, R.T., and Crawford, A.H. Slipped capital femoral epiphysis. *Instr Course Lect* 33:310–318, 1984.
60. Wenger, D.R. Slipped capital femoral epiphysis. *In* Tronzo, R.G. (Ed.), *Surgery of the Hip Joint.* New York, Springer-Verlag, 1984.

CHAPTER EIGHTEEN

PATELLOFEMORAL MECHANISM

Carl L. Stanitski, M.D.

SECTION A

Anterior Knee: Basic Considerations

The patella is an essential part of an efficient quadriceps mechanism. This quadriceps-patellofemoral complex demands precise, dynamic anatomic congruency. The patellofemoral articulation is prone to incongruities that are occasionally major but are usually minor. Patellar mechanism function is multifaceted. The primary role of the patella is to promote the efficiency of load transmission. The articular surface of the patella is more efficient in bearing compressive forces than the quadriceps tendon. The patella also acts as a bony shield to the underlying structures, and its presence adds to the cosmetic contours of the knee.

EMBRYOLOGY

At 4 weeks of gestation, the patellofemoral joint is an ectodermal sac stuffed with mesenchyme of somatic mesoderm. Mesenchymal condensations appear at 4 to 5 weeks in precartilage, and chondrification of the patella and femur begins at about 5 weeks of gestation. The joint space and ligamentum patella become evident by 6 weeks, and at 7 weeks well-established patellar and distal femoral chondral models are present. By then, the patellar retinaculum is well formed, as are the anterior and posterior cruciate ligaments, menisci, and joint capsule. The original cartilage rudiments of the joint proceed to form the articular surfaces of the femur, tibia, and patella. By 8 weeks in utero (the end of the embryonic period) the knee is present in its adult form (Fig. 18–1) [7, 9, 33]. A well-developed patellar and quadriceps mechanism is present, and active joint motion has begun. The patella is formed prior to the onset of joint

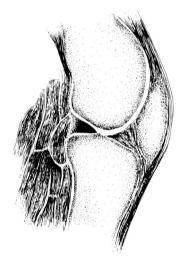

11 weeks

FIGURE 18–1
Schematic representation of knee development at 11 weeks' gestation. Note well-formed patellofemoral complex.

294

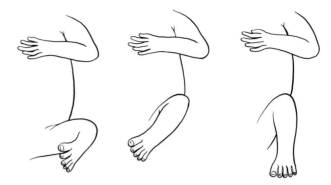

FIGURE 18–2
Progressive lower extremity in utero rotation.

motion, and the femoral sulcus is shaped embryologically in concert with it.

Concomitant with formation of the knee, lower extremity internal rotation and knee flexion begin 6 weeks after gestation. A concomitant 90-degree torsional motion about the lower extremity's longitudinal axis occurs, producing the final position of the anterior quadriceps and posterior hamstring (Fig. 18–2).

Patellar ossification is equivalent to that of an epiphysis. Patellar maturation occurs in stages. From a cartilaginous disc at birth, the patella consolidates from a variable number of ossific centers. The rate of ossification varies (Fig. 18–3). The patella usually appears roentgenographically at age 5 or 6 years but may be seen as early as the age of 2 years (Fig. 18–4). The patella appears to be roentgenographically complete at about 12 years of age. Ossification proceeds in a centrifugal manner until full patellar maturity is reached at about age 16 to 18 years.

Patellar modeling occurs in response to both voluntary and involuntary motion. This modeling occurs primarily during the first several years of life when bone renewal occurs at its highest rate (Fig. 18–5). Ossification proceeds in a manner similar to that of an epiphysis of a long bone (i.e., with articular cartilage and a well-vascularized central epiphysis). The end result of this complex antenatal and neonatal development is an intimately inter-related quadriceps-patellofemoral condylar mechanism (Fig. 18–6).

ANATOMY

The articular surface of the patella (''little plate'') is roughly triangular in shape and has superior and inferior quadrants (Fig. 18–7). The medial and lateral quadrants are separated by a thickened central ridge. The primary facets include the lateral, medial, and odd facets (medial perpendicular), the latter appearing to be developmental in origin because it is not found in the newborn but develops with the increased forces that accompany ambulation. This nonarticulating ''odd'' facet is so termed not because of its morphology but because it is not a paired structure.

In 1941 Wiberg [34] began to evaluate the relationship between the patella and joint congruity. He noted, ''. . . as might be expected, much variation in shape was exhibited by the patella, and the size also varied in

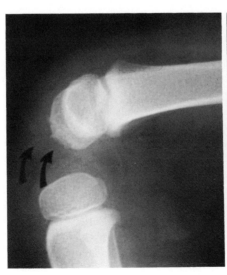
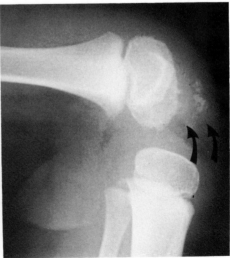

FIGURE 18–3
Accelerated patellar and femoral ossification in a 2½-year-old child with a right lower extremity hemangioma.

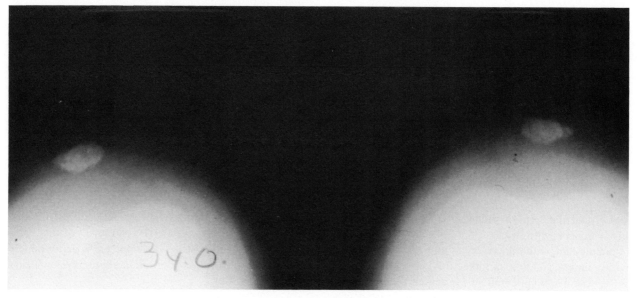

FIGURE 18–4
Early radiographic appearance of patellar ossification in a normal 3-year-old child.

different individuals.'' He classified patellae according to the size relationships between the medial and lateral facets. In type I patellae, the medial and lateral facets are equal; in type II (the most common group), the lateral facet is larger than the medial by a ratio of 1.4 :1; and in type III, little medial facet is present. He noted that the lateral patellar bone surface was usually concave, but that the medial surface could be convex, flat, or concave. Despite this broad range of patellar morphology, Wiberg was unable to find any evidence of increased articular surface changes with any particular patellar type, although the type III patella has been strongly associated with patellar instability.

ABNORMALITIES

Abnormalities of formation of the patella include absence, hypoplasia, and duplication (Fig. 18–8). Absence of the patella is rarely an isolated finding. Patellar hypoplasia (patella parva) is usually associated with a syndrome such as the nail-patella syndrome or Down syndrome and is commonly an asymptomatic state.

Patella infera may rarely occur as a developmental anomaly (Fig. 18–9). It occurs more commonly secondary to either acute traumatic injury of the quadriceps mechanism or following surgery for tibial tubercle transfer, patella fracture repair, or repair of the patellar quadriceps mechanism done with excessive tension (Fig. 18–10). It may also be a complication of anterior cruciate ligament (ACL) repair with diminished postoperative joint extension.

Patella alta may be a developmental anomaly (i.e.,

secondary to cerebral spasticity in which a patellar avulsion may result from persistent tensile forces (Fig. 18–11), or it may be acquired, for example, following trauma either directly to the patellar tendon or postsurgery following traction pin insertion, rectus femorus release, various hip procedures using an anterior lateral approach, quadriceps intramuscular injections (Fig. 18–12), or injudicious hamstring lengthening. A causal relationship between Osgood-Schlatter's disease and patella alta has been suggested [17, 19, 23]. Patella alta is most commonly noted during periods of rapid growth in the adolescent (Fig. 18–13) [27].

Determination of patella alta roentgenographically may be difficult in the skeletally immature patient because tibial tubercle and patellar development is limited, and a significant portion of the patella consists of nonossified cartilage (Fig. 18–14). Brattstrom's work [3] discredited Blumenstat's roentgenographic assessment of patella alta [2] by demonstrating its marked variance relative to the amount of knee flexion and extension on lateral radiographs. In an attempt to obviate the effect of knee position on the determination of patella alta, Insall and Salvati [18] advocated determining the ratio of the length of the patella to the length of the patellar tendon with the knee flexed between 20 and 70 degrees. In patients with patella alta a ratio of 1.3 or greater is seen (Fig. 18–15). Grelsamer and Meadows [12], in an attempt to provide more sensitivity to the vagaries of patellar morphology with skeletal immaturity, proposed a modification of the Insall-Salvati ratio using the posterior ossified patellar surface instead of the entire patellar length. Using this modified technique, they found that patella alta in a significant number of patients was under-

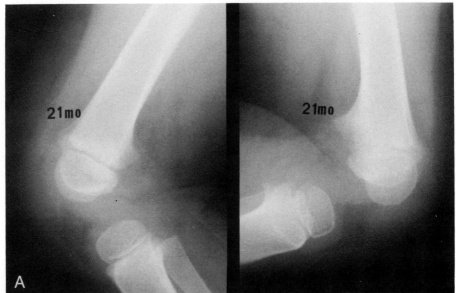

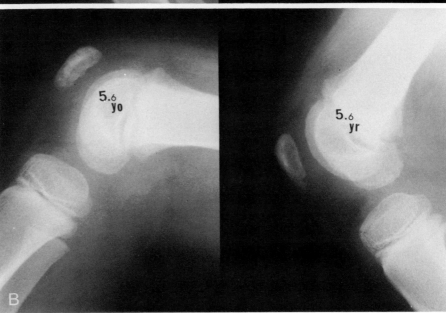

FIGURE 18–5
A and *B*, Progressive radiographic appearance of the patella. Note variance of shape and ossification pattern.

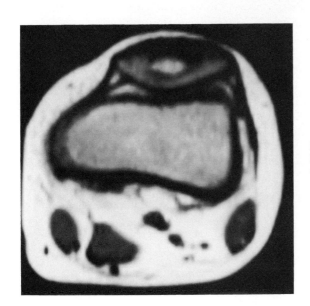

FIGURE 18–6
MRI of knee in a 5-year-old boy showing relatively large amount of unossified patellar cartilage.

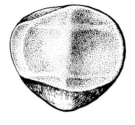

Medial   Lateral

Right patellar
articular surface

FIGURE 18–7
Patellar articular surface showing superior and inferior as well as
medial and lateral segments. Note ''odd'' medial perpendicular facet.

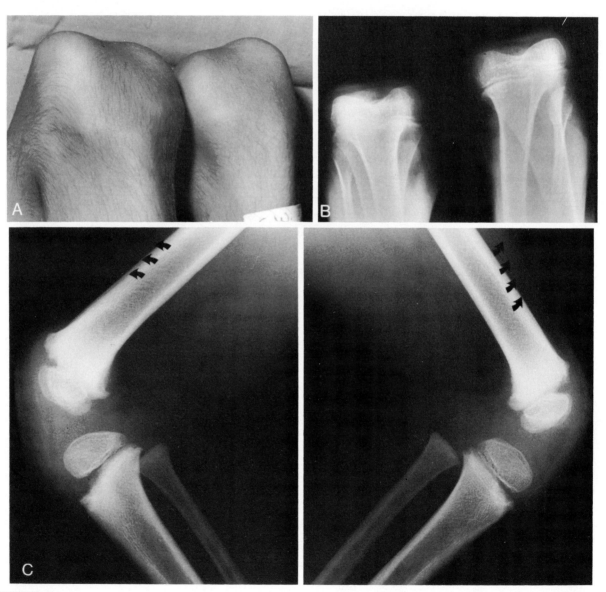

FIGURE 18–8
A and *B*, Nine-year-old boy with absent patellae clinically and radiographically. *C*, Four-year-old with clinically absent patella. Note loss of
quadriceps muscle bulk (arrows).

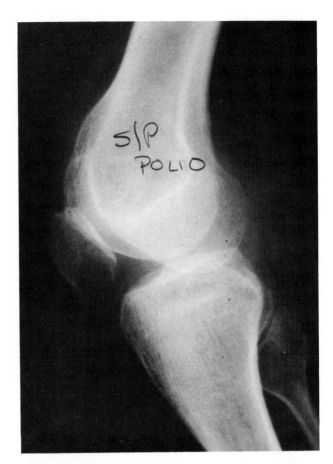

FIGURE 18–9
Patella infera in a 48-year-old man who had had polio at age 6.

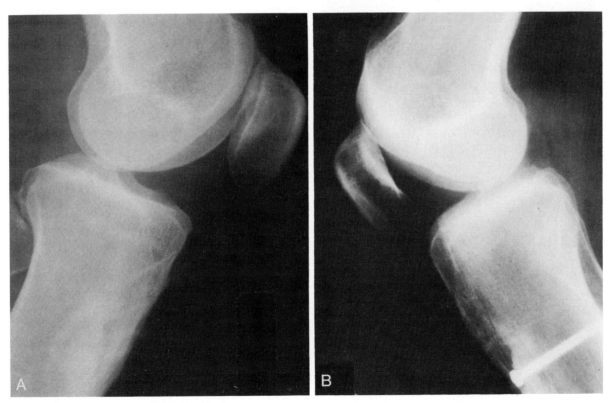

FIGURE 18–10
A, Patella infera in a 22-year-old woman who had had a Hauser transfer at age 12. *B*, Patella infera after tibial tubercle transfer 4 years previously.

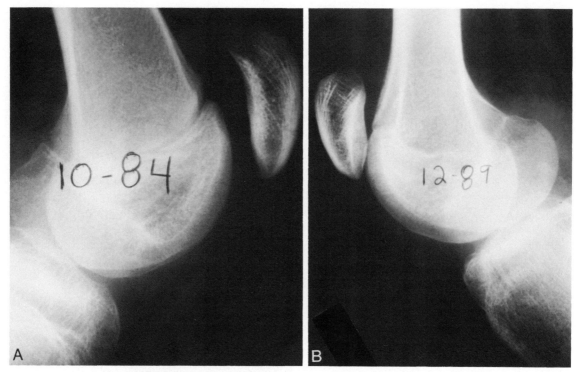

FIGURE 18–11
A and *B*, Patella alta in a child with spastic diplegia and crouched gait.

estimated with use of the more traditional ratio but could be easily identified using this modified index, in which the cut-off ratio between normal and patella alta is considered to be 2 (Fig. 18–16).

Koshino and Sugimoto [21] used ratios of patellar length, the distance from the patella to the tibial epiphysis, and femoral and tibial epiphyseal distances in an attempt to avoid the need to depend on tibial tubercle morphology as an end-point (Fig. 18–17). They believe that changes in this value are minimal with flexion of the knee between 30 and 90 degrees (Fig. 18–18). Although they did not include data on the reproducibility of their technique, this method may prove to be an attractive alternative in skeletally immature patients (Fig. 18–19).

BIOMECHANICS

The patella is acted upon by forces in four quadrants (superior, inferior, medial, and lateral) to produce a balanced system that provides centralization of the patella during knee flexion and extension (Fig. 18–20). The moment arm of the quadriceps mechanism is increased by the presence of the patella, which enhances the distance between the quadriceps and the center of rotation during knee flexion and extension. By distributing joint reaction forces by increasing the surface area of contact,

patellofemoral pressures are diminished (Fig. 18–21). With level walking, the normal patellofemoral joint reaction force approximates one-half body weight. With stair climbing, this force increases to 3.3 times body weight, and with activities demanding rapid deceleration, acceleration, and jumping, the forces at the patellofemoral junction reach 7 to 8 times body weight (Fig. 18–22) [1, 6, 20]. Patellofemoral forces are also increased with such activities as straight leg raising or, more commonly, during isokinetic exercise at midflexion [25, 26]. Møllar and colleagues [28] noted a 25% to 30% increase in the quadriceps tendon force compared with the patellar tendon force when the knee is flexed between 60 and 100 degrees. With flexion of less than 60 degrees these forces are equal. Approximately 60 degrees more tension is placed on the quadriceps during the last 15 degrees of extension than anywhere else in its range.

Goodfellow and colleagues [10, 11], in a study of cadaver knees, defined patellofemoral contact areas under load. In motion from zero to 90 degrees of flexion, a contact band progressed from the inferior to the superior patellar pole, the odd facet having no contact at this range. Increased articulation between the patella and the femur began at 10 to 20 degrees of flexion, the patellar tendon length being the main determinant of onset of contact. Continuing increases in force between the patella and its femoral groove were present at both the

Text continued on page 306

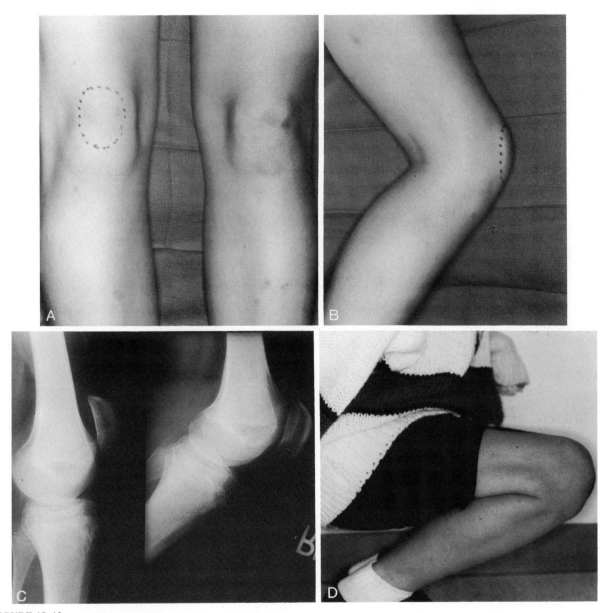

FIGURE 18–12
A and *B*, Patella alta in a 13-year-old girl. Note diminished quadriceps development. She had received more than 50 antibiotic injections in her thigh as an infant. *C*, Lateral radiographs showing maximal preoperative extension and flexion. *D*, Complete knee flexion following quadriceps-plasty.

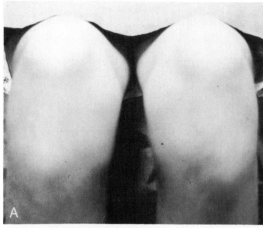

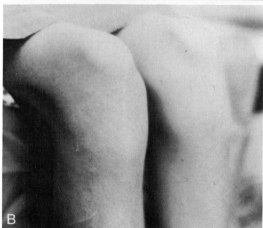

FIGURE 18–13
A and *B*, Patella alta in a 14-year-old boy who had grown 6 inches in the previous 6 months.

FIGURE 18–14
Patellar tendon (arrowheads) insertion is difficult to determine owing to the vagaries of tibial tubercle ossification (open arrows).

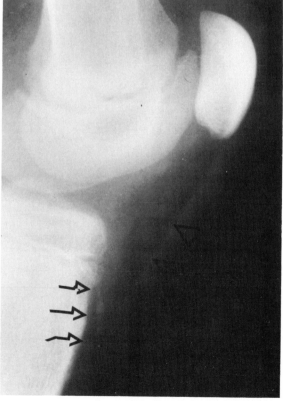

FIGURE 18–15
A and *B*, Patellar tendon–patella ratio described by Insall-Salvati to determine patella alta or infera.

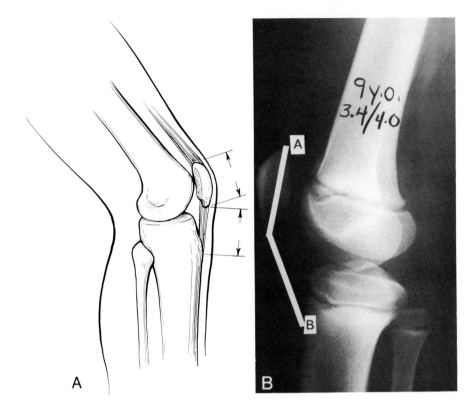

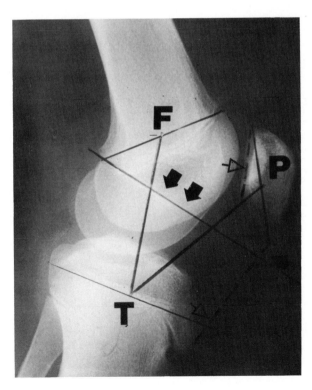

FIGURE 18–16
Modified Insall-Salvati ratio (dotted lines) using the posterior ossified patella (open arrow) (modified ratio 1.38). Other lines include Blumenstat's line (double solid arrow) and Koshino and Sugimoto patella-tibial–femoral-tibia (PT/FT) ratio (1.0.). The Insall-Salvati ratio is 1.1.

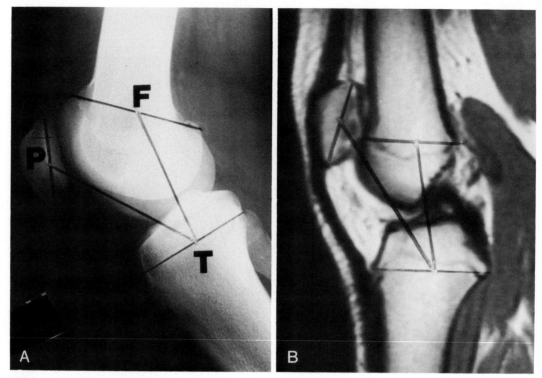

FIGURE 18–17
A and *B*, Radiograph and MRI of a 13½-year-old boy. The Koshino and Sugimoto ratio was 1.18 on radiographs and 1.35 on MRI, the latter a reflection of the improved visualization of the true patellar and epiphyseal landmarks gained by this modality.

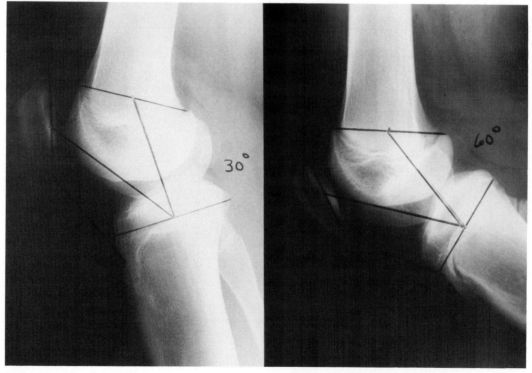

FIGURE 18–18
Ratio was insignificantly changed with knee flexion: 1.22 at 30 degrees and 1.15 at 60 degrees by the PT/FT ratio, and 0.92 and 0.95 by the Insall-Salvati technique.

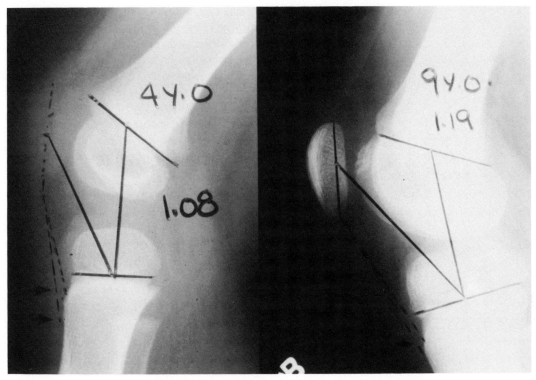
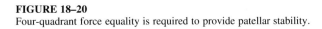

FIGURE 18–19
Growth causes a small change in the PT/FT ratio over a 5-year period.

FIGURE 18–20
Four-quadrant force equality is required to provide patellar stability.

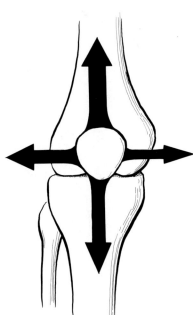

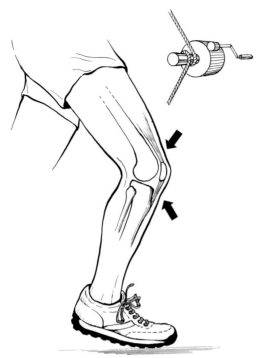

FIGURE 18-21
The windlass effect of the quadriceps with knee flexion increasing the patellofemoral forces.

medial and lateral facets with further knee flexion up to 90 degrees. From 90 degrees to full flexion at 135 degrees, the patellar border remained in full contact, and from then on femoral contact occurred by way of the quadriceps tendon. Engagement of the odd facet with the femoral condyle did not begin until well past 110 degrees of knee flexion.

The high loads to which the patellar ridges are subject may be related to the progressive changes that occur in the patellar articulation. At the insertion site for the quadriceps muscles, the patella acts as a focus for their pull, and, nestled in the trochlear groove, it aids in controlling the motion of the quadriceps mechanism at almost all positions.

PATELLAR STABILITY

Patellofemoral stability is a result of a complex series of interactions among joint congruity and static and dynamic stabilizers both local and remote. With the progressive change of quadrupeds to a more bipedal gait, the patellofemoral relationship altered, and the patella became broader and shorter and the trochlear groove more shallow with less well defined medial and lateral walls than are seen in quadrupeds, whose patellar-trochlear groove morphology and relationships are just the reverse (Fig. 18-23). In the adult human, the normal average depth of the femoral trochlear groove is 5.2 mm with a lateral femoral condyle height of 3.4 mm. The patellar articular cartilage is the thickest in the body and may be as much as 6 to 7 mm thick (three times normal) in the central ridge. This abnormal thickness may reflect the range of patellar stability throughout its flexion-ex-

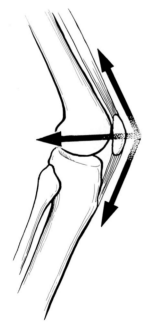

FIGURE 18-22
Patellofemoral resultant force increases with knee flexion due to position and muscle actions.

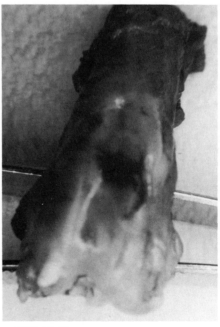

FIGURE 18-23
Elongated and deep femoral sulcus in a rabbit knee.

tension path. The articular cartilage provides a superb compressive bearing surface because it is a self-pressurized hydrostatic system lubricated by a fiber reinforced gel. As such, it is well suited to its major role, i.e., load transmission.

Abnormal lateral patellar motion is secondary to inadequate medial stabilizers, abnormal lateral tethers, joint surface incongruities, or a combination of these factors. Lower extremity alignment plays a major role in this process because the pronated foot, tibial rotation, and femoral rotation affect the quadriceps patellofemoral mechanism.

Abnormalities of sulcus formation are associated with quadriceps malalignment problems, forming a combination destined to produce patellar instability. Because the patella must follow a toroidal path from extension through full flexion, multidirectional demands on stability are placed on it (Fig. 18–24). As it traverses its course, the patella must follow a course of tilt, flexion, and rotation [22, 30, 31]. Static forces that provide patellar stability include primarily knee joint patellofemoral congruity (which varies according to amount of knee flexion), the meniscopatellar ligaments, and the medial and lateral tethers extending from the iliotibial band, vastus lateralis, and vastus medialis. Dynamic forces include the quadriceps group, specifically the tethering effects of the vastus medialis obliquus [24, 32]. The hamstring, gastrocnemius-soleus, and foot and ankle plantar flexors and dorsiflexors play important roles in maintaining patellofemoral stability and congruity through their complex interactions during gait as part of a highly sophisticated articulated and integrated linkage system. Femoral and tibial rotational abnormalities also affect patellofemoral orientation. The maximum amount of femoral anteversion or tibial torsion that can be compensated for and tolerated without symptoms is unknown but appears to be significant in view of the large number of patients with femoral and tibial torsion who are completely asymptomatic.

Lieb and Perry [24] noted that the vastus lateralis fascia is two times and the iliotibial band four times thicker than the medial restraints, specifically the vastus medialis fascia. Fulkerson and Gossling [8] found that the lateral retinaculum was formed in two layers. The superficial oblique retinacular fibers originate from the iliotibial band and travel from the vastus lateralis to the patellar tendon. A second and deeper layer, which is transverse, originates from the iliotibial band and goes to the lateral patellae with some fibers continuing on to the patellar tibial ligament from the inferior patella as well as to the anterior coronary ligament of the lateral meniscus and then on to the tibial tubercle. Discomfort originating within such fibers commonly causes a mistaken diagnosis because lateral joint line symptoms in patients with patellar disorders may be misinterpreted as lateral meniscal pathology. Hallisey and colleagues [13] noted three anatomic patterns of the vastus lateralis insertion and described a vastus lateralis obliquus whose path varied significantly from origin to insertion between men and women. Men had greater variability in this angle of insertion because of a more obtuse angle with the long axis of the patella compared with that seen in women.

In cadaveric studies, MacDonald and co-workers [25] and Perry and co-workers [29] showed that the vastus medialis longus and the vastus medialis obliquus function in different patterns, the medialis providing no extensile force but stabilizing the patella medially when the knee is in extension. These authors demonstrated that atrophy within the vastus medialis obliquus is nonselective but reflects a more generalized state of entire quadriceps atrophy [24]. Much has been written about the *Q angle*, i.e., the relationship between the tibial tubercle, the midpatella, and the anterior iliac spine as a demon-

FIGURE 18–24
Multiplanar toroidal patellar path during knee flexion.

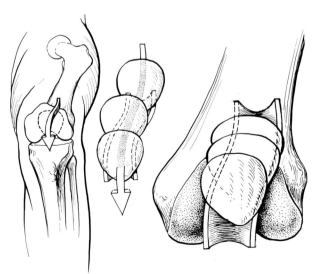

stration of less than straight line quadriceps mechanism forces. Brattstrom [3] described his version of the Q angle in 1964 and recognized its multifaceted determination, which included the effects of tibial torsion and knee angle of position. Active quadriceps contraction may change the alignment, and tibial external rotation by means of the "screw home" mechanism also alters the Q angle. Brattstrom suggested that the upper limit of the Q angle should be considered to be 24 degrees. The Q angle, also called the "deformation en baionette," was described by Trillat. Huberti and Hayes [16] assessed the influence of the Q angle on patellofemoral contact forces and noted no significant change with any of the various Wiberg patellar types. Uniform pressure across both medial and lateral facets was present throughout almost the entire range of motion. Due to uniformity of the contact area, excessive compression is avoided. Both increases and decreases in the Q angle result in enhancement of maximum contact pressures, and the authors caution against surgical diminution of the Q angle to less than its normal physiologic value because correction out of that range will increase the patellofemoral joint reaction force.

SUMMARY

In 1945 Haxton [14] was credited with the observation, "It seems likely that more has been written about the patella relative to its size than about any other bone in the human body." Fifty years before that, some authors thought that the patella was superfluous and unnecessary [4, 5, 14, 15]. They reasoned that if the patella served any useful purpose it would regenerate after being removed or else be replaced by a structure of similar size, shape, or function. These authors would be amazed at the plethora of information currently available about the patellofemoral joint. The patella plays a major role in normal knee mechanics. Alterations in any of a multitude of factors may cause pain or instability at the patellofemoral joint. Previous studies of this complex articulation were usually static assessments that were commonly done in a single plane. As appreciation is gained of the complexity of motion that occurs at the patellofemoral joint, improved data on normal function are currently being developed. These data will provide a physiologic rationale for the diagnosis and treatment of patellofemoral disorders in the future.

Multipartite Patella

A multipartite patella may present a diagnostic dilemma in an athlete with anterior knee pain (Fig. 18–25). After roentgenograms are taken of a patient with knee complaints, the patient is often told erroneously (by a nonorthopedist) that he or she has a patellar fracture when none exists in a patella that is nontender and previously was not a site of symptoms (Fig. 18–26).

Multipartite patellae are often incidental roentgenographic findings (Fig. 18–27) [43, 44]. The exact incidence is unknown, but the reported incidence of bipartite patellae ranges from 0.2% to 6% [43]. Bilaterality is uncommon (Fig. 18–28) [38]. A strong male (9:1) dominance is a consistent finding. Although the anomaly exists most commonly in two parts, three or even four segments may be seen.

The superior lateral aspect of the patella has a diminished blood flow along its margin, and this change has been hypothesized to account for abnormalities in either

formation or healing that occur in response to injury. Traction forces by the vastus lateralis insertion have also been thought to play a role in fragment production [46]. Green [46] suggested the possibility of nonunion of a previous fracture as a source of symptoms. Weaver [47] reports that bipartite patella may be a potential source of disability in early adulthood, especially during athletic endeavors. It has been suggested that the fragment results from chronic chondro-osseous tensile forces, a circumstance analogous to Osgood-Schlatter's disease or Sinding-Larsen-Johannsen's disease [44]. In Ogden and colleagues' review [44] of patellar specimens in cadavers 3 to 16 years old, only two specimens were found to have discrete supralateral ossification centers.

The normal patella is formed from the centrifugal coalition of multiple sites of ossification. This ossification is similar to that of long bone physes with production of hyaline cartilage in well-developed vascular channels. Small foci of ossification can be seen roentgenographically in the patella as early as 2 to 3 years of age, but significant ossification does not usually occur

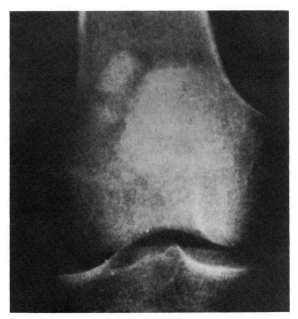

FIGURE 18–25
Incidental roentgenographic finding of a tripartite patella in a 24-year-old NFL defensive back.

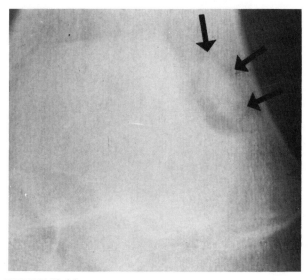

FIGURE 18–26
Asymptomatic bipartite patella misdiagnosed as an acute fracture. Note smooth edges at margins.

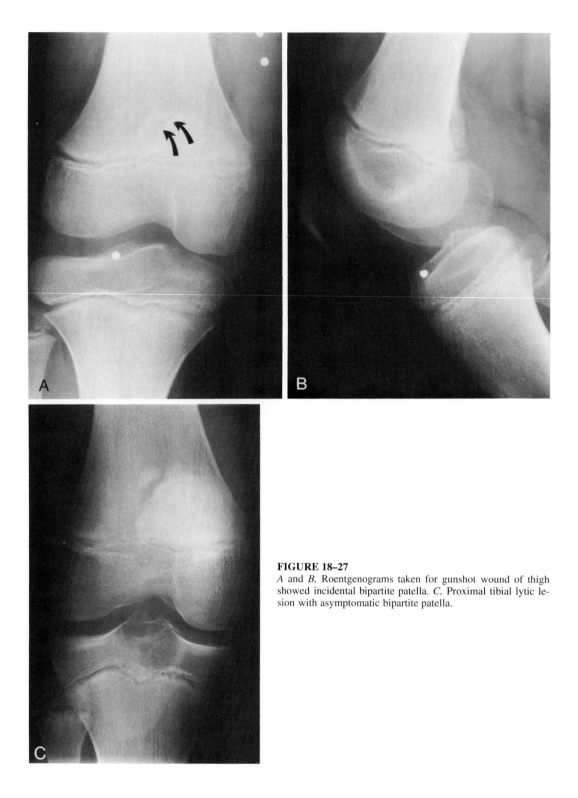

FIGURE 18–27

A and *B*, Roentgenograms taken for gunshot wound of thigh showed incidental bipartite patella. *C*, Proximal tibial lytic lesion with asymptomatic bipartite patella.

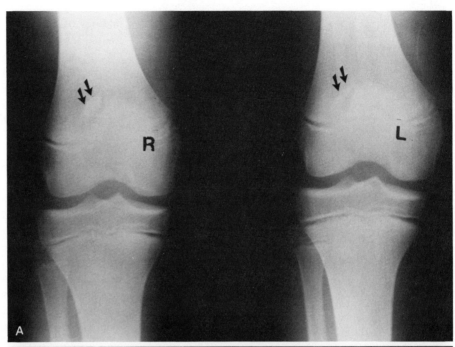

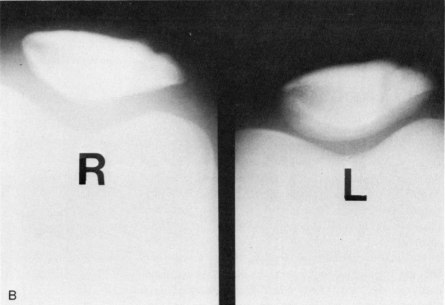

FIGURE 18–28
Asymptomatic bilateral bipartite patellae.

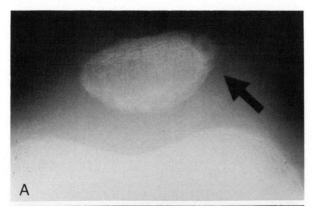

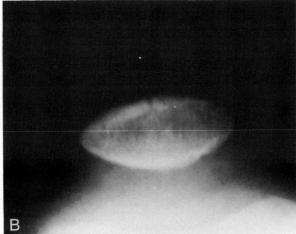

FIGURE 18–29
A and *B*, Progressive ossification pattern over a period of 1 year in a 6- and 7-year-old boy.

until age 5 or 6, at which time the patella becomes visible roentgenographically (Fig. 18–29). Abnormalities of formation may result in a bi- or tripartite patella.

Multipartite patellae were first described by Gruberin [45] in 1883. Bipartite patellar formations were classified into three roentgenographic types by Saupe [45]. (Fig. 18–30). In type I the junction of the fragment and the main patellar body is at the inferior pole (5% incidence), in type II it is at the lateral margin (20% incidence), and in type III, which is by far the most common, it is at the superior lateral quadrant (75% incidence).

The junctional sites of these patellar variants may become symptomatic after acute or chronic stress, especially in the early teen years. Eccentric quadriceps stresses that cause junctional micromotion are thought to be the sources of these symptoms at the chondral osseous junction in chronic cases, which are particularly aggravated by such activities as jumping, squatting, and kneeling. The acute situation, in which there is a history of pain following direct trauma to the site, is uncommon, but this pain may represent an acute fracture at the fragment junction (Fig. 18–31).

The patient with a symptomatic multipartite patella complains of activity-related knee pain, usually at the superolateral patellar margin. On examination, the knee is found to be normal except for a slightly enlarged patella that is tender at the junction of the main patellar body and the aberrant fragment. Patients with complaints after direct trauma to the patella may have additional findings of an acute patellar fracture, i.e., hemarthrosis, limited motion, and so on [37]. Roentgenographically, the size, location, formation, and junctional morphology of the multipartite patella vary widely. The patella is usually larger than the normal opposite patella. Tomograms, computed tomography (CT) scans, and magnetic resonance imaging (MRI) may be needed to evaluate the fragment–patellar body articular surface relationships in a symptomatic patient (Fig. 18–32).

Treatment depends on the acuity and severity of symptoms. In chronic cases, modification of activity over 3 to 4 weeks may be all that is required [40, 44]. In acute situations the pain is secondary to an acute separation between the fragment and the main patellar body, and immobilization with a cylinder cast for 3 weeks usually resolves the circumstance [37]. In the subacute or chronic case, if symptoms persist or if acute symptoms occur at the fragment site despite nonoperative measures, surgical excision of the fragment and repair of the quadriceps retinaculum are indicated (Fig. 18–33) [35, 40, 44, 47]. Following a brief postoperative period of immobilization for comfort, motion and strengthening exercises are begun. Return to play is predicated on attaining a full range of motion, strength, and endurance. An inferior patellar pole (''sleeve'') frac-

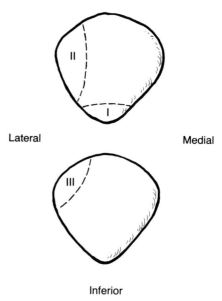

FIGURE 18–30
Saupe's classification of bipartite patellae.

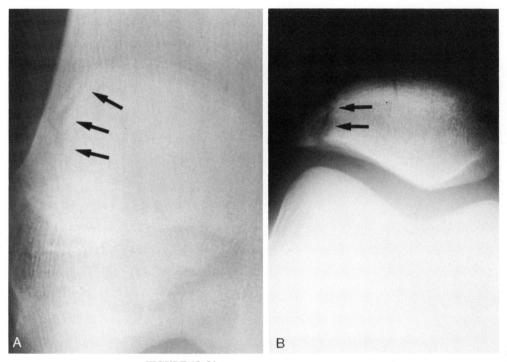

FIGURE 18–31
Acute fracture. Note irregularity and displacement.

ture may be confused with a type I bipartite patella (Fig. 18–34). Combinations of patellar injury with an incidental note of bipartite patellar formation may occur (Fig. 18–35).

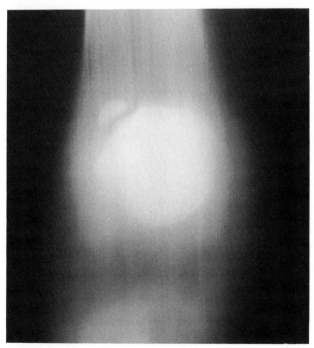

FIGURE 18–32
Tomography demonstrates extent of junction between bipartite fragment and main patellar body.

The uncommon so-called dorsal patellar defect is another incidentally noted roentgenographic curiosity [36]. In a review of 1349 consecutive knee radiographs, Johnson and Brogdon [42] found 13 lesions in 12 patients (1%). Although 10 of the 12 patients were female, most other studies cite a higher male preponderance [36, 41, 46]. The defect is most commonly located at the dorsal superolateral patella (Fig. 18–36). The dorsal defect has been noted to resolve spontaneously with further growth and may be a normal variant of ossification (Fig. 18–37). Van Holsbeeck and colleagues [46], in analyzing 2286 knee radiographs, noted six patients with dorsal defects four of whom had an associated bipartite patella. These authors suggested that the dorsal defect of the patella is a stress-induced anomaly of ossification caused by traction forces on the insertion of the vastus lateralis and patellar subluxation.

Goergen and associates [39] reviewed dorsal patellar defects in seven patients, two of whom were symptomatic. Arthrography in these patients showed that four of seven arthrograms were normal. The arthrograms were used to differentiate this condition from osteochondritis dissecans. Osteochondritic lesions are located in a significantly different position, i.e., convex, inferior (below the transverse central axis), and medial from that of the dorsal patellar defect site.

Haswell and colleagues [41], in reviewing cases of patellar defects from three centers, described 16 cases in which three patients were symptomatic. Twelve of the sixteen patients were between the ages of 10 and 19

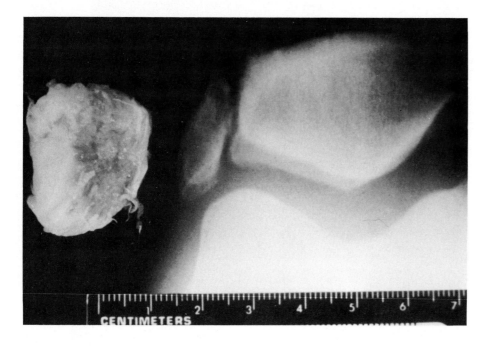

FIGURE 18–33
Chronically symptomatic, separated Saupe type II bipartite patella and surgical specimen. There had been no history of significant knee trauma.

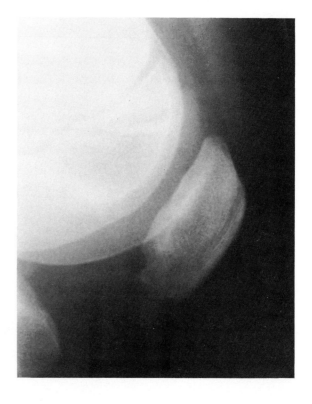

FIGURE 18–34
Type I bipartite patella. No symptoms or signs were referable to this lesion.

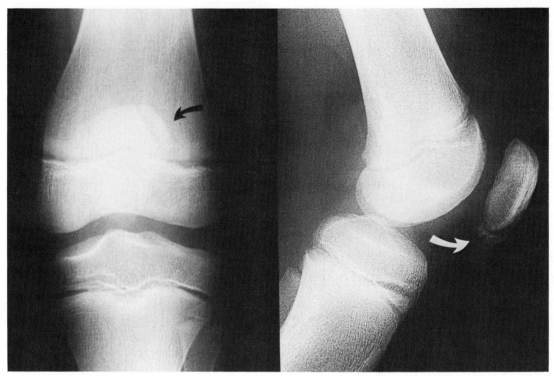

FIGURE 18–35
Left, Type III bipartite patella. *Right*, Associated minimally displaced patellar acute sleeve fracture.

FIGURE 18–36
Dorsal defect on the patella. The patient was asymptomatic, and the knee was nontender at this site.

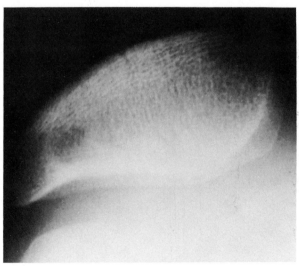

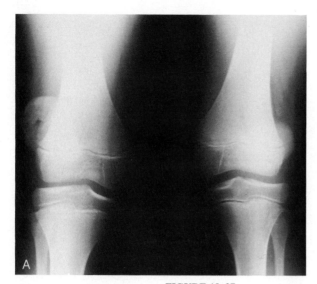 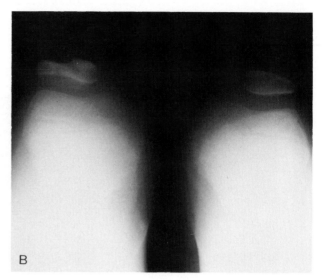

FIGURE 18–37
A and *B*, Asymptomatic dorsal patellar defect. Note normal opposite side.

years. Four had bilateral involvement. Arthrograms, including a tomoarthrogram, were normal. Defects averaged 9 mm in diameter (range 4 to 26 mm). These authors recommended an oblique external patellar view for better roentgenographic delineation. Biopsies in two patients showed the cartilage to be intact and demonstrated normal bone repair without inflammation. At follow-up, spontaneous resolution of the defect had occurred in three of the five untreated patients in the interim. Benign lesions such as stress fractures, osteoid osteoma, or subacute osteomyelitis must be considered in the differential diagnosis. Most cases of dorsal defects of the patella are radiologic curiosities that resolve spontaneously and usually require little intervention.

Plica

Knee plicae are normal synovial folds. Attention has recently focused on these arthroscopically viewed structures [48]. Pathologic conditions of the plicae have become recognizable as a cause of knee symptoms. Four plicae are considered normal in the knee synovium. The infrapatellar plica is located in the femoral notch and is better known as the ligamentum mucosum. If thickened, it may be mistaken for the anterior cruciate ligament by the unsophisticated arthroscopist (Fig. 18–38). A suprapatellar plica is present within the superior portion of the suprapatellar pouch (Fig. 18–39). A medial patellar (shelf) plica is a common finding; it varies in width, length, and thickness and usually travels from the superior or midpatella to the medial fat pad (Fig. 18–40). A rare lateral synovial plica completes the array (Fig. 18–41).

The knee's synovial anatomy was first analyzed in detail by cadaveric dissections performed by Mayda in 1918 [55] and was originally studied arthroscopically by Iino [52] in 1939. Among the names given particularly to the medial patellar plica are Iino's band, "meniscus of the patella," and plica synovialis [48, 52, 55].

The knee is thought to be formed embryologically into three compartments: medial, lateral, and suprapatellar. The synovial plicae are considered remnants of these compartment's divisions. Gardner and O'Rahilly [50] and Dosko [49] hypothesized that multiple cavitation at 8 weeks of embryologic development would eventually form a single joint space. The reported incidence of abnormally thickened plicae within the knee varies tremendously and ranges from 17% to 75% [52, 56–58, 61]. This wide range of incidence may reflect the method of study. The first authors investigated the knee plicae by means of anatomic dissection [52, 55], whereas later authors assessed them arthroscopically [56, 57, 61].

The medial patellar plica originates proximally and medially and is attached distally to the medial patellar fat pad. In Patel's series [56] the incidence of symptomatic medial patellar and suprapatellar plicae combined was 18.9%, i.e., 72 of 371 symptomatic knees, significantly less than the 35% to 55% previously reported by

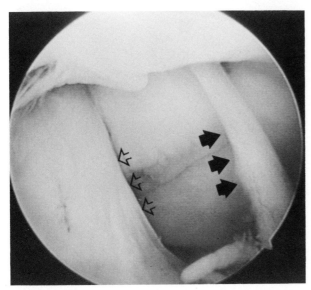

FIGURE 18–38
Dark arrows show the ligamentum mucosum compared with the anterior cruciate ligament (ACL) (open arrows).

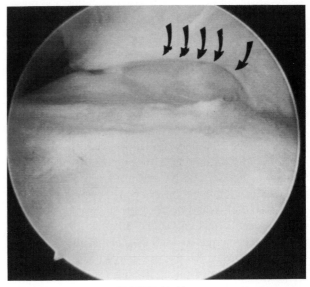

FIGURE 18–39
Suprapatellar plica.

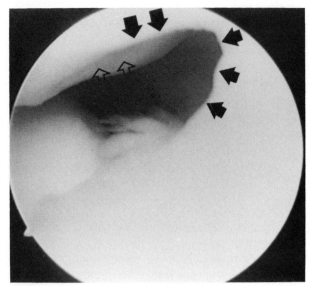

FIGURE 18–40
Medial plica (solid closed arrows) with patellar impingement (open arrows).

others. The increased incidence of symptomatic plicae in the Japanese has been ascribed to ethnic and cultural demands for prolonged squatting and kneeling.

Clinically, the diagnosis is nonspecific. Historically, the patient complains of a "pop" or "snap" in the knee at particular degrees of flexion, the "snap" and discomfort becoming progressively more symptomatic with increased levels of activity. A history of direct anterior knee trauma may be a factor. A significant increase in a sports training program, especially one requiring repetitive knee flexion and extension, may produce overuse symptoms. Anterior knee pain may follow prolonged sitting. Swelling is usually not a significant part of the complaint. Hardaker and colleagues [51] noted exercise-related snapping in two-thirds of the symptomatic plicae they reviewed.

Findings on physical examination are often limited and may consist only of localized tenderness at the site of the plica as well as a snapping sensation with increasing degrees of knee flexion. The popping or snapping may be palpated medially as the knee passes from 30 to 60 degrees of flexion, the fibrous band being occasionally palpable along the medial patella between the mid-patella and the joint line. Lateral patellar translation may cause traction on this band and increase its symptoms. Symptoms should not be attributed mistakenly to an unstable patellofemoral mechanism. The medial patellar plica's anterior extension onto the fat pad or meniscus may produce symptoms at the anterior joint line that may be misinterpreted as meniscal pathology. Pipkin [58, 59] advocated the use of a particular physical finding for diagnosis of plica. He suggested bringing the knee from flexion to extension with internal rotation of

the leg and associated medialization of the patella to produce a pop between 45 and 60 degrees of flexion.

Imaging studies have not been particularly helpful. Since this is a dynamic problem, it is difficult to assess with static images. Erosive changes of the formal condyle or patella may be noted radiographically in long-standing, severe cases. No criteria have been outlined yet for diagnosis of pathologic plicae by MRI.

The proposed pathophysiology varies with the causative mechanisms. The first mechanism is a direct blow to a synovial structure resulting in hemorrhage, edema, and progressive fibrosis. The second mechanism is overuse in which task-specific demands (often associated with minor aberrancies of knee mechanics) cause progressively increasing stress at this site leading to recurrent synovitis, edema, fibrosis, and hyalinization with further thickening of the tissue, which now becomes a space-occupying lesion that progressively abrades the surrounding tissues (Fig. 18–42).

Differential diagnoses include all circumstances that can cause snapping or popping about the knee with resultant anterior knee pain (e.g., patellar maltracking, loose bodies, meniscal instability, etc.). In most circumstances, a diagnosis of plica must be considered one of exclusion. Hardaker and colleagues [51] noted a 65% incidence of synovitis and articular cartilage erosion at the femoral condyle in patients with pathologic suprapatellar plica lesions. In Patel's series [57] 60% of patients had gross malacic changes of the medial patella, and 40% had similar changes of the medial femoral condyle when a medial pathologic patellar plica was present.

Symptoms tend to result from excessive use and may

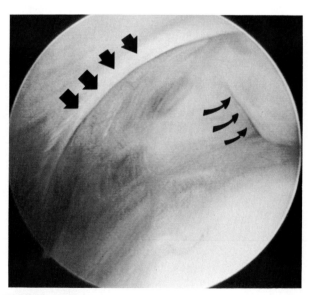

FIGURE 18–41
Lateral plica (large arrows) with suprapatellar plica above (curved arrows).

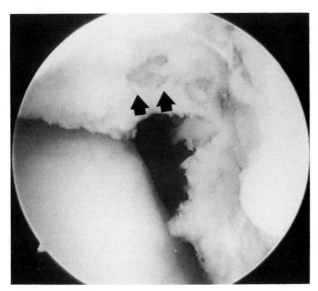

FIGURE 18–42
Patellar chondral erosion from pathologic medial plica abrasion.

be relieved by means of the basic treatment principles used for any overuse problem, i.e., identification of the attending activity, modification of that activity, relative rest, improved balance of strength and flexibility, anti-inflammatory medications, and a variety of external modalities (ice, heat). Abnormal patellofemoral mechanisms that cause excessive stress at the synovium must be ruled out. Most patients are relieved of their symptoms by use of these principles when an early diagnosis is made and treatment is started promptly [62]. In a prospective study, Rovere and Adair [60] studied 31 knees in 30 patients and found that 73% experienced complete relief of symptoms with return to full activity following injection of the plica with local anesthetic and

steroid. In 10 patients who received injections of anesthetic alone, only transient relief correlated with the action of the local anesthetic occurred. Because extremely accurate placement of this injection into a small anatomic site is required, if inadvertent intra-articular injection occurs simultaneously, a positive but nonspecific response is expected.

Arthroscopy has led to a significant incidence of diagnosis of "pathologic plicae" and subsequent surgical management. It has been suggested that in the past, open surgery for medial meniscectomy by a formal arthroscopy cut the medial plica. If the plica was abnormal, symptom reduction independent of meniscal removal or nonremoval occurred.

Because so many plicae are currently released or resected, the pathologic significance of these is in question. One must ask if this is an arthroscopic "wastebasket" diagnosis when no other obvious pathology is seen in the knee at the time of arthroscopy [48, 53, 54]. This is not to say that a condition of pathologic plica may not exist and may be cured by arthroscopic resection. However, the frequency with which the diagnosis of pathologic plica is currently being made seems perhaps out of proportion to the true number of such pathologic lesions. It must be recalled that the plica is a normal intra-articular structure. Sources of patellar overuse with resultant synovial stress must be corrected or the lesion will recur. It is important to rule out all other obvious causes of anterior knee pathology and not ascribe dominant symptoms to this often gossameric structure. Surgery should not be carried out in a plica "just because it is there" when nothing else is found at the time of arthroscopy. As Patel notes, "The relationship between the plica and disease and the relationship between the plica and symptoms remain inconclusive and unclear" [56].

Osgood-Schlatter Disease

Osgood-Schlatter "disease" is an extremely common source of sports disability. Its classic presentation in a preteen or early teenage child with activity-related discomfort, swelling, and tenderness at the tibial tubercle readily suggests its diagnosis. The ominous sounding title aggrandizes this condition by elevating it to disease status.

Boys are more commonly affected than girls, although Osgood-Schlatter disease is now being seen with more frequency in girls, a reflection of the increased levels of sports participation by girls. Girls tend to be involved at an earlier age (11 to 13 years), whereas boys tend to present with symptoms between the ages of 12 and 15. In his original paper, Osgood [77] specifically referred to the relationship between sports activity and the occurrence of symptoms. Kujala and colleagues [70] found a 21% incidence of Osgood-Schlatter disease in an athletic group of adolescents, whereas only a 4.5% incidence was seen in an age-matched nonathletic group. The condition is bilateral in 20% to 30% of cases. Tubercle prominence may be bilateral, but commonly only one side is symptomatic (Fig. 18–43).

When the condition was described concurrently by Schlatter [78] and Osgood [77] in 1908, they believed that trauma to the tibial tubercle, either directly or via a patellar tendon force, caused partial or complete avulsion at the growing tubercle. Both authors differentiated this condition from an acute tibial avulsion fracture. In discussing Osgood's paper at the time of its presentation, Codman [77] acknowledged the role of persistent chronic avulsion but felt that trauma to the distal patellar tendon or its insertion could cause periostitis and subsequent new bone formation. The condition is currently thought to result from submaximal repetitive tensile stresses acting on an immature patellar tendon-tibial tubercle-tibial junction resulting in minor avulsion and attempts at repair [66, 75] (Fig. 18–44).

Ehrenborg and colleagues [66] described four stages of tibial tubercle development. The initial stage is cartilaginous (birth to 8 to 10 years), the second apophyseal, the third epiphyseal with coalescence of the tibial tubercle and a proximal tibial ossification center, and the

fourth phase is bony and includes tibial proximal epiphyseal closure. Based on this analysis, Ehrenborg and associates [66] concluded in 1962 that the cause of this lesion was a traumatic avulsion of the patellar tendon from the tibial tubercle. Ogden and Southwick [75] described three histologic zones at the immature tibial tubercle. The proximal area is similar to the proximal tibial physis and consists of columnar cartilage. The midzone is composed of fibrocartilage, and the distal portion is fibrous tissue that blends into the tibial perichondrium. The tissues change with age, and progressive physiologic epiphysiodesis of the tubercle begins proximally and travels centrifugally and distally.

Symptoms usually begin during rapid growth at the time of tibial tubercle maturation. The patient usually complains of pain at the tibial tubercle, the pain being intermittent and aggravated by eccentric quadriceps demand activities, particularly jumping, squatting, and kneeling (Fig. 18–45). The pain rarely becomes severe enough to interrupt routine daily activity. On examination, exquisite tenderness, prominence, and swelling are found at the tibial tubercle. In some children, especially in the early teen years, the patellar tendon and peripatellar areas are also tender.

Roentgenographically, many patterns of tibial tubercle

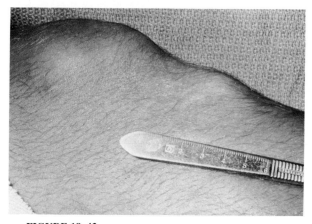

FIGURE 18–43
Tibial tubercle prominence due to Osgood-Schlatter disease.

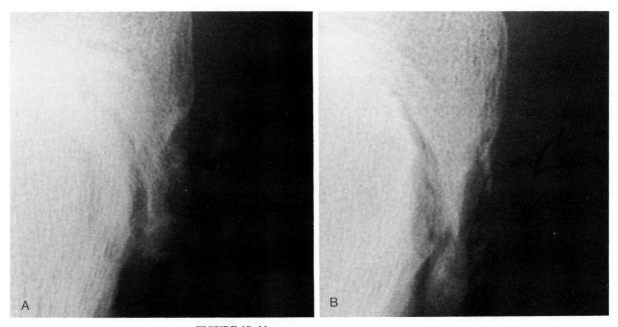

FIGURE 18–44
A and *B*, Healing chronic avulsions at tibial tubercle.

morphology may be seen depending on the child's age and skeletal development (Fig. 18–46). Fragmentation of the tubercle is common, as is partial coalescence of these fragments. In as many as 50% of the cases studied by Krause and colleagues [69] a discrete ossicle was noted, separate from the tibial tubercle. Associated soft tissue swelling was invariable regardless of the tibial tubercle configuration.

Roentgenograms are essential for completeness in the diagnostic process. One should not be lulled into complacency by the seeming obvious and mundane diagnosis, especially in unilateral cases, Lewis and Reilly [72]

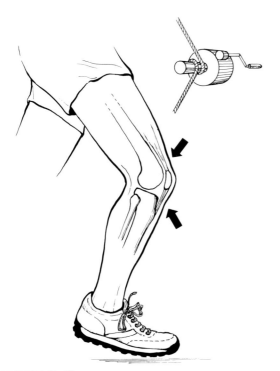

FIGURE 18–45
''Windlass'' effect of quadriceps mechanism and tibial tubercle.

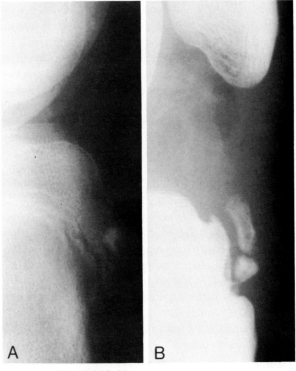

FIGURE 18–46
A and *B*, Variations in tubercle morphology.

advised caution about the misdiagnosis of a "sports tumor." D'Ambrosia and McDonald [65] have warned against pitfalls in the diagnosis of Osgood-Schlatter disease. They reported two cases presenting with clinically "obvious" Osgood-Schlatter disease that in retrospect turned out to be osteomyelitis of the tibial tubercle in one patient and an arteriovenous malformation in another. It should be kept in mind that concurrent disease can be present in patients with Osgood-Schlatter disease, and benign and malignant conditions may be masked by the more common and obvious appearance of Osgood-Schlatter symptoms and signs. Osgood-Schlatter disease may coexist with slipped capital femoral epiphysis. It must be remembered that knee pain in a child is hip pain until proved otherwise, and a hip examination is an essential part of knee examination.

In reviewing lateral roentgenograms of patients with Osgood-Schlatter disease, Lancourt and Christina [71] noted an increased incidence of patella alta. They hypothesized that chronic traction at the tibial tubercle caused proximal migration and secondary patella alta but could not determine whether this was cause or effect. It is difficult to accurately measure the patellar tendon insertion on radiographs of less skeletally mature patients. Because this landmark is lost, the patellar tendon-patella ratio may be inaccurate, and the determination of patella alta or patella infera is made more difficult.

A relationship between patella alta, Osgood-Schlatter disease, and tibial tubercle avulsion fractures has been suggested [63, 64, 67, 73, 75]. Ogden and colleagues [76] reported 14 patients with 15 tibial tubercle fractures, 13 boys and 1 girl between the ages of 12 and 16 years. The patients included one with myelodysplasia and one with skeletal dysplasia and tibial deformity. Nine patients had Osgood-Schlatter disease, but in seven the disease was on the opposite side from the avulsion fracture. One patient had bilateral asymptomatic Osgood-Schlatter disease before sustaining a unilateral avulsion fracture. In three patients Osgood-Schlatter disease was present on the side of the avulsion fracture, but the condition was asymptomatic prior to the fracture. There appeared to be no significant relationship between symptomatic preexisting Osgood-Schlatter disease and acute tibial tubercle avulsion fractures in this series. Bowers [64] reported patellar tendon avulsion fractures associated with Osgood-Schlatter disease in a series of young patients, some of whom required operative intervention. One of the six athletes in the series reported by Mirbey and associates [73] had bilateral Osgood-Schlatter symptoms prior to suffering a major tibial tubercle avulsion fracture while jumping.

Few studies have analyzed the natural history of Osgood-Schlatter disease. Krause and colleagues [69] found that the great majority of patients were asymptomatic at follow-up in adulthood except for an occasional

inability to kneel for prolonged periods. Almost half of the patients at skeletal maturity had a separate tibial tubercle ossicle. Patients in this group had not received any treatment. In a second group of 12 patients who had been treated with plaster immobilization while they were symptomatic during childhood, 8 still had epiphyseal fragmentation, and 7 of the 12 had symptoms while kneeling. These authors suggest that Osgood-Schlatter disease has two presentations. Type I, characterized by soft tissue swelling alone, tends to become roentgenographically and clinically normal with time. Type II includes roentgenographic evidence of fragmentation of the tibial tubercle and may cause persistent symptoms as well as bony abnormalities at follow-up.

Treatment is usually nonoperative. Osgood [77] noted that nonintervention resulted in progressive subsidence of symptoms in most cases. The patient and family must understand that 12 to 18 months are needed for spontaneous physiologic epiphysiodesis and symptom resolution. The variability in time must be explained to them as a function of the inexactitude of predicting skeletal maturity at this site. Based on Ehrenborg's [66] theory that this condition was an acute traumatic avulsion of the tibial tubercle, full limb immobilization for varying periods and the subsequent elimination of any activity during the next 12 to 18 months was popular during the 1960s and early 1970s. Currently, treatment with ice, anti-inflammatory medication, and a properly contoured knee pad is usually thought to control the symptoms. Maintenance of knee motion with hamstring and quadriceps flexibility exercises during the child's rapid growth phase is also helpful. Sports activity is balanced with tolerance of pain and severity of symptoms. Coaches, physical education instructors, and parents must understand and appreciate the unpredictable variability of symptom intensity. Sports requiring prolonged squatting or kneeling may not be tolerated. A change of team position, e.g., from catcher to second baseman, may be necessary. If symptoms progress to the point of being disabling during routine daily activity, a brief period (7 to 10 days) of immobilization usually resolves the discomfort. Injections of corticosteroid into the tibial tubercle should be condemned. Both child and parent must be apprised of the variable amount of tibial tubercle prominence that will persist after symptoms have resolved.

Because of the rarity of tibial tubercle avulsion fractures in patients with Osgood-Schlatter disease, carte blanche condemnation of sports activity is not indicated. Patients with persistent symptoms at the tibial tubercle not associated with a loose ossicle are at a stage just prior to tubercle closure and may be at risk for fracture if they are involved in powerful leaping activities, e.g., slam-dunking a basketball or maneuvers requiring high concentric or eccentric quadriceps loading.

Surgery for Osgood-Schlatter disease is uncommon.

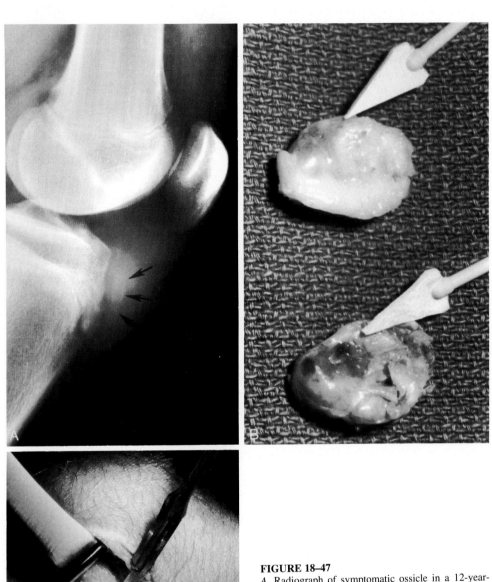

FIGURE 18–47

A, Radiograph of symptomatic ossicle in a 12-year-old boy. *B,* Bilateral ossicle specimens. Note articularlike surfaces. *C,* Ossicle bed—note facetlike changes with a bursa.

Over the years a multitude of procedures have been suggested [79, 80], including tibial ossicle excision, drilling of the tubercle, and bone pegs to encourage union at the tibial tubercle. Glynn and Regan [68] reported Osgood-Schlatter disease in 41 knees (39 patients) in whom half underwent excision of the ossicle because symptoms persisted despite management by limitation of activity for 3 months. Twenty-two other knees had had various treatments including surgical drilling. In a histologic review of six of the cases, the authors found a cartilage-bone junction within a fibrin bed but did not mention any inflammatory changes. None of their patients suffered a growth arrest of the proximal tibia or had clinical evidence of genu recurvatum. They believed that the ossicle was a site of a persistent nonunion and recommended its excision. Mital and colleagues [74] in reporting the "so-called Osgood-Schlatter lesion," found that 10% of patients with Osgood-Schlatter disease had a separate persistent ossicle at the tubercle. Ossicle resection and attendant removal of the bursa produced a cure. Histologic examination demonstrated no evidence of fragment avascularity. They agreed with the concept that Osgood-Schlatter disease is an avulsion of the proximal portion of the tibial tubercle.

If an ossicle (or ossicles) are symptomatic, one need not wait until skeletal maturity to excise them. They are easily enucleated from the patellar tendon via a longitudinal fiber-splitting incision. An articulating zone with

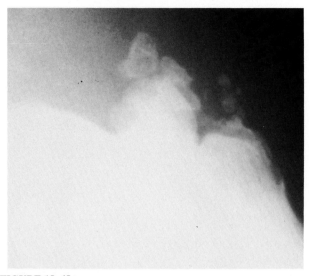

FIGURE 18–48
Large symptomatic tibial tubercle and ossicles in a 26-year-old carpet installer who had been symptomatic for 14 years.

the tubercle is commonly noted, often with a reactive capsule and fluid (Fig. 18–47). Because the tibial tubercle physis closes well before the tibial metaphyseal junction, recurvatum should not occur. In the mature patient, debulking of the prominent tubercle may be done as a cosmetic procedure at the time of ossicle excision (Fig. 18–48). The patient and family must be forewarned that some soft tissue and bony prominence may remain.

Sinding-Larsen-Johansson Disease

Anterior knee pain may be caused by Sinding-Larsen-Johansson "disease," a condition thought to result from persistent traction at the immature inferior patellar pole leading to calcification and ossification at this junction [87, 88, 90]. Symptoms at this site commonly occur in active preteen boys (10 to 12 years old), who complain of activity-related pain, especially with jumping or running. The pain is usually localized to the inferior patellar pole, the most common site of this condition. Occasionally symptoms occur at the proximal patellar-quadriceps junction but much less commonly than at the distal site.

Point tenderness is found at the patella-patellar tendon junction. The remainder of the knee examination is usually normal. One must rule out patellar sagittal alignment abnormalities (e.g., patella alta, patella infera, or limited hip or knee motion that would cause increased anterior knee stress. Roentgenograms are usually normal except for varying amounts of calcification or ossification at the patella-patellar tendon junction (Fig. 18–49). Similar roentgenographic findings may be noted in asymptomatic patients (Fig. 18–50). Medlar and Lyne [88] proposed five roentgenographic stages. Stage I is a normal patella on roentgenograms. Stage II shows irregular calcification at the inferior patellar pole. Stage III shows progressive coalition of this calcification. Stage IVA demonstrates incorporation of calcification within the patella, and stage IVB shows the calcific mass remaining separate from the main body of the patella. One occasionally sees concomitant Osgood-Schlatter disease in

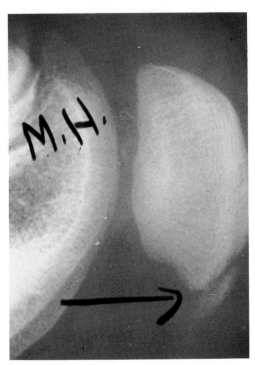

FIGURE 18–49
Sinding-Larsen-Johansson change in a symptomatic 10-year-old wrestler.

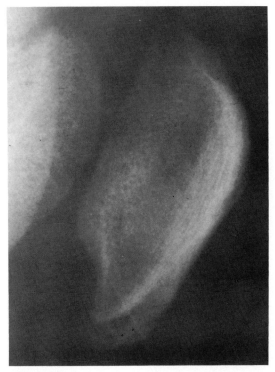

FIGURE 18–50
Sinding-Larsen-Johansson changes noted incidentally in an 11-year-old basketball player. He was asymptomatic, and the knee was nontender at the distal patella.

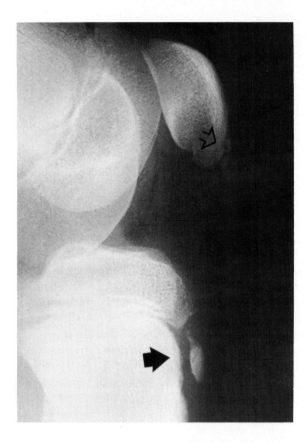

FIGURE 18–51
Concomitant Sinding-Larsen-Johannson and Osgood-Schlatter disease in an 11-year-old basketball player. Symptoms were related only to the tibial tubercle.

the older child (Fig. 18–51). Batten and Menelaus [81] reported six patients with roentgenographic fragmentation of the patellar proximal pole. Four of the patients presented with symptoms of Osgood-Schlatter or Sinding-Larsen-Johansson disease on the same or the opposite knee. None of the patients had signs or symptoms relating to the patellar proximal pole. Two of the patients had roentgen evidence of proximal pole fragmentation on the opposite knee, and both were asymptomatic. Fol-

low-up of these patients showed total resolution of the roentgenographic findings within 2 years in one patient and significant roentgenographic resolution in the other patients within 9 months of the initial evaluation.

Patellar stress or sleeve fractures and type I bipartite patella should be considered in the differential diagnosis (Fig. 18–52). In the more mature adolescent, an adult-type "jumper's knee" (i.e., chronic patellar proximal tendinitis) may be found, especially in athletes engaged

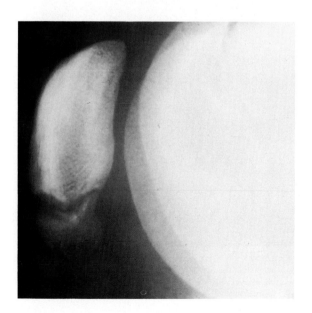

FIGURE 18–52
Type I (Saupe) bipartite patella in a 12-year-old asymptomatic gymnast.

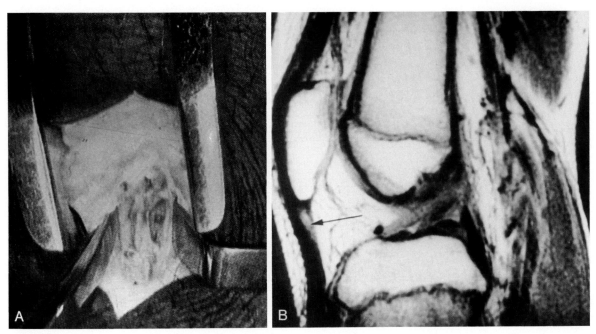

FIGURE 18–53
A, "Jumper's knee" in a 16-year-old basketball player. Note necrotic intratendinous debris. *B*, MRI of chronic patellar tendinitis in a 14-year-old high-jumper. (Courtesy George W. Gross, M.D.).

in sports demanding repetitive eccentric quadriceps loading (e.g., jumping) [83, 89].

Sinding-Larsen-Johansson disease is thought to be due to persistent traction at the immature inferior patellar pole with resultant ossification and calcification at this junction. As in Osgood-Schlatter disease, treatment

consists primarily of explaining to the patient and parents the time course needed for spontaneous resolution of the condition (12 to 18 months). Moderation of activity, a knee sleeve, ice massage, and anti-inflammatory medications are usually helpful. It is important for physical education teachers and coaches to understand the

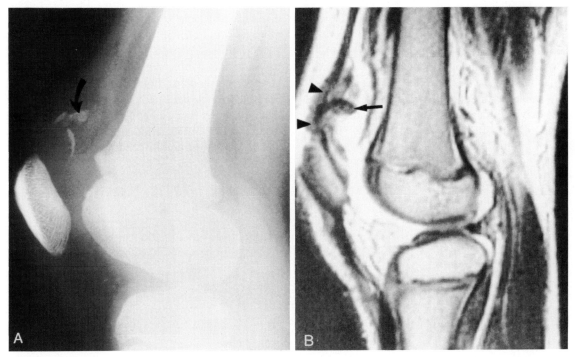

FIGURE 18–54
A, Proximal patellar "sleeve" fracture. *B*, MRI of same lesion. Note that a significant part of the fracture fragment is cartilage. (Courtesy George W. Gross, M.D.)

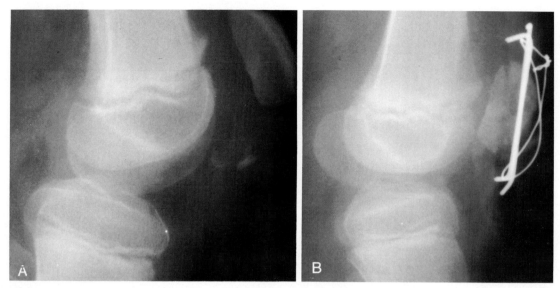

FIGURE 18–55
A, Inferior pole sleeve fracture in a 13-year-old soccer player. *B,* After open reduction and internal fixation. A significant portion of the fracture fragment is cartilage.

intermittent nature of symptoms with this entity. This condition almost always resolves without sequelae, and intervention requirements are minimal.

In the older child with jumper's knee, initial treatment is proportional to that of Sinding-Larsen-Johansson disease. Karisson and colleagues [86] recently quantified symptomatic patellar tendon involvement with ultrasound. Grade I lesions were less than 10 mm, grade II lesions were between 10 and 20 mm, and grade III lesions were more than 20 mm. Almost all grade III lesions required surgery. Histology of the tissue showed areas of necrosis and chronic inflammation. Intratendinous steroid injection is to be condemned because it carries a potential for tendon rupture. Causes of excessive patellar tendon stress (e.g., lower extremity malalignment, inappropriate training programs) must be eliminated. In recalcitrant cases, surgical debridement of the involved tissue may be necessary (Fig. 18–53) [83, 89].

A site of acute junctional stress is the inferior nonar-

ticulating patellar pole. An acute patellar "sleeve fracture" may occur in this zone [82, 84, 85]. The patient is usually between 9 and 12 years old and suffers an acute hyperflexion or deceleration moment causing a rapid quadriceps contraction. Because of pain or incompetence of the quadriceps mechanism, the knee is unable to extend fully actively. Focal tenderness is present at the inferior patellar pole, and a palpable gap is noted. A rare proximal pole avulsion may occur with loss of quadriceps mechanism continuity (Fig. 18–54). Because the distal patellar pole is largely cartilaginous at this age, minimal bony change may be seen, and the diagnosis may be missed because the avulsion is less readily apparent than in a more skeletally immature person. Roentgenograms show a high-riding patella (Fig. 18–55). Treatment is by open reduction and internal fixation to restore intra-articular alignment and quadriceps mechanism isometry. With solid fixation, rapid mobilization and rehabilitation are possible.

Acute Tibial Tubercle Avulsion Fracture

An acute avulsion fracture of the tibial tubercle is a dramatic but fortunately uncommon event. The patient is almost always a well-developed, muscular athletic boy who is near skeletal maturity and is involved in a leaping activity. Simultaneous bilateral fractures are very rare but have been reported [96, 97]. Patients with an acute tibial tubercle avulsion present with pain, usually following a vigorous athletic maneuver during which the knee is flexed against a rapidly contracting quadriceps, often during a maneuver preparatory to or during take-off. In reported series of tibial tubercle avulsion fractures [91, 99, 101], high jumping and basketball are the major sports associated with this injury.

Findings on physical examination depend on the magnitude and severity of the injury. Marked swelling and tenderness are present at the tibial tubercle, and deformity is proportional to the magnitude of the injury. The patient is unable to fully extend the knee because of both pain and loss of integrity of the quadriceps mechanism. Hemarthrosis may result from associated intra-articular structural injury (ACL, meniscus) or from intra-articular extension of the fracture.

Roentgenograms usually confirm the diagnosis. In less mature patients the avulsion may occur through unossified cartilage, and clinical findings are important for diagnosis. Osgood-Schlatter changes may be associated with the acute injury. Watson-Jones [103] catego-

rized tuberosity injuries into three types according to the extent of proximal tibial epiphyseal involvement. He described a case of a 14-year-old boy, nearly skeletally mature, who was injured during a high jump (Fig. 18–56). More recently, Ogden and colleagues [101] expanded the Watson-Jones classification to account for fragment comminution and displacement, the amount of physeal invasion, and the degree of intra-articular extension. Type III fractures in this classification should be considered Salter-Harris type IV fractures.

If the fracture is undisplaced or minimally displaced, cylinder cast immobilization for 3 to 4 weeks allows healing to occur (Figs. 18–57 and 18–58). In patients with fragment displacement (Figs. 18–59 and 18–60), especially with type II or III fractures, open reduction and internal fixation are required for anatomic alignment and restoration of isometry to the quadriceps-patellar mechanism (Fig. 18–61). Fixation may be done by direct suture, tension band wiring, or screw fixation (Fig. 18–62). Care must be taken intraoperatively to avoid creating a patella alta or patella infera (Fig. 18–63).

Since 1853, 106 cases of acute tibial tubercle avulsion fracture have been reported, and all point to a male predominance in the age range of 13 to 16 years. In a retrospective series over a period of 13 years, Bolesta and Fitsch [91] reported 15 cases of tibial tubercle avulsion in boys (average age 15.2 years at time of injury).

Text continued on page 334

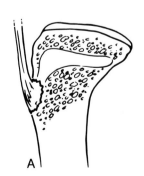 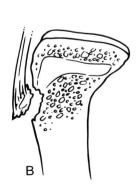 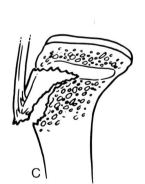 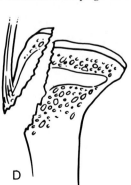

FIGURE 18–56
Classification of tibial tubercle fractures. *A*, Undisplaced. *B*, Displaced without extension. *C*, Displacement with physeal extension. *D*, Displacement with intra-articular extension.

329

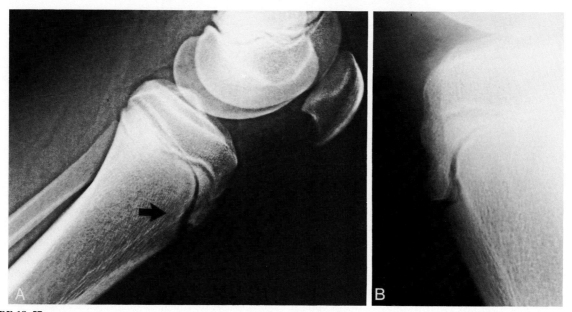

FIGURE 18–57
A, Minimally displaced tuberosity fracture. *B*, Eight weeks postinjury, 5 weeks after a 3-week period of cylinder casting. The patient returned without symptoms to high-level basketball.

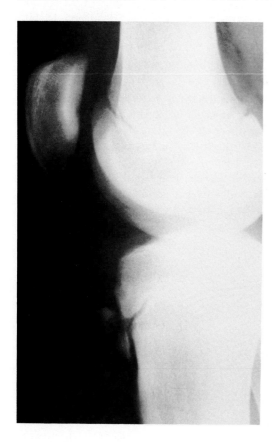

FIGURE 18–58
Displaced tuberosity fracture.

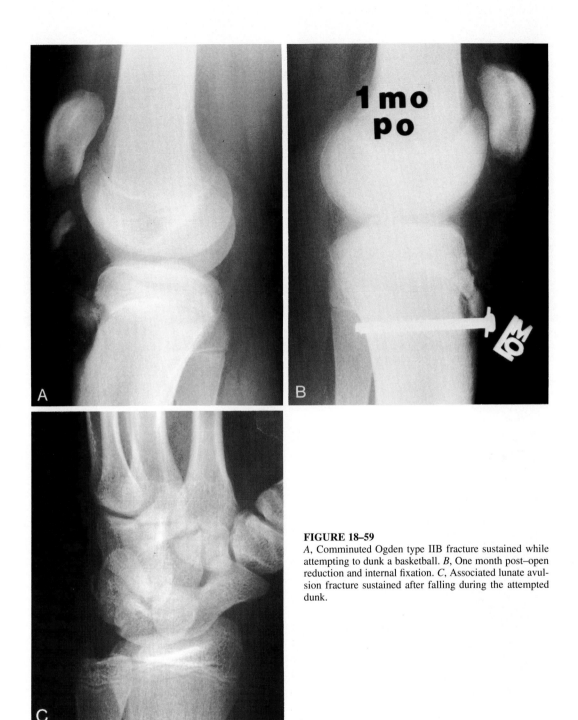

FIGURE 18–59

A, Comminuted Ogden type IIB fracture sustained while attempting to dunk a basketball. *B*, One month post–open reduction and internal fixation. *C*, Associated lunate avulsion fracture sustained after falling during the attempted dunk.

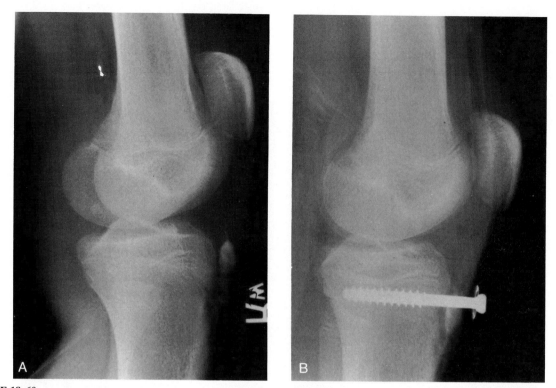

FIGURE 18–60
A, Marked type I fragment displacement with patella alta, untreated, 6 weeks postinjury. *B*, Quadriceps isometry restored postoperatively. Washer aids in force distribution on relatively small fragment. (Courtesy Greg Georgiadis, M.D.).

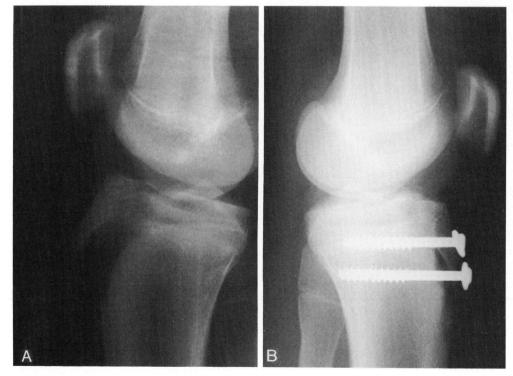

FIGURE 18–61
A, Watson-Jones type IV fracture (Ogden type IIIA) with proximal displacement. *B*, Anatomic reduction. (Courtesy Deborah F. Bell, M.D.).

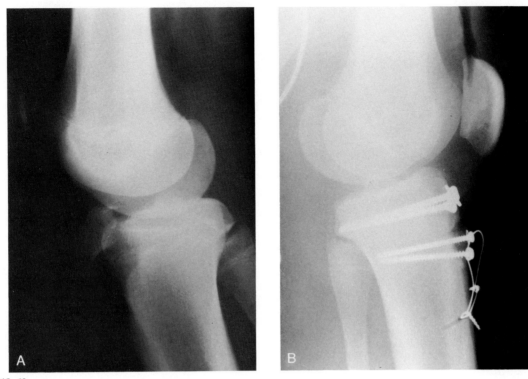

FIGURE 18–62
A, Comminuted, markedly displaced type IV (Ogden type IIIB) fracture. Note almost full closure of proximal tibial physis. *B*, Anatomic reduction requiring multiple screws plus tension band. (Courtesy Greg Georgiadis, M.D.).

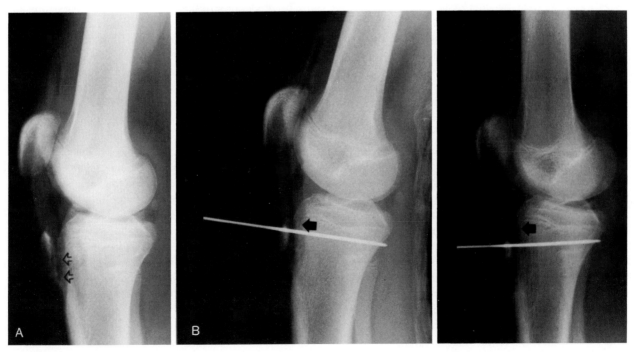

FIGURE 18–63
A, Avulsion fracture 6 weeks postinjury. *B*, Reduction with persistent patella alta. *C*, Anatomic reduction. (Courtesy Greg Georgiadis, M.D.).

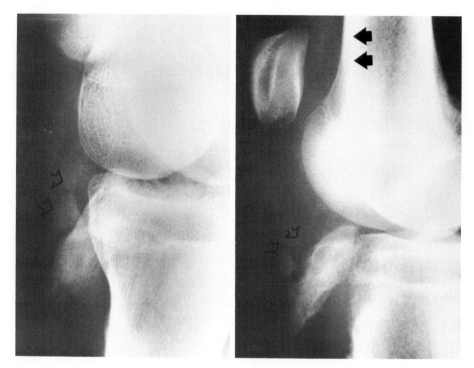

FIGURE 18–64
A, Type III fracture with associated Osgood-Schlatter change *(open arrow). B,* Note patella alta *(solid arrows).* (Courtesy of Richard H. Lamont, M.D.)

In their study, four patients with a unilateral tibial tubercle avulsion had preexisting bilateral Osgood-Schlatter disease. Among their patients treated with open reduction and internal fixation, the period of immobilization averaged 5 weeks. In short follow-up, all patients were able to return to sports without symptoms. Other authors' experience with athletes has been similar [91–94, 99–101].

The incidence of genu recurvatum following this injury is insignificant. The age at which the fracture occurs is a time when the tibial tubercle apophysis is still open and vulnerable but the proximal tibial physis is well on its way to closure [100, 101]. The exact incidence of the different types of acute tibial tubercle avulsion fracture is unknown. All previous series have been retrospective [91, 93, 95, 99, 101] and have reported a preponderance of type III injuries (30% to 75%, average 54%). Most type I fractures are treated nonoperatively and tend not to be reported, thereby falsely inflating the true proportion of reported type II and III injuries. Because of the significant forces involved in the injury (or in a fall after the fracture), associated intra-articular lesions such as ACL tears (partial or complete), medial collateral ligament injuries, and meniscal tears must be considered [91–94, 96–99, 101, 103]. In Bolesta and Fitch's series [91], two peripheral lateral meniscal tears were found. Falster and Hasselbalch [94] reported combined ACL,

superficial medial collateral ligament, and peripheral lateral meniscal tears in a 15-year-old long jumper.

In reported series, the incidence of preexisting Osgood-Schlatter disease ranged from 12% to 60%. Although the mechanism of injury in acute tibial tubercle avulsion fractures and Osgood-Schlatter disease is similar (i.e., traction forces across an immature junction), the rate and magnitude of loading are significantly different (Fig. 18–64). In Ogden and colleagues' series [102] of 14 patients with 15 acute tibial tubercle avulsion fractures, nine had Osgood-Schlatter changes, but in seven the changes were in the contralateral knee. Three patients with a fracture and roentgenographically evident Osgood-Schlatter disease had never been symptomatic before the fracture. Since the denominator of the equation, that is, the number of athletes with symptomatic or asymptomatic Osgood Schlatter disease but without tibial tubercle fracture, is unknown, there is not enough current documentation to recommend that all children with Osgood-Schlatter disease avoid jumping and deceleration sports for fear of tibial tubercle avulsion fracture. Perhaps patients who have persistent, symptomatic Osgood-Schlatter disease and are at the age just prior to tibial tubercle closure or are going through the peak height velocity phase of the adolescent growth spurt may need to curtail activity requiring powerful, rapid, eccentric quadriceps loading.

Anterior Knee Pain

Patellofemoral disorders in the pediatric and adolescent age group present a particular challenge because the unpredictable factor of growth (rate, intensity, magnitude, duration) is involved. The spectrum of such patellofemoral disorders ranges from instability due to congenital patellar dislocation or acute traumatic dislocation to the extremely common pain complaints about the anterior knee. Galen noted in 150 A.D., "The patella covers the condyles of the underlying bone in well suited depressions—some call this bone the knee cap, some the millstone." Anterior knee pain, especially during adolescence, is often perceived as a millstone about the treating orthopedist's neck. Complaints about the patellofemoral area have been called "the low back pain of knee surgeons." [162] Most past data concerning anterior knee complaints represent a series of mixed diagnoses and a broad spectrum of ages (usually adults), these problems often occur in patients following direct knee trauma [109, 113, 117, 120, 122, 128, 135, 149, 157, 160, 162, 189, 195, 212, 224–227]. This chapter will focus on the commonly encountered condition of anterior knee complaints in children and adolescents.

Budinger [115] in 1906 described fissures noted at surgery within the articular cartilage of the knee, particularly in the patella. He considered these fissures traumatic in origin and termed the condition "chondromalacia patella traumatica." In 13 of 15 patients who underwent excision of the involved articular cartilage, he noted satisfactory results (in general) in a very short follow-up. The term "chondromalacia patella" first appeared in published form in 1922 as used by Konig [162]. Karlson [162] credits Aleman with the first use of the term in his (Aleman's) laboratory as early as 1917. "Chondromalacia patella" was first used in the English literature in 1933 by Kulowski [167], who also attributed central patellar lesions to diminished blood flow in that zone. Among Budinger's original descriptions (Knorpelrisse) [115] was a report of one acute post-traumatic case that demonstrated a patellar subchondral hematoma. Owre [195] described the pain in the anterior knee due to pressure across the patellofemoral joint as being a "toothache-like pain."

During the past several decades, chondromalacia patella has been converted from a term connoting a gross pathologic observation at the time of surgery or autopsy [110, 131, 181] to an ill-defined clinical entity of anterior knee pain that is attributed to a deranged patellar articular surface. This knee ache commonly occurs during the teenage years, particularly in two types of patients, the first comprising active athletes and those involved in jumping or kneeling sports, and the second including nonathletic, inactive, often overweight adolescents, commonly girls.

Aleman [109] in 1928 used the term chondromalacia in a diagnosis of "chondromalacia post-traumatic patella" and referred to it as an articular lesion noted at surgery. He believed that the lesion was due to old trauma and found such patellar changes in one-third of 220 knees that had come to surgery for a variety of reasons. After reviewing 100 knees in adults at necropsy, Abernethy and colleagues [105] suggested that fibrillation of the medial central patellar facet was a universal finding in adults even in the third decade of life. Radin [201] observed similar findings at the time of knee arthrotomy and believed that such changes were asymptomatic and nonprogressive. Insall and colleagues [160] in 1976 assessed patients for evidence of patellar chondromalacic changes at the time of arthrotomy. Fifty percent of the patients in the group had a history of a direct blow to the knee. These latter authors' data, however, may be skewed and may not represent the true clinical picture of the symptomatic adolescent who usually has no history of significant direct knee trauma. Outerbridge [193] and Outerbridge and Dunlop [194] graded the articular surface characteristics. In this system zero is a normal surface; grade I has a change in articular luster; grade II has fissuring; grade III has fibrillation; and grade IV has subchondral bone erosion. Stougard [215], in an attempt to correlate physical findings with articular cartilage changes of the patella, studied 100 patients undergoing arthrotomy for articular disorders. Cartilaginous changes about the patella were noted in 50% of them. He was unable to correlate patellofemoral crepitus with such changes on the surface, and in most cases

335

articular surface changes were present in the absence of any positive preoperative physical signs. Fulkerson and Schutzer [141] referred to Stougard's work and noted that even gross articular surface patellar changes correlated poorly in their patients with symptoms (i.e., the opposite of pristine surfaces that have been indicted as sources of pain). In Fulkerson and Schutzer's review, only 13% of patients studied at surgery had evidence of gross articular surface changes on the patella. Goodfellow and colleagues [147, 148] noted that pathologic cartilage consisted of two types: one with age-dependent surface degradation that was usually asymptomatic, and the second with a basilar degeneration that became symptomatic and continued to progress to degenerative joint disease.

The true cause of this adolescent nontraumatic type of anterior knee pain is unknown. Examination of the synovium in patients with isolated anterior knee pain has proved it to be normal. Insall [157, 158] hypothesized that the majority of patients with such anterior knee pain have malalignment, and the malalignment rather than the articular surface abnormalities is the source of pain. The abnormal stresses that occur at the joint surface because of malalignment are thought to be the source of pain. Although this is an attractive thesis, no further specific data has been forthcoming to document this assertion. Goodfellow and colleagues [147, 148] hypothesized that anterior knee pain results from a basilar patellar cartilage lesion that interferes with the fibrous structure of the intermediate zone of collagen, which makes the subchondral osseous plates more sensitive to variations in compressive force. Darracott and Vernon-Roberts [122] believed that the initial changes in the patellar articular surface begin in the subchondral bone, and they attributed this process to changes in the bone's blood supply. Fulkerson and colleagues [136, 138] hypothesized that the primary symptoms about the anterior knee are caused by retinacular stresses. They have produced evidence in biopsies of the lateral retinaculum in patients with anterior knee pain and minor patellofemoral malalignment that showed retinacular nerve injury and histologic changes compatible with those seen in a Morton's interdigital neuroma (i.e., neurodemyelination and fibrosis (Fig. 18–65). Fulkerson and Hungerford [137] implicated an abnormal vastus lateralis insertion that produces excessive lateral tightness and increased pressure along the lateral patellar border as the cause of the "excessive lateral pressure syndrome."

Fairbank and associates [132] discussed mechanical factors affecting the incidence of knee pain in adolescents and young adults. They examined 446 patients aged 13 to 17, 136 of whom had suffered from anterior knee pain during the previous year. No differences in joint mobility, increased Q angle, knee valgus, and femoral neck anteversion were found in patients with and

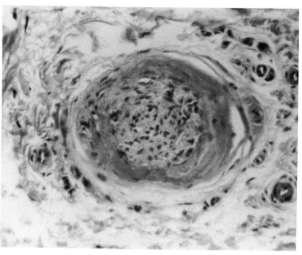

FIGURE 18–65
Retinacular nerve stress changes are hypothesized as a cause of anterior knee pain (Courtesy John Fulkerson, M.D.).

without anterior knee pain. The single differentiating point between symptomatic and asymptomatic patients was the increased level of enjoyment of sports participation in patients with symptoms compared with their symptom-free contemporaries. These authors concluded that chronic overload rather than faulty mechanics was the dominant factor in this group. Unfortunately, the tests used to assess the patellofemoral joint were static rather than dynamic. Unlike their study subjects, many patients with anterior knee complaints are semi-obese, nonathletic teens with little embracement of physical activity. In summary, many theories have been proposed to account for adolescent anterior knee pain, but no definitive proof has been forthcoming. The cause of this discomfort appears to be multi-factorial [190].

HISTORY AND PHYSICAL EXAMINATION

During history taking the patient often complains of vague, poorly localized anterior knee discomfort. When asked to indicate the focus of such discomfort, he or she encompasses the entire front of the knee with his or her hand, a sign that I call the "grab sign" (Fig. 18–66). I find this sign particularly helpful in differentiating this type of anterior knee pain from various other disorders in which the focus or discomfort is very specifically indicated. Patients commonly complain of discomfort following prolonged sitting (theater sign), with stair ascent and descent, and with increased levels of activity, although this last is an inconsistent symptom. They may complain of a feeling of locking of the knee, but on further questioning this turns out to be more of a feeling of catching or pseudolocking with no true mechanical

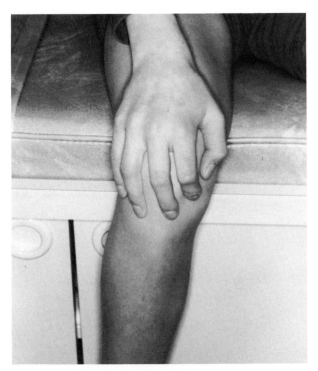

FIGURE 18–66
''Grab sign''—nonspecific localization of anterior knee pain.

block. This feeling may be associated with a sensation of knee instability and ''giving way,'' perhaps secondary to reflex quadriceps inhibition. Complaints of occasional swelling within the joint are common, although this is not often well documented by other observers. Some patients also complain of pain at the distal hamstrings. Anterior knee complaints are usually bilateral with varying intensity from side to side.

During evaluation of athletes, an accurate assessment of the training program is essential to be sure that overuse factors are not playing a significant role [185]. Running stadium steps, using exercise equipment for stair climbing, running up and down hills, performing deep squats with or without weights are all important stress factors at the patellofemoral joint [111, 134]. Previous knee injury or surgery and rehabilitation should be explored to understand better the starting point of such a patient's complaints. Program compliance may also be assessed. The knee may act as a target for somatization of complaints to avoid school, work, athletics, and so on, so functional versus true organic pathology must be kept in mind, especially in early adolescent patients. A multitude of vague nonanatomic complaints combined with incapacitating pain, especially of a burning type out of proportion to any injury or physical findings, should rapidly alert the physician to the possibility of reflex sympathetic dystrophy [104, 123]. An important cautionary finding in patients with adolescent knee pain is a parent (usually a mother) who talks more than the pa-

tient. The surgeon must be very wary of this combination.

Physical examination must be done with the patient appropriately dressed and not merely with the slacks rolled up above the knee or the skirt hiked above the patella. The physical examination must take into account the entire lower extremity in both stance and gait. Abnormal foot and ankle alignment may place undue stress on the knee resulting in knee pain, particularly in patients involved in sports requiring repetitive lower extremity stress (Fig. 18–67). It is essential to differentiate joint line tenderness from retinacular tenderness. Anterior joint line tenderness commonly occurs in patients with patellar disorders as opposed to the more often mid- to posterior joint line tenderness that is characteristic of most true meniscal pathology (Fig. 18–68). Quadriceps, hamstring, and calf muscle tone and definition should be compared with that of the opposite side. The physical examination should also provide a measure of the patient's ability to cooperate, interest in the problem, and capability of following directions, which are important in treatment protocols. A patient who is a true ''motor moron'' with limited or no kinesthetic sense or a truculent, misanthropic adolescent who will not join in an effort at improvement is often unmasked during this process. Gait, range of motion, muscle tone and bulk (Fig. 18–69), knee joint stability, patellar tracking stability, focal tenderness, and presence of effusion are assessed on physical examination [192]. ''Ordinary'' anterior knee pain produces no evidence of effusion, and tenderness is diffuse compared to that seen with a specific focal finding. Patellar tracking is best observed when the patient is seated and the knee is put through a complete passive and active range of motion. The phy-

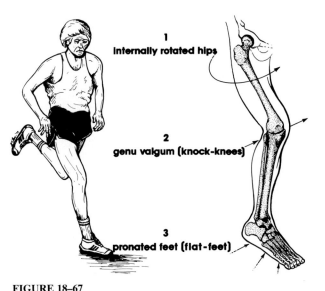

FIGURE 18–67
''Miserable malalignment syndrome,'' which can manifest itself as anterior knee pain.

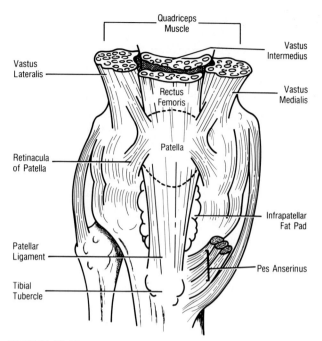

FIGURE 18–68
Patellar retinacular expansion to the anterior joint lines forming meniscopatellar ligaments.

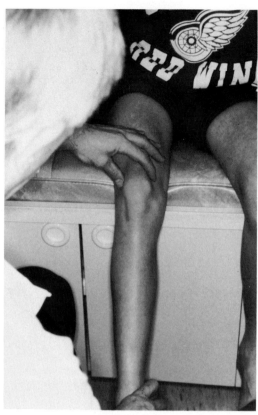

FIGURE 18–70
Direct examination of patellar tracking.

sician maintains specific, direct "en face" observation of the relationship between the patella and the femoral condyle (Fig. 18–70) [178]. Much has recently been made of the concepts of patellar tilt and patellar glide

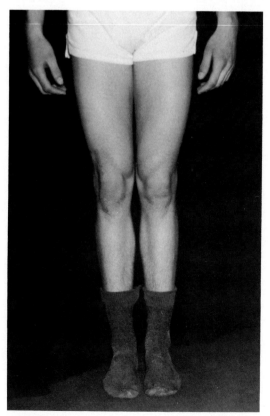

FIGURE 18–69
Note excellent quadriceps and calf definition in high-level athlete.

(Fig. 18–71) [164]. Although these are important components of patellar motion, normal values for these entities have not been agreed upon. The "normals" noted in the initial papers specifically referred to young adults. It must be remembered that the patella follows a toroidal course within the femoral groove. Its motion is not simply one of flexion-extension but more like a bobsled in a chute during its run.

Patellofemoral crepitus is not necessarily an indicator of knee pathology. Abernethy and colleagues [105], in reviewing 123 medical students under the age of 25, found asymptomatic patellofemoral crepitus in more than 60% of them. Only 29% of the patients had any previous transient patellofemoral discomfort, and only 3% had true chronic anterior knee pain. Articular surfaces are usually pristine in young patients with crepitus. The cause of such sounds in this age group remains obscure.

Attempts to elicit patellar tenderness when the patella is displaced laterally or medially while the knee is fully extended (Perkins sign) may be misleading in patients in whom synovitis is present and the synovium is trapped on the undersurface of the patella. It is usually the synovium that is painful and not the patellar surface. A variety of patellar compression tests with or without quadriceps contractions are often not reproducible and can produce significant discomfort in previously asymp-

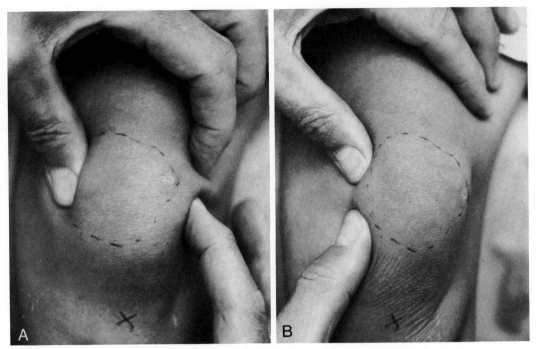

FIGURE 18–71
A, Patellar tilt—passive lateral elevation of the patella in 30 degrees of knee flexion. *B*, Patellar glide, (i.e., lateral or medial translation).

tomatic normal subjects. Excessive patellar mobility as evidenced by patient apprehension is commonly the first sign of patellar instability. Remote factors that can affect patellofemoral articulation range from excessive femoral or tibial rotation and abnormal foot and ankle mechanics, primarily excessive foot pronation, to the so-called miserable malalignment syndrome. Hip examination is essential because of referred pain from such hip disorders as Perthes disease or slipped capital femoral epiphysis. Because of the referred pathways, the pain may be misinterpreted as originating from the knee. It must be remembered that knee pain in a skeletally immature patient is hip pain until proven otherwise.

IMAGING

Standard roentgenographic views may be helpful. On a simple anteroposterior (AP) film, patellar size, location, and relationship to the femoral condyle are easily noted. Lateral knee views can be used to assess patella infera or patella alta [150, 159, 165, 221]. Unfortunately, all such views provide information in only a single plane. A variety of tangential skyline views have been suggested to ascertain the relationship between the patella and its femoral trochlear groove [127, 168, 169, 183]. Brattstrom [112] described the sulcus angle as an indicator of the relationship between the femoral condyle and the depth of the trochlea. Merchant and colleagues [183] described a technique in which the knee was in a different position of flexion and discussed the congru-

ence angle. If the apex of the patellar articular ridge is lateral to a central perpendicular line of the sulcus, the congruence angle is considered positive; if it is medial the angle is negative. In 200 knees in 100 control subjects, Merchant and associates noted an average congruence angle of minus 6 degrees with a significant standard deviation of 11 degrees. They believed a congruence angle of greater than 16 degree was abnormal at the 95% confidence limit. They noted no significant difference of the data in terms of gender, age, laterality, or patella alta. In patients with proven recurrent patellar dislocation an average congruence angle of plus 22 degrees was seen in 25 abnormal knees. Laurin and colleagues [168, 169] described a roentgen tangential view made with the knee flexed at 20 to 30 degrees with the patient supine (Fig. 18–72). A line between the femoral superior condyles and the margin of the lateral patellar facet formed the lateral patellofemoral angle which the authors found to be of diagnostic value in patients with patellar subluxation. The authors did not find this measurement helpful in patients who complained only of knee pain without a history of instability. They believed that the normal lateral patellar angle is also open laterally. In instances of abnormal patellar tilt, the angle opens medially, or the lines become parallel.

Unfortunately, most such axial patellar views are taken in the static situation whereas most patellar abnormalities occur in dynamic circumstances. Since positioning plays a major role in obtaining all of these views, reproducibility of the view may be difficult. Arthrography and arthroscopy of patellofemoral joints correlates

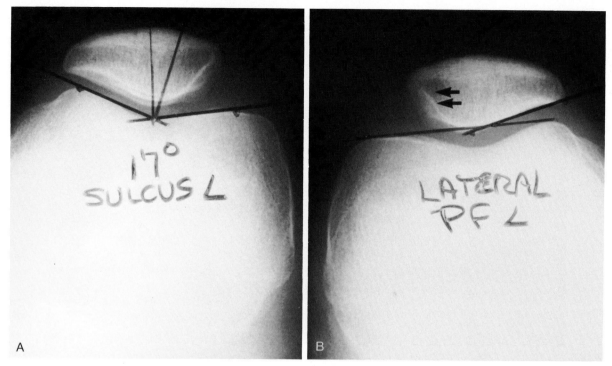

FIGURE 18–72
A, Congruence (sulcus angle). *B*, Lateral patellofemoral angle.

poorly with mechanical complaints in patients with anterior knee pain. Shellock and colleagues [210] reviewed kinematic MRI assessments of patellar stability using multiple sequential images at 5-degree increments of flexion ranging from 0 to 30 degrees. Such studies are merely computer simulations and manipulations of static images and have little to do with the true dynamic assessment of patellofemoral relationships. Although advantageous in terms of using nonionizing radiation and providing a view of the soft tissue and articular surface, MRI in this circumstance is certainly not to be considered dynamic because the test is done in a weight-bearing position with no functional force loading by the quadriceps. Maldague and Malghem [175, 176] suggest making a tangential view of the patella with the quadriceps relaxed and then a repeat view with the quadriceps contracted to assess the more dynamic relationships of the patella. Difficulty with positioning may limit the effectiveness of such views. Schutzer and colleagues [208] found no significant differences in radiographs taken with or without quadriceps contractions.

Delgado-Martins [125] reported the use of computer tomography to determine patellofemoral congruence in 50 patients, predominantly adolescents and young adults whose knees were examined in 10 to 15 degrees of flexion. He believed that CT scans had a much higher sensitivity and specificity for diagnosing minor patellar subluxation than standard Merchant or Laurin views. Fulkerson and colleagues [139, 140, 208, 209] and others [203] documented the use of CT scans of the patel-

lofemoral joint following lateral release or realignment procedures. These authors advocated the use of CT scans not as a routine test but as part of the information-gathering process in complex cases, especially those who have failed to improve following previous surgery. These authors specifically found it helpful to evaluate patellar tilt with or without subluxation [209]. They classified the views as type I, subluxation without tilt; type II, subluxation with tilt, and type III, tilt without subluxation.

Dye and colleagues [129], in a review of bone scans used to assess patellofemoral pain disorders in young adults, noted that a positive scan implied an altered homeostasis with increased osseous remodeling that may or may not necessarily be associated with changes in the knee articular cartilage surfaces. They emphasized that once the remodeling process is initiated it may be extended for a significant period of time (more than 6 months) before resolution occurs. A less favorable prognosis was indicated in scans that demonstrated diffuse uptake in the patella or femur. A negative scan, according to the authors, indicated that the pathology was likely to lie in the soft tissue areas about the knee rather than in the osseous patella.

In 1956, Wiles and associates [224] noted that "chondromalacia is a precursor of osteoarthritis." Later in the article they backed off somewhat from the stridency of this initial statement and stated that "chondromalacia sometimes progresses to osteoarthritis." Karlson [162] examined 71 adult males with anterior knee pain. At a follow-up ranging from 1 to 21 years, 10 of the knees were normal, 41 of the patients had mild knee complaints, and 16 had severe complaints. At the time of follow-up, only seven of the patients showed any evidence of radiographic degenerative changes of the patellar joint, none of which were severe. Karlson [162] and Darracott and Vernon-Roberts [122] attempted to analyze the natural history of anterior knee pain in young male military recruits. They found that the majority of patients continued to have some symptoms refererable to the patellofemoral joint. Unfortunately, in each of these series a significant number of patients had had previous knee surgery for meniscal or other lesions, so the studies were not truly assessments of the natural history of anterior knee pain. Goodfellow [145, 146] called chondromalacia a "mythical disease." He equated pain in the anterior knee in adolescents to that of a headache and suggested that arthroscopic intervention for this "condition" was no more rational than skull burr holes for a headache. He recommended instead that treatment attempts focus on establishing minor tracking abnormalities as potential sources of symptoms. At a 2- to 8-year follow-up of patients in Oxford, he noted that of those who had received no treatment at all, 94% still had some occasional mild knee complaints, but 49% had improved spontaneously, and only 13% ever required any analgesic medication [206]. As a primary management method, Goodfellow recommended reassuring the patient about the benignity of the disorder.

Once other sources of anterior knee pain have been ruled out, the physician is left with an ill-defined clinical entity that must be treated. The spectrum of suggested therapeutics ranges from nihilism to aggressive surgical intervention. In reported controlled series, nonoperative management has been extremely (75% to 90%) successful [111, 126, 133, 137, 138, 141, 142]. It must be remembered that nonoperative treatment does not mean no treatment.

The complaint of anterior knee pain in athletes is commonly a manifestation of overuse and a reflection of either training errors or sports equipment that produces unfriendly stresses at the patellofemoral joint [185]. Basic management protocol includes identification of risk factors, modification of risk factors, pain control, rehabilitation, and a maintenance program (see Chap. 8). Pain control can be achieved by a variety of medications and/or modalities such as contrast. Rehabilitation should proceed at a comfortable level with the principle of "relative rest" playing a major role. Further management should be directed toward sports-specific rehabilitation. Review and modification of training schedules and changes in lower extremity mechanics to improve the distribution of patellofemoral force have become the essence of most active nonoperative therapy proposals. Orthotics are used to control minor limb length inequality and abnormal foot and ankle mechanics, partic-

ularly pronation [134]. Improvement of quadriceps, hamstring, and gastrocnemius and soleus flexibility and strength balance are mainstays of nonoperative management. The rehabilitation prescription must be tailored individually, and a "cookbook" approach to anterior knee pain problems must be avoided. The patient must become an integral part of the treatment program, not just a passive observer. Continued participation in sports should be encouraged. A carte blanche excuse from physical education activities is frowned upon (Fig. 18–73). Coaches and physical education instructors must understand the ongoing therapy program and the patient's limits and needs.

Chronic patellofemoral complaints should not be treated with prolonged knee immobilization, which only leads to further patellofemoral joint fibrosis, loss of motion, and quadriceps and hamstring atrophy. Although the use of contrast modalities may be helpful for pain control, which will allow rehabilitation, their mechanism of action is not precisely understood in patellofemoral joint complaints, which are usually without evidence of signs of inflammation. Medications for the treatment of anterior knee disorders have been advocated by a number of authors [200, 204]. The effects of salicylate, both analgesic and anti-inflammatory, make it the drug of choice for initial management of anterior knee pain in a nonacute, nontraumatic setting. The use of nonsteroidal anti-inflammatory agents for anterior knee pain has not been looked at specifically in a controlled series, particularly in skeletally immature patients. Varied responses to these agents (e.g., a patient's condition may respond favorably to one of a family of medications and not to another) aggravate attempts to carry out such controlled evaluations. Intra-articular injection of steroids for diffuse knee complaints in children is absolutely contraindicated.

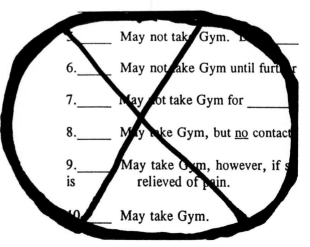

FIGURE 18–73
Athletic (and other nonsedentary) activity should be encouraged.

A variety of taping and strapping techniques have been suggested. The most popular technique recently proposed is that of McConnell [179], who advocates patellar strapping as a means of unloading patellar forces and allowing enhanced action of the vastus medialis obliquus. The taping is only part of the overall management program, which includes muscle strengthening and improvement of flexibility. McConnell claims a 90% rapid response rate with persistent good results at follow-up at 6 months. No data are presented to document the effect of taping on patellar position by objective measurements, nor are any data given that demonstrate enhancement of the vastus medialis obliquus or other portion of the quadriceps function in response to tape.

A variety of knee ''braces'' have been proposed to manage anterior knee pain. Most are of a sleeve design with inserts or straps to control patellar motion. Levine and Splain [170] describes the use of a infrapatellar strap to control anterior knee symptoms and claimed a 77% success rate in 57 adults. All patients had positive results on patellar compression tests at 20 degrees of knee flexion. With the knee extended and the patellar strap in place, patellar elevation was claimed to occur on lateral roentgenograms. The amount of elevation and the frequency with which it occurred while using this technique were not noted, nor was the reproducibility of the data recorded. Palumbo [196] used a ''dynamic patellar brace'' to treat patellofemoral symptoms in 62 patients with mixed causes of patellofemoral disorders. He claimed a 93% success rate. The exact mechanism of action of such a patellar brace is unknown. Whether the patellar ''stabilizing'' brace truly stabilizes the patella has not been objectively documented. A significant placebo effect must be considered in these workers' assessment. Lysholm and colleagues [174] attempted to evaluate the effect of patellar braces on quadriceps function as measured by isokinetic quadriceps testing. They claimed improved (10% or more) quadriceps output in 13 of 19 patients who were less than 30 years old. Unfortunately, the test was carried out at extremely slow speeds and in nonweight-bearing positions; the rate of loading was not a normal functional rate and was nowhere near the rate required for athletic pursuits.

At times of mild recurrence of symptoms, the patient must be reminded of the need to continue maintenance program emphasizing hamstring and quadriceps flexibility and strength. Return to this program usually allows resolution of symptoms. If the patient is unresponsive to a well-monitored program with which he or she is compliant, one must question the accuracy of the diagnosis and search for other causes of symptoms, including physiatric and nonorthopedic sources of pain. It must be remembered that during exercise training, effective muscle use becomes a function of limb position, limb segment velocity, joint angle, and type of contraction (e.g., concentric, eccentric).

Quadriceps exercises that incorporate long arch extension should be avoided because they involve excessive loading forces across the patellofemoral articulation (Fig. 18–74) [106, 107, 144, 151, 154, 172, 191, 218, 219, 222]. Kaufer [163] analyzed patellofemoral forces during isokinetic quadriceps exercises and showed that forces of up to five times body weight or 10 times the normal patellar force generated by walking on level ground occur during the exercise when loading occurred over 70 degrees of knee flexion. Full squat exercises with free weights or use of a weight machine requiring hyperflexion and rapid extension of the knee should be avoided because they generate abnormally high patellofemoral joint reaction forces.

In DeHaven and colleagues' [123] group of 100 consecutive college athletes with anterior knee pain (half of whom had a history of recurrence of subluxation), a four-phase treatment program was advocated, consisting of (1) symptom control, (2) isometric quadriceps and hamstring exercise, (3) gradual running, and (4) a maintenance program. Phase one, symptom control, was accomplished by eliminating or reducing activity using the concept of relative rest. Anti-inflammatory medications were used for 3 to 4 weeks for pain control, and ambulatory aids or brief periods of immobilization were carried out as needed. Once symptoms were under control, eccentric strengthening of the quadriceps and hamstrings was instituted using a gradual progressive resistance exercise (PRE) program (three sets of 10 repetitions daily) during the following 5 to 6 weeks (Fig. 18–75). Use of an exercise bike and running was prescribed when the patient was able to lift 30 pounds without difficulty with knee extension. The authors emphasized the need for a continued maintenance program with specific exercise of the quadriceps at least three times weekly. They reported full return of unrestricted activity in two-thirds of their patients. Twenty-three percent had mild restriction, and only 11% were unable to return to their previous levels of athletic activity.

Chondromalacia appears to be a disorder that awaited the invention of the arthroscope [104, 130, 143, 180]. In a prescient statement in 1933, Kulowski [167] noted, ''the arthroscope, an instrument designed for the direct visualization of joints . . . should gain a wider clinical application.'' He reported three cases of arthroscopically excised abnormal articular patellar cartilage and subchondral bone. The arthroscope has become a major factor in the diagnosis and treatment of patellofemoral disorders. Because gross changes were noted on the patellar surface at the time of arthroscopy, patellar surface shaving and trimming enjoyed a vogue in the 1970s and 1980s [186]. A great number of arthroscopic mechanical articular surface debriders of various designs were developed. The obvious simplicity of the procedure and an eagerness to remove abnormal appearing tissue led to the widespread use of arthroscopy including bilateral

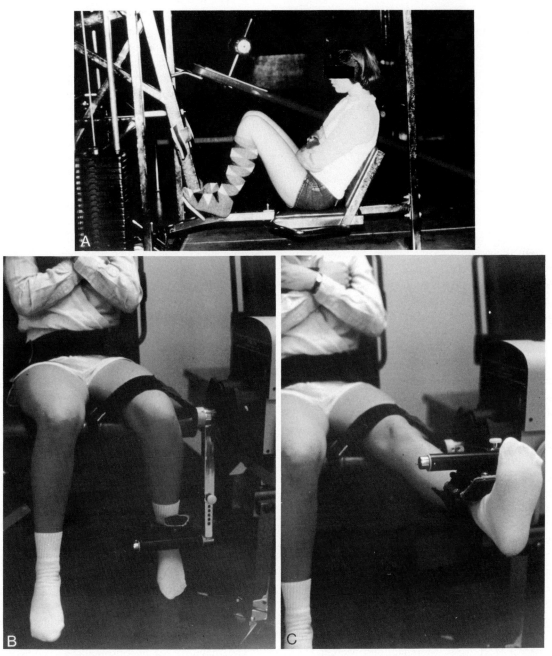

FIGURE 18–74
A–C, Excessive forces from high compressive loads may cause enough symptoms to limit a treatment phase.

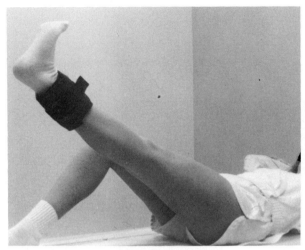

FIGURE 18–75
PRE programs with straight leg raising exercises are usually well tolerated in the initial treatment phase.

simultaneous knee arthroscopy, which had not previously been used. The thesis behind such articular cartilage removal was that by debridement of such projections of fibrillated tissue, breakdown products of this cartilage were eliminated and a subsequent synovial response avoided. Other authors emphasized that shaving provided an inexact way of removing articular debris and that only formal excision of the cartilaginous lesion to subchondral bone was appropriate for pathologic surfaces. Marks and Bentley [178] suggested that the results of patellar shaving were unreliable.

Lateral retinacular release hypothetically allows a decreased load on the vastus medialis obliquus and improves dynamic stability within the patellofemoral joint in cases of minimal lateral malalignment [153–155, 207]. Roentgenographic studies of preoperative and postoperative use have shown no effect of retinacular release on patellar location, tilt, or translation when the procedure is done for anterior knee pain alone without evidence of maltracking [209]. In patients with lateral patellar tilt and possible patellar lateral facet overload, lateral release has been noted to improve patellar tilt on postoperative roentgenograms. Lateral retinacular release became a popular surgical approach because of its simplicity, particularly when it was used with arthroscopic control [153, 164]. Merchant and Mercer [182] reported 85% good to excellent results in an earlier series of young patients undergoing nonarthroscopic lateral retinacular releases. They cautioned that the procedure should be used only in patients with incongruence of the patellofemoral mechanism and not in those with normal roentgenograms who complain only of anterior knee pain. They stated that in this latter group the results of lateral release are unpredictable. Micheli and Stanitski

[184] reported a series of patients undergoing open retinacular release, emphasizing that only 6.9% of patients with patellofemoral symptoms during the study period required surgical treatment, the remaining 92 + % responding well to nonoperative management.

Gecha and Torg [143] reported improved results following lateral retinacular release in patients without ligamentous laxity or excessive "tightness of lateral structures." Similar findings were noted by Micheli and Stanitski [184] Doucette and Goble [126] showed that a 6-week rehabilitation program emphasizing quadriceps flexibility and strength training improved the patellofemoral angle in those who demonstrated good results on follow-up. In a prospective study by O'Neil and colleagues [191] an isometric quadriceps exercise program was used to manage anterior patellofemoral discomfort. Resolution of symptoms occurred in 80% of patients who had normal lower extremity and knee alignment. In skeletally immature patients, a change in congruence angle of greater than 5 degrees was noted following this exercise program. Whether this change is statistically significant has not yet been documented. Demonstration of improved quadriceps strength may be a nonspecific finding in management of patients with patellofemoral discomfort. Moller and colleagues [187, 188] showed that despite improvements in quadriceps strength in all patients, only 15% of patients with subluxation experienced diminution of symptoms, and 28% of patients with anterior knee pain alone benefited from the exercises. In both groups, no change in the vastus medialis or vastus lateralis was noted on electromyography in response to strength training.

The long-term effect of nonoperative treatment programs (i.e., longer than 2 years) have not been well substantiated.

Tibial tubercle elevation in an attempt to diminish patellofemoral contact forces is contraindicated in skeletally immature patients [152, 177]. Patellectomy for anterior knee pain alone should be condemned, especially in skeletally immature patients. Diminution in quadriceps force and abnormal knee cosmesis are sinister sequelae of patellectomy [108, 217, 220]. Decreases in function of the quadriceps following patellectomy are commonly associated with pain, quadriceps weakness, and progressive difficulty in performing routine daily activities, much less athletics.

The diagnosis of chondromalacia patella is nonspecific, and the term should be abandoned. If the patient has pain at the anterior knee, then that is what it should be called, i.e., *anterior knee pain*, until a satisfactory etiology is established. The use of the term *chondromalacia patella* for complaints about the anterior knee is as nonspecific as *internal derangement* is for intra-articular disorders. As Radin has suggested, "Let's stop calling it chondromalacia patella" [198, 201, 202]. Diagnostic ef-

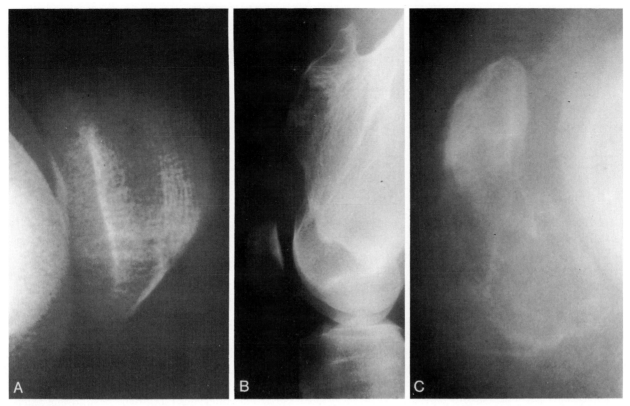

FIGURE 18–76
Anterior knee pain caused by (*A*) patellar stress fracture, (*B*) osteochondroma—quadriceps mechanism impingement, and (*C*) patellar aneurysmal bone cyst.

forts should be focused on ruling out specific causes of pain (i.e., pain secondary to patellar instability, intra-articular disorders, overuse, malalignment, referred pain, and so on) (Fig. 18–76). Diligence in history taking, physical examination, and various imaging studies is required. Not all knee pain that is unexplained should be written off as chondromalacia patella.

Anterior knee pain must be considered idiopathic until the true etiology of such pain is known. In the recent past, chondromalacia patella has been overdiagnosed and overtreated. All diagnostic efforts must be brought to bear to discover the true cause of anterior knee pain [114, 161, 166, 197, 199, 205, 216]. Care must be taken to diagnose patients with underlying reflex sympathetic dystrophy, especially in its early stages. Use of the term chondromalacia as a diagnosis for anterior knee pain should be eliminated because of its lack of specificity. Excessive treatment should be avoided. Nonoperative management using a well-designed and well-monitored therapy program allows resolution of symptoms in the

great majority of patients. The diagnosis of anterior knee pain should not be made arthroscopically. An invasive procedure such as arthroscopy should play a minor role in the management of this condition, especially in light of the fact that the highest complication rate among all arthroscopic procedures occurs in those associated with patellofemoral surgery [116, 124, 156, 173, 211, 213, 214, 228]. The most important factor in the management and rehabilitation of patients with this condition is reassurance of the patient and family of the nonfatal nature of these complaints. In athletes participating in sports with high-demand repetitive tasks requiring deceleration, acceleration, and jumping, modification of the training schedule, participation in a rehabilitation program, and an understanding of the nature of the condition will go a long way toward allowing the athlete to continue to participate. There is little evidence that adolescent anterior patellofemoral pain leads to the development of progressive articular malacic changes, early joint senescence, or patellofemoral arthritis.

Patellar Instability

Acute patellar instability is a dramatic event. It has been suggested that Casey (of popular Mudville strike-out fame) may have suffered from an acute patellar dislocation that led to such batting ineptitude that his name is associated with eternal ignominy in the sports world [273].

Patellar instability is a common source of sports disability, particularly in sports requiring jumping or rapid changes of direction. Little has been written specifically about noncongenital [325, 326] or nondevelopmental (e.g., Down's syndrome) patellar instability in children and adolescents. Most data on this topic are incorporated into series that include older populations. Patellar instability presents a spectrum ranging from minimal mal-tracking to gross and obvious loss of patellofemoral congruence (Fig. 18–77). This mal-tracking may be congenital, acquired from conditions such as Down's syndrome or Ehlers-Danlos disease, or acquired secondary to acute trauma. The mechanism of injury, frequency of occurrence, and resultant disability should be taken into account to allow the diagnosis and treatment to be specific.

In the literature, the terms malalignment and instability are commonly used interchangeably. *Malalignment* should be considered an abnormal relationship between the patella and its associated soft tissue and bony surroundings throughout the course of knee motion. *Instability* is usually manifest only at certain points within the range of motion when abnormal alignment occurs.

Initial patellar dislocations may be classified as acute and indirect following deceleration or change of direction or acute and direct following direct percussion from sports equipment or an opponent's body. Recurrent patellar instabilities can be classified as initial recurrence, second recurrence, or, after three episodes, chronic. The magnitude of force needed to precipitate the instability and the interval between episodes (with associated disability) need to be considered when treatment decisions are made (Table 18–1).

The patella follows a toroidal path (i.e., rotation, translation, and flexion) along its three axes in its normal course through the femoral sulcus. In the great majority of cases, dislocation is lateral. Medial dislocations are rare, and the intra-articular type of patellar dislocation is extremely rare [239, 261]. Anatomic factors purported to predispose patients to patellar instability include patella alta, generalized joint hypermobility, increased Q angle, increased femoral anteversion, increased external tibial torsion, abnormal iliotibial band attachments, genu valgum, genu recurvatum, femoral condylar hypoplasia, or a combination of these [229, 234, 240, 244, 249, 262, 271, 280, 282, 284, 286, 288, 290, 291, 299, 303, 307, 311, 312, 334].

Floyd and colleagues [260] hypothesized that patellar instability was due to a primary quadriceps defect that allowed recurrent dislocation and instability to occur. Among 12 patients, 11 had significant joint hypermobility, and these authors felt that this predisposed them to instability. Carter and Sweetnam [244], Heywood [279], and Beighton and Horan [234] all noted increased patellar instability in patients with increased generalized ligamentous laxity.

Jeffreys [288] reported cases of recurrent patellar dislocation due to an abnormal lateral band of the iliotibial tract in children. Recurrent patellar dislocation due to an abnormal iliotibial band had been well described previously by Ober [307, 308]. Ober's physical examination test should be done on all patients with recurrent patellar dislocation to search for such abnormal patellar-iliotibial tract connections.

Patellofemoral dysplasias present a variety of signs and symptoms associated with this disorder. In reviewing the use of CT scans before and after lateral retinacular release, Fulkerson and associates [263, 320] found

TABLE 18–1
Classification of Patellar Instability

Onset	Mechanism	Frequency	Interval
Acute	Direct	First episode	Daily
	Indirect	Initial recurrence	Weekly
	Major force	Second recurrence	Monthly
	Minor force	Chronic	Yearly

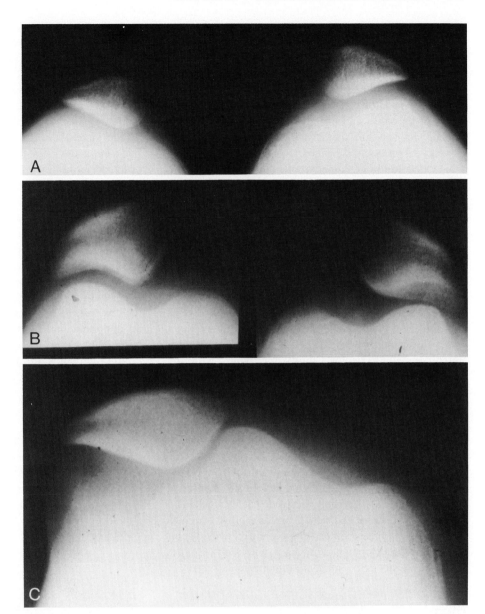

FIGURE 18–77
A–C, Spectrum of patellar instability ranging from mild dysplasia and maltracking to acute dislocation.

that lateral release was satisfactory for patients who demonstrated abnormal tilt only, without evidence of patellar subluxation. Hawkins and colleagues [277], in reviewing acute patellar dislocation in 27 patients, found that patients with abnormal patellar configurations, patellar malalignment, or a history of previous instability symptoms were prone to recurrence at a rate of 30% to 50% with persistent symptoms, redislocation, and pain.

Mariani and Caruso [299] showed that the vastus medialis and the vastus lateralis had equal amounts of activity between 0 and 30 degrees of flexion. A slight difference in these muscles was noted between 30 and 90 degrees of flexion, the lateralis being relatively more active in patients with normal knees. In seven of eight patients with patellar subluxation, EMG of the vastus medialis preoperatively showed a fall in activity compared with the lateralis over the entire range of flexion,

but an especially significant drop-off occurred between full extension and 30 degrees of flexion. Following the Elmslie-Trillat repair, EMG studies in seven of the eight patients had returned to normal. The authors surmised that the vastus medialis dysfunction was secondary to previous static alterations in the extensor mechanism that produced an insufficiency in the vastus medialis, which then added to the viscious cycle of patellar instability. Based on histochemical analysis and EMG evidence in patients with recurrent patellar dislocation, Floyd and associates [260] found a predominance of abnormal type 2C fibers in eight of nine patients. Three of six patients studied electromyographically had normal conduction velocities but abnormal EMG tracings, two of the three showing evidence of a myopathy. Eleven of twelve patients had generalized ligamentous laxity, and the authors suggested that a soft tissue and perhaps myopathic component existed in patients with recurrent patellar dislocations. Whether these changes were primary or secondary was not determined.

Patellar subluxation has been noted following excision of a medial patellar plica [236], the hypothesis being that the plica allowed a tethering effect on the medial aspect of the knee, and once released, the medial-lateral balance was lost and lateral maltracking occurred in the 12-year-old cheerleader. Limbird [295] reported patellar subluxation following a medial plica release. He hypothesized that this subluxation resulted from the loss of a medial tether that allowed further lateral patellar translation.

In a consecutive group of 15 adolescents operated on for recurrent patellar dislocation the vastus medialis insertion of the patella was compared to the insertion in 130 cadaver knees, Outerbridge [194] reported that the vastus medialis fibers inserted into the upper half of the medial patellar ridge in the cadaveric knees. In patients with recurrent dislocation, only 25% of the fibers had a similar insertion. He felt that the abnormal insertion affected the medialis vector's ability to provide a tethering counterforce to lateral displacement. Based on his dissections, Outerbridge was among the first to suggest a vastus medialis transfer for treatment of recurrent patellar instability. Such muscle changes may have been due to recurrence of the dislocation with tearing of the vastus connection and changes in its angle.

Hvid and associates [284] questioned the role of patella alta and its association with a flat, poorly developed femoral trochlea. They hypothesized that the lack of a constant presence of the patella in the normal trochlea provides less stimulation and therefore diminished femoral sulcus development compared with normal. This ''chicken versus egg'' quandary remains unanswered.

HISTORY AND PHYSICAL EXAMINATION

Evaluation consists of three phases: history, physical examination, and appropriate imaging and other studies. Hughston [282, 283] championed the concept of patellar subluxation as part of the differential diagnosis of patients with knee pain. More than two decades ago he emphasized the role of patellar instability as a source of such pain, particularly medial pain, and suggested that patellar instability be considered a diagnosis rather than the (at that time) all too common isolated diagnosis of a torn medial meniscus. The patient presents with a complaint of the knee ''giving way,'' often despite minimal precipitating factors. One must carefully assess the circumstances in which the initial instability occurred including the magnitude of force required. A history of injections into the thigh should be sought because they

may produce quadriceps fibrosis and a secondary tether. A family history may reveal such heritable conditions as nail-patella syndrome or Ehlers-Danlos syndrome with patella parva or hyperlaxity and subsequent patellar instability. Underlying conditions such as cerebral spasticity, Down's syndrome, significant congenital leg length inequality, and so on are pertinent historical points.

The patient's complaints of giving way and locking must be considered to rule out the presence of intra-articular loose bodies as sequelae of articular surface injury resulting from previous dislocations. It should be remembered that meniscal pathology may coexist with patellar disorders. The same forces (deceleration/rotation) that produce patellar dislocation may produce an associated anterior cruciate ligament injury in which the ligamentous instability is the source of the patient's complaint of giving way (Fig. 18–78).

Previous methods of treatment and compliance with that program need to be assessed. The patient should be an important part of the rehabilitation effort and not a passive observer. Precipitating factors resulting from training demands are also important. Acute patellar instability that occurs during a sport session may be due to quadriceps fatigue with resultant inability to generate appropriate vectors to ensure normal patellar anatomic tracking.

The patient's cooperation during physical examination varies according to the severity of the instability event and the patient's comfort. Associated syndromes should be looked for in terms of the patient's size, upper extremity changes, facial morphology, nail bed changes, and so on (Fig. 18–79). Generalized ligamentous laxity should be evaluated (Fig. 18–80). The entire lower ex-

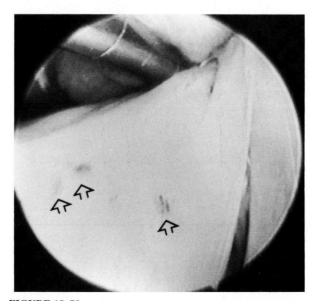

FIGURE 18–78
Anterior cruciate ligament intraligamentous hemorrhage in patient with acute patellar dislocation.

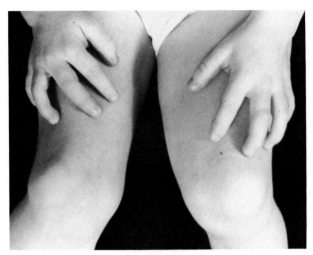

FIGURE 18–79
Patellar instability in a 3-year-old with multiple epiphyseal dysplasia.

tremity should be assessed in regard to stance and gait. Muscle bulk and tone of the quadriceps, hamstrings, and gastrocnemius should be determined using the opposite normal side (if present) as a control. Following an acute injury, an effusion may or may not be present. Diffuse swelling about the knee resulting from a capsular tear after a major patellar dislocation allows dispersal of a

hemarthrosis throughout the soft tissues of the anterior and posterior thigh.

Quadriceps retinacular tenderness should be looked for not only along the medial patellar edge but also along the quadriceps-adductor junction, which may be the site of a rent in the vastus medialis obliques. Range of motion of the hip, knee, and ankle should be part of the examination. Both active and passive patellar tracking (if patient comfort allows) should be assessed bilaterally along with patellar glide, patellar tilt, and Q angle (Fig. 18–81). True normative data are not available for tilt and glide, which must be considered in context of the opposite knee [291]. The best way to assess the true tracking of the patellar mechanism clinically is to sit in front of the patient as he or she takes the knee through a full active range of motion.

Acute patellar instability is a memorable event to the patient and serves as the source of the apprehension sign (attributed to Fairbanks [256]), a negative feeling generated by attempted or actual dislocation (Fig. 18–82). The patient will stop the overvigorous examiner from laterally translating the patella because he or she recalls the discomfort caused by this motion. Joint line tenderness medially and laterally usually occurs anteriorly in patients with patellar disorders.

IMAGING

Initial imaging begins with standard roentgen views, i.e., AP, lateral, skyline, and tunnel views. It must be appreciated that these are static examinations used to rule out broad aberrations of patellar location (alta or

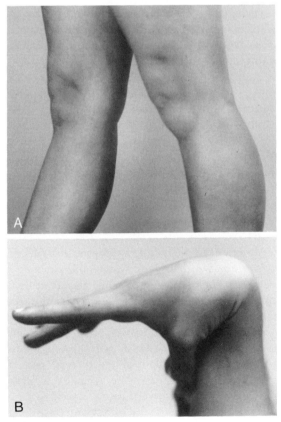

FIGURE 18–80
A and B, Generalized ligamentous laxity in a 14-year-old girl with recurrent patellar dislocations.

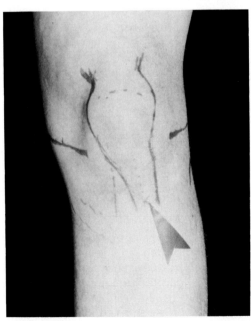

FIGURE 18–81
Increased Q angle due to tibial tubercle lateral development.

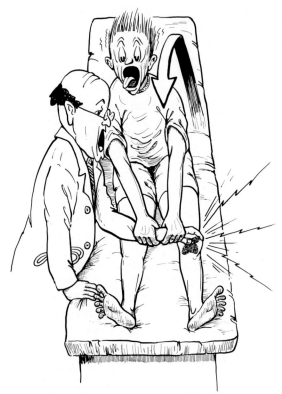

FIGURE 18–82
Apprehension sign: Patient anxiety due to awareness of unpleasantness associated with patellar dislocation.

infera), size (hypoplasia, "parva"), and morphology (multipartite) [255, 294]. Following injury, osteochondral fragments may or may not be seen on routine views. If such fragments are suspected, oblique views may be helpful (Fig. 18–83). Ossification within the medial retinaculum in chronic cases is evidence of a previous patellar-quadriceps mechanism insult (Fig. 18–84). These changes represent an avulsion of the medial retinaculum with subsequent ossification. Associated sources of pain resulting from bipartite patella, Sinding-Larsen-Johanssen disease, and Osgood-Schlatter disease may also be assessed in standard views (Fig. 18–85). Schutzer and colleagues [320] noted an inability to demonstrate malalignment consistently using routine roentgenograms despite an excellent history and physical examination findings compatible with instability. They suggested using CT scans with the knee in less than 20 degrees of flexion to document further patellofemoral malalignment.

Inoue and co-workers [285] emphasized the sensitivity and specificity of CT scanning in the evaluation of subluxation in extension. The CT study was clearly superior to routine roentgenography using a variety of patellar views. The articular surface as well as quadriceps and hamstring bulk can be evaluated by CT scans. MRI is helpful for evaluating the articular surface to detect osteochondral fragments or injury and provides information about damage to the menisci or ligaments.

Merchant and colleagues [304] described a roentgen technique used to assess patellofemoral alignment. They suggest a 45-degree flexed knee view with the patient supine. The roentgenogram is then used to construct a congruence angle, which measures the relationship of the patellar articular ridge to the intracondylar sulcus. These authors suggested that a lateral patellar angle of more than 16 degrees was abnormal. They felt that the proposed view offered improved analysis of the patellofemoral joint compared with previous views that required increased amounts of knee flexion. Roentgenographic and other imaging findings must be correlated with the physical examination findings to permit an appropriate choice of correction.

In complex cases, other tests may be required to aid in diagnosis [322] (Fig. 18–86). EMG and nerve conduction studies may help to rule out a quadriceps defect resulting from neural or primary muscle disease. Skin biopsy may be useful to evaluate abnormal collagen metabolism such as occurs in Ehlers-Danlos conditions. A glucose tolerance test may be required to rule out diabetes mellitus involving an associated femoral neuropathy and quadriceps weakness.

Assessment of treatment efficacy is difficult because evaluation of most series shows that they were not pure patient populations (i.e., a single problem treated in an isolated manner). Most series include a mixture of diagnoses including anterior knee pain alone, "mild to moderate" subluxation, acute dislocation, and dislocation in various stages of chronicity with previous treatments including surgery and rehabilitation efforts. Data in skeletally immature patients and the subsequent course of operative and nonoperative management with long-term follow-up are extremely limited [293]. Most data on skeletally immature patients have been lost in large series of primarily young adults, and it is impossible to assess their specific outcomes.

Many authors report good to excellent postoperative results in management of patellar instability in the short term, but a marked drop-off in patellar stability occurs with longer term follow-up [231, 241, 247, 250, 253, 258, 264, 265, 275, 279, 289, 296, 309, 313]. In most reported series follow-up time is extremely short, particularly considering the young age of the patients. The patients' demands both vocationally and avocationally are usually not specifically addressed in regard to sports demands.

In discussing the natural history of patellar instability in 1952, MacNab [296] noted that short-term results were rather good regardless of the type of procedure used. Longer term outcomes were generally disappointing. He suggested that surgery be done early to prevent patellar instability leading to subsequent degenerative disease. In his series of surgical procedures performed for patellar instability in adults, a significant number of patients had severe degenerative joint disease in the knee

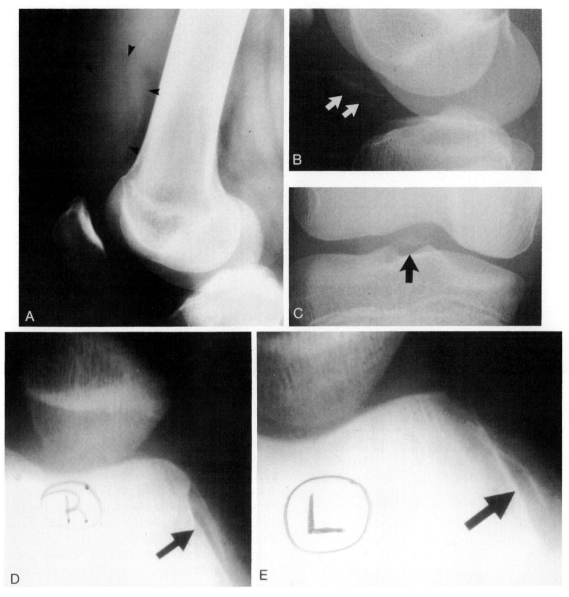

FIGURE 18–83

A, Large effusion associated with patellar dislocation with osteochondral fracture. *B* and *C,* Loose bodies after patellar dislocation. *D* and *E,* Osteochondral fragments following patellar dislocations 1 year apart.

at sites other than the patella. Many of the dislocations in his series were secondary to direct patellar trauma. Cash and Hughston [245] reviewed 103 patients who had had an acute primary dislocation and divided them into two groups. Patients in group I had physical signs in the opposite knee that the authors felt would predispose the knee to patellar dislocation whereas the second group (group II) had no evidence of such a predisposition on the opposite side. In the first group 52% of patients had a good result with nonoperative management. Those in group II had a 75% excellent nonoperative result. Although the authors suggest that nonoperative treatment of acute primary dislocation produced good results, only half of the patients in group I followed

such a course. Their series was somewhat unique in that it had a significantly higher number of males than females, the reverse of most previous reports.

In their series from the Mayo Clinic, Cofield and colleagues [248], in a retrospective review, reported on 50 patients with an acute initial patellar dislocation who had been managed nonoperatively. Forty-four percent of the patients had recurrences of the problem. If return to full activity is considered the mark of success, 52% of the patients were failures with this primary treatment. In a study of 81 knees by Crosby and Insall [251], the authors compared 26 adults treated nonoperatively for recurrent patellar dislocation with 55 adults treated operatively by tibial tubercle transfer augmented by cap-

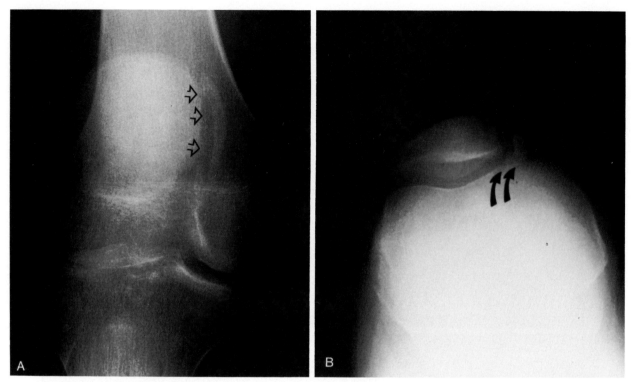

FIGURE 18–84
A and *B*, Medial patellar retinacular ossification resulting from repetitive patellar dislocations.

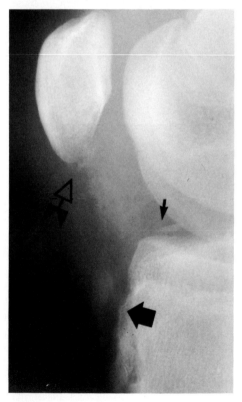

FIGURE 18–85
Intra-articular loose body (small arrow) following patellar dislocation. Note concomitant Osgood-Schlatter (large solid arrow) and Sinding-Larsen-Johanssen (open arrow) changes.

sular reefing. In the nonsurgical group, dislocations became less frequent with advancing age. Twenty percent of the patients who had undergone tibial tubercle transfer required further operative procedures. These authors suggested that patellar realignment ". . . should be recommended with caution. The patient should be managed conservatively if possible."

In a review from the Hospital of Sick Children in Toronto, McManus and Rang [302] reported on 33 children with acute patellar dislocations. Three patients underwent immediate surgery for removal of osteochondral fragments. The remainder were treated with joint aspiration and a cylinder cast. At follow-up (ranging from 6 to 61 months, average 31 months), 11 patients were asymptomatic, 10 were symptomatic, 7 required operative stabilization of the quadriceps mechanism, and 5 were lost to follow-up. Most of the patients had roentgenographic evidence of patellofemoral dysplasia. The authors stated that they could not accurately predict which knee would redislocate but concluded that most likely one of the six patients would redislocate and two in six in any group with patellar dislocation would occasionally experience patellar instability at sports. Twelve of the patients had had previous dislocations on the same side, so this series did not include only initial dislocations. Only 40% of the patients were considered asymptomatic. Sport demands and participation were not specifically assessed in this study.

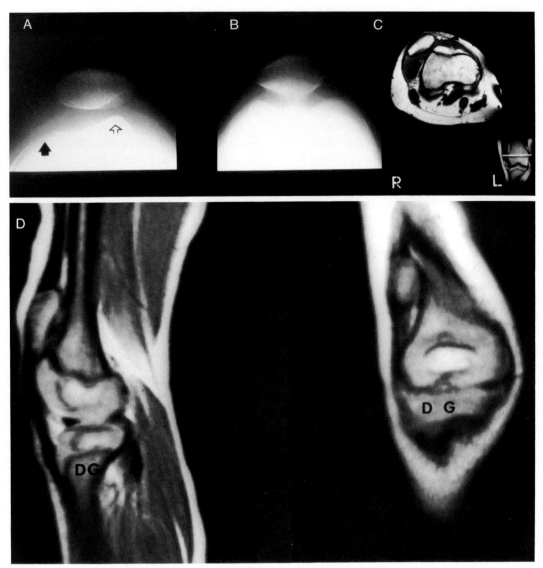

FIGURE 18–86
A and *B*, Patellar and femoral trochlear dysplasia. *C*, MRI showing patellar dislocation and retinacular attenuation (solid arrow). *D*, MRI of 20-month-old child with congenital patellar dislocation. Note superior and lateral position of patella and quadriceps mechanism.

In a unique study from Sweden, Arnbjornsson and and associates [231] reviewed the natural history of recurrent patellar dislocation and reported results in adult patients with bilateral disease who had undergone only a unilateral surgical procedure. The authors concluded that although the initial response to surgery in these young adults was satisfactory, the long-term results demonstrated that the operated knees were clinically worse and showed a higher incidence of degenerative disease. In a commentary on the paper, Jackson [287] pointed out the marked variability of operative techniques, age at surgery, and postoperative rehabilitation techniques that were variables in the study. He suggested that three groups with patellar instability should be distinguished. Lateral subluxation in extension was initially thought to be rare [252] but actually is extremely common in pa-

tients with childhood and adolescent patellar instability. The instability occurs between 0 and 30 degrees of flexion, and once the knee is past this zone, patellar femoral congruency occurs. Current roentgenographic techniques are unable to appreciate this type of instability because the views are taken in various stages of increased flexion. Clinical examination, however, easily demonstrates this instability, which is caused by quadriceps malalignment and will not be cured by lateral retinacular release. Combined lateral release and soft tissue reefing medially may produce short-term benefit, but with further growth and development, the instability will recur.

The second group of patients includes those with subluxation in flexion, which will be manifest on standard radiographic views for patellar instability, especially as patellar tilt. In these patients, lateral release will help to improve patellar tilt and should be incorporated as part of the reconstructive procedure. In the third group of patients, tilt plus lateral translation occur in flexion, and more complex reconstruction is required.

As patients age, many show evidence of patellar instability but have no gross evidence of patellar maltracking. Fortunately, these patients constitute a small group, with which generalized ligamentous laxity is often associated. In addition to surgical correction, prolonged rehabilitation as well as bracing may be required, especially during sports.

The first report of knee bracing for patellar instability was recorded by Pearson [310], an English surgeon who in 1884 fabricated a "knee cage." Patellar braces have been advocated to manage a variety of patellofemoral disorders but have had limited documentation in clinically controlled trials. Following acute patellar dislocation or surgery, improved rehabilitation techniques and an understanding of the physiology behind them have resulted in diminished time of immobilization and rapid mobilization that produces less joint stiffness, muscle atrophy, and improved function. It must be kept in mind that treatment, either operative or nonoperative, is a function of biology, not technology, and the patient is a significant factor in the effort.

Acute patellar dislocations, not unlike acute glenohumeral instability, causes significant injury to the periarticular soft tissues. The resultant tear in the quadriceps retinaculum is predisposed to heal in an attenuated position, which allows further maltracking and instability (Fig. 18–87). With each episode of recurrence, the mechanism is further disturbed, leading to continued poor patellofemoral mechanics. Athletes who place high demands on their knees should be treated aggressively following initial presentation of the instability to avoid repeated recurrences and prolonged recovery.

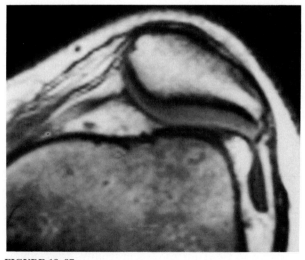

FIGURE 18–87
MRI of 13-year-old child with recurrent patellar dislocations. Note attenuation and fibrosis within the medial patellar retinaculum.

At the time of an acute patellar dislocation, tremendous shear forces are generated at the articular surface of the patella and femur, and chondral or osteochondral injury occurs [324]. With increased force, fragmentation of the surface may progress to loose body formation [233, 237, 300, 315]. Korner (1905) is given credit for recognizing the association between acute patellar instability and osteochondral injury [277]. Milgram [305] described a small number of patients with this combination of injuries and recommended aggressive surgical management of quadriceps defects. Much earlier, Harman, Klineberg, Krada, McDugal, and Miekison [277] all had described osteochondral injuries associated with acute patellar instability. With the advent of arthroscopy, an increased number of patients with osteochondral injuries have been recognized at the time of acute patellar dislocation, either primary or, less frequently, recurrent (Fig. 18–88).

In a retrospective review of 18 patients with acute patellar dislocation seen over a 12-year period at the Hospital for Sick Children in Toronto, Rorabeck and colleagues [314] found that all had suffered osteochondral fractures. The inframedial nonarticular portion of the patella was the major source of the fragments in this series. In two patients a lateral femoral condylar fragment was also found. These authors recommended either excision of the fragment or its replacement with fixation and repair of the quadriceps mechanism. In patients who underwent only fragment excision without repair of the quadriceps, continued repetitive dislocations occurred. Dandy [252] presented 29 cases of acute traumatic dislocation of the patella, among which 25 patients (86%) had a significant osteochondral free fragment. Following lateral release and fragment excision, 73% of the patients had good to excellent results in a brief follow-up.

In one of my own series of 30 patients, 13 males and 17 females, ranging in age from 12 to 16 years old, who had an initial acute noncontact lateral patellar dislocation, the patients were divided into two groups. Each group had similar history and physical examination findings with the exception of generalized ligamentous laxity in group A (15 patients), whereas in group B (15 patients) there was no evidence of generalized laxity. Thirty percent of group A patients suffered chondral damage. In group B there was an 80% (12 of 15) incidence of chondral damage. In group A there were two chondral contusions and three loose bodies, and in group B there were seven osteochondral fractures and three loose bodies, that is, a 2½ times increased incidence of articular surface injury in the nonlax patients at the time of initial noncontact acute patellar instability. This evidence of articular injury is further testimony to the significant forces associated with patellar dislocation (Fig. 18–89).

Orthopedic surgeons are commonly asked to assess patient capability for Special Olympic participation. The

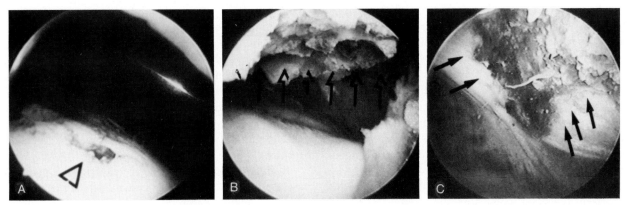

FIGURE 18–88
Arthroscopic views of post acute patellar dislocation: *A*, Femoral lateral condylar osteochondral injury (open arrow). *B*, Medial patellar facet osteochondral defect (open arrows). *C*, Medial quadriceps retinacular tear (arrows).

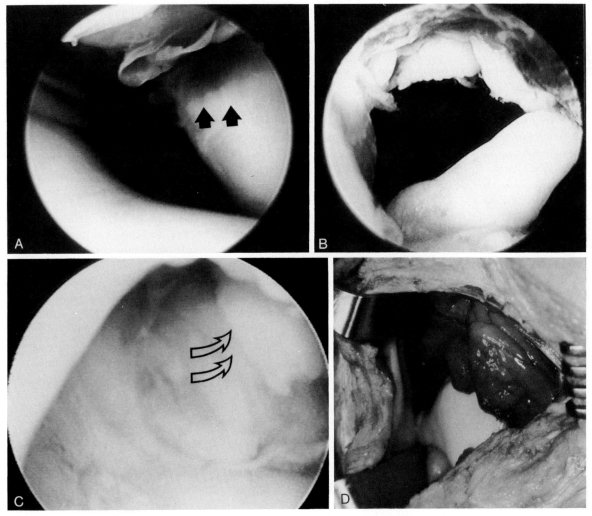

FIGURE 18–89
Arthroscopic views of changes occurring following acute patellar dislocation. *A*, Medial patellar facet—articular cartilage contusion and hemorrhage. *B*, Medial patellar facet crater after fracture. *C*, Intra-articular loose body due to medial patellar injury seen in *B*. *D*, 14-year-old boy with recurrent patellar dislocations. Marked synovitis was noted at time of patellar mechanism reconstruction.

patient with Down syndrome has particular needs about the knee because of an unstable quadriceps mechanism. Mendez and colleagues [303] studied 16 Down syndrome patients with 26 dislocatable or dislocated patellae. These patients had increased amounts of patellar instability with associated progressive deformities in the lower extremity including increased knee valgus and foot pronation. The authors also implicated patient hypermobility, hyperlaxity, and quadriceps hypotonia in association with knee flexion contractures, genu valgum, and external tibial torsion as predisposing factors to patellar instability. Patients who were independent ambulators had a good result in two-thirds of the cases with nonoperative treatment. Eight percent of the patients who were not good ambulators had a poor result with any type of management.

In an excellent review of surgical procedures used to correct an unstable patellofemoral mechanism, MacNab [296] in 1952 noted that Blumenstat, as of 1938, had recorded 79 different operative procedures for patellar instability. In 1959, Corta noted that 137 separate procedures had been advocated for resolution of patellar malalignment [265, 266]. All previously reported surgical procedures for patellofemoral instability sought, either individually or in combination, to (1) release tight lateral structures, including the retinaculum and capsule; (2) improve anatomic alignment by repositioning the patellar tendon or tibial tubercle, (3) enhance a medial tether by performing a patellar retinaculum imbrication or vastus medialis or medial hamstring transfer [230, 232, 238, 243, 249, 256–258, 272, 274, 292, 298, 301, 317, 318, 329, 333, 335].

Reconstructive procedures for management of patellar instability may consist of (1) proximal realignment by means of lateral release, medial reefing, or combined reefing and lateral release, (2) distal realignment by means of patellar tendon or tibial tubercle transfer or semitendinosus tenodesis, or (3) a combination of proximal and distal realignment. Whatever style of treatment is used, surgical correction of patellar instability must take into account the three-dimensional, toroidal path of the patella as it traverses the femoral sulcus.

Lateral retinacular release was first described by Pollard in 1891 [265], who combined it with an osteochondral chiseling of the femoral trochlea to provide patellar stability and prevent subluxation. Pollard gave credit to Haller for suggesting this release as an initial procedure for correcting patellar instability. Ober [307, 308] described release of a tight tensor band with transfer of the distally attached band of fascia to the medial knee where it could work as a tether and checkrein against lateral displacement. Lateral retinacular release under arthroscopic control has increased rapidly in popularity [235]. The release, whether done percutaneously or ''semiopen,'' is used by many as the first surgical step in the treatment of patellar instability. The procedure is attractive for its simplicity and relative noninvasiveness. A more formal open procedure, often combined with other stages, is reserved for those who fail this limited surgical approach.

Merchant and Mercer [304] in 1974 reported preliminary findings on lateral retinacular release in 16 patients (20 knees) with a broad age range and diagnoses that included patellar subluxation and dislocation. In patients without objective evidence of patellar malalignment, the authors did not recommend this procedure, particularly for those whose sole complaint was pain.

Results of lateral retinacular release have not been assessed specifically in high-demand athletes as a group, although many of the patients in Merchant's original study were athletes. The athlete may be more symptomatic because of diminished quadriceps strength secondary to violation of the lateral quadriceps mechanism.

Schoenholtz and colleagues [319], in reviewing lateral retinacular release in a small number of patients, felt that it was a reasonable preliminary step when nonoperative treatment failed. They questioned its use in the management of persistent patellar pain with no history of instability. Henry and associates [278], in reviewing 96 patients (100 knees) who had undergone arthroscopic lateral retinacular release for patellar subluxation following nonoperative management, found that the results of simple release compared favorably with more formal patellar femoral instability reconstructions. Sherman and colleagues [323], in a series of 45 knees treated with arthroscopic lateral release using elective surgery to manage recurrent patellar subluxation or dislocation, found that 75% of the knees were rated better at a short follow-up of 2 years. Patients with dislocations tended to have worse results than those with subluxation.

Cerullo and associates [246] reviewed 116 patients with extensor malalignment and noted poor results if the patient underwent surgery for pain alone if there was no evidence of patellar instability. The opposite was true (with 100% good results) if proximal and distal realignments were carried out, and there was a 75% satisfactory result if proximal realignment alone was done.

Scuderi and co-workers [321] reviewed 16 knees in 52 patients who had undergone lateral release and proximal realignment for either subluxation or dislocation. At brief follow-up, 80% of the patients had good or excellent clinical results, and only one patient had a redislocation. Outcome was unaffected by the amount of cartilage change noted at the time of surgery. In general, older patients and females had poorer results.

Fulkerson and colleagues [263] reviewed CT scans of the patellofemoral joint before and after lateral retinacular release and concluded that the release was effective in reducing patellar tilt but not maltracking. Correction of subluxation was less consistent with either lateral release or lateral release combined with tibial tubercle transfer. Fulkerson and associates [263, 266] reported that patients with a Q angle of greater than 20 degrees had a poor result following a lateral release alone for patellar instability. They noted that patients who underwent lateral release at follow-up 18 months later had results equal to those reported for more complex stabilizing procedures for patellar instability. Excellent results with absence of symptoms and return to full activity were obtained in 48% of patients.

Complications of lateral retinacular release may be multiple and include hematoma or neuroma formation, reflex sympathetic dystrophy, quadriceps rupture, medial patellar instability, phlebitis, and infection [242, 336]. In Hughston and Deese's [281] report of medial subluxation as a complication of lateral retinacular release, CT scans in three patients showed severe atrophy and retraction after overvigorous release of the vastus lateralis. Subluxation medially after lateral retinacular release surgery was reported by Hughston and Deese based on their ability to displace the patella clinically a significant amount medially following such surgery. The authors did not specify their starting point relative to medial translation (i.e., central versus lateral). Three patients had postoperative CT scans that demonstrated significant atrophy of the vastus lateralis. Since no preoperative scans were presented for comparison, the amount of atrophy that was present prior to release is unknown, and all such noted changes on CT scans may not be attributable to retinacular release alone. Complications following lateral retinacular release procedures may be as high as 7%, much higher than those associated with any other type of arthroscopic knee procedure [242, 336]. This figure emphasizes the fact that arthroscopic surgery is not "no problem" surgery and potential complications may be significant, particularly bleeding from unrecognized geniculate artery lacerations.

With arthroscopy there was a surge of interest in patellofemoral disorders. The factors producing the instability must still be well defined prior to setting up an orthopedic plan, particularly a surgical one. The question that must be asked is, Can surgery correct the involved factors to allow improved function over a prolonged time so that degenerative joint disease and premature joint senescence do not occur? This decision is especially critical when the extra factor of growth comes into play as it does in the preadolescent and adolescent. Objective measures of evaluation, e.g., range of motion, motor strength, and specific work or sport capabilities, need to be made preoperatively so that similar objective measures can be used to assess postoperative progress and results. If possible, preoperative rehabilitation should be encouraged to enhance baseline quadriceps and hamstring fitness, allowing postoperative efforts to start at a higher level.

Insall and colleagues [286] described a proximal realignment procedure including lateral release and transfer of the vastus medialis obliquus for treatment of chondromalacia and recurrent dislocation. The procedure was further modified to include a tube-type repair, and the authors claimed a 91% rate of excellent or good results at 2- to 10-year follow-up. Abraham and associates [228a] reviewed this type of procedure and divided their patients into two groups: (1) those with anterior knee symptoms related to articular surface change, and (2) those with historical and physical evidence of patellar instability. In group 1 patients, 87% had excellent results at 2 years with a decline to 55% excellent results at 5 to 11 years of follow-up. Patients in group 2, those with patellar instability, had 78% excellent results and maintained these results at 5- to 11-year follow-up. As part of their study, the authors dissected four adult knees to assess the nerve supply to the patella and found the patella to be supplied by the femoral and lateral femoral cutaneous nerves. They noted that the three incisions required to carry out the Insall procedure (skin, lateral release, and medial quadriceps retinacular repair) cut all of the nerves in question and suggested that denervation resulted in diminished symptoms. Abraham and colleagues suggested that young adults with a redislocated patella and grade III or IV patellar malaisic change were the patients who might benefit most from such a procedure.

Madigan and colleagues [297] reported possible soft tissue realignment combined with lateral retinacular release in skeletally immature patients with patellar subluxation and dislocation. In their small series of patients with limited follow-up, approximately half of the patients had associated underlying conditions (such as nail-patella syndrome) that predisposed the patient to patellar instability.

Transfer of the semitendinosus had been popularized by Galeazzi in 1925 [267], who did not feel that lateral release was required as a concomitant procedure. Baker and colleagues [232] and Hall and associates [274] reported excellent results in 80% of the patients studied following a medial hamstring transfer combined with a vastus medialis obliquus advancement.

Distal and medial transfer of the tibial tubercle was described by Roux in 1888 [316] and popularized by Hauser [276] in 1938. The Hauser procedure was commonly performed until the 1970s, when complications, particularly compartment syndrome, were recognized in a significant number of patients [247, 253, 330, 332]. It was also appreciated that a large number of patients developed symptomatic patella infera with progressive degenerative joint disease (Fig. 18–90). This was due to posterior and distal translation of the patellar axis by the transfer, which caused further compressive force between the femur and the patella. Tibial tubercle transfer

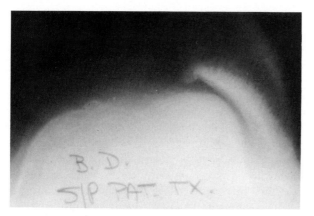

FIGURE 18–90
Patellar malposition following Hauser patellar tendon transfer.

procedures should be delayed until near skeletal maturity to prevent abnormal growth of the upper tibial physis. Recurvatum or angular deformity may result as a consequence of premature physeal arrest [259]. In 1961 Heywood [279] discussed the risks of tibial tubercle transfers and noted that significant failures occurred with procedures dealing with the soft tissues alone in children and adolescents with recurrent patellar dislocation. Chrisman and colleagues [247] compared the long-term results of the Hauser procedure with those of the Goldthwait technique in adult patients with recurrent patellar dislocation. They found the Goldthwait procedure to be significantly

better (93% versus 72% satisfactory results). Both procedures were accompanied by lateral release and medial retinacular reefing. Fourteen knees had associated torn menisci, and six had loose bodies. Almost half (46% of the patients) underwent surgeries other than those on the patella. It was thought that these procedures had no effect on results in either group. Major or minor complications were seen in 53% of the patients undergoing the Hauser technique. The Hauser procedure was also noted to cause external tibial rotation deformities, which aggravated preexisting lateral patellar translation. The authors concluded that the Goldthwait procedure was better because the potential for overcorrection was less likely.

The Roux procedure of tibial tubercle rotational transfer was popularized by Elmslie. Trillatt and associates [328] in 1964 gave Elmslie credit for furthering the conception of this tibial tubercle rotational osteotomy (Fig. 18–91). More than a century ago, Roux [316] did not recommend transfer of the tibial tubercle in skeletally immature patients. In 1888 he reported a typical correction of patellar instability in a 13-year-old girl 1 year following lateral patellar dislocation. His pertinent comments on the examination are equally true today: ''. . . aponeurotic expansion of the quadriceps on either side of the patella does not get taut when the child contracts the thigh muscles. If a dislocation occurs, it is obvious when the quadriceps contraction surprises the patella

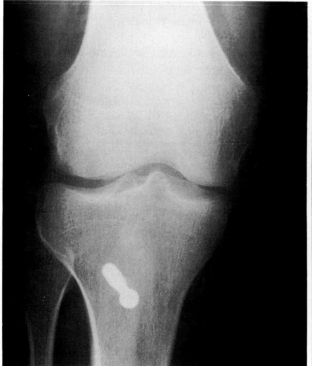
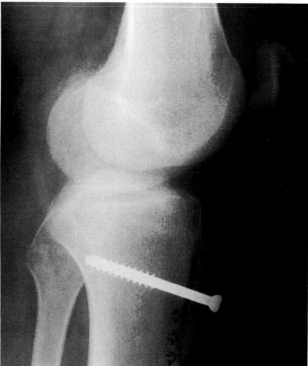

FIGURE 18–91
Elmslie-Trillat transfer.

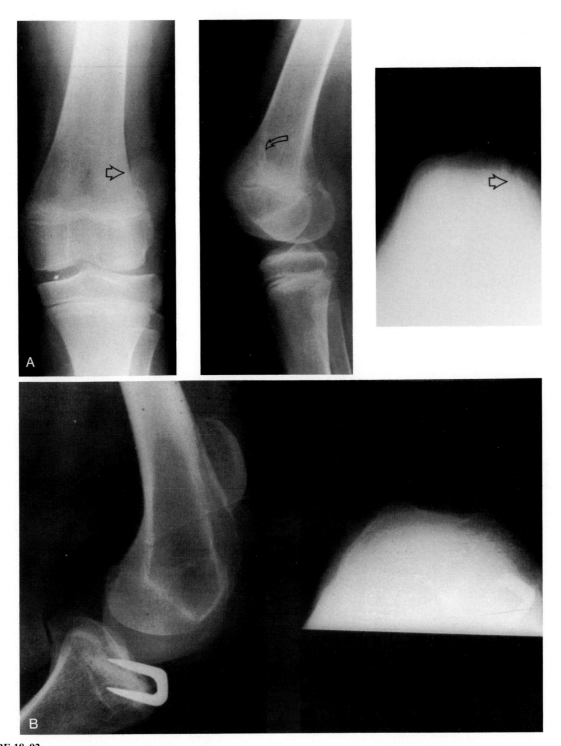

FIGURE 18–92
A, Congenital patellar dislocation. *B*, Poor results due to hardware complications following ill-fated attempt at reconstruction. The congenital nature of the dislocation was not appreciated at the initial surgery.

before its two superior half-facets arrive in contact with the anterior aspect of the condyle and are engaged in the intercondylar notch. The primary goal of the procedure was to suture the torn medial aponeurosis, exclude temporarily the perturbing axis of the vastus lateralis and insure good results by displacing medially the insertion of the patellar ligament.'' Ten days postoperatively the patient began active range of motion of the knee to prevent knee stiffness and was out of a splint at 3 weeks. An excellent result was noted 1 year later.

In a review of the Roux-Elmslie-Trillat procedure in 116 Naval midshipmen 1 year postoperatively, Cox [250] found a 7% recurrence rate. Eighty-eight percent of the results were rated as good or excellent. Cox correlated a poor result with intra-articular pathology such as hemarthrosis or malaisic change or torn or absent menisci or cruciate ligaments. Brown and colleagues [241], in further follow-up of the same group of patients at the Naval Academy at an average of 42 months postoperatively, noted that the results had diminished in quality with time. Up to 7 years following the procedure, two-thirds of the patients still had good to excellent results compared with 88% at the time of the initial study.

More than one hundred years ago Goldthwait [268–270] emphasized the concept of lateral release and medial capsular reefing in association with his hemitendon crossover transfer technique. In one patient, in 1909, he noted that a better result was obtained with a combination of proximal and distal repair than proximal repair alone.

Patellectomy as management for an unstable patella is inadequate. Removal of the osseous element of the patellofemoral quadriceps complex simply leaves one with an unstable quadriceps mechanism that is made even more unstable with the absence of the patella [327, 331]. Correction of the instability should be carried out, not patellectomy. Patellectomy for this condition in the skeletally immature patient should be unheard of.

More than 150 years ago Malgaigne observed, ''when I searched along past and present authors for the origins of the doctrines generally accepted today concerning dislocation of the patella, I was surprised to find among them such a dearth of facts with such an abundance of opinions [265]. Unfortunately, this situation has not changed significantly among current practitioners. In young children, because of the often multifaceted nature of their patellar instability (patellar size, femoral trochlear maldevelopment, abnormal lower extremity biomechanics), soft tissue surgery alone usually does not pro-

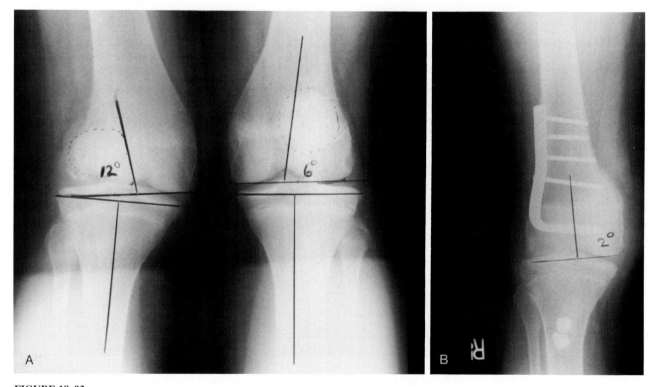

FIGURE 18–93
A, 16-year-old boy with recurrent patellar dislocations. Note distal femoral valgus. *B*, After femoral osteotomy with proximal soft tissue realignment and tibial tubercle transfer, he is asymptomatic. (Courtesy Deborah F. Bell, M.D.)

duce satisfactory long-lasting results, and the surgeon is challenged to find a technique that provides patellar stability without causing epiphyseal damage.

Management of patellar instability has spawned a multitude of procedures owing to the nonspecificity of the diagnosis, treatment variations, and obvious dissatisfaction with any one particular procedure. Surgical treatment of patellar instability requires an operation tailormade for each patient because each condition requires a unique solution based on the patient's morphologic as-

sets and liabilities (Fig. 18–92). Bilateral patellar instability may not always be secondary to identical factors (Fig. 18–93). By assiduously identifying the factors that lead to the instability and correcting all that are necessary, improved results both short-term and long-term may be possible. In a patient with a generalized ligamentous laxity, even surgical techniques cannot overcome collagen biology, and patients must be advised of this situation.

Reflex Sympathetic Dystrophy

In 1864 S. Weir Mitchell [359, 360] described "causalgia" attendant on war injuries of nerves of the upper extremity. Twenty-five years later Sudek [372] noted the difference between diffuse osteoporosis and focal bony change secondary to causalgia. He was the first to postulate an autonomic system disorder as its cause. In 1923 Leriche [356, 357] suggested that initial vasoconstriction and secondary vasodilation caused inflammatory findings and focal osteoporosis. Ficat and Hungerford [344] have described the correlation between altered interosseous hemodynamics and bony histologic findings in this condition. Evans [343], in 1946, first used the term reflex sympathetic dystrophy (RSD) and pointed out the wide range of complaints and findings associated with this condition. In a review of potential causes of this entity, Schutzer and Gossling [366] concluded that RSD seems to be due to a combination of both central and peripheral factors.

Ficat and Hungerford [344] were the first, in describing a large series, to emphasize the presence of this disorder in the lower extremity, particularly in association with knee complaints. Katz and Hungerford [349] in 1987 described 36 patients with knee complaints secondary to RSD. They suggested that the disorder was an exaggerated sympathetic autonomic response to the injured limb. Injury or surgery at the patellofemoral joint triggered the onset of symptoms in about two-thirds of the patients in their series. In a national survey of complications of arthroscopic surgery in the United States [340, 369], patellofemoral joint procedures were reported to have an inordinately high incidence of associated RSD.

Despite recent publications emphasizing the emergent recognition of RSD of the lower extremity, it is still not commonly considered in the differential diagnosis of knee pain [344, 349, 366, 371, 374]. In a retrospective study of 67 patients with unexplained knee pain, Tietjen [374] found that 14 (21%) met the criteria for reflex dystrophy.

Numerous publications during the last decade have pointed out the increased frequency with which this condition is being seen in children [337, 338, 341, 343, 345,

348, 350, 355, 362, 366, 367]. Despite such publicity, Wilder and associates[375], in a recent series of 70 patients under the age of 18 (average age 12.5 years), found an average delay of 1 year from the onset of symptoms to the time of diagnosis. Unfortunately, orthopedists uncommonly consider this diagnosis at the initial visit, especially in children and adolescents who have unexplained knee pain either pre- or postoperatively. The diagnosis is usually not made until the manifestations of the condition have become much more florid, a stage at which treatment is more difficult.

RSD is a clinical condition marked by a disproportionate pain response with autonomic sequelae affecting the skin, muscles, vessels, and bone. Classically, three temporally arranged stages have been described: acute, onset less than 3 months; dystrophic, onset 3 to 6 months; and atrophic, onset greater than 6 months. The acute stage is characterized primarily by pain. Stiffness, pain, swelling and osteoporosis are manifestations of the dystrophic phase. The atrophic stage is characterized by continued pain, nail and skin changes, cyanosis of the extremity, and bony demineralization noted roentgenographically. Gradations of these stages exist because a spectrum of findings is seen in any one patient depending on the duration and magnitude of the disorder. Such stages are not to be considered absolute guideposts but rather points within that spectrum.

Historically, complaints of pain out of proportion to the magnitude of the initiating event and associated swelling, stiffness, and cutaneous manifestations may be present. In addition to the disproportionate pain associated with minor trauma or surgery, the absence of expected improvement with specific treatment for a previously diagnosed disorder should raise the question of a possible sympathetic dystrophy. Ficat and Hungerford [344] suggested that "a high suspicion is probably the best weapon" in recognizing and diagnosing RSD. Wilder and colleagues [375] suggest that a carefully done history and physical examination are the best diagnostic tools. Physical findings are a function of the status of the condition and also are stage dependent; they may include limitation of motion, abnormal gait, sweat gland and skin trophic changes, and manifestations of atrophy. Radiographic findings include focal patchy demineralization or osteoporosis, or both.

Schutzer and Gossling [366] described the manifestations of RSD as intense, prolonged pain, disturbances of vasomotor function, delay in functional recovery, and associated trophic changes. Cooper and colleagues [339] found that knee limitation of motion was common, particularly restriction of flexion. In his series, 11 of 14 patients had had a patellar operation prior to the diagnosis of RSD. On further retrospective analysis, the history in nine of those patients suggested a diagnosis of sympathetic dystrophy preoperatively.

Extreme sensitivity to slight touch (allodynia) is the most common finding on physical examination and is noted in over 90% of patients with reflex sympathetic dystrophy. Vasomotor signs and symptoms fluctuate, and findings differ at each examination. Dietz and associates [341] emphasized the physical sign *tache cerebral* as an indication of vasomotor dysfunction. A positive sign is elicited by lightly stroking the skin of the affected area and that of the contralateral limb as control. The sign is positive if an erythematous line appears at the involved site within 15 to 30 seconds. This line may last for as long as 15 minutes and may precede other signs of autonomic dysfunction.

Technetium bone scanning has been recommended by several authors to aid in diagnosis [347, 349, 352, 354, 358] Katz and Hungerford [349] found a 61% positive incidence of delayed scintigraphic images in patients with chronic RSD. Wilder and colleagues [375] recommended bone scanning to rule out underlying disorders such as osteoid osteoma, infection, or stress fracture. They do not place great emphasis on isotopic imaging as an aid in diagnosing RSD because the scan varies at different stages of RSD, particularly in children and adolescents.

Ogilvie-Harris and Roscoe [361] studied 19 patients with lower extremity sympathetic dystrophy associated with knee disorders. In their patients, if the diagnosis was made within the first 6 months of onset of symptoms, a much more predictable, rapid, and sustained response to treatment occurred than in patients who were diagnosed and treated at a later stage. Ladd and associates [353] described the condition of ''reflex sympathetic imbalance'' in 11 patients. They concluded that this entity was an incomplete manifestation of classic RSD because one or more of the cardinal classic features was missing. Dietz and associates [341] reported five cases of pediatric sympathetic dystrophy and summarized 80 cases of pediatric sympathetic dystrophy from the literature. In one previous study [368] 21 patients with RSD were thought to have significant psychological stress within the family unit. Other authors have observed ac-

ademic, athletic, social, and familial stresses in children and adolescents with RSD [364, 373].

The difference between the patterns and course of the condition in children and adolescents compared with adults is becoming recognized. These include differences in gender, diminished frequency of trophic changes, limited imaging study abnormalities, more poorly defined symptom complex, and less predictable response to both invasive and noninvasive treatment protocols; there is, however, overall a more optimistic outcome (Table 18–2). Dietz and co-workers [341] noted that preadolescent girls (average age 11 years) tended to be characteristic patients with reflex sympathetic dystrophy in the pediatric age group. A similar observation was made by Wilder and colleagues [375] in 70 patients in their study. In contrast, there is an almost equal male-female ratio in adult RSD. The presentation as a sequela of surgery or trauma is noted in only about half of the cases in children compared with a much higher number in adults.

Radiographically evident osteopenia is much less common in children than adults. Isotopic bone scans are commonly not helpful in adults and are extremely variable in children. In a literature review of RSD in children, Dietz and colleagues [341] noted that in 35 reported bone scans one-third were normal, one-third had diffuse increased uptake, and one-third had diffuse diminished uptake. Because the scan findings are a function of the stage of the disease, sequential scan findings may produce a difference in data.

Treatment of RSD is extremely difficult and frustrating for both patient and physician. Ficat and Hungerford [344] have commented that ''it is a disorder not to be beaten into submission, but rather seduced.'' Treatment may consist of a variety of paths. A recently emerging treatment concept is to manage the pain in such a way that other therapeutic interventions such as physical therapy and functional use may be carried out simultaneously. In children, noninvasive management techniques produce satisfactory results as the initial form of treatment in over 50% of cases [341, 375]. Use of sympa-

TABLE 18–2

Reflex Sympathetic Dystrophy in Children and Adults

	Children	Adults
Gender	Female	Male = female
Trauma history	<50%	Almost all
Upper extremity	Rare	Common
Lower extremity	Common	Common
Radiographic changes	Not significant	Significant
Response to treatment	Rapid	Slow
Need for invasive treatment	Less common	Common
Recurrence	≤ 5%	≥ 20%

thetic block or other invasive management methods may occasionally be necessary. The almost pathognomonic response to sympathetic block makes a nonresponse to a properly executed block reason to question the diagnosis of RSD [342, 344, 346, 350, 363, 370]. It is important to establish control of the RSD constellation before surgery is contemplated. Injury to the inferior patellar branch of the saphenous nerve should be considered as a diagnostic point in patients with localized nerve findings.

Transcutaneous nerve stimulation, physical therapy, psychological counseling, and antidepressant medication may all play roles in management. [340, 341, 350, 375]. Resolution of juvenile RSD tends to occur sooner than in adults, but this is by no means a universal finding [341, 375]. Sympathectomy for RSD in children is rarely required and theoretically may have the unpredictable side effect of affecting limb growth due to changes in vascular flow.

RSD must be considered in any patient with knee pain especially when the complaints seem out of proportion to the inciting incident. Pertinent physical and radiographic findings and response to treatment complete the assessment. Any patellofemoral joint surgery, particularly arthroscopy, is contraindicated for pain alone without objective evidence, by either physical examination or imaging techniques, documenting a specific preoperative diagnosis of a surgically correctable lesion.

References

Basic Considerations

1. Ahmed, A.M., et al. Force analysis of the patellar mechanism. *J Orthop Res* 5(1):69 –85, 1987.
2. Blumenstat, C. Die Lageabweichungen und Verrenkungen der Kniescheibe. *Ergebn Chir Orthop* 31:149, 1938.
3. Brattstrom, H. Patella alta in non-dislocating knee joints. *Acta Orthop Scand* 41:578, 1970.
4. Brooke, R. The treatment of fractured patella by excision. A study of morphology and function. *Br J Surg* 24:733–747, 1936.
5. Bruce, J., and Walmsley, R. Excision of the patella. Some experimental and anatomical observations. *J Bone Joint Surg* 24:311–325, 1942.
6. Buff, H.U., et al. Experimental determination of forces transmitted through the patello-femoral joint. *J Biomech* 21(1):17–23, 1988.
7. Dosko, C.L. Formation of the femoral patellar part of the human knee. *Folia Morphol* 33:38–47, 1985.
8. Fulkerson, J.P., and Gossling, H.R. Anatomy of the knee joint lateral retinaculum. *Clin Orthop* 153:183–188, 1980.
9. Gardner, E., and O'Rahilly, R. The early development of the knee joint in staged human embryos. *JANAT*, 102:289–299, 1968.
10. Goodfellow, J., et al. Patellofemoral joint mechanics and pathology: Functional anatomy of the patellofemoral joint. *J Bone Joint Surg* 58B:287, 1976.
11. Goodfellow, J., et al. Patellofemoral joint mechanics and pathology: Chondromalacia patellae. *J Bone Joint Surg* 58B:291, 1976.
12. Grelsamer, R.P., and Meadows, S. The modified Insall-Salvatti ratio for assessment of patellar height. *Clin Orthop* 253:170–176, 1990

13. Hallisey, M., et al. Anatomy of the junction of the vastus lateralis tendon and the patella. *J Bone Joint Surg* 69A:545, 1987.
14. Haxton, R. The function of the patella and the effects of excision. *Surg Gynecol Obstet* 80:389–395, 1945.
15. Hey Grovers, E.W. A note on the extension apparatus of the knee-joint. *Br J Surg* 24:747–748, 1936.
16. Huberti, H., and Hayes, W. Contact pressures in chondromalacia patellae. *J Orthop Res* 6:499–508, 1988.
17. Hvid, I., Andersen, L.I., and Schmidt, H. Patellar height and femoral trochlear development. *Acta Orthop Scand* 54:91, 1983.
18. Insall, J., and Salvati, E. Patellar position in the normal knee joint. *Radiology* 101:101, 1971.
19. Jacobsen, K., and Bertheussen, K. The vertical location of the patella. *Acta Orthop Scand* 45:436, 1974.
20. Kaufer, H. Patellar biomechanics. *Clin Orthop* 144:51–54, 1979.
21. Koshino, T., and Sugimoto, K. New measurement of patellar height in the knees of children. *J Pediatr Orthop* 9:216–218, 1989.
22. Kujala, U.M., et al. Patellar motion analyzed by magnetic resonance imaging. *Acta Orthop Scand.* 60(1):1306, 1989.
23. Lanscourt, J.E., and Cristini, J.A. Patella alta and patella infera. *J Bone Joint Surg* 57A:1112–1114, 1985.
24. Lieb, F.J., and Perry, J. Quadriceps function: An electromyographic study under isometric conditions. *J Bone Joint Surg* 83A:749–758, 1971.
25. MacDonald, D.A., et al. Maximal isometric patellofemoral contact force in patients with anterior knee pain. *J Bone Joint Surg* 71B:296–299, 1989.
26. Maquet, P.G.J. *Biomechanics of the Knee with Applications to the Pathogenesis and the Surgical Treatment of Osteoarthritis.* Berlin, Springer-Verlag, 1976, p. 204.
27. Micheli, L.J., et al. Patella alta and the adolescent growth spurt. *Clin Orthop* 213:159–162, 1986.
28. Møller, B.N., et al. The quadriceps function in patellofemoral disorders. A radiographic and electromyographic study. *Arch Orthop Trauma Surg* 106:195–198, 1987.
29. Perry, J., Antonelli, D., and Ford, W. Analysis of knee-joint forces during flexed-knee stance. *J Bone Joint Surg* 57A:961, 1975.
30. Reider, B., Marshall, J., and Rink, B. Patellar tracking. *Clin Orthop* 157:143–148, 1981.
31. Reider, B., Marshall, J.L., et al: The anterior aspect of the knee joint: Anatomic study. *J Bone Joint Surg* 63A:351–356, 1981.
32. Reynolds, L., et al. EMG activity of the vastus medialis oblique and the vastus lateralis retinacular release. *Clin Orthop* 134:158, 1987.
33. Walmsley, R. Development of the patella. *J Anat* 74:360–368, 1940.
34. Wiberg, G. Roentgenographic and anatomic studies on the femoropatellar joint, with special reference to chondromalacia of the patella. *Acta Orthop Scand* 12:319–410, 1941.

Multipartite Patella

35. Bourne, M.H., et al. Bipartite patella in the adolescent: Results of surgical excision. *J Pediatr Orthop* 10(2):255–260, 1990.
36. Denham, R.H. Dorsal defect of the patella. *J Bone Joint Surg* 66A:116, 1984.
37. Echeverria, T.S., and Bersani, F.A. Acute fracture simulating a symptomatic bipartite patella. *Am J Sports Med* 8:48–50, 1980.
38. George, R. Bilateral bipartite patella. *Br J Surg* 22:555, 1935.
39. Goergen, T.G., Resnick, D., Greenway, G., et al. Dorsal defect of the patella (DDP): A characteristic radiographic lesion. *Radiology* 130:333, 1979.
40. Green, W.T., Jr. Painful bipartite patellae. *Clin Orthop* 110:197–200, 1975.
41. Haswell, D.M., Berne, A.S., and Graham, C.B. The dorsal defect of the patella. *Pediatr Radiol* 4:238, 1976.
42. Johnson, J.F., and Brogdon, B.G. Dorsal defect of the patella: Incidence and distribution. *AJR* 139:339, 1982.
43. Lawson, J.P. Symptomatic radiographic variants in extremities. *Radiology* 157:625, 1985.
44. Ogden, J.A., McCarthy, S.M., and Jabl, P. The painful bipartite patella. *J Pediatr Orthop* 2:263–269, 1982.

45. Saupe, E. Beitrag zur Patella bipartitia. *Fortschr Ged Ront* 28:37, 1921.
46. van Holsbeeck, M., Vandamme, B., Marchal, G., et al. Dorsal defect of the patella: Concept of its origin and relationship with bipartite and multipartite patella. *Skel Radiol* 16:304, 1987.
47. Weaver, J.K. Bipartite patella as a cause of disability in the athlete. *Am J Sports Med* 5:137–143, 1977.

Plica

48. Broom, M.J., and Fulkerson, J.P. The plica syndrome: A new perspective. *Orthop Clin North Am* 17:279, 1986.
49. Dosko, C.L., Formation of the femoral patellar part of the human knee. *Folia Morphol* (PRAHA), 33:38–47, 1985.
50. Gardner, E., and O'Rahilly, R. The early development of the knee joint in staged human embryos. *JANAT* 102:289–299, 1968.
51. Hardaker, W.T., Whipple, T.L., and Bassett, F.H., III. Diagnosis and treatment of the plica syndrome of the knee. *J Bone Joint Surg* 62A:221, 1980.
52. Iino, S. Normal arthroscopic findings in the knee joint in adult cadavers. *J Jap Orthop Assoc* 14:467–523, 1939.
53. Kinnard, P., Levesque, R.Y. The plica syndrome: A syndrome of controversy. *Clin Orthop* 183:141, 1984.
54. Mital, M.A., and Hayden, J. Pain in the knee in children; The medial plica shelf syndrome. *Orthop Clin North Am* 10:713, 1979.
55. Mizumachi, S., Kawashima, W., and Okamura, T. So-called synovial shelf in the knee joint. *J Jap Orthop Assoc* 23:22–25, 1948.
56. Patel, D. Arthroscopy of the plicae-synovial folds and their significance. *Am J Sports Med* 6(5):217, 1978.
57. Patel, D. Plica as a cause of anterior knee pain. *Orthop Clin North Am* 17:273, 1986.
58. Pipkin, G. Knee injuries. The role of suprapatellar plica and suprapatellar bursa in simulating internal derangements. *Clin Orthop* 74:161, 1971.
59. Pipkin, G. Lesions of the suprapatellar plica. *J Bone Joint Surg* 32A(2):363–369, 1950.
60. Rovere, G.D., and Adair, D. Medial synovial shelf plica syndrome: Treatment by intraplical steroid injection. *Am J Sports Med* 13:383, 1985.
61. Sakakibara, J. Arthroscopic study on Iino's band (plica synovialis mediopatellaris). *J Jap Orthop Assoc* 50:513–522, 1976.
62. Stanitski, C.L. Common injuries in preadolescent and adolescent athletes: Recommendations for prevention. *Sports Med* 7(1):32–41, 1989.

Osgood-Schlatter's Disease

63. Bolesta, M.J., and Fitch, R.D. Tibial tubercle avulsions. *J Pediatr Orthop* 6:186, 1986.
64. Bowers, K.D. Patellar tendon avulsion as a complication of Osgood-Schlatter's disease. *Am J Sports Med* 4:253, 1976.
65. D'Ambrosia, R., and MacDonald, G. Pitfalls in the diagnosis of Osgood-Schlatter's disease. *Clin Orthop* 110:206–209, 1975.
66. Ehrenborg, G. The Osgood-Schlatter's lesion: A clinical and experimental study. *Acta Clin Scand* (Suppl) 288:1, 1962.
67. Falster, O., and Hasselbalch, H. Avulsion fracture at the tibial tuberosity with combined ligament and meniscal tear. *Am J Sports Med* 20:82, 1992.
68. Glynn, M.K., and Regan, B.F. Surgical treatment of Osgood-Schlatter's disease. *J Pediatr Orthop* 3:216–219, 1983.
69. Krause, B.L., et al. Natural history of Osgood-Schlatter's disease. *J Pediatr Orthop* 10:65–68, 1990.
70. Kujala, U.M., et al. Osgood-Schlatter's disease in adolescent athletes. *Am J Sports Med* 13(4):236–241, 1985.
71. Lancourt, J.E., and Christina, J.A. Patella alta and infera: Etiologic role in patellar dislocation, chondromalacia and apophysitis of the tibial tubercle. *J Bone Joint Surg* 57:1112, 1975.
72. Lewis, M.M., and Reilly, J.F. Sports tumors. *Am J Sports Med* 15(4):362–365, 1987.

73. Mirbey, J, et al. Avulsion fractures of the tibial tuberosity in the adolescent athlete. *Am J Sports Med* 16:336, 1988.
74. Mital, M.A., et al. The so-called unresolved Osgood-Schlatter's lesion. *J Bone Joint Surg* 62A:732–739, 1980.
75. Ogden, J.A., and Southwick, W.O. Osgood-Schlatter's disease and tibial tubercle development. *Clin Orthop* 116:180–189, 1976.
76. Ogden, J.A., et al. Fractures of the tibial tuberosity in adolescents. *J Bone Joint Surg* 62A:205, 1980.
77. Osgood, R.B. Lesions of the tibial tubercle occurring during adolescence. *Boston Med Surg J* 148:114–7, 1903.
78. Schlatter, C. Verletzungen des Schnabelförmingen fortsatzes der oberen Tibiaepiphyse. *Beitr Klin Chir Tubing* 38:874–878, 1903.
79. Thomson, J.E.M. Operative treatment of osteochondritis of the tibial tubercle. *J Bone Joint Surg* 38A:142, 1956.
80. Uhrey, E., Jr. Osgood-Schlatter's disease. *Arch Surg* 48:406, 1944.

Sinding-Larsen-Johanssen Disease

81. Batten, J.M., and Menelaus, M. Fragmentation of the proximal pole of the patella. *J Bone Joint Surg* 67B:249–251, 1985.
82. Beddow, F.H., et al. Avulsion of the liagmentum patellae from the lower pole of the patella. *J R Coll Surg Edinb* 4:66, 1963.
83. Blazina, M.E., Kerllan, R.K., Jobe, F.W., et al. Jumper's knee. *Orthop Clin North Am* 4:665–678, 1973.
84. Grogan, D.D., et al. Avulsion fractures of the patella. *J Pediatr Orthop* 10:721–730, 1990.
85. Houghton, G.R., and Ackroyd, C.E. Sleeve fractures of the patella in children. *J Bone Joint Surg* 61B:165, 1979.
86. Karisson, J., et al. Partial rupture of the patellar ligament. *Am J Sports Med* 20(4):390, 1992.
87. Johanssen, S. En forut icke beskriven sjukdom i patella. *Hydiea* 84:161–162, 1922.
88. Medlar, R.D., and Lyne, E.D. Sinding-Larsen-Johnssen disease. *J Bone Joint Surg* 60A:1112–1116, 1978.
89. Roels, J., Martens, M., Mulier, J.C., et al. Patella tendinitis (jumper's knees). *Am J Sports Med* 6:362–368, 1987.
90. Sinding-Larsen, M.F. A hitherto unknown affection of the patella. *Acta Radiol* 1:171–174, 1921.

Acute Tibial Tubercle Avulsion Fracture

91. Bolesta, M.J., and Fitch, R.D. Tibial tubercle avulsions *J Pediatr Orthop* 6:186, 1986.
92. Bowers, K.D. Patellar tendon avulsion as a complication of Osgood-Schlatter's disease. *Am Med J Sports Med* 4:253, 1976.
93. Christie, M.J., and Dvonch, V.M. Tibial tuberosity avulsion fracture in adolescents. *J Pediatr Orthop* 1:391, 1981.
94. Falster, O., and Hasselbalch, H. Avulsion fracture of the tibial tuberosity with combined ligament and meniscal tear. *Am J Sports Med* 20:82, 1992.
95. Hand, W.L., et al. Avulsion fractures of the tibial tubercle. *J Bone Joint Surg* 53A:1579, 1971.
96. Lepse, P.S., et al. Simultaneous bilateral avulsion fracture of the tibial tuberosity. *Clin Orthop* 229:232–235, 1988.
97. Maar, D.C., et al. Simultaneous bilateral tubercle avulsion fracture. *Orthopaedics* 11(11):1599–1601, 1988.
98. Meyba, A. II. Avulsion fracture of the tibial tubercle apophysis with avulsion of the patellar ligament. *J Pediatr Orthop* 2:303, 1982.
99. Mirbey, J., et al. Avulsion fractures of the tibial tuberosity in the adolescent athlete. Risk factors, mechanism of injury and treatment. *Am J Sports Med* 16(4):336–340, 1988.
100. Nimityungskul, P., et al. Avulsion fracture of the tibial tubercle in late adolescence *J Trauma* 28(4):505, 1988.
101. Ogden, J.A., et al. Fractures of the tibial tuberosity in adolescents. *J Bone Joint Surg* 62A:205, 1980.
102. Polakoff, D.R., et al. Tension band wiring of displaced tibial tuberosity fractures in adolescents. *Clin Orthop* 209:161, 1986.
103. Watson-Jones, R., et al. *Fractures and Joint Injuries* Vol. 2. 4th ed. Baltimore, Williams & Wilkins, 1955, p. 786.

Anterior Knee Pain

104. American Association of Orthopedic Surgeons, Department of Health Policy and Research. *Orthopaedic Practice in the United States 1990–1991.* Chicago, American Association of Orthopaedic Surgeons, 1991.

105. Abernethy, P.J., et al. Is chondromalacia patellae a separate clinical entity. *J Bone Joint Surg* 60B:205–210, 1978.

106. Ahmed, A.M., Burke, D.L., et al. In-vitro measurement of static pressure distribution in synovial joints, part 2. Retropatellar surface. *Trans ASME* 105:226–236, 1983.

107. Ahmed, A.M., et al. Force analysis of the patellar mechanism. *J Orthop Res* 5(1):69–85, 1987.

108. Albanese, S.A., et al. Knee extensor mechanics after subtotal excision of the patella. *Clin Orthop* 285:217–222, 1992.

109. Aleman, O. Chondromalacia posttraumatic patellae. *Acta Chir Scand* 63:149–189, 1928.

110. Axhausen, G. Die umschriebenen Knorpel-Knochenlasionen des Kniegelenks. *Berl Klin Wochnschr* 56:265–269, 1919.

111. Bennet, J.G., and Stauber, W.T. Evaluation and treatment of anterior knee pain using eccentric exercises. *Med Sci Sports Exerc* 18:526, 1986.

112. Brattstrom, H. Shape of the intercondylar groove normally and in recurrent dislocation of the patella. *Acta Orthop Scand* 68:1–48, 1964.

113. Bronitsky, J. Chrondromalacia patellae. *J Bone Joint Surg* 29:931–945, 1947.

114. Broom, M.J., and Fulkerson, J.P. The plica syndrome: A new perspective. *Orthop Clin North Am* 17:279, 1986.

115. Budinger, K. Ueber Ablosung von Gelenkteilen und verwandte Prozzess. *Dtsch Z R Chir BD,* 1984.

116. Busch, M.T., and DeHaven, K.E. Pitfalls of the lateral retinacular release. *Clin Sports Med* 8:279–290, 1989.

117. Carson, W.G., et al. Patellofemoral disorders: Physical and radiographic evaluation: 1. Physical examination. *Clin Orthop* 185:165–177, 1984.

118. Cave, E.F., and Rowe, C.R. The patella. Its importance in derangement of the knee. *J Bone Joint Surg* 32A:542, 1950.

119. Cox, J.J. Chondromalacia of the patella: A review and update, Part I. *Contemp Orthop* 6:6, 1983.

120. Cox, J.J. Chondromalacia of the patella: A review and update, Part II. *Contemp Orthop* 7:1, 1983.

121. Cox, J.S. Patellofemoral problems in runners. *Clin Sports Med* 4:699–715, 1985.

122. Darracott, J., and Vernon-Roberts, B. The bony changes in chondromalacia patellae. *Rheum Phys Med* 11:175, 1971.

123. Dehaven, K.E., Dolan, W.A., and Mayer, P.J. Chondromalacia patellae in athletes: Clinical presentation and conservative management. *Am J Sports Med* 7:5–11, 1979.

124. DeLee, J. Reflex sympathetic dystrophy following arthroscopic surgery. *Arthroscopy* 1:214, 1985.

125. Delgado-Martins, H. A study of the position of the patella using computerized tomography. *J Bone Joint Surg* 61B:443–444, 1979.

126. Doucette, S.A., and Goble, E.M. The effect of exercise on patellar tracking in lateral patellar compression syndrome. *Am J Sports Med* 20:434, 1992.

127. Dowd, G.S., et al. Radiographic assessment in patellar instability and chondromalacia patellae. *J Bone Joint Surg* 68B:297–300, 1986.

128. Dugdale, T.W., and Barnett, P.R. Historical background: Patellofemoral pain in young people. *Orthop Clin North Am* 17(2):211, 1986.

129. Dye, S.F., et al. Radionuclide imaging of the patellofemoral joint in young adults with anterior knee pain. *Orthop Clin North Am* 17:249–262, 1986.

130. Dzioba, R.B. Diagnostic arthroscopy and longitudinal open lateral release. A four year follow-up study to determine predictors of surgical outcome. *Am J Sports Med* 18(4):343–348, 1990.

131. Emery, I.H., and Meachim, G. Surface morphology and topography of patello-femoral cartilage fibrillation in Liverpool necropsies. *J Anat* 116:103–120, 1973.

132. Fairbank, J.C., et al. Mechanical factors in the incidence of knee pain in adolescents and young adults. *J Bone Joint Surg* 1984;66B:685–693.

133. Fisher, R.L. Conservative treatment of patellofemoral pain. *Orthop Clin North Am* 17:269–272, 1986.

134. Frederick, E.C. Biomechanical consequences of sports shoe design. *Exerc Sports Sci Rev* 14:375–400, 1986.

135. Fulkerson, J.P. Current concept review: Patello-femoral alignment. *J Bone Joint Surg* 72A:1424–1428, 1990.

136. Fulkerson, J.P., Tennant, R., Jaivin, J.S., et al. Histologic evidence of retinacular nerve injury associated with patellofemoral malalignment. *Clin Orthop* 197:196–205, 1985.

137. Fulkerson, J., and Hungerford, D. *Disorders of the Patellofemoral Joint* (2nd ed.). Baltimore, Williams & Wilkins, 1990.

138. Fulkerson, J.P. The etiology of patellofemoral pain in young, active patients: A prospective study. *Clin Orthop* 179:129–133, 1983.

139. Fulkerson, J.P., et al. Computerized tomography of the patellofemoral joint before and after lateral release. *Arthroscopy* 3:19–24, 1987.

140. Fulkerson, J.P., et al. Disorders of patellofemoral alignment. *J Bone Joint Surg* 72A:1424–1429, 1990.

141. Fulkerson, J.P., and Schutzer, S.F. After failure of conservative treatment for painful patellofemoral malalignment: Lateral release or realignment? *Orthop Clin North Am* 17:283, 1986.

142. Fulkerson, J.P., et al. Patellofemoral pain. *Instr Course Lect* 40:52, 1991.

143. Gecha, S.R., et al. Clinical prognosticators for the efficacy of retinacular release surgery to treat patellofemoral pain. *Clin Orthop* 253:203–208, 1990.

144. Goldstein, S.A., et al. Patellar surface strain. *J Orthop Res* 4(3):372–377, 1986.

145. Goodfellow, J.W. Chondromalacia patella: A mythical disease. *J Bone Joint Surg* 66B:455–458, 1984.

146. Goodfellow, J.W. Knee prostheses—one step forward, two steps back. (Editorial). *J Bone Joint Surg* 74B:1–2, 1992.

147. Goodfellow, J.W., Hungerford, D.S., et al. Patello-femoral joint mechanics and pathology. I: Functional anatomy of the patellofemoral joint. *J Bone Joint Surg* 58B:287–290, 1976.

148. Goodfellow, J.W., Hungerford, D.S., et al. Patello-femoral joint mechanics and pathology. II. Chondrolamalcia patellae. *J Bone Joint Surg* 58B:291–299, 1976.

149. Grana, W.A., and Kriegshause, L.A. The scientific basis of extensor mechanism disorders. *Clin Sports Med* 4:247–257, 1985.

150. Grelsamer, R.P., and Meadows, S. The modified Insall-Salvati ratio for assessment of patellar height. *Clin Orthop* 170–176, 1990.

151. Hallisey, M.J., et al. Anatomy of the junction of the vastus lateralis tendon and the patella. *J Bone Joint Surg* 69A:545–549, 1987.

152. Heatley, F.W., et al. Tibial tubercle advancement for anterior knee pain. A temporary or permanent solution. 208:215–224, 1986.

153. Hille, E., et al. Pressure and contact surface measurements within the femoropatellar joint and their variations following lateral release. *Arch Orthop Trauma Surg* 104:275–282, 1985.

154. Huberti, H.H., and Hayes, W.C. Patellofemoral contact pressures: The influence of Q angle and tendofemoral contact. *J Bone Joint Surg* 66A:715, 1984.

155. Huberti, H.H., et al. Contact pressures in chondromalacia patellae and the effects of capsular reconstructive procedures. *J Orthop Res* 6(4):499–508, 1988.

156. Hughston, J.C., and Deese, M. Medial subluxation of the patella as a complication of lateral retinacular release. *Am J Sports Med* 16:22, 1988.

157. Insall, J. Current concepts review: Patellar pain. *J Bone Joint Surg* 64A:147–152, 1982.

158. Insall, J. Chrondromalacia patellae: Patellar malalignment syndrome. *Orthop Clin North Am* 10:117–127, 1979.

159. Insall, J., and Salvati, E. Patella position in the normal knee joint. *Radiology* 101:101, 1971.

160. Insall, J., Falvo, K.A., and Wise, D.W. Chondromalacia patellae—a prospective study. *J Bone Joint Surg* 58A:1–8, 1976.

161. Joyce, M.J., and Mankin, H.J. Caveat arthroscopos: Extra-artic-

ular lesion of bone stimulating intra-articular pathology of the knee. *J Bone Joint Surg* 65A:289–292, 1983.

162. Karlson, S. Chondrolmalacia patellae. *Acta Chir Scand* 83:347, 1940.

163. Kaufer, H. Mechanical function of the patella. *J Bone Joint Surg* 53A:1551, 1971.

164. Kolowich, P.A., Paulos, L.E., Rosenberg, T.D., et al. Lateral release of the patella: Indications and contraindications. *Am J Sports Med* 18:359–365, 1990.

165. Koshino, T., and Sugimoto, K. New measurement of patellar height in the knees of children. *J Pediatr Orthop* 9:216–218, 1989.

166. Krandsdorf, M.J., et al. Primary tumors of the patella. *Skel Radiol* 18:365–371, 1989.

167. Kulowski, J. Chondromalacia of the patella. Fissural cartilage degeneration; traumatic chondropathy: Report of three cases. *JAMA* 100:1837–1840, 1933.

168. Laurin, C.A., Dusault, R., and Levesque, H.P. The tangential x-ray investigation of the patellofemoral joint, x-ray technique, diagnostic criteria and their interpretation. *Clin Orthop* 144:16–26, 1979.

169. Laurin, C.A., Dusault, R., and Levesque, H.P. The abnormal lateral patello-femoral angle: A diagnostic roentgenographic sign of recurrent patellar subluxation. *J Bone Joint Surg* 60A:55, 1978.

170. Levine, J., and Splain, S. Use of the infrapatellar strap in the treatment of patellofemoral pain. *Clin Orthop* 139:179–181, 1979.

171. Lewis, M.M., and Reilly, J.F. Sports tumors. *Am J Sports Med* 15(4):362–365, 1987.

172. Lieb, F.J., and Perry, J. Quadriceps function: An electromyographic study under isometric conditions. *J Bone Joint Surg* 53A:749–758, 1971.

173. Limbird, T.J. Patellar subluxation following plica resection. *Orthop Rev* 17:168, 1988.

174. Lysholm, J., et al. The effect of a patellar brace on performance in a knee extension strength test in patients with patellar pain. *Am J Sports Med* 12:110–112, 1984.

175. Maldague, B., and Malghem, J. Chondromalacia patella: A radiological approach. *Acta Rheum Belg* 1:109–114, 1977.

176. Maldague, B., and Malghen, J. The true lateral view of the patellar facets. A new radiological approach to the femoral-patellar joint. *Ann Radiol* 19:573–581, 1976.

177. Maquet, P. Mechanics and osteoarthritis of the patellofemoral joint. *Clin Orthop* 144:70–73, 1979.

178. Marks, K.E., and Bentley, G. Patella alta and chondromalacia. *J Bone Joint Surg* 60B:71, 1978.

179. McConnell, J. The management of chondromalacia patellae: A long-term solution. *Aust J Physiother* 32:215, 1986.

180. McGinty, J.B., Johnson, L.L., et al. Current concepts review— Uses and abuses of arthroscopy. A symposium. *J Bone Joint Surg* 74A:1563, 1992.

181. Meachim, G. Age-related degeneration of patellar articular cartilage. *J Anat* 132:365–371, 1982.

182. Merchant, A.C., and Mercer, R.L. Lateral release of the patella: A preliminary report. *Clin Orthop* 103:40–45, 1974.

183. Merchant, A.C., et al. Roentgenographic analysis of patellofemoral congruence. *J Bone Joint Surg* 56A:1391, 1974.

184. Micheli, L.J., and Stanitski, C.L. Lateral patellar retinacular release. *Am J Sports Med* 9:330–336, 1981.

185. Milgrom, C., Kerem, E., et al. Patellofemoral pain caused by overactivity. *J Bone Joint Surg* 73A:1041–1043, 1991.

186. Mitchell, N., et al. Effect of patellar shaving in the rabbit. *J Orthop Res* 5(3):388–392, 1987.

187. Moller, B.N., Jurik, A.G., et al. The quadriceps function in patellofemoral disorders: A radiographic and electromyographic study. *Arch Orthop Trauma Surg* 106:195–198, 1987.

188. Moller, B.N., Krebs, B., and Jurik, A.G. Patellofemoral incongruence in chondromalacia and instability of the patella. *Acta Orthop Scand* 57:232, 1986.

189. Moller, B.N., et al. Chondromalacia induced by patellar subluxation in the rabbit. *Acta Orthop Scand* 60(2):188–191, 1989.

190. Mori, Y., Kuroki, Y., et al. The relationship between arthroscopic findings and clinical features in chondromalacia patellae. *Arthroscopy (Jpn)* 6:41–45, 1991.

191. O'Neil, D.B., et al. Patellofemoral stress. *Am J Sports Med* 20:151–156, 1992.

192. Ober, F.R. Recurrent dislocation of the patella. *Am J Surg* 43:497, 1939.

193. Outerbridge, R. The etiology of chondromalacia patella. *J Bone Joint Surg* 43A:752–757, 1961.

194. Outerbridge, R.E., and Dunlop, J.A.Y. The problem of chondromalacia patellae. *Clin Orthop* 110:177, 1975.

195. Owre, A. Chondromalacia patella. *Acta Chir Scand* (Suppl) 41, 1936.

196. Palumbo, P.M., Jr. Dynamic patellar brace: Patellofemoral disorders: A preliminary report. *Am J Sports Med* 9:45–49, 1981.

197. Patel, D. Plica as a cause of anterior knee pain. *Orthop Clin North Am* 17:273, 1986.

198. Pickett, J.G., and Radin, E.L. (Eds.). *Chondromalacia of the Patella.* Baltimore, Williams & Wilkins, 1983.

199. Pipkin, G. Lesions of the suprapatellar plica. *J Bone Joint Surg* 32A(2):363–369, 1950.

200. Raatikainen, T., et al. Effect of glycosaminoglycan polysulfate on chondromalacia patellae. A placebo-controlled 1-year study. *Acta Orthop Scand* 61(5):443–448, 1990.

201. Radin, E.L. Anterior knee pain: The need for a specific diagnosis: Stop calling it chondromalacia! *Orthop Rev* 14:128–134, 1985.

202. Radin, E.L. A rational approach to the treatment of patellofemoral pain. *Clin Orthop* 144:107–109, 1983.

203. Reikeras, O., et al. Patellofemoral relationships in normal subjects determined by computed tomography. *Skel Radiol* 19(8):591–592, 1990.

204. Roach, J.E., Tomblin, W., and Eyring, E.J. Comparison of the effects of steroid, aspirin and sodium salicylate on articular cartilage. *Clin Orthop* 106:350–356, 1975.

205. Roy, D.R., Green, W.B., and Gamble, J.G. Osteomyelitis of the patella in children. *J Pediatr Orthop* 11:364–366, 1991.

206. Sandow, M.J., and Goodfellow, J.W. The natural history of anterior knee pain in adolescents. *J Bone Joint Surg* 67B:36–38, 1985.

207. Schonholtz, G.J., et al. Lateral retinacular release of the patella. *J Arthroscopy Rel Surg* 1:92, 1985.

208. Schutzer, S.F., et al. The evaluation of patellofemoral pain using computerized tomography. A preliminary study. *Clin Orthop* 204:286–293, 1986.

209. Schutzer, S.F., Ramsby, G.R., and Fulkerson, J.P. Computed tomographic classification of patellofemoral pain patients. *Orthop Clin North Am* 7:235–248, 1986.

210. Shellock, F.G., et al. Patellofemoral joint: Evaluation during active flexion with ultrafast spoiled grass MR imaging. *Radiology* 180:581–585, 1991.

211. Simpson, L.A., and Barrett, J.P. Factors associated with poor results following arthroscopic subcutaneous lateral retinacular release. *Am J Sports Med* 12:251, 1984.

212. Slowick, F.A. Traumatic chondromalacia of the patella. Report of two cases. *N Engl J Med* 213:160–161, 1935.

213. Small, N. An analysis of complications in lateral retinacular release procedures. *J Arthroscopy* 5:282–286, 1989.

214. Small, N.C. Complications in arthroscopic surgery performed by experienced arthroscopists. *Arthroscopy* 4:215–221, 1988.

215. Stougard, J. Chondromalacia of the patella. Incidence, macroscopical and radiographical findings at autopsy. *Acta Orthop Scand* 46:809, 1975.

216. Sugiura, Y., Ikuta, Y., and Muroh, Y. Stress fractures of the patella in athletes. *J Jpn Orthop Assoc* 51:1421–1425, 1977.

217. Sutton, F.S., Jr., and Thompson, C.H., et al. The effect of patellectomy on knee function. *J Bone Joint Surg* 58A:537–540, 1976.

218. Townsend, P.R., Rose, R.M., Radin, E.L., et al. The biomechanics of the human patella and its implications for chondromalacia. *J Biomech* 10:403–407, 1977.

219. Voight, M.L., and Wieder, D.L. Comparative reflex response times of vastus medialis obliquus and vastus lateralis in normal subjects and subjects with extensor mechanism dysfunction. *Am J Sports Med* 19:131–137, 1991.

220. Watkins, M.P., and Harris, B.A., et al. Effect of patellectomy on the function of the quadriceps and hamstrings. *J Bone Joint Surg* 1983;65A:390.

221. Wiberg, G. Roentgenographic and anatomic studies on the femoropatellar joint, with special reference to chondromalacia of the patella. *Acta Orthop Scand* 1941;12:319–410.

222. Wild, J.J., Franklin, T.D., and Woods, G.W. Patellar pain and quadriceps rehabilitation. An EMG study. *Am J Sports Med* 1982;10:12–15.

223. Wilder, R.T., Berde, C.B., Wolohan, M., et al. Reflex sympathetic dystrophy in children. *J Bone Joint Surg* 74A:910–919, 1992.

224. Wiles, P., Andrews, P.S., Devas, M.B. Chondromalacia of the patella. *J Bone Joint Surg* 38B:95–113, 1956.

225. Wilppula, E., and Vahvanen, V. Chondromalacia of the patella. *Acta Orthop Scand* 42:521, 1971.

226. Yates, C., and Grana, W.A. Patellofemoral pain—A prospective study. *Orthopaedics* 9:663–667, 1986.

227. Yates, C.K., et al. Patellofemoral pain in children. *Clin Orthop* 255:36–43, 1990.

228. Youmans, W.T. Surgical complications of the patellofemoral articulation. *Clin Sports Med* 8:331–342, 1989.

228a. Abraham, E., Washington, E., and Huang, T.L. Insall proximal realignment for disorders of the patella. *Clin Orthop* 248:61, 1989.

Patellar Instability

229. Ahstrom, J.P. Osteochondral fracture in the knee joint associated with hypermobility and dislocation of the patella. *J Bone Joint Surg* 47A:1491–1502, 1965.

230. Albee, F.H. The bone graft wedge in the treatment of habitual dislocation of the patella. *Med Rec* 88:257, 1915.

231. Arnbjornsson, A., Egund, N., Rydling, O., et al. The natural history of recurrent dislocation of the patella—long-term results of conservative and operative treatment. *J Bone Joint Surg* 74B:140–142, 1992.

232. Baker, R.H., Caroll, N., Dewar, P., et al. Semitendinosus tenodesis for recurrent dislocation of the patella. *J Bone Joint Surg* 54B:103–109, 1972.

233. Bassett, F.H. Acute dislocation of the patella, osteochondral fractures, and injuries to the extensor mechanism of the knee. *Instr Course Lect* 25:40–45, 1976.

234. Beighton, P., and Horan, F. Orthopaedic aspects of the Ehlers-Danlos syndrome. *J Bone Joint Surg* 51B:444, 1969.

235. Bigos, S.J., and McBride, G.G. The isolated lateral retinacular release in the treatment of patellofemoral disorders. *Clin Orthop* 186:75–80, 1984.

236. Blasier, R.B., and Cuillo, J.V. Rupture of the quadriceps tendon after acute and recurrent dislocation of the patella—a preliminary report (Abstract). *Arthroscopy: J Arthroscopy Rel Surg* 2:68, 1986.

237. Boring, T.H., and O'Donoghue, D.H. Acute patellar dislocation: Results of immediate surgical repair. *Clin Orthop* 136:182–185, 1978.

238. Bradford, E.H. Slipping patella. *Boston Med J* 134, 1896.

239. Brady, T.A., et al. Intraarticular horizontal dislocation of the patella. A case report. *J Bone Joint Surg* 47A:1393, 1965.

240. Brattstrom, H. Shape of the intercondylar groove normally and in recurrent dislocation of the patella. *Acta Orthop Scand* 68:1–48, 1964.

241. Brown, D.E., Alexander, A.H., et al. The Elmslie-Trillat procedure: Evaluation in patellar dislocation and subluxation. *Am J Sports Med* 12, 1984.

242. Busch, M.T., and DeHaven, K.E. Pitfalls of the lateral retinacular release. *Clin Sports Med* 8:279–290, 1989.

243. Canton, D.D. Operation for recurrent dislocation of the patella. *Lancet*, March, 1860.

244. Carter, C., and Sweetnam, R. Familial joint laxity and recurrent dislocation of the patella. *J Bone Joint Surg* 40B:664, 1958.

245. Cash, J.D., and Hughston, J.C. Treatment of acute patellar dislocation. *Am J Sports Med* 16:244–249, 1988.

246. Cerullo, G., Puddu, G., Conteduca, F., et al. Evaluation of the results of extensor mechanism reconstruction. *Am J Sports Med* 16:93–96, 1988.

247. Chrisman, O.D., et al. A long-term prospective study of the Hauser and Roux-Goldthwait procedures for recurrent patellar dislocation. *Clin Orthop* 144:27, 1979.

248. Cofield, R.H., et al. Acute dislocation of the patella. Results of conservative treatment. *J Trauma* 17:526, 1977.

249. Cox, J.S. Evaluation of the Roux-Elmslie-Trillat procedure for knee extensor realignment. *Am J Sports Med* 9, 1982.

250. Cox, J.S. An evaluation of the Elmslie-Trillat procedure for management of patellar dislocations and subluxations: A preliminary report. *Am J Sports Med* 4, 1976.

251. Crosby, E.B., and Insall, J. Recurrent dislocation of the patella. Relation of treatment to osteoarthritis. *J Bone Joint Surg* 58A:9–13, 1976.

252. Dandy, D.J. Recurrent subluxation of the patella in extension of the knee. *J Bone Joint Surg* 53B:483–487, 1971.

253. DeCesare, W.F. Late results of Hauser procedure for recurrent dislocation of the patella. *Clin Orthop* 140:137, 1979.

254. Delgado-Martins, H. A study of the position of the patella using computerized tomography. *J Bone Joint Surg* 61B:443–444, 1979.

255. Dowd, G.S., and Bentley, G. Radiographic assessment in patellar instability and chondromalacia patellae. *J Bone Joint Surg* 68B:297–300, 1986.

256. Fairbanks, M.S. Internal derangement of the knee in children and adolescents. *Proc R Soc Med* 30:427, 1937.

257. Ficat, R.P., and Hungerford, D.S. *Disorders of the Patellofemoral Joint.* Paris, Masson, 1977.

258. Fielding, J.W., Liebler, W.A., Urs, N.D.K., et al. Tibial tubercle transfer: A long-range follow-up. *Clin Orthop* 144:43–44, 1979.

259. Fielding, J.W., et al. The effect of a tibial-tubercle transplant in children on the growth of the upper tibial epiphysis. *J Bone Joint Surg* 42A:1426, 1960.

260. Floyd, A., et al. Recurrent dislocation of the patella. Histochemical and electromyographic evidence of primary muscle pathology. *J Bone Joint Surg* 69B:790–793, 1987.

261. Frangakis, E.K. Intra-articular dislocation of the patella: A case report. *J Bone Joint Surg* 56A:423, 1974.

262. Fulkerson, J.P. Current concept review: Patello-femoral alignment. *J Bone Joint Surg* 72A:1424–1428, 1990.

263. Fulkerson, J.P., Schutzer, S.F., Ramsby, G.R., et al. Computerized tomography of the patellofemoral joint before and after lateral release or realignment. *Arthroscopy* 3:19–24, 1987.

264. Fulkerson, J.P. Anteromedialization of the tibial tuberosity for patellofemoral malalignment. *Clin Orthop,* 1983.

265. Fulkerson, J.P., and Hungerford, D. *Disorders of the Patellofemoral Joint* (2nd ed.). Baltimore, Williams & Wilkins, 1990.

266. Fulkerson, J.P., and Shea, K.P. Disorders of patellofemoral alignment. *J Bone Joint Surg* 72A:1424–1429, 1990.

267. Galeazzi, R. Nuove applicazion del trapianto muscolare e tendineo (XII Congress Societa Italiana de Ortopedia). Archivio de Ortopedia, 1922.

268. Goldthwait, J.E. Permanent dislocation of the patella. *Ann Surg* 29:62, 1899.

269. Goldthwait, J.E. Slipping or recurrent dislocation of the patella, with the report of eleven cases. *Boston Med J* 150:169, 1905.

270. Goldthwait, J.E. Dislocation of the patella. *Trans Am Orthop Assoc* 8:237–238, 1895.

271. Grana, W.A., and Kriegshauser, L.A. The scientific basis of extensor mechanism disorders. *Clin Sports Med* 4:247–257, 1985.

272. Grana, W.A., and O'Donoghue, D.H. Patellar-tendon transfer by the slot-block method for recurrent subluxation and dislocation of the patella. *J Bone Joint Surg* 59A:736–741, 1977.

273. Gross, R.M. Acute dislocation of the patella: The Mudville Mystery. *J Bone Joint Surg* 68A, 1986.

274. Hall, J.E., Micheli, L.J., and McNanama, G.B., Jr. Semitendinosus tenodesis for recurrent subluxation or dislocation of the patella. *Clin Orthop* 144:31–35, 1979.

275. Hampson, W.G.J., and Hill, P. Late results of transfer of the tibial tubercle for recurrent dislocation of the patella. *J Bone Joint Surg* 57B:209–213, 1975.

276. Hauser, E.D.W. Total tendon transplant for slipping patella. A new operation for recurrent dislocation of the patella. *Surg Gynecol Obstet* 66:199, 1938.

277. Hawkins, R.J., et al. Acute patellar dislocations. The natural history. *Am J Sports Med* 14:117–120, 1986.

278. Henry, J.H., et al. Lateral retinacular release in patellofemoral subluxation. Indications, results, and comparison to open patellofemoral reconstruction. *Am J Sports Med* 14:121–129, 1986.

279. Heywood, A.W.B. Recurrent dislocation of the patella: A study of its pathology and treatment in 106 knees. *J Bone Joint Surg* 43B:508, 1961.

280. Hoffa, H.Z. Habitual luxation of the patella. *Arch Klin Chir* 59:543, 1899.

281. Hughston, J.C., and Deese, M. Medial subluxation of the patella as a complication of lateral retinacular release. *Am J Sports Med* 16:383–388, 1988.

282. Hughston, J.C., and Stone, M.M. Recurring dislocations of the patella in athletes. *South Med J* 57:623, 1964.

283. Hughston, J.C. Subluxation of the patella. *J Bone Joint Surg* 50A: 1003–1026, 1968.

284. Hvid, I., Andersen, L.I., and Schmidt, H. Patellar height and femoral trochlear development. *Acta Orthop Scand* 54:91, 1983.

285. Inoue, M., Shino, K., Hirose, H., et al. Subluxation of the patella: Computed tomography analysis of patellofemoral congruence. *J Bone Joint Surg* 70A:1331–1337, 1988.

286. Insall, J., et al. Recurrent dislocation and the high-riding patella. *Clin Orthop* 88:67, 1972.

287. Jackson, A.M. Recurrent dislocation of the patella. *J Bone Joint Surg* 74B:2–4, 1992.

288. Jeffreys, T.E. Recurrent dislocation of the patella due to abnormal attachment of the ilio-tibial tract. *J Bone Joint Surg* 45B:740, 1963.

289. Kettlekamp, D.B. Current concepts review. Management of patellar malalignment. *J Bone Joint Surg* 63A:1344–1348, 1981.

290. Kirk, J.A., Ansell, B.M., and Bywaters, E.G.L. The hypermobility syndrome. *Ann Rheum Dis* 26:419, 1967.

291. Kolowich, P.A., Paulos, L.E., Rosenberg, T.D., et al. Lateral release of the patella: Indications and contraindications. *Am J Sports Med* 18:359–365, 1990.

292. Kummel, B.M., et al. Stabilization of the subluxating patella by semitendinosus transfer to the lateral third of the infrapatellar tendon. *Am J Sports Med* 5:194, 1977.

293. Larsen, E., and Lauridsen, F. Conservative treatment of patellar dislocations. *Clin Orthop* 171:131–135, 1982.

294. Laurin, C.A., Levesque, H.P., et al. The abnormal patellofemoral angle. *J Bone Joint Surg* 60A:55–60, 1978.

295. Limbird, T.J. Patellar subluxations following plica resection. *Orthop Rev* 17, 1988.

296. MacNab, I. Recurrent dislocation of the patella. *J Bone Joint Surg* 34A:957–967, 1952.

297. Madigan, R., et al. Preliminary experience with a method of quadricepsplasty in recurrent subluxation of the patella. *J Bone Joint Surg* 57A:600, 1975.

298. Maquet, P. Advancement of the tibial tuberosity. *Clin Orthop* 115:225–230, 1976.

299. Mariani, P.P., and Caruso, I. An electromyographic investigation of subluxation of the patella. *J Bone Joint Surg* 61B:331, 1979.

300. Mayer, G., et al. Chondral and osteochondral fractures of the knee joint—treatment and results. *Arch Orthop Trauma Surg* 107:154–157, 1986.

301. McCarrol, H.R., and Schwartzmann, J.R. Lateral dislocation of the patella: Correction by simultaneous transplantation of the tibial tubercle and semitendinous tendon. *J Bone Joint Surg* 27:446–452, 1945.

302. McManus, F., Rang, M., et al. Acute dislocation of the patella in children. The natural history. *Clin Orthop* 139:88–91, 1979.

303. Mendez, A.A., Ketet, D., and MacEwen, G.D. Treatment of patellofemoral instability in Down's syndrome. *Clin Orthop*, 1988.

304. Merchant, A.C., and Mercer, R.L. Lateral release of the patella. *Clin Orthop* 103:40–45, 1974.

305. Milgram, J.E. Tangential osteochondral fracture of the patella. *J Bone Joint Surg* 25:271–280, 1943.

306. Moller, B.N., Krebs, B., et al. Patellofemoral incongruence in chondromalacia and instability of the patella. *Acta Orthop Scand* 57:323, 1986.

307. Ober, F.R. Slipping patella or recurrent dislocation of the patella. *J Bone Joint Surg* 17:774–779, 1935.

308. Ober, F.R. Recurrent dislocation of the patella. *Am J Surg* 43:497, 1939.

309. Orr, H.W. Review of the surgical treatment of congenital dislocation, recurrent dislocation, and slipping patella. *Clin Orthop* 3:3, 1954.

310. Pearson: Pad for recurrent dislocation of the patella. *Lancet* 2:12, 1884.

311. Reider, B., Marshall, J., and Rink, B. Patellar tracking. *Clin Orthop* 157:143–148, 1981.

312. Reider, B., Marshall, J.L., Koslin, B., et al. The anterior aspect of the knee joint: Anatomic study. *J Bone Joint Surg* 63A:351–356, 1981.

313. Riegler, H.F. Recurrent dislocations and subluxations of the patella. *Clin Orthop* 227:201–209, 1988.

314. Rorabeck, C.H., et al. Acute dislocation of the patella with osteochondral fracture. A review of 18 cases. *J Bone Joint Surg* 58B:237–240, 1976.

315. Rosenberg, N.J. Osteochondral fractures of the lateral femoral condyle. *J Bone Joint Surg* 46A:1013–1026, 1964.

316. Roux, C. Recurrent dislocations of the patella—operative treatment. *Clin Orthop* 144:4–8, 1979.

317. Runow, A. The dislocating patella. *Acta Orthop Scand* (Suppl) 201:54, 1983.

318. Sargent, J.R., and Teipner, W.A. Medial retinacular repair of acute and recurrent dislocation of the patella—a preliminary report. *J Bone Joint Surg* 53A:386, 1971.

319. Schoenholtz, G.J., et al. Lateral retinacular release of the patella. *Arthroscopy: J Arthroscopy Rel Surg* 3:27, 1987.

320. Schutzer, S.F., Ramsby, G.R., and Fulkerson, J.P. Computed tomographic classification of patellofemoral pain patients. *Orthop Clin North Am* 17:235–248, 1986.

321. Scuderi, G., Cuomo, F., and Scott, N. Lateral release and proximal realignment for patellar subluxation and dislocation. *J Bone Joint Surg* 70A:856–861, 1988.

322. Shellock, F.G., Mink, J.H., et al. Patellar tracking abnormalities: Clinical experience with kinematic MR imaging in 130 patients. *Radiology* 172:799–804, 1989.

323. Sherman, O.H., Fox, J.M., et al. Patellar instability: Treatment by arthroscopic electrosurgical lateral release. *J Arthroscopic Rel Surg* 3:152–160, 1987.

324. Simon, W.H., et al. The effect of shear fatigue on bovine articular cartilage. *J Orthop Res* 8(1):86–93, 1990.

325. Stanisavljevic, S. Congenital, irreducible permanent lateral dislocation of the patella. *Clin Orthop* 116:190, 1976.

326. Stanisavljevic, S., Zemincik, G., and Miller, D. Congenital, irreducible, permanent lateral dislocation of the patella. *J Bone Joint Surg* 116:190, 1976.

327. Sutton, F.S., et al. The effect of patellectomy on knee function. *J Bone Joint Surg* 58A:537, 1976.

328. Trillat, A., Dejour, H., and Couette, A. Diagnostic et traitement des subluxations récidivantes de la rotue. *Rev Chir Orthop* 50:813, 1964.

329. Vainionpaa, S., Laasonen, E., Patiala, H., et al. Acute dislocation of the patella. *Acta Orthop Scand* 57:331, 1986.

330. Wall, J.J. Compartment syndrome as a complication of the Hauser procedure. *J Bone Joint Surg* 61A:185–191, 1979.

331. West, F.E. End results of patellectomy. *J Bone Joint Surg* 44A:1089, 1962.

332. Wiggins, H.E. Anterior tibial compartment syndrome. A complication of the Hauser procedure. *Clin Orthop* 113:90–94, 1975.

333. Wilber, M.C. Recurrent lateral dislocation of the patella: Preliminary results of pes anserinus transfer. *South Med J* 67:531–533, 1974.

334. Wilberg, G. Roentgenographic and anatomic studies on the femoral patellar joint. *Acta Orthop Scand* 12:319, 1941.

335. Yamamoto, R.K. Arthroscopic repair of the medial retinaculum and capsule in acute patellar dislocations. *Arthroscopy: J Arthroscopic Rel Surg* 2:125–131, 1986.

336. Youmans, W.T. Surgical complications of the patellofemoral articulation. *Clin Sports Med* 8:331–342, 1989.

Reflex Sympathetic Dystrophy

337. Aftimos, S. Reflex neurovascular dystrophy in children. *NZ Med J* 99:761, 1986.

338. Bernstein, B.H., Singsen, B.H., Kent, J.T., et al. Reflex neurovascular dystrophy in childhood. *J Pediat* 93:211–215, 1978.

339. Cooper, S.L., et al. RSD following knee surgery. *Am J Sports Med* 15:525, 1987.

340. DeLee, J. RSD following arthroscopic surgery. *Arthroscopy* 1:214, 1985.

341. Dietz, F.R., et al. Reflex sympathetic dystrophy in children. *Clin Orthop* 258:225, 1990.

342. Ehrlich, M.G., and Zaleske, D.J. Pediatric orthopaedic pain of unknown origin. *J Pediatr Orthop* 6:460, 1986.

343. Evans, J.A. Reflex sympathetic dystrophy. *Surg Gynecol Obstet* 82:36–43, 1946.

344. Ficat, R.P., and Hungerford, D.S. Disorders of the patellofemoral joint. Baltimore, Williams & Wilkins, 1977.

345. Forster, R.S., and Fu, F.H. Reflex sympathetic dystrophy in children. A case report and review of literature. *Orthopedics* 8(4):475, 1985.

346. Fulkerson, J., and Hungerford, D. Disorders of the patellofemoral joint. Baltimore, Williams & Wilkins, 1990.

347. Goldsmith, D.P., Vivino, F.B., Eichenfield, A.H., et al. Nuclear imaging and clinical features of childhood reflex neurovascular dystrophy: Comparison with adults. *Arthritis Rheum* 32:480–485, 1989.

348. Greipp, M.E., Thomas, A.F., and Renkum, C. Children and young adults with adults reflex sympathetic dystrophy syndrome. *Clin J Pain* 4:217–222, 1988.

349. Katz, M.M., and Hungerford, D.S. Reflex sympathetic dystrophy affecting the knee. *J Bone Joint Surg* 69B:797–803, 1987.

350. Kesler, R.W., Saulsbury, F.T., Miller, L.T., et al. Reflex sympathetic dystrophy in children: treatment with transcutaneous electric nerve stimulation. *Pediatrics* 82:728–732, 1988.

351. Kozin, F., McCarty, D.J., Sims, J., et al. The reflex sympathetic dystrophy syndrome. *Am J Med* 60:321–331, 1976.

352. Kozin, R., Ryan, L.M., Carrera, G.F., et al. The reflex sympathetic dystrophy syndrome (RSDS): III. Scintigraphic studies, further evidence for the therapeutic efficacy of systemic corticosteroids, and proposed diagnostic criteria. *Am J Med* 70:20–30, 1981.

353. Ladd, A.L., DeHaven, K., et al. Reflex sympathetic imbalance (RSI). *Am J Sports Med* 17:660, 1989.

354. Laxer, R.M., Allen, R.C., Malleson, P.N., et al. Technetium 99m-methylenediphosphonate bone scans in children with reflex neurovascular dystrophy. *J Pediatr Orthop* 106:437, 1985.

355. Lemahieu, R.A., Van Laere, C., and Verbruggen, L.A. Reflex sympathetic dystrophy: An under reported syndrome in children? *Eur J Pediatr* 147:47–50, 1988.

356. Leriche, R. *Surgery of Pain*. Translated and edited by A. Young. Baltimore, Williams & Wilkins, 1939.

357. Leriche, R. Desequilibres vaso-moteurs postz-traumatiques primitifs des extremities. *Lyon Chir* 20:746, 1923.

358. Mackinnon, S.E., and Holder, L.E. The use of three-phase radionuclide bone scanning in the diagnosis of reflex sympathetic dystrophy. *J Hand Surg* 9A:556, 1984.

359. Mitchell, S.W., Morehouse, G.R., and Keen, W.W. *Gunshot Wounds and Other Injuries of Nerves*. New York, J.B. Lippincott, 1864.

360. Mitchell, S.W. *Injuries of Nerves and Their Consequences*. Philadelphia, J.B. Lippincott, 1892, p. 11.

361. Ogilvie-Harris, D.J., and Roscoe, M. Reflex sympathetic dystrophy of the knee. *J Bone Joint Surg* 69B(5):804–806, 1987.

362. Olsson, G.L., Arner, S., and Hirsch, G. Reflex sympathetic dystrophy in children. *In* Tyler, D.C. and Krane, E.J. (Eds.), *Advances in Pain Research Therapy*. New York, Raven Press, 1990, pp. 323–331.

363. Patman, R.D., Thompson, J.E., and Persson, A.V. Management of post-traumatic pain syndromes: Report of 113 cases. *Ann Surg* 177:780–787, 1973.

364. Pillemer, F.G., and Micheli, L.J. Psychological considerations in youth sports. *Clin Sports Med* 7:679–689, 1988.

365. Ruggeri, S.B., Athreya, B.H., Doughty, R.G., et al. Reflex sympathetic dystrophy in children. *Clin Orthop* 163:225–230, 1982.

366. Schutzer, S.F., and Gossling, H.R. Current concepts review. The treatment of reflex sympathetic dystrophy syndrome. *J Bone Joint Surg* 66A:625–629, 1984.

367. Schwartsman, R.J., and McLellan, T.L. Reflex sympathetic dystrophy. A review. *Arch Neurol* 44:555–561, 1987.

368. Sherry, D.D., and Weisman, R. Psychologic aspects of childhood reflex neurovascular dystrophy. *Pediatrics* 81:572–578, 1988.

369. Small, J.S.: Arthroscopic lateral release. *Arthroscopy* 5:282, 1989.

370. Spurling, R.G. Causalgia of upper extremity: Treatment by dorsal sympathetic ganglionectomy. *Arch Neurol Psychiat* 23:784–788, 1930.

371. Sudeck, P. Über die akute (reflectorische) Knochenatrophie nach Entzundungen und Verletzungen an den Extremitaten und ihre klinische Erscheninungen. *Fortschr Reontgenstr Nuklearmed* 5:277, 1901–1902.

372. Sudeck, P. Über die acute Entzundliche Knochenatrophie. *Arch Clin Chir* 62:147, 1890.

373. Ter Meulen, D.C., and Weisman, R. Psychologic stresses in the evaluation of children with obscure skeletal pain. *Pediatrics* 79:587–592, 1987.

374. Tietjen, C. Reflex sympathetic dystrophy of the knee. *Clin Orthop* 209:234, 1986.

375. Wilder, R.T., Berde, C.B., Wolohan, M., et al. Reflex sympathetic dystrophy in children. *J Bone Joint Surg* 74A:910–919, 1992.

MENISCAL LESIONS

Carl L. Stanitski, M.D.

The knee menisci are biconcave, C-shaped wedges of fibrocartilage on the medial and lateral aspects of the femoral-tibial articulation. The medial meniscus is semilunar in shape, whereas the lateral meniscus tends to be more circular and could be considered similar in appearance to a doughnut with a bite taken from it. Both menisci are well attached to the intracondylar eminence and along the tibia by the coronary ligament and, for the medial meniscus, by the medial collateral ligament as well. Lateral collateral ligament attachment to the lateral meniscus is variable.

Only recently have the knee menisci been documented to be of significant importance to normal and prolonged knee function. In the 1800s they were considered functionless remains of intra-articular muscle origin, atavistic remnants that served no functional use. It is not surprising, given their perceived lack of importance to normal knee function, that their extirpation was felt to produce no significant consequence and no untoward sequelae.

EMBRYOLOGY

By the end of the embryonic period (8 weeks), the menisci have formed from the interzone or intermediate layer of the knee blastema and appear in almost adult form. The menisci form in concert with the anterior cruciate ligament (ACL), capsule, and patella and respond to intrauterine forces and active fetal motion. As intrauterine life progresses, the meniscal vascularity gradually diminishes, and there is continued progressive loss of vascularity from the postnatal period to preadolescence. This diminution in vascularity proceeds from the central area toward the periphery with retention of vascular segments at the periphery. Adult meniscal morphology is evident by 14 weeks of fetal life [27].

It has recently been hypothesized by Bird and Sweet [18] that nutrient canals through fenestrated capillaries in the periphery of the meniscus allow central meniscal perfusion and also supply nutrients, remove metabolic byproducts, and maintain the hydrostatic properties of the meniscus. Obstruction within such a system would lead to secondary meniscal degenerative changes.

During fetal life the menisci undergo changes of configuration to accommodate alterations in the femoral and tibial contact areas. Although the lateral meniscus may show more developmental variation, it is never normally discoid in shape at any time during its development. Clark and Ogden [27] showed that the ratio of meniscal to tibial surface areas on both the lateral and medial menisci and tibial plateaus is constant, demonstrating a uniform development with intimate concordant maturation of the tibia and meniscus.

The meniscal blood supply comes from a rich anastomosis from five constant arteries that include the superior (medial and lateral), middle (posterior), and inferior (medial and lateral) geniculate arteries [91]. In adults, Akeson and colleagues noted no intrinsic abnormal vasculature in menisci that were abnormal [29].

Over 50 years ago King [62], in a study of the vascularity of dog menisci, noted in the first sentence of his classic paper that "the semilunar cartilages have a very limited blood supply." He also proposed that canine menisci provide shock absorption, lubrication, and joint stability [63].

In a study of older adult cadavers, Arnoczky and Warren [10] demonstrated an excellent perimeniscal capsular vascular plexus through synovial and capsular tissues by way of the lateral, medial, and middle geniculate vessels. The peripheral 10% to 25% of menisci were well vascularized with the middle geniculate providing the main blood supply to the horn attachments. In the popliteal hiatus, the posterior lateral meniscus was devoid of any peripheral vessels.

Meniscal cellularity diminishes with increasing age. The superficial meniscal layers contain cells similar to fibroblasts, and the cells in the deeper layer appear to be more related to chondrocytes [27].

ULTRASTRUCTURE AND BIOMECHANICS

The decrease in vascularity and cellularity of the developing meniscus is accompanied by an increase in collagen density; the adult stage of meniscal vascularity and collagen concentration is reached at age 10 years. Approximately 75% of the organic matrix of the meniscus is composed of type I collagen [34, 71]. The ratio of collagen to noncollagen protein increases with increasing age, and the effect is most marked in the neonatal and early childhood periods. Collagen bundles in the more central portions are arranged radially, and the peripheral bundles are arranged longitudinally (circumferentially), the latter bundles being of a larger diameter [13, 21, 23]. Vertical and oblique fibers also are present, producing a mesh structure that provides improved compressive resistance centrally and tension resistance peripherally [37]. Peripheral compression displacement is resisted by the circumferential peripheral fibers that are attached to the intercondylar area [16]. Mucopolysaccharides, proteoglycans, and water further enhance protection against hydrostatic viscoelastic compression [71]. The entire system, however, is susceptible to shear and tensile forces. A change in orientation of the collagen fibers to the adult form of the meniscal infrastructure is seen with the increase in weight-bearing function that occurs during the early developmental years [27]. The most common type of meniscal tear in young people, the longitudinal tear, appears to be a function of the resistance provided by radial and vertical fibers.

Menisci also aid joint lubrication by producing a windshield washer effect on distribution of synovial fluid. Articular cartilage nutrients are thought to be wrung out of the menisci during weight bearing [64].

In canine and cadaveric human menisci, compression testing caused actual meniscal deformation, not just meniscal displacement. Krause and colleagues [64] believed that hoop stresses were generated following compression for a given load, and compressive articular deformation was two times that in meniscectomized knees compared with normal knees, illustrating the articular surface sparing effect provided by the menisci.

It is estimated that knees flex between 2 and 4 million times annually. By providing a balanced position of the tibia on the femur, the menisci provide load-bearing capabilities. Forty to eighty percent of the load transmission in the knee is taken up by the menisci [14, 15, 19, 39, 45, 64, 66, 68, 81, 88, 89, 107]. They also are an important anterior and posterior joint stabilizer [28]. DeHaven [30] noted a 30% failure rate for repaired medial menisci if a torn ACL was not also addressed. In Tria, Johnson, and Zawadsky's [101] study of 40 adult cadaver knees, 82.5% had no lateral meniscal attach-

ments to the popliteus, and these authors believed that the popliteus played no role in either meniscal retraction or meniscal protection. In contrast, the medial meniscus is well fixed to the deep layers and capsule of the medial collateral ligament.

Using three-dimensional magnetic resonance imaging (MRI) in cadaveric knees, Thompson and associates [100] demonstrated an average meniscal excursion of 5 mm for the medial meniscus and 11 mm for the lateral meniscus, a ratio of 1:2.3. Displacement was greater in an anterior to posterior direction than medial to lateral (Fig. 19–1).

Seedhom and Hargreaves [88, 89], in studying load transmission across menisci, noted a diminution in load sharing from 85% to 35% after partial medial meniscectomy and from 75% to 50% after partial lateral meniscectomy.

Baratz and colleagues [14, 15], in a study of adult cadaveric models, used pressure-sensitive film to study compression effects and the relationship of various types of meniscectomy to contact area stresses. Excision of a surgically created bucket-handle tear caused a 10% diminution of contact area and increased peak local compressive stress by 65%. In contrast, complete meniscectomy reduced the contact area by 75% and resulted in a 235% increase in peak local contact stress. With surgically created peripheral meniscal lesions that were repaired either by open or arthroscopic techniques, duplication of the test after the repair showed a normal peak stress distribution.

Contact stress was thought to be proportional to the

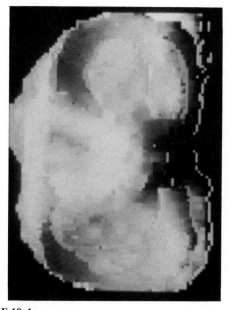

FIGURE 19–1
Top view 30 degrees of dynamic MRI of menisci. (Courtesy of Dr. Freddie Fu.)

amount of meniscus removed. Meniscal tears changed the normal joint mechanics. The instant centers of rotation and surface (tibial-femur) velocities were altered, the forces becoming less tangential and more compressive.

The functional need for the meniscus emphasizes that it is not an "appendix" of the knee awaiting extirpation at the first sign of pain. Meniscal preservation in young patients, if possible, should be a goal of all orthopedists.

INCIDENCE

In the United States, due to the increased number of children in organized competitive athletics and in individual unorganized sports, meniscal injuries are no longer considered uncommon. Football, basketball, and soccer seem to be the most significant sources of meniscal injuries. Several factors may account for this: (1) increased participation and competition; (2) increased body weight, speed, and strength; and (3) vascular and ultrastructural meniscal changes. When a sufficient change in meniscal properties is combined with increased demand, a rise in meniscal injury rate follows.

In the past, meniscal injuries in children were considered very uncommon [67]. The exact incidence of childhood meniscal injury is not known. Fairbank [35] thought that such tears in children all occurred in congenitally abnormal menisci. Meniscal tears were considered rare in anyone under 10 years of age. Smillie [94] reported a 3-year-old with a torn rudimentary medial meniscus. Saddawi and Hoffman [85] reported the youngest patient with a tear in a previously normal meniscus, a peripheral detachment in a 4-year-old. Volk and Smith [105] presented a case of a 5-year-old with a bucket-handle medial meniscal tear.

Stanitski and colleagues [95a] noted a significant number of isolated meniscal injuries in children in the preadolescent age group who presented with knee hemarthrosis. The frequency of combined meniscal and anterior cruciate ligament injury increases with age as the child approaches adolescence. The old attitude that children do not sustain meniscal injuries still persists, resulting in misdiagnosis and significant treatment delay.

If one reviews meniscal injuries in children, injuries of the lateral and medial menisci seem to occur with equal frequency if all discoid meniscal injuries are included. If discoid meniscal injuries are eliminated, the medial meniscus is injured significantly more often compared to the lateral.

HISTORY

A history of meniscal injury in children can be difficult to ascertain. Many times in school-age children,

especially those below high school age, the exact mechanism of injury is vague, and the usual complaints of delayed onset of effusion, mechanical signs of obstruction, and other historical points are often lacking. Care must be taken to differentiate pseudolocking from true mechanical blocking, that is, a limitation of motion within the joint that is alleviated by a specific maneuver about the knee that allows free motion by eliminating the offending mechanical block.

PHYSICAL EXAMINATION

Determination of the location, frequency, and magnitude of the pain should become a major interest and focus in taking the history. As Sir William Osler once said, "Pain is the enemy of the patient and the friend of the physician. Listen to the patient—he is telling you his disease." It is this complaint that commonly brings the patient to the physician's office and can serve as an excellent channel for determining many factors concerning the patient's knee.

Questions about changes of function should be asked to gain an appreciation of the magnitude of interference in the child's activities caused by the meniscal injury. Routine daily activities such as stair climbing, sitting, kneeling, and squatting should be investigated as well as symptoms that may occur only with increased stress such as athletic activities. A spectrum of the time of occurrence of symptoms needs to be kept in mind, one end being represented by symptoms that are present at a constant level even when at rest and the other end being represented by symptoms that occur only with vigorous athletic demands.

Knee symptoms occur in proportion to meniscal stability (e.g., pain versus locking) and to altered function (e.g., joint stability, articular cartilage lubrication and nutrition, and load bearing or sharing).

The mechanism of injury is usually a decelerating contact or noncontact force causing a compressive load with rotation that results in shear forces on the meniscal fiber. The exactitude of such a force will produce a specific pattern and magnitude of meniscal tear.

Symptoms vary with the acuity of the injury. Pain and giving way may be present in the early stages, whereas effusion, diminished range of motion, and intermittent pain are common complaints in more chronic meniscal injuries. The complaint of a pop at the time of acute injury, especially when coupled with immediate onset of significant effusion, is usually associated with an ACL tear with or without a meniscal lesion. In contrast, the onset of a delayed and smaller effusion is more commonly associated with an isolated meniscal injury that is not in the meniscal-synovial junction. Snapping, especially in a young child, may be the only complaint in someone with a discoid meniscus.

A history of past injury to the knee as well as its diagnosis, treatment, and recovery scheme should be evaluated. Any injury, treatment, and recovery of the opposite knee should also be assessed. Disorders such as Osgood-Schlatter's disease may co-exist with intra-articular pathology from a meniscal tear.

Clinical assessment still plays a major role in the diagnosis of meniscal injuries in children. Although the history of many knee complaints may be somewhat nonspecific in children, a meniscal injury is usually a memorable event with a precipitating single factor. Children sometimes are reluctant to divulge the exact situation in which such an injury may have occurred. In Vahvanen and Aalto's [102] series, 95% of patients presented with pain, 71% with intermittent complaints of effusion, 66% with snapping, 63% with giving way, and 54% with intermittent locking. Only 7% presented with a locked knee due to a meniscal lesion.

Determining the exact site of knee pain is an important historical point. This is particularly true in trying to differentiate a meniscal injury from a patellofemoral complaint because the former tends to have a more specific joint line focus, whereas the latter has a more diffuse distribution of discomfort. It should be remembered, however, that patients may have combined patellofemoral and meniscal injury secondary to similar mechanism of injury, that is, a deceleration and rotation injury, which also may cause an ACL injury.

Physical examination must be done in a situation that allows ease of observation. The patient should wear shorts. Assessment of knee problems should not be attempted by allowing the patient simply to roll up a pants leg.

Physical examination of the injured knee also may not reveal specific clues to meniscal injury. Joint line tenderness, either medially, laterally, or both, must be sought with precision. Anterior joint line tenderness, either laterally or medially, may be related to patellofemoral disorders that place stress on the patellomeniscal ligaments. The classic McMurray hyperflexion rotation test is commonly negative in children with meniscal tears. A truly locked knee resulting from displacement of a meniscal tear is uncommon. Effusion, knee instability, and range of motion also must be assessed, keeping in mind that without full motion, true instability of the knee may be masked and difficult to evaluate. Immediately following an acute injury, significant guarding will be present that will limit the efficacy of the initial examination.

The patient's gait should be observed to rule out a limp or other abnormality. In stance, varus, valgus, and recurvatum deformities should be noted. Range of motion of the entire lower extremity including hip, knee, ankle, and subtalar joint should be done and compared to the opposite normal side. Thigh girth and contour provide information about disuse or misuse with resultant atrophy. Knee joint effusion and synovial thickening should be sought. Tenderness about the knee should be assessed in a systematic manner not unlike that of playing a stringed instrument wherein small changes over short distances can be significant—specifically, joint line versus physeal versus collateral ligament tenderness. Tenderness about the anterior joint line as opposed to the mid to posterior joint line is often a helpful diagnostic sign of patellar versus meniscal pathology. A variety of described flexion-rotation maneuvers are often of little value in children and are rather nonspecific. Ligamentous stability about the involved knee compared to the opposite normal knee also needs to be assessed. It is interesting that in Vahvanen and Aalto's series of documented meniscal tears [102], up to one-third of patients had no significant findings on physical examination. In Harvell and colleagues' study [48], the initial physical findings and preoperative clinical diagnosis were poorly correlated with lesions documented arthroscopically, particularly in the preadolescent age group (Fig. 19–2).

IMAGING

Knee imaging techniques have markedly improved during the past decade and can aid significantly in the diagnosis of knee complaints and injuries in children. Each technique carries its own particular advantages and disadvantages. All imaging procedures depend on the sophistication of the equipment and the image interpreter.

Plain radiographs remain the standard of initial knee imaging and help to rule out other lesions that may mimic a meniscal disorder. It should be recognized that knee pain in children may be a consequence of hip disease, and appropriate hip roentgenograms should be obtained when clinical suspicion warrants. Nathan and Cole [76] suggest that hypoplastic femoral condyles and lateral tibial spines and an increased lateral joint space may be helpful in diagnosing a discoid meniscus on routine roentgenograms (Fig. 19–3).

Standard views include weight-bearing anteroposterior (AP) lateral, tunnel, and some type of skyline view to assess the patellofemoral relationships. Stress roentgenograms are required if ligamentous as opposed to physeal injury is suspected.

Double-contrast arthrography has been reported to be 60% to 97% accurate in assessing meniscal tears, especially medial meniscal tears [44]. Arthrographic findings of discoid menisci are considered notoriously inaccurate, especially as commented on by Vandermeer and Cunningham [104]. Hall [47] proposed an arthrographic classification of discoid types into six varieties and suggested that abnormal and inferior fascicles were present at the lateral meniscus or the entire popliteal sheath.

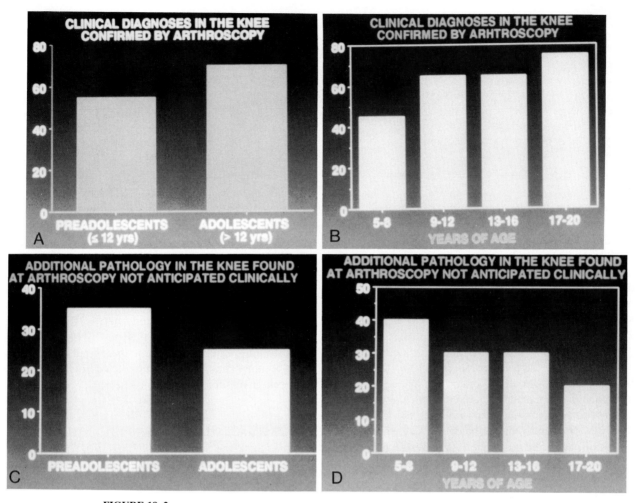

FIGURE 19–2
A–D, Children's Hospital of Pittsburgh arthroscopy study. Note age-dependent diagnostic accuracy.

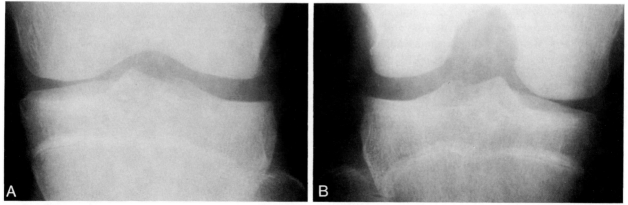

FIGURE 19–3
A and *B,* Discoid lateral meniscus. Note tibial spine changes and significant increase in width of lateral compartment space.

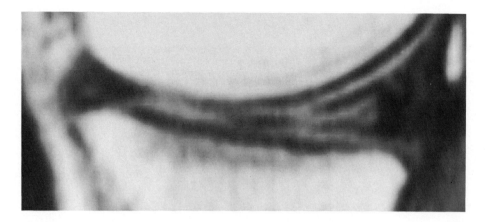

FIGURE 19–4
MRI of a medial meniscal tear in a 14-year-old basketball player.

Patient cooperation and the interest and experience of the arthrographer contribute significantly to the value of this test. Arthrography in children is invasive, often unreliable, and has largely been supplanted by MRI.

Computed tomography has never been of very much help with meniscal lesions, and it carries with it an increased amount of radiation exposure. It too has been supplanted by MRI, which is noninvasive and does not expose the child to ionizing radiation.

Interest in the use of MRI for knee disorders has expanded during the past several years [57, 109]. There is a limited amount of experience in the use of this technique in assessment of children's articular disorders. Diagnostic accuracy seems to vary with the technology involved, the primary factor being the size of the magnetic coil, with the larger coil (1.5 Tesla) having an advantage over smaller ones. Polly and associates [80] reported a 90% accuracy rate for the diagnosis of lateral meniscal tears and 98% accuracy for medial meniscal tears using MRI (Fig. 19–4). Silva and Silver [92] reported only a 45% diagnostic accuracy when assessing meniscal tears, but they used a significantly smaller coil in their study.

The advantages associated with MRI are its lack of ionizing radiation, its noninvasiveness, and enhanced resolution of intra-articular soft tissue images. Its expense and prolonged imaging time may be prohibitive in certain children. With the increased enhancement of images by MRI, the specter of a false-positive diagnosis arises from the misinterpretation of normal intra-articular structures such as the meniscofemoral ligament. Dynamic three-dimensional MRI may provide information about the stability of meniscal lesions and appears to be a promising technique for knee assessment (Fig. 19–5). MRI may also be valuable in follow-up studies of the fate of menisci that have been repaired or sculpted.

Diagnosis of a meniscal lesion still must be done using a combination of data including careful assessment of pertinent historical points, physical examination findings, and associated studies. Imaging findings must be correlated with the clinical picture. Diagnosis of knee pathology must be as specific as possible through use of clinical and imaging findings. The term "internal derangement of the knee" [5, 35, 53, 67] is imprecise and should be abandoned.

The differential diagnosis of a meniscal tear in a child, particularly a preadolescent, may be difficult and should include patellar instability, osteochondritis dissecans, loose body, juvenile rheumatoid arthritis, "plica," pigmented villonodular synovitis, synovial osteochondromatosis, and primary hip disease that mimics knee pain. Less common sources of such knee pain include benign and malignant tumors about the knee.

SURGICAL RESULTS

Approximately 50 years ago, under the influence of Smillie [94, 95] and Watson-Jones, total meniscectomy

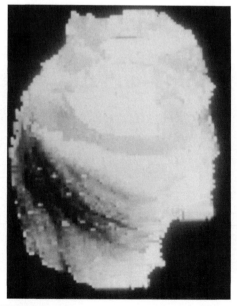

FIGURE 19–5
Three-dimensional dynamic MRI. (Courtesy of Dr. Freddie Fu.)

became the vogue. Almost "ritualistic genuclasis" (as noted by Goodfellow) was widespread. A totally removed meniscus was the goal and was a sought after surgical trophy. Much of this philosophy was based on the fear of allowing a torn posterior horn to go unnoticed. It was also believed that such complete removal of the meniscus enhanced the chances of formation of a new meniscal analog [20]. Unfortunately, using arthrotomy with limited visualization, a significant number of normal menisci were removed as well. As longitudinal follow-up studies were presented, the evidence became more compelling that meniscectomy was not a benign procedure, and the sequelae of the force-sparing effect of the meniscus became manifest.

Previous studies [1–4, 9, 26, 28, 36, 46, 55, 58, 61, 69, 72, 73, 77–79, 82, 83, 85, 86, 94, 95, 98, 102, 106, 112] reporting 40% to 90% satisfactory rates following meniscectomy included a mixed bag of injuries, nonspecific diagnoses (e.g., internal derangement of the knee), limited follow-up, absence of control groups, wide age ranges, and a multitude of treatment protocols. There are no studies following the more contemporary arthroscopic techniques of meniscal management in children with any significant follow-up. One must remember that a 10-year follow-up for an adolescent simply puts him or her in the early adult years with a significant portion of functional demands remaining on the knee.

In 1948 Fairbank [36] published a classic article on the roentgen changes that occurred following meniscectomy. A decrease in medial joint space with flattening of the femoral condyle and medial arthritic ridge formation were thought by him to be due to the loss of the weight-bearing function of the meniscus (Fig. 19–6). As he commented, "meniscectomy is not wholly innocuous: it interferes, at least temporarily, with the mechanics of the joint." He also believed it likely that these roentgenographic changes would predispose the patient to early

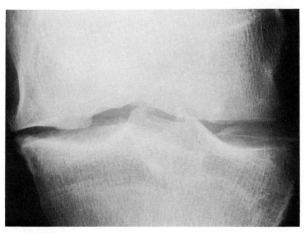

FIGURE 19–6
Fairbank's changes in a 20-year-old man who had had a complete medial meniscectomy at 10 years of age.

degenerative disease, but any connection between these appearances and later arthritis was not well established—"It was too indefinite to justify any clinical deductions," he suggested.

Cave and Staples [25] suggested that an uncomplicated medial meniscal tear should produce a 100% surgical cure. If not, the patient had an associated ligament tear or traumatic articular cartilage change that was unrecognized. In Tapper and Hoover's study [98], overall only 40% of knees were normal clinically at a 10-year follow-up. Interestingly, these authors felt that a long duration of preoperative symptoms did not prejudice the result and may actually have improved the result by allowing enough locking episodes to occur to enhance precision of diagnosis. The smallest percentage of excellent or good results was recorded in the under 28-year-old age group who had total meniscectomies. The authors ascribed this result to the more violent nature of the injury from sport and continued athletic abuse. Tapper and Hoover [98] also found that in patients under 28 years of age who underwent a partial meniscectomy (i.e., excision of only the bucket-handle fragment), there was an 80% success rate at follow-up. The poorer results noted in females were thought to be a result of misdiagnosis of meniscal tears instead of patellar instability in this group.

Abrams [3], in reviewing 10 children 12 years of age or younger who had meniscectomies from 1945 to 1955, thought that results were good but offered no follow-up. In 1953 Volk and Smith [105] reported on a 5-year-old with a bucket-handle tear who underwent a total meniscectomy and at follow-up 2 years and 3 months later complained of occasional slight pain when playing baseball or kneeling. Vahvanen and Aalto [102] reviewed 42 knees in 41 children with an average follow-up of 5.6 years following meniscectomy. In 12 of these knees a normal meniscus was removed. Seventy-one percent of the patients were reported to be symptom-free, but the patients had been followed for less than 5 years. Medlar and colleagues [73], in a review of 26 patients with an average follow-up of 8 years after total meniscectomy, found that only 42% had good or excellent results and 15 of the 26 patients had not returned to competitive athletics. Only 6 of 26 patients were totally asymptomatic, and all of the patients showed evidence of Fairbank's roentgenographic changes at follow-up. Rang [82], in reporting 96 meniscectomies performed at Toronto's Hospital for Sick Children over a 10-year period, found that the bucket-handle medial meniscal tear was the most common type, but classic meniscal symptoms and signs of positive McMurray tests, locking, or effusion were absent in more than half of the patients. In review of 61 cases after "several years follow-up," most were thought to have excellent results. Unfortunately, this follow-up was rather short.

Zaman and Leonard [111] reviewed meniscectomy results in 59 knees in 49 children whose surgery was done at an average age of 13 years and who were followed for an average of 7.5 years postoperatively. Twenty-five knees were asymptomatic in young adulthood, 11 knees were symptomatic only during sport participation, and 22 knees (40%) were symptomatic with any normal activity. Interestingly, 16 of these 22 knees had normal menisci that were removed at surgery. Roentgen changes were noted in 43 of the 59 knees, and only 27% of knees had normal roentgenograms at follow-up. The authors commented on the poor results in females and in knees that had undergone removal of a normal meniscus. They summed up this experience by noting that "the chance to do a meniscectomy is not a chance to cure, it is more like a visit to a loan shark."

Manzione and colleagues [69] studied 20 children between the ages of 5 and 16 years 3 to 14 years (average 5.5 years) after excision of an isolated meniscal tear through an open meniscectomy. Twelve medial and eight lateral menisci underwent excision, fifteen by total meniscectomy and five by partial meniscectomy. Sixty percent of these showed unsatisfactory results. There was no correlation of results with the procedure, whether lateral versus medial meniscectomy, type of tear, or partial versus total meniscectomy. Sixteen of twenty (80%) demonstrated Fairbank's x-ray changes, but the authors found no correlation between these changes at this stage and satisfactory or unsatisfactory clinical results. A statistically significant decrease in hip abduction strength was noted in patients with unsatisfactory results. Failure to achieve full rehabilitation produced compromised results even in these young children.

Abdon and associates [1] in a 1985 study reported on 89 children who underwent meniscectomy between the ages of 7 and 18 years (average 16.2 years) with a follow-up of 10 to 28 years (average 16.8 years). Medial and lateral meniscectomies were equally distributed, and males had each type of tear more often than females. By questionnaire, 74% of the patients reported satisfactory results, but only 52% had excellent or satisfactory results

by objective measurements. Patients who had had medial meniscectomies had a much better outcome than those who had had lateral meniscectomies. These authors noted no change in results with gender. Of the 23 patients who were displeased with their results 19 also showed significantly decreased objective scores.

At follow-up, 40% of patients had grade I instability, and 15% had grade II to III instability. This was especially true following lateral meniscectomy. Eighty-nine percent of knees showed roentgenographic evidence of diminution of joint space regardless of the type of injury or meniscal tear.

All the patients had been operated on by arthrotomy, and none were treated by partial meniscectomy. Because the patients at follow-up were only in their late twenties and early thirties, it was too soon to project exact outcomes, but with almost 90% of these patients demonstrating roentgenographic evidence of diminished joint space, progressive degenerative disease would seem to be not far behind, although roentgen changes and clinical status are not always exactly correlated (Table 19–1).

In a prospective study by Noble and Erat [77] on 200 knees, the risk of removal of a normal meniscus was thought to far exceed that of leaving a tear of the posterior third in the prearthroscopic era.

ARTHROSCOPY

Arthroscopy has revolutionized the diagnosis and management of meniscal injury in adults as well as children. A much more accurate diagnosis is possible, and precise corrective surgery is readily available. Most important, enhanced visualization of almost all parts of the knee virtually eliminates the fear of allowing posterior horn lesions to go unrecognized. Despite arthroscopy's accuracy, a diagnosis of medial meniscal tear is still commonly made preoperatively but is not confirmed arthroscopically.

Most authors of papers on children's knee arthroscopy note the difference between a correct clinical preopera-

TABLE 19–1
Comparison of Children's Meniscectomy Results

	Abdon [2]	Manzione [69]	Zaman [111]	Medlar [73]	Vahvanen [102]
No. of patients	89	20	49	26	41
Mean age at surgery	16.2	14.8	13.0	15.0	12.2
Mean follow-up	16.8	5.5	7.5	8.3	5.6
Publication year	1990	1983	1981	1980	1979
Normal (%)	34	25	19	15	—
Symptomatic (%)	66	—	58	77	29
Roentgen changes (%)	48	80	73	84	20

Note low percentage of normals, especially with increasing time of follow-up.

TABLE 19–2
Children's Preoperative and Postarthroscopy Diagnosis Correlation and Its Direct Relationship to Patient Age

	Morrissey [75]	Ziv [112]	Bergstrom [17]	Juhl [59]	Suman [97]	Angel [7]	Harvell [48]
Total number	32	156	71	76	72	205	310
Number of preadolescents	11	43	20	12	20	49	29
Number of adolescents	21	113	51	64	48	156	71
Percentage of correct preadolescent diagnosis	27			37.3	42		55
Percentage of correct adolescent diagnoses	61			45.4	55	56	70
Additional findings (%)							35/25

tive diagnosis and findings noted at time of arthroscopy (Table 19–2). Incorrect diagnoses in the preadolescent (i.e., less than 13 years old) range from 36% to 73%. Morrissy and colleagues [75], in the first article that specifically reviewed arthroscopy in the preadolescent, found only a 25% correlation between preoperative clinical assessment and arthroscopic findings. By comparison, there was a 61% correlation in adolescents over 13 years of age.

Angel and Hall [7] noted a 56% overall accuracy rate in clinical assessment as opposed to a 99% accuracy rate with arthroscopic diagnosis and arthroscopic findings. In their study, which comprises the largest series of arthroscopies to date in children, Harvell and co-workers [48] reported that of 310 knees in 285 children preoperative clinical diagnosis achieved an accuracy rate of only 55% in the preadolescent group (85 knees) compared with a 70% accuracy of clinical diagnosis in the adolescent 13- to 18-year-old age group (225 knees). At time of arthroscopy, an additional 35% of the preadolescent and 25% of the adolescent patients had intra-articular pathology not anticipated on preoperative clinical evaluation.

In all series, a high frequency of meniscal injury was noted in preoperative clinical diagnosis, whereas at arthroscopy no such injury was noted. All authors caution about the routine overdiagnosis of meniscal tears in children [7, 17, 33, 48, 50, 59, 70, 75, 97, 109].

Hopkinson and colleagues [54] and Terry and associates [99] reported isolated articular fractures of the femoral condyles that may mimic medial meniscal tear signs and symptoms. Arthroscopy in such a circumstance allows a precise diagnosis and eliminates unnecessary meniscal surgery.

Mariani and colleagues [70] followed 75 patients who had initial negative findings on arthroscopy (despite the fact that 28 of the patients experienced significant preoperative locking symptoms). They noted that 68 patients had complete resolution of symptoms following arthroscopy alone. In Angel and Hall's [7] study of arthroscopy in children less than 18 years of age, 38% of the knees were noted to be normal. The most commonly

disproved diagnoses were those of medial meniscal tear and chondromalacia patella. In only 36 of 76 patients older than 14 years of age was a meniscal tear confirmed. In six patients younger than 14 years old with a preoperative diagnosis of medial meniscal tear, all had normal knees at the time of arthroscopy. Juhl and Boe [59] found that out of a group of 76 patients only three who underwent arthroscopy and had had a preoperative diagnosis of meniscal tear required meniscal surgery. It must be remembered that clinical examination still plays a major role in preoperative assessment, and imprecise clinical evaluation is to be avoided as much as inappropriate surgery.

In a review of arthroscopic patients at Children's Hospital of Pittsburgh, Stanitski and colleagues [95a] found that 88 of 310 knees presented with significant knee hemarthroses. At follow-up, 70 patients were reviewed, and it was found that the majority had suffered a knee injury while involved in sports. In the preadolescent age group (12 years of age or under), 47% of patients had a meniscal tear (of these, 57% were peripheral medial and 43% were central longitudinal). Forty-seven percent of patients had an ACL tear, and one patient had a combined ACL and medial meniscal tear. In the adolescent age group (13 to 18 years old) 45% of patients had meniscal tears equally divided between peripheral and central types. Forty percent had ACL tears associated with meniscal tears, and 70% had isolated ACL tears (Table 19–3).

TABLE 19–3
Children's Hospital of Pittsburgh Arthroscopic Data in Acute Knee Hemarthrosis

	Meniscal Tear	Isolated ACL Tear	Meniscal + ACL Tear
Preadolescent (<12 years old)	47%	47%	6%
Adolescent (13 to 18 years old)	45%	70%	40%

With hemarthrosis, meniscal tear is as common as ACL tear, even in preadolescents.

Combining both groups, 46% of patients with acute knee hemarthrosis had a meniscal tear (23% isolated medial tears and 7% isolated lateral tears). An ACL tear was present in 67% of the patients either as an isolated entity (47%) or with an associated medial meniscal tear (20%). Hemarthrosis must be recognized as a harbinger of major intra-articular injury.

Associated meniscal and ligamentous injuries are not as uncommon in children as previously thought, particularly in the "never-never land" of adolescence. Increased sophistication in the diagnosis of acute tears of the anterior cruciate ligament, knowledge of its role in normal knee function, and management of its injury may provide improved data on meniscal injuries. Poor results following meniscal surgery in the past may have been due to unrecognized ACL instabilities, especially when these were coupled with total meniscectomy, which further destabilized the joint.

Interestingly, hemarthrosis in the early days of arthroscopy was considered a contraindication because of the attendant diminished visibility. Because hemarthrosis is such a beacon of significant knee injury, an accurate diagnosis is required to allow institution of specific treatment. Arthroscopy allows the physician to make such a precise diagnosis and to formulate a treatment plan, thus preventing the sequelae of delay in diagnosis and specific treatment. One should not condemn a knee by performing simple hemarthrotic aspiration and casting because these diagnoses are not specific enough for appropriate postcasting management.

It must be remembered that the result of meniscal surgery is a function of biology, not technology. The previous fear of knee surgery and its attendant sequelae should be diminished in this modern era of arthroscopic management, with the hope that delays in diagnosis and treatment will be reduced.

Meniscal function is directly related to its ultrastructure, and rational treatment for meniscal lesions must be based on this microanatomy and physiology. The most common meniscal tear in children is a longitudinal tear. Its position relative to the vascular junction as well as its size and stability are the primary criteria for treatment. One must rule out other meniscal or ACL injuries and take these factors into account when formulating a treatment plan.

Treatment protocols of meniscal injuries fall into five groups [31, 109]. In the first group, no treatment is required, and the meniscal tear is left alone if it is less than 5 mm in size, is in a peripheral zone, and is stable. Weiss and colleagues [109] noted in a 1989 multicenter study that only 12% of patients with such a lesion required surgery at a 2- to 8-year follow-up, with two-thirds requiring partial meniscectomy and one-third requiring meniscal repair.

The second group includes those patients who require immobilization for a larger stable peripheral meniscal tear measuring up to 1 cm in size. A gradual return to increased levels of activity is allowed during the 3 to 4 months following a 4- to 6-week period of immobilization and guarded weight bearing.

Group three comprises patients with meniscal lesions that are amenable to repair (i.e., tears of between 6 and 30 mm in an unstable meniscus). Tears occurring in the meniscus synovial (red-red) or red-white zones have the potential for healing because of the improved vascularity in these areas. A variety of techniques that augment healing such as the rasp or fibrin clot, among others, may be of value, but no specific data in children for such techniques are present. The body of the remaining meniscus must be undamaged to allow success of such reconstruction.

Group four includes patients with meniscal lesions that are not amenable to meniscal preservation and must undergo partial meniscectomies. These lesions most commonly include a variety of flap tears that are present within the body of the meniscus at the free margin. Such tears should be excised with only a small margin of normal tissue while preserving as much normal meniscus as possible. Small meniscal cysts may resolve with excision of such small partial tears [90].

Total meniscectomy should be a rare event in children. Complex tears within the body of the meniscus that are unrepairable and significant cystic degeneration within menisci with large associated meniscal cysts [90] are two circumstances that would require total meniscectomy. Total meniscectomy is often difficult, especially in the hands of an inexperienced arthroscopic surgeon, and the articular surface may be at risk.

TREATMENT

Meniscal preservation has become much more popular as data on normal meniscal vascularity have been gained [10, 22, 51, 62]. Repair physiology is based on the three zones of vascularity in the normal meniscus: the red-red junction at the periphery with vascularity on each side; the red-white junction between the peripheral vascular zone and the more avascular central zone; and a white-white zone characteristic of a tear (i.e., an avascular central area) (Fig. 19–7). Healing of peripheral lateral meniscal tears remains problematic because of the absent vascularity in the popliteal hiatus.

The first report of a meniscal repair was published in 1885 by Annandale [8], who repaired an anterior peripheral meniscal horn tear in a 30-year-old miner; excellent function was reported at follow-up.

Arthroscopic and open meniscal repair of peripheral tears gained popularity in the 1980s [11, 22, 24, 30, 51]. As techniques have improved, the complications of neu-

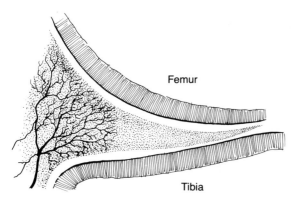

FIGURE 19–7
Meniscal vasculature diminishing from peripheral to central.

rovascular compromise and infection have diminished but still must be kept in mind in the course of arthroscopic meniscal repair [87]. Current procedures allow repair under arthroscopic control using a limited exterior incision to improve visualization of the stabilizing sutures and protect the neurovascular structures (Fig. 19–8). Use of an autologous fibrin clot, a meniscal rasp, and other stimuli for improved vascularity seems to enhance the results of meniscal repair. The frequency of fully healed meniscal repairs is higher in those who undergo simultaneous ACL repairs. Whether this improvement is due to the increased synovitis or to guarded prolonged immobility following the ligament repair is unknown.

Chronic tears may require increased preparation of the vascular zone compared to acute tears [11, 22]. A variety of techniques (outside-in and inside-out) have recently been advocated; the outside-in technique seems to be more appropriate for tears of the anterior meniscal horns, whereas the inside-out technique is more amenable to

posterior horn involvement (Fig. 19–9) [11, 22, 30, 51].

Scott and colleagues [87] reported on 178 repairs made in patients aged 9 to 52 years old (average 22.2 years). Sixty-eight of the patients were less than 19 years old, and 57 of those 68 were 15 to 18 years old. Of the lateral meniscal tears 73% healed, whereas 60% of the medial meniscal tears healed. Gershuni and colleagues [41] performed experimental studies in mature dogs and noted that vascularity could be encouraged from the periphery into the central area via a core made from the periphery to the central tear portion and transfer of a synovial flap. Keeping the dogs nonweight-bearing and immobilized enhanced meniscal healing.

All meniscal tears in children need not be either excised or repaired. Because of the improved vascularity and healing potential in children, peripheral meniscal tears of less than 1 cm that are stable (i.e., have less than 2 mm of motion when probed arthroscopically) do not need to be surgically treated but will respond to immobilization for 4 to 6 weeks and further rehabilitation. Return to agility sports in 4 to 6 months can be expected. The peripheral rim of the meniscus is assuredly vascular within its first 3 mm, but there is less assurance of vascularity from 3 to 5 mm, and all menisci in later childhood, adolescence, and adulthood, appear to be avascular beyond 5 mm.

When necessary, the damaged meniscal segment should be excised with preservation of a stable, well-balanced remaining meniscus to allow weight-sharing function. Whether this meniscal surgery is done arthroscopically or by the more formal arthrotomy depends on the surgeon's expertise. A well-executed partial meniscal excision via arthrotomy is a much better option than a poorly performed arthroscopic procedure with attendant significant articular damage.

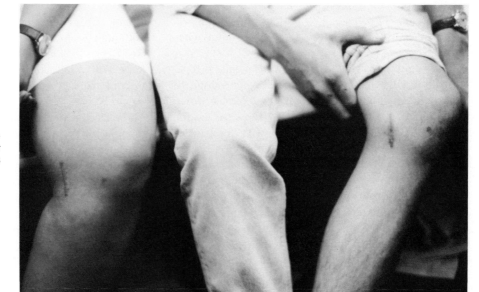

FIGURE 19–8
A brother and sister after medial meniscal repairs were performed for identical lesions from sports injuries 2 weeks apart.

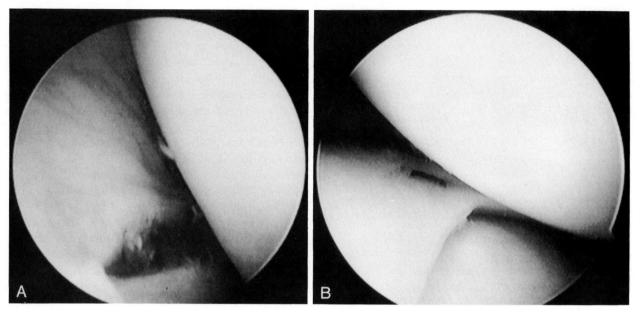

FIGURE 19–9
A, Unstable midposterior medial meniscal red-red junction tear. *B,* Repair of this tear under arthroscopic control.

Total meniscectomy, although performed significantly less frequently than in past decades, is still a viable management option for certain very specific types of meniscal lesions. If the meniscus has a large and complex tear including radial and longitudinal fibers and is unstable, or if a major meniscal tear and an associated parameniscal cyst are present, then total meniscectomy is indicated. Although uncommon, total meniscectomy still is indicated in very specific conditions.

Current attempts, both experimental and in very limited research clinical trials, to use meniscal replacements with allographic materials are in the preliminary stages with short follow-up [12, 96]. These substitutes may in the future provide a successful alternative to meniscal excision alone in patients with prolonged demands who would otherwise be destined to premature joint senescence.

Postoperative management following meniscal repair must protect the repair site while allowing motion for joint lubrication and physiologically tolerable forces across the junction for 4 to 6 weeks. The exact healing time needed for complete maturation of such repair, especially in children, has not been established. Rehabilitation efforts to maintain muscle strength and endurance as well as joint range of motion should be considered throughout the postoperative course.

Children require post-treatment rehabilitation as much as adults. Manzione and colleagues [69] correlated poor results with diminished hip abductor strength. It is incorrect to assume that these children will rapidly return to full function without any guided program. Children often become their own worst enemies during rehabili-

tation because of peer pressure, excessive expectations (professional athlete role models), and a feeling on the part of coaches and parents that children require less rehabilitative effort than adults. Maximum function following meniscal treatment is not possible until the child's lower extremity has normal strength, endurance, and agility. It is only at that point that sport-specific tasks and demands can be assessed prior to return to athletic endeavor.

DISCOID MENISCI

A discoid lateral meniscus was first discovered by Young [110] over 100 years ago in a cadaver specimen. Although he first described this entity anatomically, it was Kroiss [65] in 1910 who first attributed a "snapping knee" in childhood to this anomaly. The frequency of discoid menisci varies worldwide from 3% to 5% in Anglo Saxons [25, 32, 74, 93] to 20% in Japanese [6]. The exact incidence of bilateralness is unknown but is thought by Watanabe and colleagues [108] to be about 10% in Japanese.

In 1948, Smillie [93] suggested that three types of discoid lateral menisci exist: primitive, intermediate, and infantile. He hypothesized that the discoid meniscus was due to an arrest of embryologic development, a lack of resorption of the central portion of the meniscus that resulted in a persistent fetal state [94]. In Kaplan's [60] as well as Clark and Ogden's [27] studies a discoid configuration was not seen at any stage of fetal development. Kaplan [60] thought that, because of a lack of a posterior tibial attachment, stress caused the development of an increased thickness of the meniscus that produced the discoid morphology.

Watanabe and colleagues [108] suggested the possibility of three types of discoid lateral meniscus: (1) complete, (2) incomplete, and (3) Wrisberg (i.e., when the posterior meniscal attachment is attached solely by the meniscal-femoral attachment of Wrisberg and there is an absence of any tibial capsular attachment, leading to abnormal meniscal motion) (Fig. 19–10). This classification combines the elements of those of both Smillie [93] and Kaplan [60], that is, there is a varying increase in size compared with normal but with a posterior attachment versus size alone criteria. Such size assessment may be extremely subjective because the normal nondiscoid lateral meniscus covers 80% to 90% of the lateral tibial surface.

Gebhardt and Rosenthal [40] reported 14-year-old twin girls with bilateral discoid menisci with associated cystic changes. Ritchie [83] believed that lateral menisci were much more abnormal in children and presented a higher risk than in adults. In a study by Harvell and colleagues [48] of 310 knees that underwent arthroscopy, discoid menisci were found in only three knees (1%).

Meniscectomies of discoid menisci are reported infrequently. Of over 8000 meniscectomies reported by Smillie [94], 4.2% were discoid lateral and 0.06% were discoid medial menisci. Past teaching about discoid menisci held that total or subtotal meniscectomy produced the best results. It was thought that the meniscus was thickened, poorly vascularized, and poorly attached.

Vandermeer and Cunningham [104] reviewed six patients under the age of 20 years with an average follow-up of 54 months following discoid lateral complete meniscectomy. In this group of patients, only one-third had received the correct diagnosis preoperatively. Harvell and associates [48] noted only a 20% to 25% accuracy rate of preoperative diagnosis of discoid lateral meniscal tear in adolescents and preadolescents.

Dickhaut and DeLee [32] reported 12 patients with discoid lateral menisci, 10 of whom were asymptomatic because the meniscus had been noted incidentally at the time of arthroscopy for another reason. These patients' ages averaged 34 years. Six other patients studied by these authors had a symptomatic Wrisberg-type discoid meniscus and underwent total meniscectomy; the average age of these patients was 14 years.

The arthroscope offers the potential in patients with Watanabe type I and II discoid menisci for sculpting the abnormal meniscus while preserving a stable peripheral meniscal rim that can maintain some weight-bearing function (Fig. 19–11) [49]. Ikeuchi [56] questioned the abnormal collagen fiber arrangement present in discoid menisci and recommended leaving a 6- to 8-mm rim following such sculpturing. The average width of the normal nondiscoid lateral meniscus is between 12 and 13 mm.

Fujikawa and colleagues [38] recommended sculpting the lateral discoid meniscus if it was a stable type I or II. During a 6-year period 32 of 39 knees undergoing arthroscopy had discoid menisci in patients ranging from 3 to 15 years. Almost all of the findings were equal bilaterally, including a significant number of silent discoid lateral menisci. Following meniscal reshaping in seven children at a 1- to 2-year follow-up (including arthroscopic assessment), results were reported as excellent.

Rosenberg and colleagues [84] recently reported an arthroscopic repair of a Wrisberg-type discoid lateral meniscus; the patient returned to full athletic function 1 year later. Val [103] reported excellent results in 19 knees in 16 children with discoid lateral menisci (at follow-up of less than 3 years) following meniscal reshaping. These authors thought that the most common site of tear was the posterior central area, whereas Smillie believed that the horizontal cleavage-type tear was the most common kind of discoid menisci. Smillie's patients were primarily adults.

It must be remembered that the mere presence of a

FIGURE 19–10
Watanabe classification of discoid menisci. Type I: stable, complete; type II: stable, incomplete; type III: unstable due to lack of meniscotibial ligament continuity.

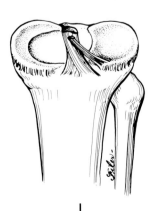
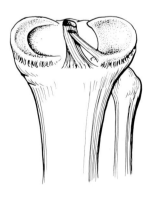
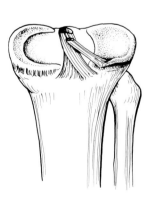

I

II

III

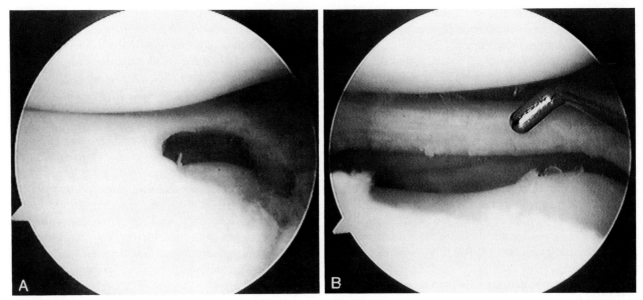

FIGURE 19–11
A, Incomplete, stable Watanabe type II symptomatic discoid meniscus. *B,* After sculpting to more normal meniscal configuration. (Courtesy of Dr. James Bradley.)

discoid meniscus is not an indication for its excision or surgery. Such menisci are often asymptomatic and are incidental findings at the time of arthroscopy for other lesions.

Meniscal injuries may occur in concert with other knee injuries, particularly ACL injuries, even in skeletally immature patients [26]. In nine patients under the age of 14 years with knee ACL injuries reported by Juhl and Boe [59], six had detached medial menisci, one had detached lateral and medial menisci, and one had a tear of the anterior lateral meniscal horn. In Angel and Hall's [7] series of arthroscopies in children under 18 years old, acute hemarthrosis was the herald of an ACL tear in 36% of patients. Harvell and associates [48] noted concomitant meniscal and ACL injuries in preadolescent and adolescent patients with hemarthrosis.

Arthroscopy remains the definitive evaluation technique of meniscal injury because it allows dynamic assessment of both the magnitude and the stability of the meniscal tear. The impact of arthroscopy and its attendant precise diagnosis is yet to be fully assessed in relation to children's meniscal injuries. There are no significant follow-up studies of arthroscopic meniscectomy or meniscal repair in children over a major period of time. Although partial meniscectomy (i.e., buckethandle or flap excision) versus total meniscectomy has been studied in adults [72, 98] and the former found to be preferable for long-term maintenance of knee function, such data are not yet available in children. Previous data on meniscectomy in children dealt with total meniscectomies done by arthrotomy, in most cases with woeful long-term results. The decreased morbidity fol-

lowing arthroscopy compared with previous results with formal arthrotomy has revolutionized postoperative management and significantly decreased atrophy, weakness, and stiffness, which were common following arthrotomy and meniscectomy in children.

The previous fear of knee surgery and the dreaded postoperative complications often led to delays in diagnosis and treatment. This enlightened era of meniscal management in children will, we hope, produce a generation of patients who will understand that knee surgery is not something to fear in either its acute or long-term stages but a procedure that will return life-long function. The meniscal preservation techniques with their associated postoperative immobilization requirement may not appear immediately palatable to a scholastic athlete. It must be emphasized to the patient and parent that the goal is for long-term, asymptomatic knee function, particularly in the workplace; it is not a quick fix that allows rapid return to pressing scholastic athletic competition at the risk of life-long vocational and avocational activities.

Ghosh and Taylor [43] described the meniscus as a "fibrocartilage of some distinction." It is essential that orthopedists continue to respect it as just that.

References

1. Abdon, C. P., Swanson, A. G., and Turner, M. S. Meniscectomy in children. *J Bone Joint Surg* 67B:847, 1985.
2. Abdon, P., Turner, M. S., Pettersson, H., et al. A long-term follow-up study of total meniscectomy in children. *Clin Orthop* 257:166, 1990.

3. Abrams, R. C. Meniscus lesions of the knee in young children. *J Bone Joint Surg* 39A:194, 1957.

4. Allen, P. R., Denham, R. A., and Swan, A. V. Late degenerative changes after meniscectomy. *J Bone Joint Surg* 66B:666, 1984.

5. Allingham, H. W. *Treatment of Internal Derangement of the Knee by Operation.* London, 1889.

6. Amako, T. On the injuries of the menisci in the knee joint of Japanese. *J Jpn Orthop Surg Soc* 33:1289, 1960.

7. Angel, K. R., and Hall, D. J. The role of arthroscopy in children and adolescents. *Arthroscopy* 5:192, 1989.

8. Annandale, T. An operation for displaced semilunar cartilage. *Br Med J* 1:779, 1885.

9. Appel, H. Late results after meniscectomy in the knee joint. A clinical and roentgenologic follow-up investigation. *Acta Orthop Scand* (Suppl) 133:1, 1970.

10. Arnoczky, S. P., and Warren, R. F. Microvasculature of the human meniscus. *Am J Sports Med* 10:90, 1982.

11. Arnoczky, S. P., Warren, R. F., and Spivak, J. M. Meniscal repair using an exogenous fibrin clot. *J Bone Joint Surg* 70A:1209, 1988.

12. Arnoczky, S. P., Warren, R. F., and McDevitt, C. A. Meniscal replacement using a cryopreserved allograft. *Clin Orthop* 252:121, 1990.

13. Aspden, R. M., Yarker, Y. E., and Hukins, D. W. L. Collagen orientations in the meniscus of the knee joint. *J Anat* 140:371, 1985.

14. Baratz, M. E., Fu, F., and Mengato, R. Meniscal tears: The effect of meniscectomy and of repair on intraarticular contact areas and stress in the human knee. *Am J Sports Med* 14:270, 1986.

15. Baratz, M. E., Rehak, D. C., Fu, F. H., et al. Peripheral tears of the meniscus. The effect of open versus arthroscopic repair on intraarticular contact stresses in the human knee. *Am J Sports Med* 16:1, 1988.

16. Beaupre, A., Choukroun, R., Guidouin, R., et al. Knee menisci. *Clin Orthop* 208:72, 1986.

17. Bergstrom, R., Gilquist, J., Lysholm, J., et al. Arthroscopy of the knee in children. *J Pediatr Orthop* 4:542, 1984.

18. Bird, M. R. C., and Sweet, M. B. E. A system of nutrient canals in the semilunar menisci. *Arthroscopy* 4:5, 1988.

19. Bourne, R. B., Finlay, J. B., Papadopoulos, P., et al. The effect of medial meniscectomy on strain distribution in the proximal part of the tibia. *J Bone Joint Surg* 66A:1431, 1984.

20. Bruce, J., and Walmsley, R. Replacement of the semilunar cartilages after operative excision. *Br J Surg* 25:17, 1937.

21. Bullough, P. G., Muneura, L., Murphy, J., et al. The strength of the menisci of the knee as it relates to their fine structure. *J Bone Joint Surg* 52B:564, 1970.

22. Cabaud, H. E., Rodkey, W. G., and Fitzwater, J. E. Medial meniscus repairs. An experimental and morphologic study. *Am J Sports Med* 9:129, 1981.

23. Cameron, H. U., and MacNab, I. The structure of the meniscus of the human knee joint. *Clin Orthop* 89:215, 1972.

24. Cassidy, R. E., and Shaffer, A. J. Repair of peripheral meniscus tears: A preliminary report. *Am J Sports Med* 9:209, 1981.

25. Cave, R. F., and Staples, O. S. Congenital discoid meniscus. A cause of internal derangement of the knee. *Am J Surg* 54:371, 1941.

26. Clanton, T. O., DeLee, J. C., Sanders, B., et al. Knee ligament injuries in children. *J Bone Joint Surg* 61A:1195, 1979.

27. Clark, C. R., and Ogden, J. A. Development of the menisci of the human knee joint. Morphological changes and their potential role in childhood meniscal injury. *J Bone Joint Surg* 65A:538, 1983.

28. Cox, J. S., Nye, C. E., Schaefer, W. W., et al. The degenerative effects of partial and total resection of the medial meniscus in dogs' knees. *Clin Orthop* 109:178, 1975.

29. Danzig, L., Resnick, D., Gonsalves, M., and Akeson, W. H. Blood supply to the normal and abnormal menisci of the human knee. *Clin Orthop* 172:271, 1983.

30. DeHaven, K. E. Peripheral meniscus repair. An alternative to meniscectomy. *Orthop Trans* 5:399, 1981.

31. DeHaven, K. E. Decision-making factors in the treatment of meniscus lesions. *Clin Orthop* 252:49, 1990.

32. Dickhaut, S. C., and DeLee, J. C. The discoid lateral-meniscus syndrome. *J Bone Joint Surg* 64A:1068, 1982.

33. Eilert, R. E. Arthroscopy of the knee joint in children. *Orthop Rev* 9:61, 1976.

34. Eyre, D. R., Koob, T. J., and Chun, L. E. Biochemistry of the meniscus: Unique profile of collagen types and site dependent variation in composition. *Trans Orthop Res Soc* 8:56, 1983.

35. Fairbank, H. A. T. Internal derangement of the knee in children and adolescents. *Proc R Soc Med* 30:427, 1934.

36. Fairbank, T. J. Knee joint changes after meniscectomy. *J Bone Joint Surg* 30B:664, 1948.

37. Fithian, D. C., Kelly, M. A., and Mow, V. C. Material properties and structure-function relationships in the menisci. *Clin Orthop* 252:19, 1990.

38. Fujikawa, K., Iseki, F., Mikura, Y. Partial resection of the discoid lateral meniscus of the child's knee. *J Bone Joint Surg* 63B:391, 1981.

39. Fukubayashi, T., and Kurosawa, H. The contact area and pressure distribution pattern of the knee. *Acta Orthop Scand* 51:871, 1980.

40. Gebhardt, M. C., and Rosenthal, R. K. Bilateral lateral discoid meniscus in identical twins. *J Bone Joint Surg* 61:1110, 1979.

41. Gershuni, D. H., Skyhar, M. J., Danzid, L. A., et al. Experimental models to promote healing of tears in the avascular segment of canine knee menisci. *J Bone Joint Surg* 71A:1363, 1989.

42. Ghadially, F. N., Wedge, J. H., and Lalonde, J.-M. A. Experimental methods of repairing injured menisci. *J Bone Joint Surg* 68B:106, 1986.

43. Ghosh, P., and Taylor, T. K. F. The knee joint meniscus: A fibrocartilage of some distinction. *Clin Orthop* 224:52, 1987.

44. Gillies, H., and Seligson, D. Precision in the diagnosis of meniscal lesions: A comparison of clinical evaluation, arthrography, and arthroscopy. *J Bone Joint Surg* 61A:343, 1979.

45. Grood, E. S. Meniscal function. *Adv Orthop Surg* 7:193, 1984.

46. Gross, R. H., and Grana, W. A. Meniscus injuries in children. *Adv Orthop Surg* 8:95, 1984.

47. Hall, F. M. Arthrography of the discoid lateral meniscus. *Am J Roentgen* 218:993, 1977.

48. Harvell, J. C., Fu, F. H., and Stanitski, C. L. Diagnostic arthroscopy of the knee in children and adolescents. *Orthopaedics* 12:1555, 1989.

49. Hayashi, L. K., Yamaga, H., Ida, K., et al. Arthroscopic meniscectomy for discoid lateral meniscus in children. *J Bone Joint Surg* 70A:1495, 1988.

50. Hayes, A. G., and Nageswar, M. The adolescent painful knee: The value of arthroscopy in diagnosis. *J Bone Joint Surg* 59B:499, 1977.

51. Henning, C. E., Lynch, M. A., and Clark, J. R. Vascularity for healing of meniscus repairs. *Arthroscopy* 3:13, 1987.

52. Henry, J. H., and Craven, P. R. Traumatic meniscal lesions in children. *South Med J* 74:1336, 1981.

53. Hey, W. Internal derangement of the knee. *In Practical Observations in Surgery.* London, 1803, Chap. 6.

54. Hopkinson, W. J., Mitchell, W. A., and Walton, W. C. Chondral fractures of the knee. Cause for confusion. *Am J Sports Med* 13:309, 1985.

55. Huckell, J. R. Is meniscectomy a benign procedure? A long-term follow-up study. *Can J Surg* 8:254, 1965.

56. Ikeuchi, H. Arthroscopic treatment of the discoid lateral meniscus: Technique and long-term results. *Clin Orthop* 167:19, 1982.

57. Jackson, D. W., Jennings, L. D., Maywood, R. M., et al. Magnetic resonance imaging of the knee. *Am J Sports Med* 16:29, 1988.

58. Johnson, R. J., Kettelkamp, D. B., Clark, W., et al. Factors affecting late results after meniscectomy. *J Bone Joint Surg* 56A:719, 1974.

59. Juhl, M., and Boe, S. Arthroscopy in children, with special emphasis on meniscal lesions. *Injury* 17:171, 1986.

60. Kaplan, E. B. Discoid lateral meniscus of the knee joint. *J Bone Joint Surg* 39A:77, 1957.

61. King, A. G. Meniscal lesions in children and adolescents: A review of the pathology and clinical presentation. *Injury* 15:105, 1985.

62. King, D. The healing of semilunar cartilages. *J Bone Joint Surg* 18:333, 1936.

63. King, D. The function of semilunar cartilages. *J Bone Joint Surg* 18:1069, 1936.

64. Krause, W. R., Pope, M. H., Johnson, R. J., et al. Mechanical changes in the knee after meniscectomy. *J Bone Joint Surg* 58A:599, 1976.

65. Kroiss, F. Die Verletzungen der Kniegelenkoszwischenk-Norpel und ihrer Verbindungen. *Beitr Lkin Chir* 66:598, 1910.

66. Kurosawa, H., Fukubayaski, T., and Nakajima, H. Load-bearing mode of the knee joint. *Clin Orthop* 149:283, 1980.

67. Lipscomb, P. R., and Henderson, M. S. Internal derangements of the knee. *JAMA* 135:827, 1947.

68. Lutfi, A. M. Morphological changes in the articular cartilage after meniscectomy. *J Bone Joint Surg* 57B:525, 1975.

69. Manzione, M., Pizzutillo, P. A., Peoples, A. B., et al. Meniscectomy in children: A long-term follow-up study. *Am J Sports Med* 11:111, 1983.

70. Mariani, P. P., Gigli, G., Puddu, G., et al. Long-term assessment of negative arthroscopies. *J Arthros Rel Surg* 3:53, 1987.

71. McDevitt, C. A., and Webber, R. J. The ultrastructure and biochemistry of meniscal cartilage. *Clin Orthop* 252:8, 1990.

72. McGinty, J. B., Geuss, L. F., and Marvin, R. A. Partial or total meniscectomy. A comparative analysis. *J Bone Joint Surg* 59A:763, 1977.

73. Medlar, R. C., Manidberg, J. J., and Lyne E. D. Meniscectomies in children—Report of long term results. *Am J Sports Med* 8:87, 1980.

74. Middleton, D. S. Congenital disc-shaped lateral meniscus with snapping knee. *Br J Surg* 24:246, 1936.

75. Morrissy, R. T., Eubanks, R. G., Park, J. P., et al. Arthroscopy of the knee in children. *Clin Orthop* 162:103, 1982.

76. Nathan, P. A., and Cole, S. C. Discoid meniscus. A clinical and pathological study. *Clin Orthop* 64:107, 1969.

77. Noble, J., and Erat, K. In defense of the meniscus. A prospective study of 200 meniscectomy patients. *J Bone Joint Surg* 62B:7, 1980.

78. Northmore-Ball, M. D., and Dandy, D. J. Long-term results of arthroscopic partial meniscectomy. *Clin Orthop* 167:34, 1982.

79. Northmore-Ball, M. D., Dandy, D. J., Jackson, R. W. Arthroscopic, open partial and total meniscectomy. A comparative study. *J Bone Joint Surg* 65B:400, 1983.

80. Polly, D. W., Callagnhan, J. J., Sikes, R. A., et al. The accuracy of selective magnetic resonance imaging compared with the findings of arthroscopy of the knee. *J Bone Joint Surg* 70A:192, 1988.

81. Radin, E. L., Delamotte, F., and Maquet, P. Role of the menisci in the distribution of stress in the knee. *Clin Orthop* 185:290, 1984.

82. Rang, M. *Children's Fractures.* Philadelphia, J. B. Lippincott, 1974, p. 186.

83. Ritchie, D. M. Meniscectomy in children. *Aust NZ J Surg* 35:239, 1965.

84. Rosenberg, T. D., Paulos, L. E., Parker, R. D., et al. Discoid lateral meniscus: Case report of arthroscopic attachment of a symptomatic Wrisberg-ligament type. *J Arthros Rel Surg* 3:277, 1987.

85. Saddawi, N. D., and Hoffman, B. K. Tear of the attachment of a normal medial meniscus of the knee in a four-year-old child. *J Bone Joint Surg* 52A:809, 1970.

86. Schlonsky, J., and Eyring, E. J. Lateral meniscus tears in young children. *Clin Orthop* 97:117, 1973.

87. Scott, G. A., Jolly, B. L., and Henning, C. E. Combined posterior incision and arthroscopic intraarticular repair of the meniscus. *J Bone Joint Surg* 68A:847, 1986.

88. Seedhom, B. B. Transmission of the load in the knee joint with special reference to the role of the menisci. Part 1: Anatomy, analysis and apparatus. *Eng Med* 8:207, 1979.

89. Seedhom, B. B., and Hargreaves, D. J. Transmission of the load in the knee joint with special reference to the role of the menisci. Part II: Experimental results, discussion and conclusions. *Eng Med* 8:220, 1979.

90. Seger, B. M., and Woods, G. W. Arthroscopic management of lateral meniscal cysts. *Am J Sports Med* 4:105, 1986.

91. Shim, A.-S., and Leung, G. Blood supply of the knee joint: A microangiographic study in children and adults. *Clin Orthop* 208:119, 1986.

92. Silva, I., and Silver, D. Tears of the meniscus as revealed by magnetic resonance imaging. *J Bone Joint Surg* 70A:199, 1988.

93. Smillie, I. S. The congenital discoid meniscus. *J Bone Joint Surg* 30B:671, 1948.

94. Smillie, I. S. Surgical pathology of the menisci. *In Injuries of the Knee Joint* (3rd ed.). Baltimore, Williams & Wilkins Co., 1962, pp. 51–90.

95. Smillie, I. S. *Injuries of the Knee Joint* (4th ed.). Edinburgh, Churchill Livingstone, 1970.

95a. Stanitski, C., Harvell, J. C., and Fu, F. Observations on acute knee hemarthroses in children. *J Pediatr Orthop* 13:510, 1993.

96. Stone, K. R., Rodkey, W. G., Webber, R. J., et al. Future directions. Collagen-based prostheses for meniscal regeneration. *Clin Orthop* 252:129, 1990.

97. Suman, R. K., Stother, I. G., and Illingworth, G. Diagnostic arthroscopy of the knee in children. *J Bone Joint Surg* 66B:535, 1984.

98. Tapper, E. M., and Hoover, N. W. Late results after meniscectomy. *J Bone Joint Surg* 51A:517, 1969.

99. Terry, G. C., Flandry, F., Van Manen, J. W., et al. Isolated chondral fractures of the knees. *Clin Orthop* 234:170, 1988.

100. Thompson, W. O., Theate, F. L., Fu, F. H., et al. Tibial meniscal dynamics using 3D reconstruction of MR images. Personal communication. In press, 1993.

101. Tria, A. J., Johnson, C. D., and Zawadsky, J. P. The popliteus tendon. *J Bone Joint Surg* 71A:714, 1989.

102. Vahvanen, V., and Aalto, K. Meniscectomy in children. *Acta Orthop Scand* 50:791, 1979.

103. Val, H. E. Discoid lateral menisci in children. *Arthroscopy* 4:122, 1988.

104. Vandermeer, R. D., and Cunningham, F. K. Arthroscopic treatment of the discoid lateral meniscus: Results of long-term follow-up. *Arthroscopy* 5:101, 1989.

105. Volk, H., and Smith, F. M. ''Bucket-handle'' tear of the medial meniscus in a five-year-old boy. *J Bone Joint Surg* 35A:234, 1953.

106. Walker, P. S., and Erkman, M. J. The role of the menisci in force transmission across the knee. *Clin Orthop* 109:184, 1975.

107. Watanabe, A. T., Carter, B. C., Teitelbaum, G. P., et al. Common pitfalls in magnetic resonance imaging of the knee. *J Bone Joint Surg* 71A:857, 1989.

108. Watanabe, M., Takeda, S., and Ikeuchi, H. *Atlas of Arthroscopy* (3rd ed.). Tokyo, Igaku-Shoin, 1978, p. 88.

109. Weiss, C. B., Lundberg, M., Hamberg, P., et al. Non-operative treatment of meniscal tears. *J Bone Joint Surg* 71A:811, 1989.

110. Young, R. B. The external semilunar cartilage as a complete disc. *In* Cleland, J., Mackay, J. Y., and Young, R. B. (Eds.), *Memoirs and Memoranda in Anatomy.* London, Williams and Norgate, 1889, p. 179.

111. Zaman, M., and Leonard, M. A. Meniscectomy in children: Results of 59 knees. *Injury* 12:425, 1978.

112. Ziv, I., and Carroll, N. C. The role of arthroscopy in children. *J Pediatr Orthop* 2:243, 1982.

OSTEOCHONDRITIS DISSECANS OF THE KNEE

Carl L. Stanitski, M.D.

Osteochondritis dissecans is a lesion of bone and articular cartilage of uncertain etiology that results in delamination of subchondral bone with or without articular cartilage mantle involvement. This lack of continuity may result in partial or complete separation of the fragment with significant effects on normal joint mechanics. Juvenile osteochondritis dissecans has a peak appearance in early adolescence with a male predominance of 3:1 or 4:1. It is rare in children under 10 years of age. Bilaterality has been reported to range between 20% and 30% [25, 32, 68]. When bilateral, the magnitude and course of the disorder are seldom equal (Fig. 20–1).

Originally described in adults, Green and Banks [32] four decades ago pointed out the frequent occurrence of osteochondritis dissecans in the skeletally immature patient. It is only in the past decade, however, that major efforts have been made to separate the juvenile form from the adult type. Previous data had combined the juvenile, adolescent, and adult types [9, 25, 39, 46, 68]. Based on physeal maturity, the differences in natural history, prognosis, and varied treatment demands of the particular types of knee osteochondritis dissecans are now recognized [10, 17, 18, 32, 56, 77].

ETIOLOGY

Although Sir James Paget first described osteochondritis dissecans in significant detail in 1867 [55] and termed it "quiet necrosis," it was Köenig in 1885 [5, 40, 41] whose name is associated with the term osteochondritis dissecans. He referred to it as "corpora mobile," a reflection of the osteochondral loose fragment that resulted from the process.

Since its initial description, there has been controversy regarding its etiology, and a variety of hypotheses have been proposed. The major ones suggest that the lesion is due to abnormal trauma or vascular configuration or reflects a normal ossific variant. Despite a variety of attempts to deduce the etiology of osteochondritis dissecans, no definite proof of its origin has been forthcoming.

Paget [55] differentiated osteochondritis dissecans from acute traumatic osteochondral fracture and asked, "How can such pieces of articular cartilage be detached from bone? They cannot be chipped off; no force can do this." Each of his patients had a history of injury, some at sport. He believed that the loose bodies in the joints were "sequestra, exfoliated after necrosis of injured portions of cartilage . . . without inflammation . . . its substance being without blood vessels." He also gave credit for the concept that localized necrosis causes loose bodies to previous authors including Broca, Lebert, and Klein, who had advocated the idea of spontaneous bone necrosis with subsequent fragment loosening.

In some cases, Köenig noted that the lesion occurred "without force worth mentioning" and raised the possibility of a spontaneous cause of separation. Despite this suggestion, he remained an advocate of trauma as the etiologic agent and hypothesized three levels of injury: (1) acute severe trauma, (2) lesser trauma causing a contusion, and (3) minimal trauma at the site of a preexisting lesion, which would cause what we now recognize as osteochondritis dissecans. He postulated that the secondary trauma and subsequent inflammation led to loose body formation.

Paget [55], Köenig [40], and later Fairbanks [24] and Smillie [68] advanced the concept of trauma as the source of the osteochondritic lesion. Fairbanks suggested that "the typical lesion is a fracture and nothing else." In 1933 he proposed that impingement of the tibial spine caused rotatory and shear stresses on the femoral condyle, producing a subchondral fracture. With increased

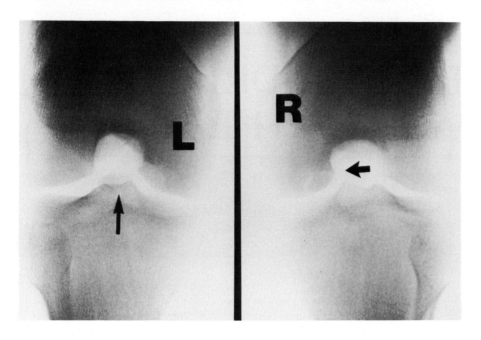

FIGURE 20–1
Unequal presentation of bilateral disease. Right knee is asymptomatic. Left knee's loose body caused locking.

use, the fracture would extend through the articular surface. Smillie [68], in 1960, supported this theory as a method of production of an osteochondritis defect in adults. Unfortunately, this theory does not explain other sites in the knee that can be affected (patella, lateral femoral condyle, lateral femoral patellar sulcus), nor does it recognize that impingement of the tibial spines does not occur during normal activity in a stable knee with full motion. In 75 patients reviewed by Carroll and Mubarak [14], no relationship was noted between osteochondritis dissecans and trauma, abnormally tall tibial spines, or patellar dislocation.

Most authors emphasize the need to differentiate between osteochondritic lesions from acute osteochondral fractures [1, 3, 4, 9, 11, 17, 18, 21, 24, 32, 39, 40, 43, 53, 54, 65, 77, 79, 81]. Repetitive microtrauma has been suggested as a cause of osteochondritis dissecans in children [6, 10, 14, 18, 53]. Other authors have suggested that sequential acute trauma might cause the lesion, the initial trauma producing necrosis and the secondary one a vascular injury leading to cartilage damage and separation [1, 9, 11, 17, 18, 39, 43, 56, 61, 73, 77, 79, 81]. In more mature children and young adults, the lesion usually appears as a concentric expanding zone. In the presence of such an area, trauma may precipitate an acute osteochondral fracture at an already weakened joint surface junction. Various authors [3, 8, 17, 21, 25, 43, 56] have suggested that up to 40% of patients with osteochondritis dissecans have a history of knee trauma ranging from mild to moderate, the initial event being far enough removed from the presenting complaint that it is almost forgotten unless an extremely accurate history is taken. Repetitive injury with subsequent denial of such is common in athletic patients. Aichroth [1] noted

that 61% of his patients with osteochondritis dissecans were classified as either excellent or good at school sports, and he believed that the lesion was secondary to a chondral or subchondral fracture that remained ununited and became a separate fragment.

Köenig [40] believed that necrosis in a part of the articular surface was followed by "dissecting inflammation," which caused separation of the fragment. When no inflammatory changes following primary fracture were found on further investigation (by himself or others), he admitted his error [41], but the term osteochondritis dissecans was by then firmly entrenched in the medical lexicon. Köenig admitted that at examination all signs of inflammation had disappeared. Most authors now think that, when it presents clinically, the lesion is in its reparative phase, not the inflammatory one.

The histopathology of human osteochondritis dissecans reflects the stages of the disease [5, 15, 51, 74]. Loose bodies are composed of dead subchondral bone of varying thickness with variable vascularization partially covered with viable articular cartilage. The femoral base shows thickened subchondral bony trabeculae with avascular changes. Normal metaphyseal bone is present below this bed. A fibrocartilaginous scar appears at the fragment junction indicating the chronicity of the problem, and in adults and older adolescents this scar mimics the tissue seen at nonunion. Reports of hemosiderin in fragments have been inconsistent. In Milgrim's study [51] only 23 of 47 loose body fragments had attached subchondral bone. He questioned the site of the original delamination and suggested that trauma and not avascular necrosis was the etiologic agent.

Acute, direct trauma on articular surfaces produced by a variety of experimental techniques results in osteochondritic-like lesions [43, 73]. Langenskjold [43] produced lesions in skeletally immature rabbits that histologically and radiographically resembled the clinical lesions of osteochondritis dissecans. The lesion was produced by cutting a segment of articular cartilage but leaving it attached to the synovium present in the notch. In a study using adult rabbits, Aichroth [1] produced osteochondral fragments that were replaced in either a stable or unstable fashion and followed for 6 to 12 weeks. Those that were fully separated and unstable led, not surprisingly, to nonunions in seven of eight fragments. Those that were completely separated but were stable united to some degree in 8 of 13 cases, the nonunited fragments having the histologic appearance of osteochondritis dissecans. The separated fragments that were stably pinned all went on to union with a thin bridge of bone. About half of them showed evidence of osteochondritic change. Aichroth concluded that the fragments that were stable would go on to union and those that were unstable would produce a nonunion compatible with osteochondritis dissecans in this lapin model.

The ischemic etiologic theory was proposed in 1920 by Rieger [65] who felt that fat caused obstruction to the vascular tree and subsequent articular and bone necrosis. Axhausen [3], in 1922, suggested that vascular obstruction by tubercle bacilli underlay the ischemia. Enneking [22] drew an analogy between the vascularity of the femoral subchondral metaphysis and that of the bowel mesentery. He suggested that the arcades in both are present with diminution of anastomoses at those zones. Infarction in this area causes wedged necrosis, resorption, and formation of granulation tissue between ne-

crotic and viable bone. Articular cartilage fracture could be caused by trauma with subsequent nonunion. Growth of articular cartilage that is nourished in synovial fluid would be unaffected. Rogers and Gladstone [66] assessed the blood supply of the distal femur in cadavers and showed that an excellent subchondral supply existed with multiple anastomoses. They believed that bone ischemia of the femur as a cause of osteochondritis dissecans was an extremely unlikely possibility.

Originally, Sontag and Pyle [69] in 1941 and later Caffey and associates [12], Ribbing [64], and others [44] suggested that the osteochondral lesion was nothing more than a normal ossific variant. Unfortunately, they did not offer follow-up in most patients to discover whether full resolution with growth occurred in these variants. Sontag and Pyle [69] thought that such epiphyseal irregularities were particularly notable in early adolescence and correlated this with the period of rapid growth. Caffey and colleagues [12] suggested that the irregular femoral chondral ossification margin is a normal feature of enchondral bone formation. With increasing maturity, such marginal abnormalities diminish (Fig. 20–2). In a review of roentgenograms of children without a history of symptoms, Caffey and associates [12] found that marginal irregularities were common and divided the patients into three groups. Group I showed some areas of calcification beyond the irregular ossific margin. Group II patients had large irregularities in the margins, and group III patients showed a true osteochondritic area with an independent zone surrounding an island of bone within a crater. These investigators suggested that this last group was similar to patients with classic osteochondritis dissecans. No formal follow-up

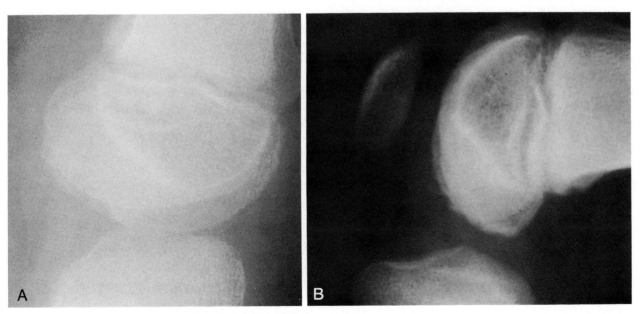

FIGURE 20–2
A and B, Normal radiographic ossific variants in 9- and 10-year-old boys.

was reported, although one of two patients had a roent-genographically normal-appearing femoral condyle 27 months later. In the other patient, at a follow-up of 18 months, roentgenographic resolution of the defect was seen. Ribbing [64], after reviewing roentgenograms of the knees of almost 300 children, suggested that osteo-chondritis dissecans was an accessory ossific nucleus that separated in childhood and did not fully reattach. He hypothesized that major or minor trauma caused fur-ther separation of the fragment, leading to subsequent clinical osteochondritis dissecans.

In 1977 in Scotland, Petrie [58] found an index patient with an autosomal dominant pedigree of osteochondritis dissecans, and he analyzed the first, second, and third degree relatives. No evidence of a familial pattern of osteochondritic defects was found. Some of the members studied had significant short stature and some had mul-tiple joint involvement, raising the question of a possible skeletal dysplasia. Patients with large weight-bearing ar-ticular defects commonly have a family history of such lesions. The incidence of such patients is unknown, and the frequency of the defect within families is likewise uncertain. Osteochondritis dissecans has been associated with Legg-Calvé-Perthes disease [78, 79], various types of dwarfism [78], and tibia vara [76]. To date, genetic factors have not been definitively shown to play a role in the development of osteochondritis dissecans [2, 26, 28, 52, 59, 60, 64, 70, 71].

The location of the lesions may vary, but the most common site is the lateral nonweight-bearing mid to posterior portion of the medial femoral condyle. The precise number of patients with significant involvement of the weight-bearing surface is unknown. In Carroll and Mubarak's [14] series of adolescents with osteochondri-tis dissecans, 72% had lateral involvement of the medial femoral condyle, 20% had lateral femoral condylar in-volvement, and 15% had patellar changes. Linden [46] reported an incidence of 57% of lesions located on the lateral portion of the medial femoral condyle in adoles-cents, and Green and Banks [32] found changes in that zone in 83% of their patients. The lateral femoral troch-lea [42] may be involved in a minor number of patients, usually young adults.

DIAGNOSIS

Historically, patients present with a vague knee ache that seems to be aggravated and precipitated with activ-ity. A history of intermittent knee swelling associated with activity is common. A patient rarely presents with an acutely locked knee due to a loose fragment as the initial manifestation of osteochondritis dissecans (Fig. 20–3).

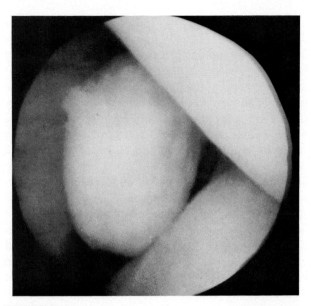

FIGURE 20–3
Intra-articular loose body from osteochondritis dissecans causing lock-ing.

Physical examination is nonspecific. Antalgic gait, loss of thigh circumference, diminished range of motion, effusion, or synovitis may be present. Wilson [80] de-scribed a helpful sign. He noted that five symptomatic children with medial femoral condylar osteochondritis dissecans all walked with external tibial rotation. In the second phase of this sign, when the tibia is internally rotated with knee extension in those with external rota-tion gait, pain is produced at the osteochondral site. The five children had intracondylar eminences of varying heights. Fairbanks [24] credits Axhausen with describing a sign of tenderness to palpation at the affected femoral condyle as the knee is brought into progressive degrees of flexion. This sign is particularly positive if the frag-ment is unstable.

A variety of imaging techniques have been suggested for diagnosis [49, 50, 51, 62, 63]. Routine plain roent-genograms remain the standard initial study. A tunnel view with the knee in flexion commonly demonstrates a lesion that is not as easily seen on a standard weight-bearing anteroposterior (AP) roentgenogram (Fig. 20–4). Lateral knee roentgenograms usually demonstrate the osteochondritic lesions between the lines proposed by Harding [34], that is, an area bounded by a line formed by the intracondylar notch at its superior recess and a line extended from the posterior femoral cortex. Lesions involving the lateral femoral cortex tend to be more posteriorly located than their medial femoral condylar counterparts (Fig. 20–5). Arthrography has been sug-gested as a means of demonstrating loss of articular continuity and fragment separation. In lesions with an intact articular mantle, arthrograms are of little value.

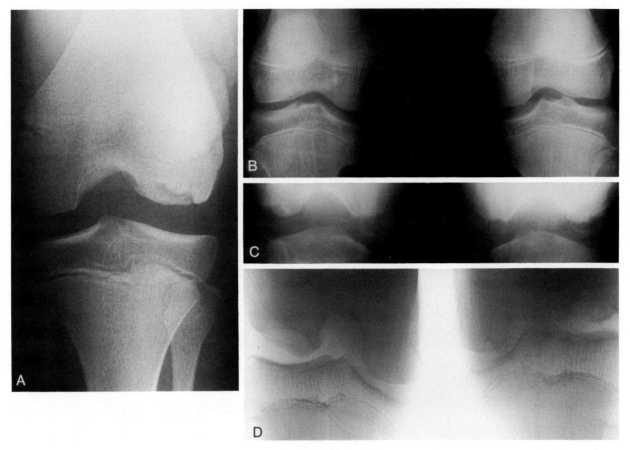

FIGURE 20–4
A, Tunnel view showing lesion in profile. *B,* Same patient as in *A* but with less defined lesion on weight-bearing AP view. *C,* Medial and lateral ossific variants seen on tunnel view in 10-year-old boy. *D,* Huge lateral condyle defects best noted on tunnel view.

Computed tomography (CT) scanning or thin film tomography may be helpful to assess the morphology of the lesion. As more experience is gained with magnetic resonance imaging (MRI) it may serve as a definitive

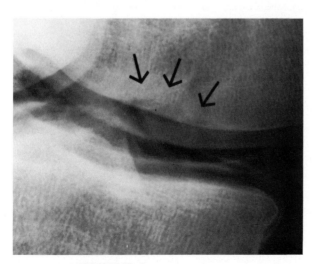

FIGURE 20–5
Posterior location of lateral OCD.

imaging tool not only for assessing the state of the articular mantle but also for evaluating the size and viability of the subchondral fragment and stages of healing (Fig. 20–6). As currently done, however, none of the imaging techniques provide information about fragment stability (Figs. 20–7 and 20–8).

In an attempt to improve assessment of the healing potential of osteochondritis dissecans, Litchman and colleagues [49] reported on the use of dynamic technetium-99 bone scintigraphy in 12 knees. Six of the patients were 11 to 18 years old. The authors thought that although this was a small series with a short follow-up, this method of quantitative analysis of regional blood flow allowed early differentiation of healing and was prognostic of a lesion that would not heal (Fig. 20–9). Symptoms in three of the patients resolved with observation. Two patients had no evidence of a fragment at surgery, and one patient, an 18-year-old boy who had experienced preoperative locking, had a loose fragment. Cahill and Berg [13] performed static bone scans every 6 weeks until there was evidence of healing in 18 adolescent patients. They correlated radionucleotide activity in the lesion with healing potential and divided bone

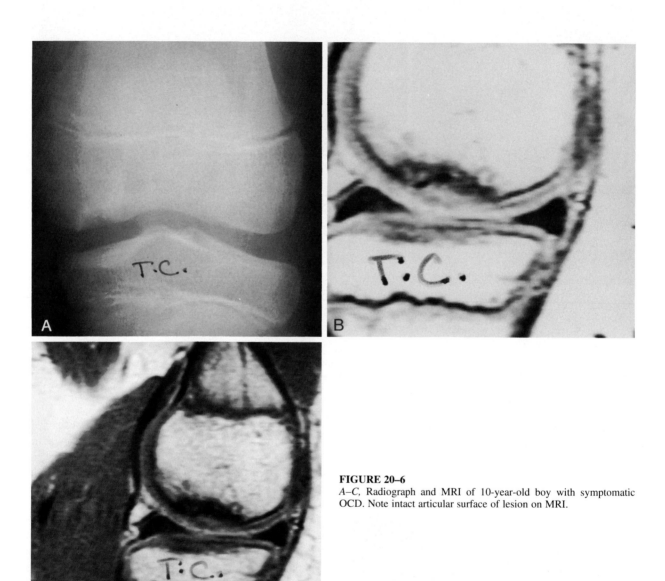

FIGURE 20–6
A–C, Radiograph and MRI of 10-year-old boy with symptomatic OCD. Note intact articular surface of lesion on MRI.

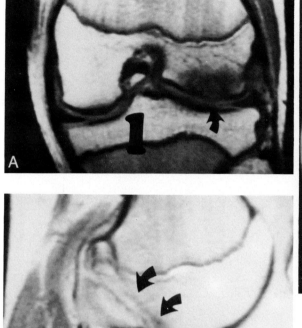

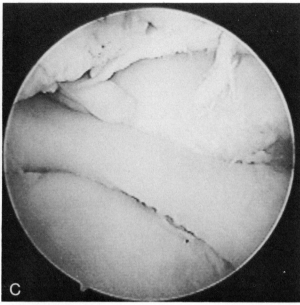

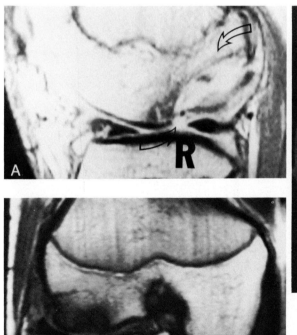

FIGURE 20–7
A and *B*, MRI of left knee with symptomatic lateral femoral OCD. *C*, Arthroscopic view of lesion showing displacement not appreciated on MRI.

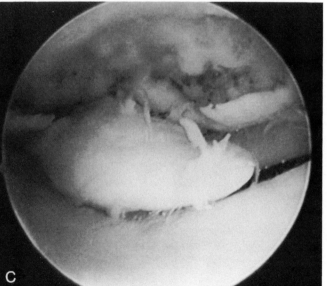

FIGURE 20–8
A–C, Findings similar to Figure 20–7 in 14-year-old boy.

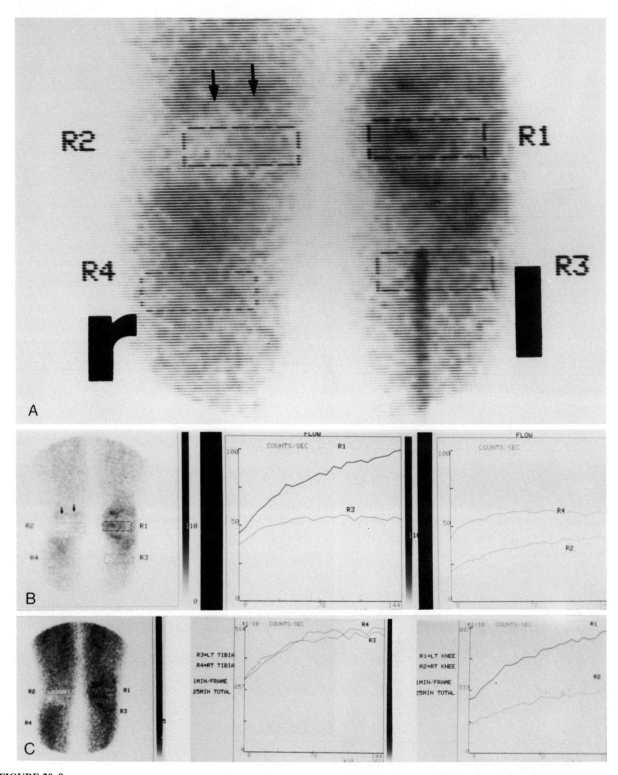

FIGURE 20–9
A, Dynamic bone scan of a 13-year-old boy with bilateral OCD that was symptomatic on the left and asymptomatic on the right. *B* and *C,* Graphic demonstration of flow and uptake at 1 and 25 minutes. With decreased right uptake, questionable healing potential exists.

scans and roentgenograms into five stages. Stage 0 was equivalent to a normal radiogram and a normal bone scan. In stage I, despite its radiographic appearance, the lesion demonstrated no bone scan activity. Stages II and III show progressive increases in nucleotide uptake, indicating increased vascularization of the area. In stage IV there was an increase in activity at the site of the defect on bone scan and some juxta-articular tibial changes as well. These authors suggested that in stage I, diminished healing potential was shown by a reduced amount of activity at the fragment. As the stage numbers increased, the predictability of healing potential increased because adequate vascularity was demonstrated by the scan.

The basic diagnostic approach should consist of a thorough history and physical examination, appropriate imaging techniques including routine roentgenograms and MRI if indicated to assess articular status, and, if adequate determination of fragment stability or articular surface status cannot be achieved by the above methods, arthroscopic assessment. In patients who have a loose body, imaging may allow assessment of the size of the fragment and the viability of the fragment bed as a preoperative planning measure.

The diagnosis of osteochondritis dissecans is commonly made as an incidental finding on roentgenograms. These previously "silent" lesions in asymptomatic patients need no other treatment than observation. In symptomatic patients, treatment proposals must take into account the natural history of the disease in this age group (i.e., children and adolescents).

In the only significant study done so far that includes long-term follow-up of juvenile and adult osteochondritis dissecans, Linden [46] reviewed 23 patients with juvenile osteochondritis dissecans in Malmo, Sweden. At an average follow-up of 33 years and an average age at follow-up of 45.5 years, he concluded that, in these untreated patients, "no complications later in life which could with certainty be associated with osteochondritis dissecans were found." Only two of these patients had minimal roentgenographic changes, and none of the patients had pain, diminished motion, change of stability, or loss of function. In contrast, those with adult-onset osteochondritis dissecans showed significant progression to early degenerative joint disease.

The primary prognostic factor is age, but other considerations such as lesion size, progression, location, and stability must be considered. Response to previous treatment and method of treatment should also be assessed. The ultimate goal is an anatomic, congruous, stable articular surface that does not progress to premature joint senescence. All recent authors agree that children with open physes have a much higher frequency of spontaneous resolution of this condition than adults (Fig. 20–10). Pappas [56] suggested a classification based on age at presentation. Category I encompasses children in early adolescence (girls less than 11 years old and boys less than 13). This group has an excellent prognosis. In category II, comprising children with a skeletal age of 12 to 20 for girls and 14 to 20 for boys, although physeal areas may still be open during some phase of this time period, the prognosis is less certain in these patients. In category III all patients are over the age of 20, and the adult form is evident with its diminished prognosis and increased need for surgical intervention.

The status of the articular cartilage mantle determines whether the lesion is open or closed (Fig. 20–11). Once the underlying bone is exposed to synovial fluid, the stability of the osteochondral fragment is compromised, and spontaneous resolution is unlikely. An open, unstable lesion is on its way to becoming a loose body. Nonoperative management in these circumstances is fu-

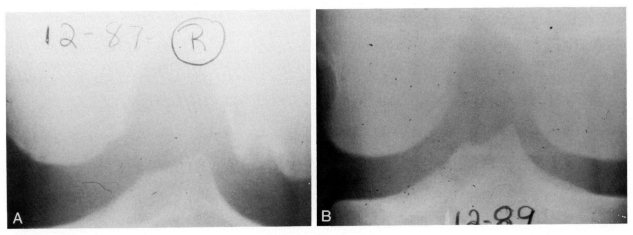

FIGURE 20–10
A and *B*, Medial femoral condylar OCD with progressive resolution over 2 years when activity was restricted in this boy who was 10 +7 years old at onset of symptoms.

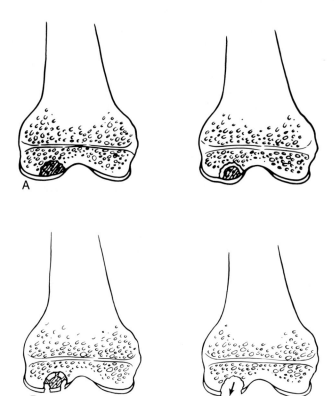

FIGURE 20–11

A and *B,* Schema of open vs. closed lesions, which are stable or unstable based on subchondral continuity.

tile. Roentgenographic evidence of sclerosis about the base fragment margin is a poor prognostic sign for spontaneous resolution (Tables 20–1 and 20–2).

TREATMENT

Nonoperative

Nonoperative treatment by a variety of means may allow spontaneous healing [6, 14, 32, 46, 77, 79]. Brief periods of immobilization or activity modification usually produce resolution. In the 1958 study by Green and Banks [32], 19 cases of osteochondritis dissecans in children under 15 years of age were reported. The great

majority of patients had medial femoral condylar involvement (83%). Nonweight-bearing treatment was achieved by plaster immobilization or bracing with ambulatory aids for an average of 7 months. It usually took at least 3 months before roentgen changes of healing became evident. Because it is essential to differentiate patients with knee pain due to other causes but with roentgen changes proportional to osteochondritis dissecans secondary to normal variance, overtreatment claims of cure for that specific treatment are avoided. The role of joint motion in articular cartilage nutrition is important, and prolonged immobilization is to be avoided.

Surgical Treatment

In 1558, Ambrose Paré [57] described the removal of a loose body (''stone, the size of an almond'') from the knee of one Jean Bourlier, the fragment due to what we now recognize as osteochondritis dissecans. Paré commented that the patient made a satisfactory recovery. More than three decades ago, Smillie [68] outlined the basic concepts underlying surgical treatment of osteochondritis dissecans. He recommended that unstable lesions that were multiple, fragmented, deformed, or necrotic be debrided. He also cautioned that the lesion's surface size often belied its true extent. In symptomatic patients (regardless of age) with closed lesions he recommended transarticular drilling. For open lesions, he recommended curettage of the base via a perilesional window. For large fragments he suggested removal, debridement of the bed, and replacement and fixation of the fragment. A subchondral bone graft can be done if required to eliminate any articular depressions.

These basic surgical principles are still pertinent with modifications to accommodate current technology. Arthroscopy has become a dominant force in evaluating the size, location, and stability of the fragment. Direct probe under arthroscopic control of the affected area reveals the change in turgor of the articular surface at the lesion margins and allows appreciation of the underlying bone's stability (Figs. 20–12 to 20–14). If required, articular transgression is avoided, and drilling or fixation [38, 45, 47] of the fragment is commonly ac-

TABLE 20–1
Symptomatic Osteochondritis Dissecans

	Closed	
Stable		Unstable
Immobilize; Activity restriction		Arthroscopic retrograde drill or fixation
Healed	Not healed	
Resume activity	Assessment and management	

TABLE 20–2
Symptomatic Osteochondritis Dissecans

	Open	
In situ stable	In situ unstable	Loose body
Retrograde fixation in situ	Retrograde fixation in situ	Anatomic reduction[a]
Healed Unhealed: Excision	Healed Unhealed: Excision	Excision[b]
		Secondary reconstruction[c]

[a]Following acute displacement of previous in situ unstable fragment
[b]Minimal or nonweight-bearing zone; fragment too large (i.e., nonanatomic fit); inadequate fragment osseous base
[c]Osteocartilaginous graft

complished retrograde via the nonarticular route using imaging guidance (Fig. 20–15). A multitude of fixation devices have been advocated including bone pegs and metallic pins and screws [10, 31, 35, 36, 37, 38, 47, 48, 75]. Replacement and fixation of a displaced fragment or excision of an anatomically loose body may also be carried out. Excision of fragments in a nonweight-bearing zone is appropriate. Recently, absorbable "pins" have been advocated to provide transarticular fixation [7, 16]. No data have yet been generated on the long-term outcome of these devices in the skeletally immature patient. Preliminary data [27] indicate that sterile synovitis secondary to pin degradation products may be of some concern. Each case must be decided on an individual basis depending on the patient's age, healing potential, fragment size, and fragment location (in terms of percentage of weight-bearing surface, amount of subchon-

dral bone remaining on the fragment, and the status of the articular portion of the fragment) (Fig. 20–16). It has been my experience that lateral femoral condylar lesions tend to be more posterior, larger, less stable, and more fragmented, and that smaller segments of subchondral bone are present on the fragment (Fig. 20–17).

Regardless of which fixation and treatment techniques are used, all current authors recommend gaining immediate stability after fragment fixation so that unimpeded range of motion exercises may begin, allowing the salutary effects of motion on articular cartilage to aid recovery.

Guhl [33] suggests that arthroscopic management of the condition is best in patients over 12 years of age with lesions of more than 1 cm and involvement of the weight-bearing surface. Fragment stability and the rationale for age and size criteria were not well defined in his manuscript. Advocates of surgical drilling of the

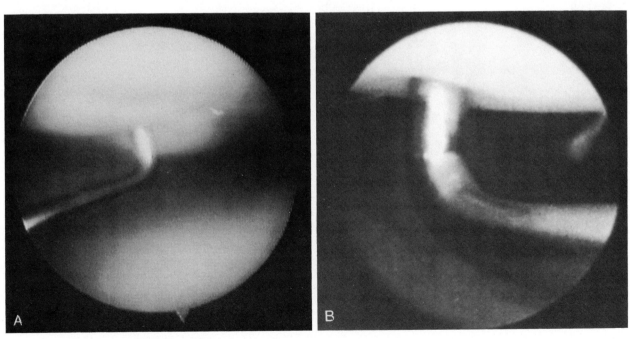

FIGURE 20–12
A and B, Intact articular mantle with soft "blister" demonstrated by arthroscopic probe.

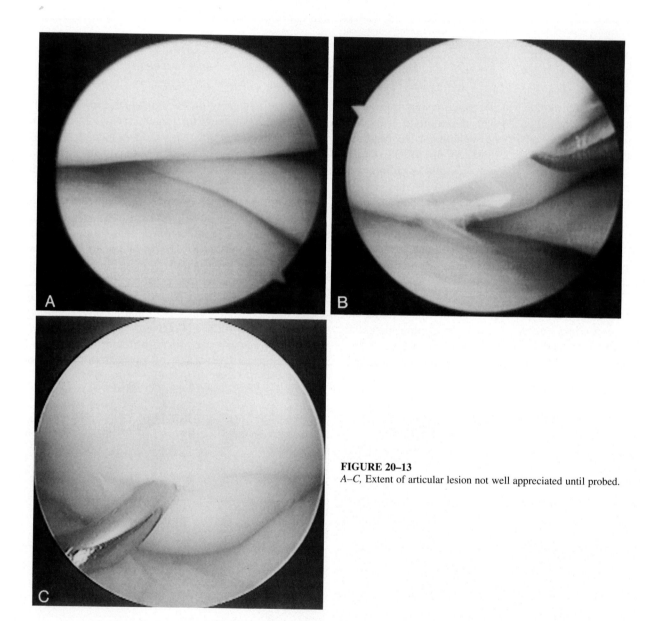

FIGURE 20–13
A–C, Extent of articular lesion not well appreciated until probed.

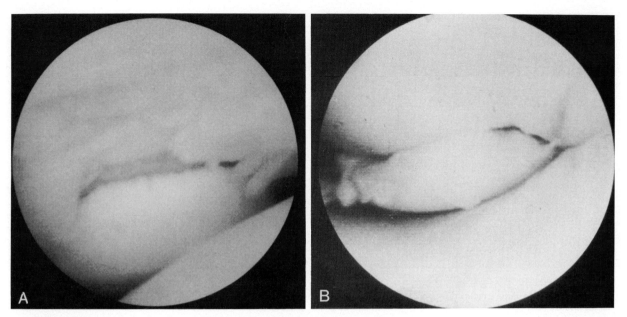

FIGURE 20–14

A, Open, unstable lesion with partial separation of subchondral zone. *B*, Open, unstable lesion fully separated from underlying bone.

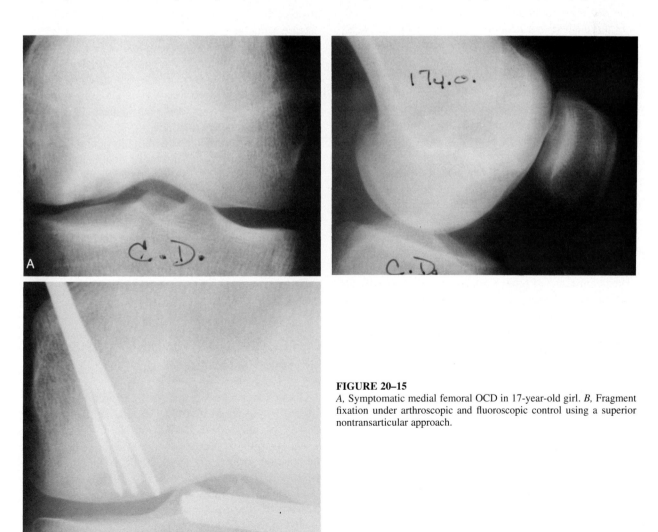

FIGURE 20–15

A, Symptomatic medial femoral OCD in 17-year-old girl. *B*, Fragment fixation under arthroscopic and fluoroscopic control using a superior nontransarticular approach.

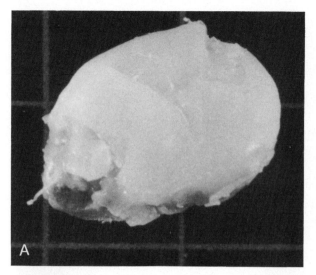 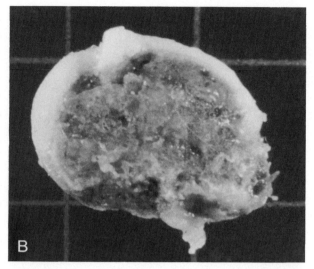

FIGURE 20–16

A and B, Loose body resulting from medial femoral OCD. Bone base had essentially no viable cells. The fragment caused locking as the primary presenting complaint.

lesion and rapid motion of the knee believe that morbidity is diminished and healing enhanced with this technique. Bradley and Dandy [8] reported on arthroscopic treatment of 11 knees in 10 patients; patient age averaged 12.7 years. Six transarticular holes were drilled via arthroscopic guidance into stable lesions on a non-weight-bearing zone of the medial femur. They allowed immediate return to activity and resumption of sport activity 2 months later. In nine of the ten patients, not surprisingly in this age group, union of the fragment occurred within 12 months. In one patient in whom union did not occur, a loose body was removed 5 years later. In all patients the authors noted rapid pain relief within a week postoperatively. Whether these lesions would have healed spontaneously over a longer time period without intervention remains questionable. Their symptomatic course was certainly diminished postsurgery.

The coexistence of other interarticular pathology must be suspected and recognized and appropriate treatment given. Large osteochondral lesions in weight-bearing zones commonly have associated meniscal tears that are usually irreparable (Fig. 20–18). Meniscal fragment excision and loss of articular surface stability are harbingers of a rapid onset of degenerative joint disease. Arthroscopic fragment excision with drilling or curettage of the lesion bed may provide satisfactory results in nonweight-bearing areas (Fig. 20–19). Ewing and Voto [23] reported excellent results following such crater debridement and drilling in 29 patients with an average age of 25 years and an average follow-up of 3 years. Five of the patients had associated meniscal tears. Aichroth [1] and Linden [46] felt that debridement and spongelization of the lesion were essential. Despite these

efforts, these authors reported that degenerative joint disease sequelae were common in adults.

For patients with a significant loss of femoral weight-bearing surface, secondary reconstruction with a composite bone–articular surface allograft may offer a solution. Although the preliminary data are very promising [29, 30], no long-term data, particularly in skeletally immature patients, are available.

The patient's compliance with a physical therapy program is essential for the success of treatment be it non-operative or operative. Swimming and biking provide excellent alternative forms of exercise and are a welcomed sports substitute by most children. Parental understanding of the time course needed for resolution of the condition is also vital to complete the patient-parent-surgeon triad for a successful outcome. Return to active sport must be judged on a case-by-case basis according to the patient's age, fragment stability, and previous treatment.

OSTEOCHONDRITIS DISSECANS OF THE PATELLA

Osteochondritis dissecans of the patella was first described by Rombold in 1933 [20] and is uncommon. It usually occurs in the second and third decades. The lesion is primarily located in the inferior patella below the midequatorial zone (Fig. 20–20). Dejour and colleagues [19] reported 25 cases in 19 patients, a 33% incidence of bilaterality. These authors believed that progression of the disease caused a sequestrum that proceeded to loose body formation. Seventy percent of their

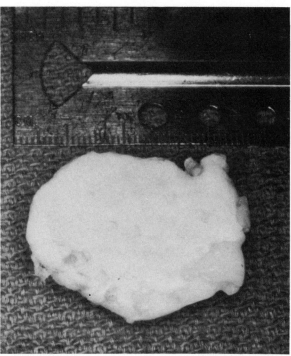

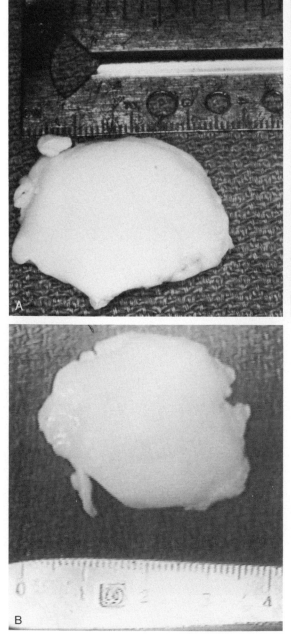

FIGURE 20–17
A and *B,* Large lateral OCD fragment in a patient with bilateral disease. Note paucity of subchondral bone.

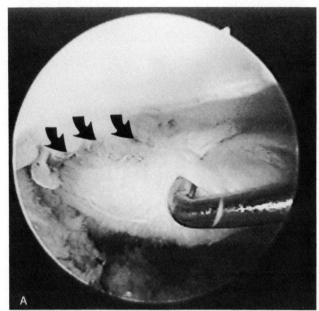

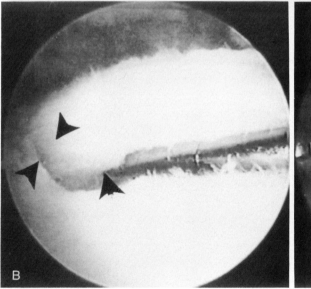

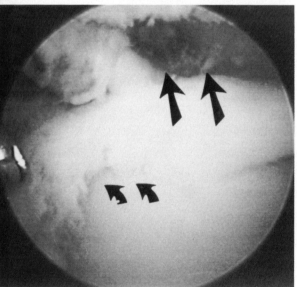

FIGURE 20–18
A and *B,* Lateral meniscal tears associated with OCD lesion. Note crater of lesion.

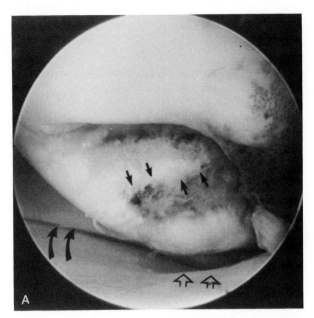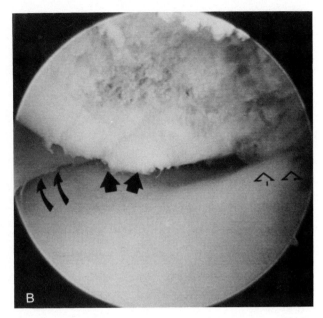

FIGURE 20–19
A and *B*, Pre- and postdebridement of crater after loose body removal.

patients obtained excellent results following fragment excision, curettage, and drilling of the crater. Desai and associates [20] reported 11 athletes with osteochondritis dissecans of the patella from a multicenter study. Seven of the athletes were between the ages of 10 and 15 years, and two had bilateral involvement. Average age at presentation was 16 years. Two patients treated nonoperatively by diminution of activity had an excellent result in two of the three knees. Eleven of the 13 knees were treated operatively by fragment excision, curettage and fragment excision, or curettage and drilling. Six of the patients had excellent postoperative results, four had good results, and one had a fair outcome. These authors thought that in the patella the prognosis was based on lesion size. In 12 patients, lesions measuring from 5 to 10 cm had satisfactory outcomes. One patient with a 20-cm lesion had only a fair result despite reoperation. Two of the patients treated nonoperatively had lesions with-

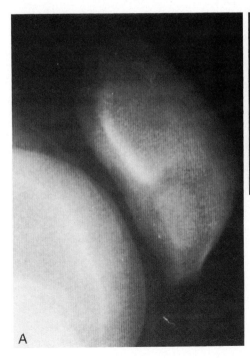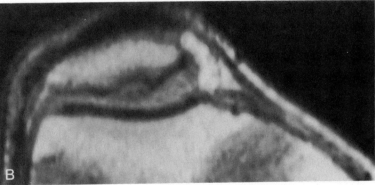

FIGURE 20–20
A, Radiograph of patellar OCD. Note lesion location below midequatorial plane. *B*, MRI of same patient showing intact articular surface.

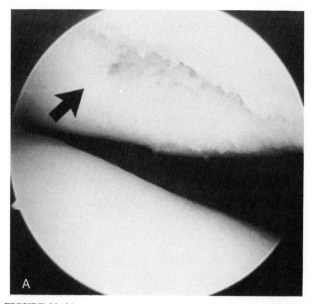 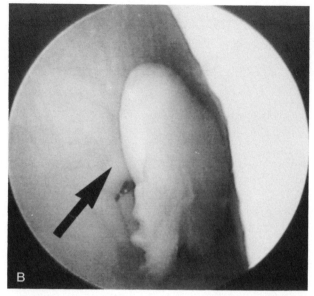

FIGURE 20–21

A, Patellar OCD crater in 16-year-old basketball player. *B,* Loose body from patellar lesion fragment was completely cartilaginous and caused no history of knee injury. The patient presented with symptoms of locking.

out radiographic marginal sclerosis. The authors suggested that if sclerosis is present at the lesion margin or if a loose body is evident roentgenographically or clinically, surgical treatment is indicated. They believed that the lesion's location in the lower third of the patella correlated with increased patellofemoral contact force during knee flexion and that this repetitive minor force caused the lesion. They believed that repetitive minor injuries of the articular surface were responsible for causing the lesion. None of their patients had a history of major injury (Fig. 20–21).

Stougaard [70] reported nine cases of patellar osteochondritis dissecans; eight were treated by fragment excision and curettage. Half of the patients still had significant patellofemoral pain at long-term follow-up, and the author suggested that osteochondritis dissecans of the patella in the older patient was a prelude to progressive patellofemoral degenerative disease. Schwartz and colleagues [67] had a similar experience. Management principles for patellar osteochondritis dissecans are similar to those described for femoral lesions. The relationship between skeletal maturity and prognosis is currently less clear for patellar lesions.

References

1. Aichroth, P. Osteochondritis dissecans of the knee. *J Bone Joint Surg* 53B:440, 1971.
2. Andrew, T. A., Spivey, J., and Lindebaum, R. H. Familial osteochondritis dissecans and dwarfism. *Acta Orthop Scand* 52(5):519–523, 1981.
3. Axhausen, G. Die Aetiologie der kohlerschan Erkrankung der Metatarsalkopfehen. *Beitr Klin Chir* 126:451, 1922.
4. Axhausen, G. Ueber dem Abgrenzungsvorgang am epiphysaren Knochen. *Virchows Arch Pathal Anat* 252:458–518, 1924.
5. Barrie, H. J. Osteochondritis dissecans 1887–1987. A centennial look at Koenig's memorable phrase. *J Bone Joint Surg* 69B:693, 1987.
6. Bigelow, D. R. Juvenile osteochondritis dissecans. *J Bone Joint Surg* 57B:530, 1975.
7. Bostman, O., Hirvensalo, E., Vainionpaa, S., et al. Degradable polyglycolide rods for the internal fixation of displaced bimalleolar fractures. *Int Orthop* 14(1):1–8, 1990.
8. Bradley, J., and Dandy, D. J. Osteochondritis dissecans and other lesions of the femoral condyles. *J Bone Joint Surg* 71B:518–522, 1989.
9. Bratsttstrom, A. J. Osteochondritis dissecans. *Acta Orthop Scand* (Suppl) 35, 1964.
10. Brucki, R., Rosemeyer, B., and Thiermann, G. Osteochondritis dissecans of the knee. Results of operative treatment in juveniles. *Arch Orthop Trauma Surg* 102:221–224, 1984.
11. Buchner, L., and Rieger, H. Könnon freie Golenkkorper durch Trauma entstehen? *Arch Klin Chir* 116:460, 1921.
12. Caffey, J., Madell, S. H., Rover, C., et al. Ossification of the distal femoral epiphysis. *J Bone Joint Surg* 40A:647, 1958.
13. Cahill, B., and Berg, B. 99m-Technetium phosphate compound joint scintigraphy in the management of juvenile osteochondritis dissecans of the femoral condyles. *Am J Sports Med* 11:329–335, 1983.
14. Carroll, N. C., and Mubarak, S. J. Juvenile osteochondritis dissecans of the knee. *J Bone Joint Surg* 59B:506, 1977.
15. Chiroff, R. T., and Cooke, P. C. Osteochondritis dissecans: A histologic and microradiographic analysis of surgically excised lesions. *J Trauma* 15:689–696, 1975.
16. Claes, L., Burri, C., Kiefer, H., et al. Resorbierbare Implantate zur Refixierung von osteochondralen Fragmenten in Gelenkflachen. *Aktuel Traumatol* 16(2):74–77, 1986.
17. Clanton, T. O., and DeLee, J. C. Osteochondritis dissecans: History, pathophysiology and current treatment concepts. *Clin Orthop* 167:50, 1982.
18. Crawford, E. J., et al. Stable osteochondritis dissecans—does the lesion unite? *J Bone Joint Surg* 72B:320, 1990.
19. Dejour, D. D., et al. Osteochondritis patella. *Clin Orthop* 158:59, 1981.
20. Desai, S. S., Patel, M. R., Michelli, L. J., et al. Osteochondritis dissecans of the patella. *J Bone Joint Surg* 69A:320, 1987.

21. Ehrenborg, G. The Osgood-Schlatter's lesion: A clinical and experimental study. *Acta Clin Scand* (Suppl) 288:1, 1962.
22. Enneking, W. *Clinical Musculoskeletal Pathology.* Gainesville, FL, Shorter Printing, 1977, p. 147.
23. Ewing, J. W., and Voto, S. J. Arthroscopic surgical management of osteochondritis dissecans of the knee. *Arthroscopy* 4:37, 1988.
24. Fairbanks, H. A. T. Osteochondritis dissecans. *Br J Surg* 21:67, 1933.
25. Federico, D. J., Lynch, J. K., and Jokl, P. Osteochondritis dissecans of the knee: A historical review of etiology and treatment. *Arthroplasty* 6(3):190–197, 1990.
26. Fraser, W. N. C. Familial osteochondritis dissecans. *J Bone Joint Surg* 48(B):598, 1966.
27. Friden, T., and Rydholm, U. Severe aseptic synovitis of the knee after biodegradable internal fixation: A case report. *Acta Orthop Scand* 63(1):94–97, 1992.
28. Gardiner, T. B. Osteochondritis dissecans in three members of one family. *J Bone Joint Surg* 37(B):139, 1955.
29. Garrett, J. Treatment of osteochondral defects of the distal femur with fresh osteochondral allografts: A preliminary report. *Arthroscopy* 2:222–226, 1986.
30. Garrett, J. Osteochondritis dissecans. *Orthop Clin North Am* 10:569, 1991.
31. Gillespie, H. W., and Day, B. Bone peg fixation in the treatment of osteochondritis dissecans of the knee joint. *Clin Orthop* 143:125, 1979.
32. Green, W., and Banks, H. Osteochondritis dissecans in children. *J Bone Joint Surg* 14A:26, 1958.
33. Guhl, J. Arthroscopic treatment of osteochondritis dissecans. *Clin Orthop* 167:66–74, 1982.
34. Harding, W. G., III. Diagnosis of osteochondritis dissecans of the femoral condyles. *Clin Orthop* 123:25, 1977.
35. Jakob, R. P., and Miniaci, A. A compression pinning for osteochondritis dissecans of the knee. *Acta Orthop Scand* 60:319, 1989.
36. Johnson, E. W., and McLeod, T. L. Osteochondral fragments of the distal end of the femur fixed with bone pegs. *J Bone Joint Surg* 59A:677–679, 1977.
37. Johnson, L. L., and Uitvlugt, G., et al. Osteochondritis dissecans of the knee: Arthroscopic compression screw fixation. *Arthroscopy* 6(3):179–189, 1990.
38. Johnson, R. P., and Aaberg, T. M. Use of retrograde bone grafting in the treatment of osseous defects of the lateral condyle of the knee. A preliminary report of three knees in two patients. *Orthopedics* 10:291–297, 1987.
39. King, D. Osteochondritis dissecans. *J Bone Joint Surg* 14:535, 1932.
40. Köenig, F. Über freie Korper in den Gelenken. *Dtsch Chir* 27:90, 1888.
41. Köenig, F. Tagung deutsche Gesellschaft für Chirurgie. *Langenbecks Arch Klin Chir* 142, 1926.
42. Kurzwell, P. R., et al. Osteochondritis dissecans of the lateral patello-femoral groove. *Am J Sport Med* 16:308, 1988.
43. Langenskjold, A. Can osteochondritis dissecans arise as a sequel of cartilage fracture in early childhood? *Acta Chir Scand* 109:204, 1955.
44. Langer, F., and Percy, E. C. Osteochondritis dissecans and anomalous centres of ossification: A review of 80 lesions in 61 patients. *Can J Surg* 14:208, 1971.
45. Lee, C. K., and Mercurio, C. Operative treatment in osteochondritis dissecans in situ by retrograde drilling and cancellous bone graft: A preliminary report. *Clin Orthop* 158:129–136, 1981.
46. Linden, B. Osteochondritis dissecans of the femoral condyles: A long-term follow-up study. *J Bone Joint Surg* 59A:769, 1977.
47. Lindholm, T. S., and Osterman, K. Long-term results after transfixation of an osteochondritis dissecans fragment to the femoral condyle using autologous bone transplants in adolescent and adult patients. *Arch Orthop Trauma Surg* 97:225, 1980.
48. Lipscomb, P. R., Jr., Lipscomb, P. R., Sr., and Bryan, R. S. Osteochondritis dissecans of the knee with loose fragments. Treatment by replacement and fixation with readily removed pins. *J Bone Joint Surg* 60A:235–240, 1978.
49. Litchman, H. M., et al. Computerized blood flow analysis for decision making in treatment of osteochondritis dissecans. *J Pediatr Orthop* 8:208, 1988.
50. Mesgarzadeh, J., et al. Osteochondritis dissecans: Analysis of mechanical stability with radiography, scintigraphy, and MR imaging. *Radiology* 165:775–780, 1987.
51. Milgram, J. Radiological and pathological manifestations of osteochondritis dissecans of the distal femur. *Radiology,* 126:305–311, 1978.
52. Mubarak, S., and Carroll, N. N. Familial osteochondritis dissecans of the knee. *Clin Orthop* 140:131, 1979.
53. Mubarak, S., and Carroll, N. N. Juvenile osteochondritis dissecans of the knee: Etiology. *Clin Orthop* 157:200–211, 1980.
54. Nagura, S. The so-called osteochondritis dissecans of König. *Clin Orthop* 18:100, 1960.
55. Paget, J. On the production of some of the loose bodies in joints. *St Barth Hosp Rep* 6:1, 1870.
56. Pappas, A. Osteochondritis dissecans. *Clin Orthop* 158:59, 1981.
57. Paré, A. *Oeuvres Completes.* Vol. 3. Paris, Balliere, 1941, p. 32.
58. Petrie, P. W. Aetiology of osteochondritis dissecans—failure to establish a familial background. *J Bone Joint Surg* 59B:366–367, 1977.
59. Phillips, H. O., IV, and Grubb, S. A. Familial multiple osteochondritis dissecans. *J Bone Joint Surg* 67:155, 1985.
60. Pick, M. P. Familial osteochondritis dissecans. *J Bone Joint Surg* 37B:142–145, 1955.
61. Rehbein, F. Die Entstechung der osteochondritis dissecans. *Arch Klin Chir* 265:69, 1950.
62. Reicher, M. A., Bassett, L. W., and Godl, R. H. High-resolution magnetic resonance imaging of the knee joint: Pathologic correlations. *AJR* 145:903, 1985.
63. Reiser, M. F., et al. Magnetic resonance in cartilaginous lesions of the knee joint with three-dimensional gradient-echo imaging. *Skel Radiol* 17(7):465–471, 1988.
64. Ribbing, S. The hereditary multiple epiphyseal disturbance and its consequences for the aetiology of local malacias—particularly the osteochondritis dissecans. *Acta Orthop Scand* 24:286–299, 1955.
65. Rieger, H. Zür Pathogenese von Gelenkmausen. *Münch Med Wochsch* 67:719, 1920.
66. Rogers, W. M., and Gladstone, H. Vascular foramina and arterial supply of the distal end of the femur. *J Bone Joint Surg* 32A:867, 1950.
67. Schwartz, C., Blazina, M. E., Sisto, D. J., et al. The results of operative treatment of osteochondritis dissecans of the patella. *Am J Sports Med* 16(5):522–529, 1988.
68. Smillie, I. S. *Osteochondritis Dissecans.* London, E & S Livingstone, 1960.
69. Sontag, L., and Pyle, S. Variations in the calcification pattern in epiphyses. *AJR* 45:50, 1941.
70. Stougaard, J. The hereditary factor in osteochondritis dissecans. *J Bone Joint Surg* 43B:256–258, 1961.
71. Stougaard, J. Familial occurrence of osteochondritis dissecans. *J Bone Joint Surg* 46B:542–543, 1964.
72. Stougaard, J. Osteochondritis dissecans of the patella. *Acta Orthop Scand* 45:11, 1974.
73. Tallqvist, G. The reaction to mechanical trauma in growing articular cartilage. *Acta Orthop Scand* (Suppl) 53, 1962.
74. Telhag, H. Osteochondritis dissecans: A histologic and autoradiographic study in man. *Acta Orthop Scand* 48:682, 1977.
75. Thomson, N. L. Osteochondritis dissecans and ostochondral fragments managed by Herbert compression screw fixation. *Clin Orthop* 224:71, 1978.
76. Tobin, W. J. Familial osteochondritis dissecans with associated tibia vara. *J Bone Joint Surg* 39A:1091, 1957.
77. Van Demark, R. E. Osteochondritis dissecans with spontaneous healing. *J Bone Joint Surg* 34:143–148, 1952.
78. White, J. Osteochondritis dissecans in association with dwarfism. *J Bone Joint Surg* 39B:248–260, 1957.
79. Wiberg, G. Spontaneous healing of osteochondritis dissecans in the knee joint. *Acta Orthop Scand* 14:270–277, 1943.
80. Wilson, J. N. A diagnostic sign in osteochondritis dissecans of the knee. *J Bone Joint Surg* 49A:477, 1967.
81. Zeman, S., and Nielsen, M. Osteochondritis dissecans of the knee. *Orthop Rev* 9:101, 1978.

LIGAMENTOUS INJURY OF THE KNEE

Jesse C. DeLee, M.D.

K nee ligament disruptions in the skeletally immature athlete, once thought to be rare, are being reported with increasing frequency [10, 12, 16, 18, 28, 29, 33, 36, 49, 52, 71, 75, 76, 77, 79, 84, 86, 87, 92, 108, 115] because more children are participating in athletic events [50, 60, 79, 117, 128] and motor vehicle accidents are also increasing [28, 29, 119]. The purpose of this chapter is to present an approach to the epidemiology, diagnosis, and treatment of ligamentous injuries of the knee in skeletally immature patients.

Historical Background

Acute traumatic injuries about the knee in children have classically been thought to cause disruptions of the physis [26, 34, 52, 79, 105, 114, 115] because the physes were believed to be the weak link when stressed [12, 13, 18, 22, 28, 33, 34, 52, 79, 87, 108, 114, 115, 117, 123]. This opinion was so widely held that, in 1974, Rang wrote that ligamentous injuries about the knee do not occur in children [105]. He retracted this statement in 1983 and acknowledged that knee ligament injuries do occur in the skeletally immature [106]. Although bony avulsions of ligaments were noted on radiographs, they too were believed to be relatively uncommon [105, 108].

Injured knees in children were, therefore, treated in one of two ways: (1) immobilization of nondisplaced physeal plate injuries and avulsions, and (2) open reduction and internal fixation of displaced fractures and bony avulsions [34]. Few data were available on disruption of the collateral or cruciate ligament. In those few patients who were recognized to have true ligamentous injury, further growth was believed to alleviate the instability [79].

More recently, it has become evident that children do injure their knee ligaments and that they may fare no better than do adults with conservative (nonoperative) treatment, particularly those who have injuries of the anterior cruciate ligament (ACL) [18, 29, 36, 71, 72, 75, 78, 79, 84, 87, 115] if alterations in activity and lifestyle do not occur.

Epidemiology

The increased interest in children's knee injuries stems from three factors. First, increased numbers of children are participating in organized sports [50, 60, 66, 79, 108, 123, 128]. Goldberg [50] estimated in 1984 that 25% of girls and 50% of boys between the ages of 8 and 16 years old are engaged in competitive athletics in any one year. Gallagher and colleagues [45], in a statewide study, reported that 1 in 14 children presenting to emergency rooms in Massachusetts were injured in sporting activities, whereas only 1 in 50 were injured in motor vehicle accidents. In football it has been estimated that up to 81% of the children participating will suffer an injury, usually minor in nature. This represents 300,000 to 1,215,000 injured athletes per year in football alone [128]. The knee is the anatomic area most frequently involved in these sports injuries, and there is a definite tendency toward increased severity of injury with increasing age [90, 92]. The higher incidence of knee injuries is related to the various demands and stresses applied to its supporting structures during a sporting event [58]. The knee is also exposed to direct trauma leading to injury.

The second factor contributing to the increased incidence of children's knee injuries is the heightened awareness of the medical community of ligament injuries in skeletally immature patients and consequently a more frequent recognition of such injuries [79]. The third factor producing an increased incidence of knee ligament injuries in children is the improved technology available for the diagnosis of ligamentous disruptions in all age groups (e.g., KT-1000 and magnetic resonance imaging [MRI]) [18, 28, 49].

Embryology and Anatomy

Congenital anomalies of the knee occur early in fetal development [4]. The knee develops embryologically as a cleft between the mesenchymal rudiments of the femur and tibia in about the eighth week of fetal development. Vascular mesenchyme becomes isolated within the joint and is the precursor tissue of the cruciate ligaments and menisci. These tissues become immature fibroblasts, which soon develop into the cruciate ligaments. By the tenth week the anterior and posterior cruciate ligaments are separate structures that become independent of each other by the eighteenth week of development [4].

Developmental ligament abnormalities can lead to congenitally unstable knees. The cruciates and menisci help to shape the femoral condyles and tibial plateau of the knee, and in their absence the intercondylar eminence of the tibia is aplastic (see Fig. 21–4) [47, 130]. The knee abnormality usually does not exist alone but is associated with other ipsilateral limb deformities such as femoral or tibial hemimelia, congenital short femur, and other limb anomalies [28, 29].

Eilert [35] states that most knee problems in children younger than 12 years of age are congenital. One must be aware, therefore, of these congenital anomalies when evaluating the child with an unstable knee. In the child with clinical instability, a developmental anomaly must be considered if there is (1) no history of significant trauma; (2) an associated limb anomaly such as hemimelia, leg length discrepancy, or a ball-and-socket ankle joint [24, 28, 74]; or (3) aplasia of the intercondylar eminence of the tibia on an anteroposterior radiograph [47] (Fig. 21–1). Only after a congenital malformation or anomaly has been excluded as the cause of instability can traumatic ligamentous instability be considered. One must also consider an underlying congenital anomaly combined with sequela from a traumatic event.

Anatomy

The anatomic relationship of the origins and insertions of the ligament to the femoral, tibial, and fibular physeal plates increases stress on the physis by concentrating force on it that leads to its failure [18, 22, 28, 29]. All knee ligament origins and insertions, except the tibial collateral ligament insertion, are within the confines of the physeal plates of the distal femur and proximal tibia and fibula [18, 28] (Fig. 21–2). Therefore, when any stress is applied to the knee of the patient with open physes, it is concentrated at the physeal plate of the distal femur or proximal tibia and fibula by the collateral or central ligaments [28, 29, 33, 99, 108]. The stress may also be a direct blow to the physis independent of the effects of the ligaments.

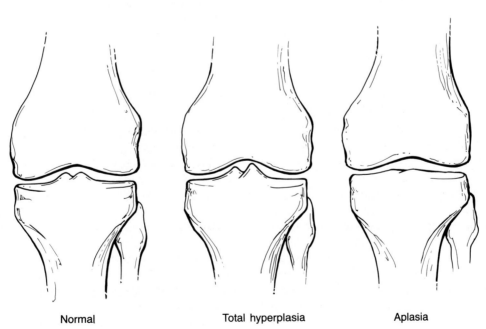

Normal   Total hyperplasia   Aplasia

FIGURE 21–1
Variations in the morphologic appearance of the intercondylar eminence of the tibia. Total aplasia of the eminence suggests congenital absence of the anterior cruciate ligament.

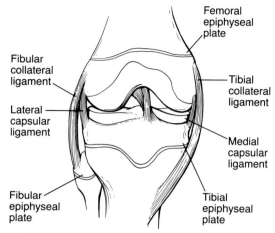

FIGURE 21–2
The capsular and cruciate ligaments insert *within* the epiphysis of the tibia and femur, respectively. Only the insertion of the tibial collateral ligament crosses the tibial physeal plate. Because of the ligaments' relationship to the physeal plates and the relative strength of the ligaments, stress concentrates at the physeal plates, producing physeal separation rather than ligament failure.

BIOMECHANICS

Strength of the Physeal Plate

Two factors help to explain the higher incidence of physeal plate disruptions compared with pure ligament injuries [10, 12, 18, 28, 33, 76, 101, 105, 114, 129]: (1) the weaker strength of the physeal plate compared with that of knee ligaments, and (2) the anatomic location of the ligament origins and insertions, which concentrates forces at the physeal plate [10, 12, 18, 28, 33, 76, 101, 105, 114, 129]. The weakest area in the physis is the zone of hypertrophy, which is the zone through which physeal disruption usually occurs [12, 93, 101, 114].

Mechanics of Physeal Plate Failure

The physeal plate is protected from disruption by mamillary processes and undulations along its surface as well as by the distal attachment of the periosteum [13]. However, it is still the weak point when stress is applied to immature bone [13]. Bright and associates [13] demonstrated that the cartilage in the physeal plate has viscoelastic properties. Therefore, the strength of the plate depends on the total strain *and* the rate at which the strain is applied. Due to the property of viscoelasticity, it takes twice the force to disrupt the physis at a rapid-loading rate than when the growth plate is loaded slowly [12]. Also, Bright and associates [13], Harris [62], and Tipton and colleagues [129] found reduced ductility of the cartilage with age. In addition, physeal plate strength

is affected by various hormones [62, 129]. Growth hormone produces a thicker physeal plate that is weaker in transverse loading at nonphysiologic strain rates, whereas estrogens cause a thinner growth plate that is stronger [62, 129].

Mechanics of Ligament Failure

Ligaments about the knee in the child undergo the same pathodynamic sequence of disruption as they do in the adult [79]. Like the physeal plate, ligaments have viscoelastic properties, and their strength is determined by the total strain and the rate at which it is applied. According to Cochran [20], at slow-loading rates, ligament failures tend to occur at the ligament-bone junction, usually with a bony avulsion, whereas at rapid-loading rates, failure occurs within the body of the ligament. These findings suggest that the strength of corticocancellous bone increases more rapidly than does the strength of ligaments as the loading rate increases. Rapid loading of ligaments seems to be the common denominator in injuries to adults as well as children [20]. Skak and colleagues [119] in 1987, in a series of 91 children under age 14, concluded that low-energy trauma was associated with ligamentous injuries, whereas high-energy trauma was associated with physeal damage [20]. Therefore, the two studies support the concept that pure ligamentous injuries occur secondary to low-energy, rapid-loading events, whereas injuries to the physis or tendon-bone junction occur with high-energy, slow-loading events. During the rapid physiologic changes characteristic of adolescence, ligament and physeal properties are progressively altered as the child reaches skeletal maturity. The morphology of the injury is a reflection of this status.

DIAGNOSIS: GENERAL PRINCIPLES

Careful evaluation of the history of the injury, the physical examination, and imaging studies is essential for accurate diagnosis of knee ligament injuries in skeletally immature patients.

History

History taking is the primary method of evaluating knee injuries. In the acute setting, the circumstances surrounding the injury (type of sport, contact versus noncontact) are critical pieces of the puzzle. Hyperextension of the knee—for example, landing with the knee extended in basketball—is frequently associated with an ACL injury. An external rotation force applied to the knee when in a valgus position can result in disruption of the medial collateral ligament (MCL) first, then the ACL. An audible "pop" heard at the time of the injury by the patient strongly suggests disruption of one of the major knee ligaments, usually the ACL [38, 49, 118]. The rapid development of an effusion, usually within 6 to 12 hours, suggests a hemarthrosis associated with disruption of the ACL, a peripheral meniscal detachment, or an osteochondral fracture [38, 39, 49, 66, 108, 118]. Development of an effusion over a longer period of time, 24 to 48 hours, suggests synovial effusion and is usually a less sinister prognosticator of knee injury.

A history of instability with weight-bearing at the time of injury is usually associated with significant ligamentous injury. These patients may have minimal pain immediately following the injury and may attempt to return to play only to find that instability prevents participation. On the other hand, if severe pain is present initially, a partial ligament disruption or physeal plate injury may be present; this situation demands removal of the patient from participation to prevent further damage to the torn ligament or fracture.

In the patient with a chronically unstable knee, the history provides additional information. A history of the knee giving way during a particular activity is important. The patient relates that the knee feels unstable when placed in certain positions. In the classic description the knee "slips out," which may be due to pathologic anterior cruciate laxity or to quadriceps inhibition from pain.

The symptom of giving way may also be related by the patient with a meniscal lesion. If both ligamentous (ACL) instability and a meniscal lesion are present, the physical examination is essential to determine which is responsible for the patient's symptoms. The severity of instability is often suggested by the history. A knee that gives way during normal walking is more unstable than one that gives way only with sports activity.

Locking, a passive restraint to knee motion, is often given as a complaint. This history is suggestive of an unstable meniscal lesion, an osteochondral flap, or a loose body. This complaint must be differentiated from "pseudolocking," in which pain, not a mechanical block, prevents knee extension.

In patients with chronic symptoms, pain may be due to episodes of ligament or patellar instability or to articular surface damage. By the history, if pain is associated with giving way, ligament laxity, patellofemoral instability, or meniscal pathology is the most likely cause. However, if pain is noted only after weight bearing and prolonged activity, chondral damage is more likely to be the problem. Distinguishing pain with instability from pain with weight bearing is critical in evaluating patients with ligamentous instability because ligament reconstruction will not improve the pain of weight bearing in patients who have chondral disease. Children and adolescents have usually not had sufficient time post-injury to produce the articular wear that precedes degenerative disease. Loss of motion in the injured knee compared to the normal knee may be due to a structural problem such as a loose body, torn meniscus, effusion, muscle spasm, or chronic guarding with secondary muscle-tendon contracture.

Physical Examination

Physical examination of the injured knee is the best diagnostic tool available for evaluating the location and severity of a knee injury. Examination of a child's knee is more difficult than examination in an adult [96]. Especially in the acute injury setting, children are often frightened and are unable to relax the muscles about the knee, making evaluation of laxity and range of motion quite difficult [40, 49]. In children one must distinguish a physeal plate injury from a ligament injury. Evaluation of the point of maximum tenderness is essential when attempting to distinguish ligament or meniscal injury from a physeal plate injury.

The uninjured extremity is examined first. This generally helps to relax the patient by giving him or her an idea of how the examination of the injured knee will be performed [49, 66, 118]. It also gives the physician an idea of the physiologic laxity of the patient when the injured knee is examined. This is extremely important because many children have *physiologic* joint laxity, which may be a manifestation of generalized ligamentous laxity. When this normal laxity is noted in the "injured knee," the observation can lead to a mistaken diagnosis of pathologic ligamentous laxity. Therefore, physiologic laxity must be distinguished from pathologic laxity by examination of the contralateral knee and other joints [28, 29, 54]. Hyperextension of the elbows, laxity of the shoulders, and hyperextension of the knees may also be present in patients with physiologically increased knee laxity [54].

Following the examination of the uninjured extremity, a visual inspection of the injured knee is undertaken. The presence of deformity usually suggests bony or physeal plate injury rather than ligament disruption. The alignment of the noninjured limb during weight bearing (i.e., varus, valgus, hyperextension) is recorded if the patient can stand. Palpation of the dorsalis pedis and posterior tibial pulses is *essential* because children with an injury to the distal femoral or proximal tibial physis may have an associated limb-threatening vascular injury [66, 108]. Motor and sensory assessment is also mandatory to rule out associated neural compromise. If ecchymosis is present, it indicates the specific ligament and the exact location of the injury [47, 100]. A large effusion is also evident on visual inspection. Prepatellar swelling may be confused with intra-articular findings.

Palpation of the knee is performed after inspection. Each capsular ligament origin, course, and insertion is palpated. Small distances separate the ligaments, menisces, and physes, and focal tenderness allows specificity of the diagnosis. The physeal plates and joint lines are palpated, noting the specific points of tenderness, which help to differentiate ligament, meniscal, and physeal plate injuries. If palpation suggests a physeal plate injury, anteroposterior (AP) and medial-lateral stress radiographs should be performed before proceeding with the clinical laxity examination. If the growth plates are not tender, the knee is tested for pathologic ligamentous laxity before radiographs are obtained.

Hip range of motion is examined to detect those pathologic conditions of the hip (e.g., slipped capital femoral epiphysis) that can present as knee pain. Passive and active knee ranges of motion are recorded as well as any associated crepitance or pain with motion. The order in which the laxity tests are performed is not important, but the same order of testing should be followed routinely. The degree of laxity is recorded as recommended by the Committee on the Medical Aspects of Sports of the American Medical Association [21]. The degree of laxity in any given direction is expressed as 0, equal to a normal knee, mild (1 +), indicating that the joint surfaces are less than 5 mm separate; moderate (2 +), indicating a separation of 5 to 10 mm; and severe (3 +), indicating a separation of more than 10 mm. In this chapter these standards will be used to express the degree of knee laxity.

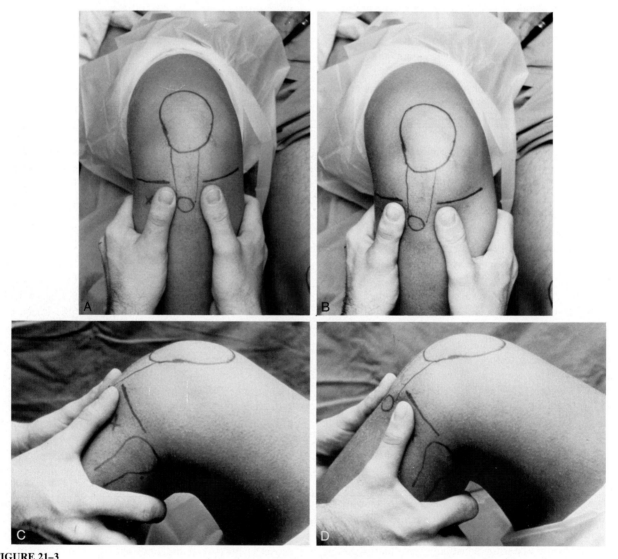

FIGURE 21–3
Posterolateral drawer test. A posterior force is applied to the tibia with the knee at 90 degrees of flexion. The foot is free. As the tibia displaces posteriorly, it also rotates laterally, indicating a positive posterolateral drawer test sign. *A,* Starting position for posterolateral drawer test. *B,* The tibial tubercle rotates posteriorly and laterally. *C,* Lateral view of posterolateral drawer test. *D,* Note the posterior and lateral displacement of the tibial tubercle.

The knee is evaluated in extension and at 30 degrees of flexion for varus or valgus laxity. The central pivot ligaments are evaluated next. Positive results on the anterior Lachman and flexion rotation drawer tests indicate ACL injury. A positive pivot shift, jerk, or Losee's test, which in a chronic case reproduces the patient's symptoms, suggests that an ACL injury is responsible for symptoms of instability. The anterior drawer test performed in 90 degrees of knee flexion that is positive in external or neutral rotation indicates the presence of ACL and collateral ligament laxity.

The posterior Lachman (Lachman-Trillat) test (see Fig. 21–16) and the quadriceps active drawer test (see Fig. 21–15) are then performed to evaluate the posterior cruciate ligament (PCL). These tests are quite sensitive even after an acute injury. The posterior sag and posterior drawer tests are more accurate determinants of PCL injury in patients with a chronically unstable knee. The posterior lateral drawer test (Fig. 21–3) and increased passive external rotation at 30 degrees of flexion indicate damage to the posterolateral structures (Fig. 21–4A and B) [57, 70]. Although increased external rotation at 30 degrees of flexion indicates injury to the posterolateral structures, increased external rotation at 90 degrees of flexion indicates injury to the posterior cruciate *and* posterolateral corner (Fig. 21–4C).

Next, the patellofemoral mechanism is evaluated for malalignment and instability. The menisci are examined by evaluating point tenderness, which may indicate a meniscal tear. Tenderness at the anterior joint line may be due to patellar disorders and should not be confused with meniscal lesions alone. Pain or crepitus with varus stress during range of motion suggests medial meniscal or chondral surface injury, whereas pain or crepitus with valgus stress on range of motion suggests lateral meniscal or chondral surface injury. McMurray's test or Apley's test may also help to detect meniscal injury, although they are difficult to perform in acute situations.

Radiographic Examination

Anteroposterior, lateral, tunnel, and skyline (patellar profile) radiographs of the knee are viewed to identify physeal plate fracture, osteochondral injury, or bony avulsion [131]. Oblique views may be required to eval-

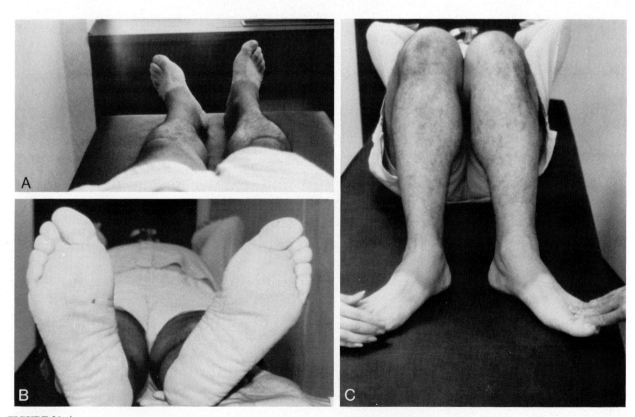

FIGURE 21–4
The dial test. Increased external rotation of the foot with the knee in 30 degrees of flexion indicates injury to the posterolateral corner. Increased external rotation of the foot with the knee in 90 degrees of flexion indicates injury to the posterior cruciate *and* the posterolateral corner. *A*, Increased external rotation with the knee in 30 degrees of flexion. This indicates injury to the posterolateral corner of the right knee. *B*, Increased external rotation of the left foot with the knee slightly flexed, indicating posterolateral injury to the left knee. *C*, Increased external rotation with the knee in 90 degrees of flexion indicates injury to the posterior cruciate *and* the posterolateral corner.

uate osteochondral fragments. Radiographs of the hip should be obtained if (1) knee films are normal, (2) knee films are not compatible with the symptoms found in the knee examination or (3) hip physical examination is abnormal [22]. If no abnormality is noted on plain radiographs in patients with an acute injury and associated clinical findings, varus-valgus and anterior-posterior stress films are obtained [18, 22, 28, 131]. Stress radiographs, which are used to *confirm* ligmentous injury in the adult, are essential to distinguish physeal disruptions from ligamentous injuries in the child (Fig. 21–5). In the mature or late adolescent, collateral ligamentous injury does occur without physeal damage and is manifest on stress views.

Specialized radiographic studies may be utilized to further clarify the diagnosis [18, 22, 73]. These include arthrograms, CT scans, polytomograms, and MRI. Care must be taken not to over- or underinterpret MRI study results. Each imaging modality has limitations, and MRI

is no exception, especially in patients with partial cruciate ligament injuries. Stress radiographs and some specialized x-ray studies may require patient sedation either by local injection or general anesthesia [18, 131]. If general anesthesia is needed, the physician should be ready to proceed with operative treatment if indicated.

Treatment

Once a physeal plate injury has been excluded, treatment of the specific ligament injury is instituted. Treatment of physeal plate injuries is beyond the scope of this chapter. There is no difference in the treatment of physeal plate injuries in children whether they are the sequelae of sport or nonathletic activity.

According to Kennedy [79] and Bradley and colleagues [10] knee ligament injuries in children respond to surgical repair in the same way as in adults, and they

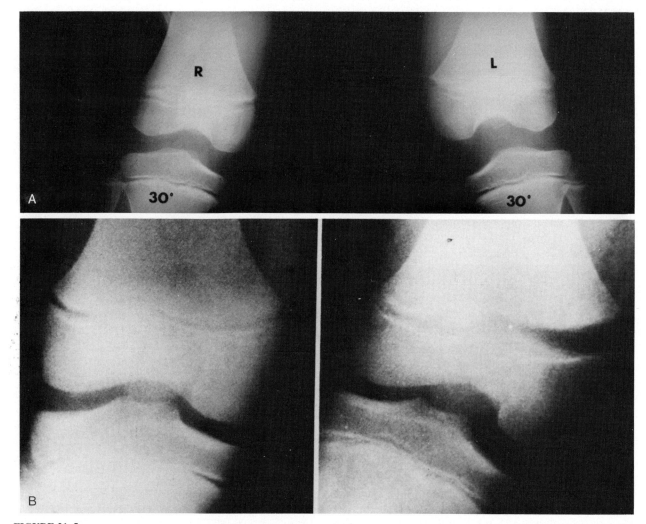

FIGURE 21–5
A, Valgus stress in 30 degrees of flexion, indicating medial collateral ligament injury. *B,* Stress radiograph with the knee in 30 degrees of flexion, indicating distal femoral physeal plate disruption rather than collateral ligament injury.

recommend treating ligamentous injuries in the child's knee in the same manner as in the adult. These series are too small and have too short a follow-up to support the authors' position strongly. The major concern in operative management of ligamentous injuries in the child is to avoid causing iatrogenic damage of the physis by the surgical repair [28]. Because of the potential for physeal plate injury with resultant limb shortening or angulation, operative procedures are sometimes delayed, or a procedure of lesser magnitude is selected to avoid damage to the physis [28, 84, 87]. Assessment of physiologic maturity by history and physical examination (e.g., menarche in girls, axillary hair development in boys) provides clues to the amount of growth remaining at the femoral and tibial physes. Tomogram mapping of the extent of physeal closure also assists in decision-making. Once the growth plate closes (or nearly so) if further operative treatment is needed, procedures proved to be effective in adults may be utilized [28].

MEDIAL COLLATERAL LIGAMENT

Medial collateral ligament injuries are usually the result of a valgus or external rotation stress to the knee when the foot is stationary, thus placing stress on the medial joint line [66, 78, 118]. After physeal injuries have been excluded by the location of point tenderness and stress radiographs [22, 28, 29], the diagnosis is confirmed, and a treatment plan is instituted.

Diagnosis

The mechanism of injury is a valgus or external rotation stress to the knee; if this stress involves contact, it is a very memorable event. The patient presents with a painful knee. A large effusion is not *usually* present unless other intra-articular injury has occurred as well. Clinical laxity examination shows no instability in incomplete lesions, and these athletes may be able to return to play immediately postinjury.

Examination of the knee may reveal a slight effusion. Hamstring spasm due to medial collateral ligament pain causes the knee to be held in slight flexion [118]. The medial aspect of the knee is tender to palpation at the femoral or tibial bony attachment of the MCL or in its midsubstance, depending on the site of injury [40, 66, 100, 118]. The knee is stable to valgus stress in full extension [40, 66, 118]. The same stress applied at 30 degrees of flexion (which relaxes the posterior capsule) causes increased discomfort and demonstrates medial opening if the MCL is injured [66, 118]. The quality of the end-point noted with this valgus stress is recorded, as is the grade of injury [21].

Careful examination for injury to the other ligamentous structures, particularly the ACL, is essential. The presence of an associated meniscal injury is suggested by tenderness at the joint line in addition to tenderness at either the tibial or femoral ligament attachment site. If the ligament is injured in its midsubstance, it is also tender at the joint line, making meniscal evaluation difficult. Meniscal injury in conjunction with an isolated MCL injury is uncommon in my experience. Routine radiographs are obtained to detect bony avulsions at the attachment of the MCL. Oblique views may be useful. If routine films are negative and guarding prevents evaluation, stress films with the patient sedated are taken to rule out ligament injury (see Fig. 21-5).

Treatment

After the location and severity of injury to the MCL have been determined and injury to the ACL, PCL, and lateral collateral ligament has been excluded, a treatment plan can be instituted. Isolated MCL injuries of grades I to III (those without associated laxity of the central pivot [ACL/PCL] or lateral collateral system) should be treated nonoperatively. Isolated bony avulsion of the MCL requires open reduction and internal fixation only if the ligament is markedly displaced from its origin; otherwise, these injuries may also be treated nonoperatively [39, 118]. Jones and colleagues [75] described 24 skeletally mature high school football players ranging in age from 14 to 18 years with isolated grade III MCL injuries that were treated nonoperatively. After treatment with a nonoperative protocol of protected motion and strengthening exercises, the athletes returned to play in an average of 34 days. They reported that all patients had stable knees and all denied symptoms of MCL instability at follow-up.

Treatment consists of an initial period in a knee immobilizer to diminish pain and to protect the repair response. Due to the low incidence of meniscal injuries in patients with isolated MCL injuries [78], arthroscopy is not recommended unless the physical examination points to associated meniscal pathology. MRI is a useful, noninvasive method of performing meniscal evaluation in questionable cases. In 5 to 7 days full knee motion is allowed in a hinged brace. Strengthening exercises, including straight leg raising, and progression to isotonic and isokinetic hamstring and quadriceps exercises, are started. Weight bearing is allowed and encouraged as soon as the knee feels comfortable in the brace. The brace is discontinued when a full range of painless motion is possible and muscle control of the limb is present.

Straight-ahead running may be started when the knee is pain-free, a full range of motion is present, and muscle strength is adequate by objective testing. When the area of ligament disruption becomes nontender to palpation and the knee has normal valgus stress stability at 30 degrees of knee flexion, full-speed running progressing to cutting is allowed. The athlete may return to full sports activity when the strength of the quadriceps and hamstrings (measured isokinetically) of the injured leg equals that of the normal leg [72, 75]. A functional brace may be used to provide perceived additional varus-valgus stability, although no evidence supporting its protective value has been presented [118].

Operative repair of an *isolated* MCL disruption is rarely indicated [39, 72, 75]. It is needed only when there is a major displaced bony avulsion of the MCL. Surgical treatment is indicated if there are other associated ligamentous or reparable meniscal injuries [39, 72, 77, 78, 118]. Critical to the success of nonoperative treatment is accurate determination of damage to the cruciate ligament and meniscal structures.

Author's Preferred Method of Treatment

Patients with isolated injury to the MCL are treated conservatively. If there is a question of associated meniscal or cruciate ligament injury, MRI or arthroscopy is performed to exclude injury to these structures.

Patients are given a postoperative knee brace with the knee fixed in extension, and immediate weight bearing is allowed. After 2 to 3 days the hinges in the brace are unlocked, and the patient begins range of motion exercises. Hip abductor, adductor, flexor, quadriceps, hamstring, and ankle dorsiflexion and plantarflexion flexibility and strengthening exercises begin immediately to prevent disuse.

A functional brace is recommended if the patient's limb is large enough to accept one of the currently available models. Straight-ahead running in the functional brace is allowed when a full range of motion is possible, quadriceps strength measured isokinetically is symmetrical, and the knee is pain-free. Slide board exercises in a functional brace are permitted when the patient can run without difficulty. The patient is allowed to run and cut when the slide board is mastered and the knee has a firm end-point to valgus stress.

Return to sports participation is allowed in the functional brace when full knee motion is possible, strength is normal, ligaments are nontender, and the patient is asymptomatic when performing specific sports activity. For patients with grade I to II lesions, this requires 10 to 14 days, whereas grade III lesions require 3 to 4 weeks.

LATERAL COLLATERAL LIGAMENT

Injuries to the lateral ligaments of the knee are uncommon and usually consist of injury to the lateral collateral ligament, the arcuate ligament complex, and the popliteal tendon [67, 79]. Isolated injury of one of these three structures is rarely recognized.

Diagnosis

The mechanism of injury is a varus stress or hyperextension injury to the knee [67]. An effusion may develop, and the range of motion is usually limited by pain, hamstring spasm, or the effusion. Palpation is helpful in determining which of the three structures is injured and where, along the course of the specific ligament, the injury is located.

Gollehon and associates [51], Kennedy [79], and Hsieh and Walker [65], in serial cutting studies of the lateral and posterior structures of the knee, demonstrated that the lateral collateral and arcuate complex function together as the principal structures resisting varus and external rotation of the tibia. The lateral collateral ligament is easily palpated when the injured leg is crossed over the opposite leg in a ''figure four'' position (Grant's Test) [79]. The popliteal tendon attachment is located anterior to the fibular collateral ligament on the femur. The tendon passes posteriorly beneath the fibula to attach on the tibia. The popliteus can also be palpated in the figure four position. The popliteal tendon appears to function as both a static and dynamic restraint to external rotation of the tibia [51].

Varus stress at 30 degrees of knee flexion is used to evaluate the integrity of the lateral collateral ligament. With a varus stress applied, the amount of laxity is graded using the same system as that used for MCL injuries [21]. The posterolateral drawer test [70] and passive external rotation at 30 degrees are used to evaluate the popliteal and arcuate ligaments [67]. The examiner must consider the amount of physiologic laxity present in the uninjured knee when testing these structures, especially in the patient with genu varum.

Treatment

Treatment of these injuries is not always easy, and the outcome is not predictable [79]. Isolated grade I and II injuries of the lateral collateral ligament, popliteal ligament, or arcuate ligament are treated nonoperatively with immobilization until the patient is comfortable and then with controlled motion in a hinged brace. Muscle strengthening exercises and protected weight bearing begin immediately. Protection is maintained until the knee is pain-free, has a full range of motion, and has strength comparable to that of the uninjured limb. Isolated grade III lesions of the lateral collateral ligament or popliteus are treated in a similar fashion.

Surgical repair is indicated for major displaced bony

avulsions of the lateral collateral ligament or popliteus and for combined ligament injuries to the fibular collateral, popliteus, and arcuate systems [77]. Arthroscopy is indicated if the physical examination, radiographic evaluation, and MRI suggests associated meniscal pathology.

Author's Preferred Method of Treatment

Isolated lesions of the lateral collateral ligament, popliteus, or arcuate complex are treated in the same manner as isolated MCL lesions (see earlier section on the MCL). Return to sports is allowed when the criteria listed earlier under MCL treatment are achieved.

Displaced bony avulsions of the lateral collateral ligament or popliteus and any injuries of the arcuate, popliteal, or lateral collateral ligaments combined with central pivot (ACL/PCL) or medial collateral injury are treated by primary surgical repair of the involved ligaments. In skeletally immature patients, reconstruction requiring drill holes through the physes should be avoided. Postoperatively, patients are treated in a knee brace with range of motion exercises beginning in the first 2 to 3 days. The patient begins weight bearing in a functional brace 5 to 7 days postoperatively. Rehabilitation of the lower extremity is the same as that described for the MCL. Running is allowed at 8 weeks, cutting at 16 weeks. Return to sports usually occurs 6 months after surgical repair.

ANTERIOR CRUCIATE LIGAMENT

Stanitski and colleagues [121] reported on 70 patients between the ages of 7 and 18 years with acute hemarthrosis of the knee who underwent arthroscopy. Of these 70 patients, 38 were truly skeletally immature and had significant growth remaining. Of these skeletally immature patients, 47% had ACL tears, 62% of which were partial.

Isolated disruption of the ACL in children is unusual, especially in children less than 14 years old [18, 28, 29, 33, 34, 108, 109, 130]. The frequency of diagnosis of this injury has increased during recent years because of (1) increased participation of children in sports, (2) improved diagnostic techniques, and (3) the profession's knowledge and subsequent recognition that children do sustain adult-type injuries of the knee ligaments [10, 18, 28, 35, 45, 50, 60, 79, 119].

Anterior cruciate laxity is present in two distinct groups of children [28, 29]. The first group comprises those with nontraumatic anterior cruciate laxity, which can be due to a generalized nonpathologic joint laxity or to congenital absence of the ACL. The second group includes those with post-traumatic anterior cruciate lax-

ity. This laxity is due to avulsion of either the femoral or tibial attachment of the ACL or to a midsubstance tear.

Nontraumatic Cruciate Insufficiency

Many young children have inherent (physiologic) joint laxity in the knee, most of which resolves with growth and physical development. This physiologic laxity may produce an erroneous suggestion of anterior cruciate laxity in the knee. It involves not only the knee but also other joints of the body such as the shoulders and elbow [54]. These children have a positive anterior drawer test with the foot in neutral rotation and a positive Lachman's test. The Lachman's test, however, has a firm end-point. Associated with these findings are a detectable pivot shift, a flexion-rotation drawer test, and hyperextension of the knee. These positive findings are bilateral, again emphasizing the importance of examining both extremities in the patient with an injured knee [22].

Congenital absence of the ACL is rare [130]. Giorgi [47] reported an absence on radiographs of the intercondylar eminence in knees that lack the ACL. He theorized that the ACL supplied traction on the tibial plateau during development and the traction then created the intercondylar eminence. When the ACL is absent, the eminence does not form, leading to the appearance of aplasia radiographically [47, 64] (see Fig 12–1).

Developmental absence of the ACL is usually associated with other congenital abnormalities of the involved limb, such as proximal focal femoral deficiency, congenital dislocation of the knee, and leg length discrepancy [24, 28, 74]. Because of the associated significant limb anomalies, athletic participation in these patients may be limited, so that the absent ACL with its associated instability is not stressed and therefore is asymptomatic.

Post-Traumatic Anterior Cruciate Insufficiency

The second group of patients with anterior cruciate laxity, a much larger group, comprises those with post-traumatic anterior cruciate instability [28, 29]. This group can be subdivided according to the location of the ACL injury—tibial or femoral avulsion, or midsubstance tear.

Avulsion of the Tibial Eminence

Most ACL injuries in children are usually avulsions of the ligament insertion at the tibial eminence [28, 44, 99, 108]. Recently, Stanitski and colleagues [121] reported finding equal incidence in children of proximal, distal, and midsubstance injury to the ACL. The ACL is attached to the tibia in a depressed area in front of and lateral to the anterior tibial spine. There is a fibrous attachment to the base of the anterior spine and a slip to the anterior horn of the lateral meniscus [48] (Fig. 21–6). This anatomic arrangement and the relative strength of the ligament compared to that of the adjacent bone and physeal plate explains the propensity for tibial avulsions. Rinaldi and Mazzarella [107] showed that, prior to fusion of the tibial growth plate, the intercondylar eminence offers less resistance to traction forces than the ligament. Injuries that result in stretching or progressive disruption of the ACL in adults may result in an avulsion (either partial or complete) of the tibial eminence in children [10, 18, 28, 29, 81, 82, 89, 90].

Meyers and McKeever, [90, 91] in their initial report of 45 cases, classified fractures of the tibial eminence into four types (Fig. 21–7). In a follow-up report 21 years later, they added 25 cases. Of the 70 reported cases, 47 were in children. In their classification, type I fractures are nondisplaced whereas type II fractures have some elevation of the tibial eminence. Type III fractures show elevation of the entire tibial eminence with displacement, and in type III+ injuries there is rotation of the completely displaced eminence. Zaricznyj [135] added an additional category IV (or III-C), which included comminution of the displaced fragment.

Avulsion of the ACL at the intercondylar eminence is often associated with damage to other supporting structures, such as the collateral ligaments and menisci [46, 71, 90, 91, 135]. It was initially noted by Garcia and Neer [46] that tibial eminence fractures or avulsions may have associated collateral ligament injury. This was confirmed by Hyndman and Brown [71] as well as by Zaricznyj [135]. Injuries to the collateral ligaments in conjunction with tibial spine avulsion produce a degree of ligamentous laxity that is greater than that following

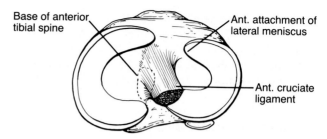

FIGURE 21–6
Anterior cruciate ligament inserts anterior and slightly lateral to the anterior tibial spine. It sends fibrous attachments to the base of the anterior spine and a slip to the anterior horn of the lateral meniscus.

either injury occurring as an isolated event. For this reason, it is essential to perform a complete evaluation of all knee ligaments in children in whom a tibial spine avulsion is diagnosed [6, 46, 71, 90, 91].

Treatment. Garcia and Neer [46] recommend that these tibial avulsions be treated by closed reduction by hyperextension of the knee. Meyers and McKeever [90, 91] treated type I and II fractures with closed reduction and immobilization and type III and III+ fractures with open reduction and internal fixation. In Zaricznyj's series of 13 fractures, half were type IV injuries and the other half were type III injuries. All patients required open reduction and internal fixation. The literature supports closed reduction for type I and II avulsions. As the knee is brought into the last 5 degrees of extension, the femoral condyles impinge on the fragment, resulting in adequate reduction. Type III, III+, and IV fractures require open reduction and internal fixation using sutures, pins, or screws. In his study of 10 children less than 15 years old with tibial eminence fractures, Zaricznyi [135] warned against residual displacement of the eminence following attempted closed reduction. A displaced eminence can block knee extension mechanically and cause relative lengthening of the ACL. Meyers and McKeever [90] reported 86% excellent results, but

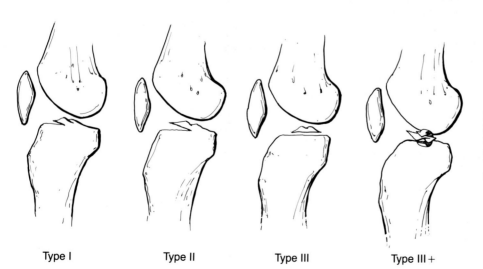

| Type I | Type II | Type III | Type III+ |

FIGURE 21–7
Meyers and McKeever classified intercondylar eminence fractures based upon the degree of displacement. Type III+ fracture is Zaricznyj's classification [135].

Smith [120] reported that only 47% of patients were asymptomatic following treatment for an avulsion of the tibial eminence.

The incidence of *residual* ACL laxity following treatment of tibial eminence avulsions is drawing more attention. Meyers and McKeever [90] found that only 1 of 35 patients had residual AP instability, and Garcia and Neer [46], in a review of 20 patients, found none with residual instability. Molander and colleagues [94] found no patients with residual ACL laxity after tibial eminence avulsion. On the other hand, Smith [120] reported that 87% of patients had anterior laxity and 27% had functional instability, and Gronkvist and associates [56] reported functional instability in 34% of patients after tibial eminence avulsion.

Baxter and Wiley [6], in 1988, used the GenuCom (Faro Medical Technologic) instrumented test system to evaluate laxity after tibial spine avulsion. Using Meyers and McKeever's classification system, they found that patients with type I injuries had minimal residual laxity, whereas those with type II and III injuries had mean differences of 3 mm (at 90 degrees of flexion) and 4 mm (at 20 degrees of flexion), respectively, between the injured and uninjured limbs. All of their patients had a measurable loss of extension in the injured knee. None of them, however, complained of knee instability. The authors concluded that in spite of anatomic reduction, these injuries lead to a measureable degree of cruciate laxity and that although the laxity seems to be "asymptomatic," a significant number of patients quit sports. Whether this laxity becomes manifest with increased vocational or avocational demands is unknown because follow-up in all studies has been brief.

More recently, Blokker and Fowler [7] reviewed 35 patients after tibial eminence avulsion. The magnitude of trauma was not specified, but the significance of injury may be a reflection of severe trauma. Twenty percent of the patients had associated collateral ligament injuries, and 12% had meniscal injuries. The authors reported that only 45% of patients had an asymptomatic knee at follow-up, whereas 55% had either pain or symptomatic instability. Twelve patients had a positive Lachman test result, and 10 had positive findings on the pivot shift test. Using the KT-1000 arthrometer, the authors found that anterior translation averaged 2.75 mm greater (range −1 mm to +11 mm) in the injured knee. There was no correlation between functional and objective test results. The authors concluded that despite an anatomic reduction patients do have cruciate laxity after tibial eminence fractures. The authors suggested that prior to tibial eminence avulsion sequential failure of the ligament fibers may result in healing of the ligament in a slightly elongated state [56, 99]. The authors reported that despite measurable laxity, significant functional in-

stability or joint deterioration does not occur frequently. However, the follow-up in these series is quite short, and few data are given about return to sports.

Author's Preferred Method of Treatment. In patients with major trauma, due to the significant incidence of associated collateral ligament and meniscal injuries, arthroscopy and examination under anesthesia are performed. Unstable meniscal injuries (those that can be displaced) are treated by meniscal repair when technically possible. Type I tibial eminence fractures are treated by reduction with immobilization for 4 weeks. Type II injuries that can be reduced are also treated closed, but fractures in which an anatomic reduction is not obtained are surgically reduced and fixed [90, 91]. Associated collateral ligament injuries with type I and reduced type II injuries are treated closed. All type III and III+ fractures undergo open reduction and internal fixation [90, 91, 111]. The physeal plate is not violated when these fragments are fixed (Fig. 21–8). Associated collateral ligament injury is treated by primary repair, and meniscal injury by repair and rarely by removal. As always, especially in children, preservation of the meniscus is desirable.

Avulsion of the Femoral Insertion

Avulsion of the anterior cruciate ligament from the femur is very rare. A single case was described by Eady and colleagues [33] in 1982. The bony femoral avulsion was seen radiographically on the tunnel view. This 7-year-old child underwent suture repair of the avulsed origin through drill holes in the medial femoral condyle without involvement of the physeal plate (Fig. 21–8). Fifteen months postoperatively the patient had a stable joint. No long-term follow-up was reported.

Author's Preferred Method of Treatment. If a displaced femoral avulsion is detected by arthroscopy or MRI, primary repair as described above is undertaken. Care must be taken to be certain that this is an avulsion and not a very proximal substance tear. Associated collateral ligament and meniscal injury are managed as described above.

Midsubstance Tear—Isolated and Combined

Midsubstance tear of the ACL, alone or associated with other ligament disruptions, is distinctly unusual in the athlete with open physes [10, 18, 28, 29]. Primary repair of this injury has been shown to produce no better results in the child than in the adult [10, 18, 28, 29].

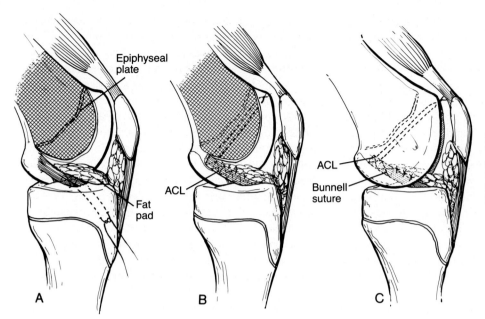

FIGURE 21–8
Three methods of repair of the anterior cruciate ligament: *A*, Repair of tibial avulsion. *B*, Repair of femoral avulsion. *C*, Repair of midsubstance tear.

Diagnosis

The keys to the diagnosis of an ACL injury in the child are the history, physical examination, and specific imaging studies just as in the adult. The history relates a contact or noncontact, twisting or hyperextension deceleration injury followed by a loud "pop" [38, 49, 118]. Isolated anterior cruciate injuries are usually noncontact injuries that occur during a rapid change of position. Any accompanying varus or valgus stress on the knee may result in associated medial or lateral collateral ligament injury. After an acute ACL injury a tense hemarthrosis usually accumulates rapidly (within 24 hours) [28]. The effusion usually subsides in a few days, leading the patient to believe that the knee is only slightly damaged. There may be associated ecchymosis at the site of associated collateral ligament injury. Range of motion may be limited by the effusion or pain caused by an associated collateral ligament or meniscal injury.

The Lachman, Losee, and flexion-rotation drawer test signs are positive and can be elicited in the cooperative patient [28, 66, 118]. The pivot shift test sign is easily detected in the chronic anterior cruciate deficient knee. It may be difficult to produce the pivot shift in patients with an acute injury owing to muscle pain and spasm. Tenderness at the mid or posterior medial or lateral joint line suggests associated meniscal pathology. Palpation of the course of the medial and lateral collateral ligaments will detect injury of these structures. A positive anterior drawer test should suggest collateral ligament injury *in addition to* anterior cruciate disruption [28, 66].

The radiographic examination is important in skeletally immature patients. It is critical to obtain routine and stress radiographs in order to demonstrate avulsions and to distinguish physeal separation from ligament disruption (Fig. 21–5) [18, 22, 24, 28]. MRI may provide valuable information about the location of an ACL injury, the presence of associated meniscal damage, and the presence of associated bony injury [73]. Fowler [42] demonstrated a significant incidence of bony injury ranging from subchondral hemorrhage to fracture noted on MRI in patients with acute ACL injury (Fig. 21–9). The significance of these injuries is not yet known.

The role of diagnostic arthroscopy is to extend the possible diagnoses by evaluating the menisci and articular surfaces and to confirm the location and extent of the ACL injury. Arthroscopy should not be substituted for adequate historical, physical, and imaging evaluation.

Treatment of "Isolated" ACL Injuries

An "isolated" ACL injury assumes that there is no significant associated meniscal, bony, or collateral ligament injury. Patients with an isolated partial ACL tear, defined clinically as a slightly increased anterior translation on the Lachman test but negative results on the pivot shift test, and confirmed (by MRI or arthroscopy) as a lesion in which some fibers are intact and functional, are treated conservatively. In my experience MRI is usually unable to determine which ACL injuries are partial (anatomically and functionally) and which are complete. MRI is useful to establish the anatomic location of the injury but usually cannot determine its extent.

Children with a complete ACL injury can be divided into two groups according to the functional significance of the laxity. The first group has no evidence of functional instability. These patients are able to participate in

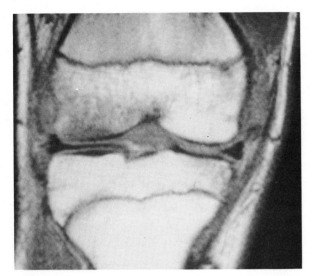

FIGURE 21–9
MRI of an ACL injury in a patient with open growth plates. Note the "bone bruise" in the lateral femoral condyle.

sports with no symptoms of giving way. In the second group the knee gives way either during activities of daily living or when participating in sports. Because the activity level of a child is difficult to curtail, these patients have significant disability.

Initially, one cannot determine whether or not the child will have functional instability. Repair of acute midsubstance tears of the ACL heal no better in the child than in the adult [29]. Also, primary reconstruction or augmentation of a primary repair by the standard methods used in the adult carries a risk of physeal plate damage. A young patient with an acute isolated midsubstance tear of the ACL should be given a trial of nonoperative treatment. It is essential to inform the child and the parents that each episode of instability with resultant swelling reflects injury to the menisci and articular cartilage. DeLee and Curtis [29] showed that many children with a chronic anterior cruciate deficient knee and concomitant episodes of instability are not functionally limited. However, episodes of instability cause progressive meniscal and articular cartilage damage that can produce a poor long-term result. Kannus and Jarvinen [77] reported 32 adolescent patients, 25 with partial ACL tears and 7 with complete ACL tears, who were treated nonoperatively by cast immobilization for 3 to 5 weeks. Treatment of partial ACL tears resulted in excellent or good Lysholm scores, and no patient had gross instability. However, Lysholm scores for patients with complete ACL injuries were significantly poorer than in those with partial tears. Also, 70% of patients with complete ACL disruption were forced to decrease their physical activity because of their knee injury, and four of the seven patients had radiographic evidence of post-traumatic arthritis. Associated injuries (i.e., meniscal and

articular) were not discussed. Angel and Hall [2] reviewed 27 patients (average age 14.3 years) with ACL tears. Partial tears were more common than complete tears. Forty-one percent of patients had associated meniscal pathology at the time of injury. Seven patients had either undergone or were awaiting knee reconstruction because of instability. The authors concluded that an ACL disruption in the skeletally immature patient is not a benign lesion when coupled with meniscal injury. Since children who undergo meniscectomy have poor long-term results [28, 83, 104], the approach to the child patient who has episodes of clinical instability should be to stabilize the knee early to reduce the incidence of progressive articular cartilage and meniscal damage. An attempt to control giving-way episodes by altering the child's lifestyle (i.e., sports participation) can be considered, but this approach has not been successful in my hands.

The child with an ACL-deficient knee presents a major problem in reconstruction. Any surgical procedure that is designed to restore the pivot control function of the ACL can violate the physeal plate [28, 29, 77]. Violation of the physeal plate in a child (the physeal plate is defined as having *significant* growth remaining) can result in angular deformity and/or leg length discrepancy.

Several authors have reported success in patients with open physeal plates following surgical reconstruction in which graft tissue is used to cross the physeal plate [77, 84, 87]. Most of these patients had minimally open physeal plates and were older and near skeletal maturity. In addition, as emphasized by Stanitski [122], bone age, Tanner classification, and stage of tibial and femoral physeal plate closure were not correlated in these patients. Also, the follow-up of these patients was extremely short, and, as Stanitski has pointed out, any surgical procedure performed in a skeletally immature patient must withstand the rigors of growth, time, and use, and these are not available in the series reported to date [122].

Lipscomb and Anderson [84] reported 24 patients with open physes who underwent ACL reconstruction. The patients ranged in age from 12 to 15 years at the time of surgery. Nine of the twenty-four patients were under the age of 14 at surgery, but only three were as young as 12 years. The authors passed the semitendinous and gracilis tendons through a ¼-inch drill hole across the tibial physis and through a ⁵⁄₁₆-inch hole through the femoral epiphysis (distal to the physeal plate). The authors reported that 11 patients had completely open physes, but 13 of the 24 were near the time of physeal closure. At follow-up, limb lengths were equal in seven patients, and 10 patients had less than 5 mm difference between the two limbs; in one patient the operated limb was 1.3 cm longer and in another it was 2 cm shorter.

Rush and Steiner [113] reported that 77% of the population have an average leg length discrepancy of 7 mm, and Nichols [97] reported that 7% to 8% of adults have a limb length discrepancy of 1.25 cm or more. Lipscomb and Anderson [84] concluded, based on the above reports, that only one of their patients had significant deformity. However, they do not recommend this procedure for patients under the age of 12 years. Graf and colleagues [53] reported on 12 patients with open physes (average age 14.5 years) with acute midsubstance ACL tears. Six patients had eight associated meniscal tears confirmed by arthroscopy. Eight patients were treated nonoperatively and wore a brace to return to sports. Four patients underwent ACL reconstruction (two extra-articular procedures and two semitendinosus over-the-top procedures). All eight patients treated conservatively (including those with meniscal tears) had repeated episodes of giving way, and seven of the eight had further meniscal damage. The patients with intra-articular reconstruction did well (after a very brief follow-up), whereas the patients who underwent extra-articular reconstruction became unstable and sustained new meniscal tears. The authors concluded that acute ACL tears in skeletally immature patients are frequently associated with meniscal tears, and hence the patients need to undergo evaluation by MRI or arthroscopy in the acute situation. Also, the authors concluded that brace management is unsuccessful in preventing instability and further meniscal damage in young active patients.

Capra and Fowler [15] reviewed 29 patients with open physes (average age 14.3 years, range 13.6 to 15.6 years) who had acute ACL tears. All were treated operatively using either hamstring tendon or patellar-quadriceps tendon passed through a 6-mm drill hole in the tibia and over the top of the femur. All patients returned to preoperative activities. There were no cases of leg length discrepancy. The authors provided no data on skeletal age, Tanner stages, or remaining growth of the patients.

Bergfeld [8], in an effort to avoid physeal plate damage during ACL reconstruction in skeletally immature patients, introduced the so-called tomato stake repair (Fig. 21–10). This is a method of intra-articular reconstruction that avoids the physis [8]. The graft is brought over the front of the tibia and over the top of the femur to avoid the physeal plate (Fig. 21–10). Drez [32] modified this technique to improve isometricity (Fig. 21–11). In this modification, the graft is brought through a groove in the tibial physis that displaces the graft posteriorly in an attempt to approach its point of isometricity on the tibia. The graft is brought ''over the top'' of the femur through a groove (in the over-the-top position) below the femoral physis. This displaces the femoral origin anteriorly and hence is more isometric than the over-the-top technique. The author reports excellent stability and no growth disturbances at short-term follow-up.

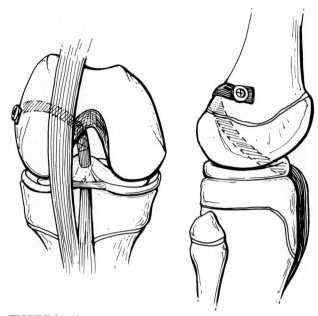

FIGURE 21–10
''Tomato stake'' procedure. The patellar tendon is left attached to the tibial tubercle or hamstring tendon or is left attached to the proximal tibia and passed over the front of the tibia beneath the transverse ligament, and then ''over the top'' of the femur. The stump of the anterior cruciate ligament may be used to augment the graft.

Associated Meniscal Lesions

Because of the frequency of meniscal tears associated with acute and chronic ACL tears, the management of meniscal tears in skeletally immature patients is pivotal in a discussion of management of ACL injuries. Numerous reports document the poor clinical and radiographic results of total meniscectomy in adults. In children, total meniscectomy is followed by pain, limited activity, and arthritic changes at long-term follow-up [27, 28, 83, 104]. Therefore, preservation of as much meniscal tissue as possible must be the goal of treatment in skeletally immature patients.

The meniscus in the young patient up to age 10 years has a better blood supply and greater cellularity, suggesting a greater potential for healing than in the adult [27]. Arnoczky and Warren [5] described blood flow in the adult meniscus. Branches of the geniculate arteries form a capillary plexus at the synovial meniscal junction. The plexus penetrates into the peripheral 10% to 30% of the meniscus. Shin and Leung [116] reviewed adult and child cadavers and reported that a circumeniscal anastomosis supplied the outer one-third to one-half of the meniscus. They noted no difference in menisci between adults and children. Clark and Ogden [19] noted a gradual decrease in the cellularity and vascularity of the meniscus from birth to age 10, at which time the vessels were located primarily in the outer third of these menisci, i.e., in the adult pattern. In adolescents, occasional

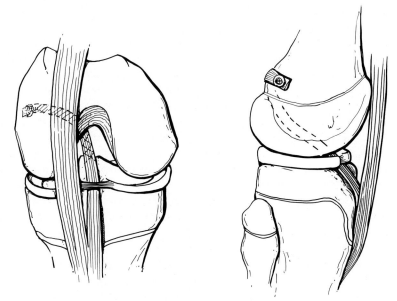

FIGURE 21–11
Modification of tomato stake repair. A groove is created in the epiphysis of the proximal tibia. The graft is then passed through the groove (which displaces its origin posteriorly), more closely approximating the tibial insertion of the ACL. The graft is then passed through the over-the-top position on the femur.

vessels were located in the inner zones, whereas in adults vessels were seen only in the outer third. The menisci also undergo a gradual decrease in cellularity and an increase in collagen fiber content between the ages of 3 and 9 years. These studies support the concept that meniscal injuries in the pediatric group have a greater potential for healing.

Any stable meniscal tissue should provide some joint stability and assist in load sharing. Hargreaves and Seedhom [61] reported that load transmission across the meniscus dropped from 85% to 35% after partial medial meniscectomy and from 75% to 50% after partial lateral meniscectomy. This finding supports the concept of preserving as much meniscal tissue as possible. DeHaven and Wascher [27] reported that not all meniscal tears require treatment because some peripheral ones heal and others are not symptomatic. For this reason, they recommended that tears of questionable significance be left alone. Weiss and colleagues [134] reported that all partial tears and all completely stable peripheral tears (less than 5 mm long and stable to probing) heal if treated conservatively.

Finally, recent interest in meniscal repair has further extended the surgeon's ability to salvage meniscal tissue [27]. The topic of meniscal repair is beyond the scope of this chapter. However, current recommendations of reparable menisci range from repairing only those in the outer vascular zones to repairing radial tears in the central avascular areas. Although long-term results of meniscal repair are not available, early reports regarding meniscal preservation are quite favorable [27]. Hence, the probable increased potential for meniscal healing in children (both with and without suturing), the possibility that a meniscal tear may be asymptomatic, and finally, the salvage of some load transmission capability by performing partial rather than total meniscectomy all support a very conservative approach to meniscal removal in skeletally immature patients.

Treatment—Combined Lesions

Disruptions of the ACL associated with complete disruption of either collateral ligament are distinctly unusual in the patient with open physes [18, 77]. Clanton and colleagues [18] demonstrated that ligament injuries in patients with open physes fared no better than those in patients who had completed growth. Indeed, Kannus and Jarvinen [77], in a review of 32 patients with open physes and combined knee ligament injuries, demonstrated that patients with complete ligament disruptions did poorly when managed nonoperatively. However, 25 patients with grade II (incomplete) ligament tears were treated successfully without surgical repair [77]. This finding parallels similar experience in adult patients. In this report seven patients had grade III (complete) tears. All seven were treated nonoperatively, and at follow-up all had marked instabilities that were no different from those noted at the time of injury. In addition, four of the seven patients had radiographic evidence of degenerative joint disease in the involved knee. The authors concluded that partial tears, like those in the adult, should be treated nonoperatively and that complete tears required primary surgical repair. The authors did concede that, as reported by Clanton and associates [18], the ACL did not heal well following primary repair and suggested that some augmentation of the ACL is required. They discussed drilling holes across the physis to pass augmenting tissue but concluded that further research in this area is necessary before the technique can be recommended.

Author's Preferred Method of Treatment

Acute ACL Disruption

I again emphasize that skeletal maturity, as noted by the absence of open physes, is a radiographic diagnosis and is age and gender dependent. The treatment of an acute ACL disruption in a patient with open physes is at best controversial. For this reason, I prefer to attempt to delay surgical treatment until growth at the distal femur and proximal tibia is near completion and an isometric reconstruction can be safely performed.

Operative repair of the ACL in a child follows two principles. The primary reason for ACL repair is to preserve the meniscal and articular cartilage because children who lose their menisci progress to degenerative arthritis [79, 83]. Second, the surgical procedure must avoid damage to the physeal plates if there is significant growth potential remaining. It is for this reason that the age of the child and the growth remaining in the limb must be known before the type of surgical treatment can be selected.

Accurate determination of growth remaining in the distal femoral and proximal tibial epiphyses requires evaluation of several factors. I obtain a wrist film and use the Greulich-Pyle atlas to determine skeletal age, appreciating the 6- to 12-month variability inherent in this system [59]. The Greulich-Pyle atlas is based on a group of "well-off" North American children in the 1930s, and the Green-Anderson tables are based on Anglo-Saxon children living in New England. Because these tables were based on Anglo-Saxon children, alterations in maturity of children from differing ethnic backgrounds must be considered when using the tables. This skeletal age is applied to the Green-Anderson tables [55] to estimate future growth.

In addition, radiographs are reviewed to determine whether the tibial and femoral physeal plates are open or closed. If there is any doubt about whether the physeal plate is open or closed, an MRI can further clarify the issue. I also carefully review the family history to determine the height of the parents and the siblings. The presence or absence of secondary sex characteristics gives important information about the status of skeletal maturity. The Tanner-Whitehouse method of determining bone age is more detailed and more accurate than the Greulich-Pyle atlas [127]. In the Tanner-Whitehouse method the development of secondary sex characteristics produces a "maturity score," which determines for each patient whether skeletal growth is advanced or delayed. This score helps to evaluate the accuracy of estimations of remaining growth taken from growth tables. Alternatively, the maturity score can be converted into a bone age, which includes the effect of secondary sex characteristics on the bone age.

I treat patients determined to have less than 1 cm of growth remaining at the distal femur and proximal tibia as adults and drill holes across the growth plates with no concern about the development of significant limb deformity. Patients with more than 1 cm of growth remaining must be treated very carefully. It is important to remember that 75% of the normal population have a leg length discrepancy of 7 mm [113], and one can make up a centimeter of leg length discrepancy with a shoe lift. Therefore, if after all these studies are completed, there appears to be more than 1 cm of growth remaining in the limb, I choose not to violate the growth plate in a reconstructive procedure.

Once the diagnosis of an acute ACL disruption is suspected in a patient with significant growth remaining (> 1 cm), complete evaluation of the knee is essential. I prefer to obtain an MRI study to (1) determine the location of the ACL disruption, (2) detect subclinical secondary restraint damage, and (3) detect possible "silent" injury to the physeal plate and the extent of physeal plate closure. If these data are not available and accurate physical examination is not possible, an examination under anesthesia is performed to confirm the ACL injury and to evaluate injury of the secondary restraints. Arthroscopy is performed to confirm the site and magnitude of the ACL disruption and to inspect the meniscal status. If an unstable peripheral detachment of the meniscus is demonstrated, repair is indicated [104]. If the meniscus has a tear in its substance and repair is technically possible, even in the so-called "white-on-white" tear, repair is recommended. Only when the meniscal tear is unrepairable is excision of the fragment the treatment of choice.

If, at arthroscopy, the ACL is found to be avulsed from the tibia or femur (with or without bone), a primary repair is performed (see Fig. 21–6) [85, 100, 109]. This repair is performed using a Bunnell-type stitch through the ligament, passing it through drill holes in the tibial or femoral epiphysis without violating the physeal plate. These patients are immobilized with the knee flexed 10 to 30 degrees for 4 to 6 weeks, followed by limited range of motion exercises in a hinged brace at 30 to 60 degrees for an additional 1 to 2 weeks. Full range of motion is then permitted.

If a midsubstance tear without collateral ligament injury is found in a patient with significant growth remaining, conservative treatment is recommended. If there is an associated repairable meniscal lesion in such a patient, meniscus is repaired and the cruciate ligament is treated nonoperatively. The meniscal pathology is treated by meniscal repair or by protecting the lesion while healing occurs by immobilization.

Nonoperative treatment of ACL injuries consists of immobilization of the knee for 7 to 10 days in a postoperative knee brace. Progressive increased range of motion is then allowed from −30 to 140 degrees. The last 30 degrees of extension is restored after 4 weeks. Once a full range of motion is possible, hamstring, quadriceps (90 to 60 degrees), and hip muscle strengthening exercises are allowed. Progressive increased activity is allowed with return to running at 12 weeks. The use of a functional brace, if one can be made that will accommodate the child's limb size, is recommended. A maintenance program is then instituted. Activity modification is encouraged once the patient has recovered from the initial injury. Certain activities place an unstable knee at risk. Acceleration and deceleration sports (football, basketball, gymnastics, soccer) are not recommended even with a brace. Swimming, biking, and softball are permitted. It is emphasized that the brace is not a substitute for a stable knee.

In my practice an acute repair for an isolated midsubstance ACL tear in a child is indicated only when there is marked pathologic laxity (grade 3(+) on the Lachman and pivot shift tests). Patients with an ACL injury or an associated complete collateral ligament injury also are treated by ACL repair. The method of repair of a midsubstance ACL tear is that of Marshall and colleagues [85] (Fig. 21–6A). Three sutures are placed in the distal portion of the ligament and are brought out through the femoral epiphysis using two small Kirschner wires for drill holes. The proximal end of the ligament is then sutured to the distal portion using simple interrupted sutures. No sutures cross the physeal plates. The fat pad is then sutured to the cruciate ligament repair. An extra-articular augmentation may be performed using a strip of iliotibial (IT) band 2.5 cm in width and 15 cm long. This strip is detached proximally but is left attached at Gerdy's tubercle. It is then passed beneath the fibular collateral ligament and fixed to the femur, beneath an osteoperiosteal tunnel but tbove the physis, with a 4.0 cancellous screw and a spiked washer. The remaining IT band is brought back over the fibular collateral ligament and reattached to bone below Gerdy's tubercle, fixed with a 4.0 cancellous screw and a spiked washer (Fig. 21–12). The patient is then placed in a long-leg brace. Motion from 30 to 70 degrees of flexion is allowed for 4 weeks, followed by progressive mobilization and muscle rehabilitation.

Chronic ACL Instability

In the child with chronic ACL laxity and instability in daily activity, the decision in favor of surgical treatment is based upon the frequency of giving way. Each episode of giving way or "slipping" produces articular cartilage shearing and potential meniscal injury. I have not been successful in treating patients in this age group by limiting their daily activities. Initial treatment consists of bracing and muscle rehabilitation. Fitting a brace in this age group is difficult. I have found that the OTI brace (Orthotech) can be fitted to the child's knee. The brace

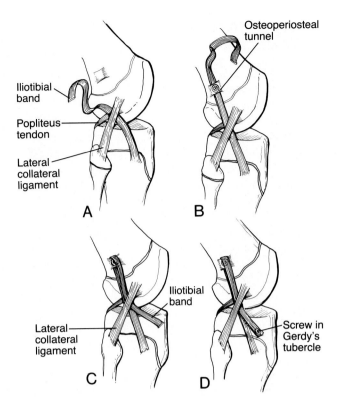

FIGURE 21–12
Technique of extra-articular reconstruction. *A,* A 2.5-cm wide strip of iliotibial band 15 cm in length is harvested. It is left attached to Gerdy's tubercle and is passed beneath the fibulocollateral ligament. *B,* After passing beneath the fibulocollateral ligament, it is passed through an osteoperiosteal tunnel *proximal* to the physeal plate and fixed in this tunnel with a ligament screw and washer. *C,* The iliotibial band is passed distally again beneath the fibulocollateral ligament. *D,* A ligament screw and washer are then used to fix the band back down to Gerdy's tubercle.

is worn during modified sports activities. If the brace is ineffective or if the patient's knee continues to give way during activities of daily living, surgical reconstruction is indicated. One must be certain that the patient has complied with wearing the brace and muscle rehabilitation (as documented by isokinetic strength testing) before surgery is undertaken.

In patients with chronic ACL instability of a mild degree (grade I to II or III) who have significant growth remaining (more than 2 cm) and in whom conservative treatment has failed, an extra-articular reconstruction is performed as outlined earlier. I have found this extra-articular procedure effective in protecting the menisci from further damage and preventing the pivot shift phenomenon in adults and children [30]. I caution against performing any extra-articular procedure that simply passes the iliotibial band around the fibular collateral ligament because this concentrates stress at the distal femoral physeal plate and can produce disruption of the plate during postoperative rehabilitation or sports participation (Fig. 21–13). It is important to close the IT band

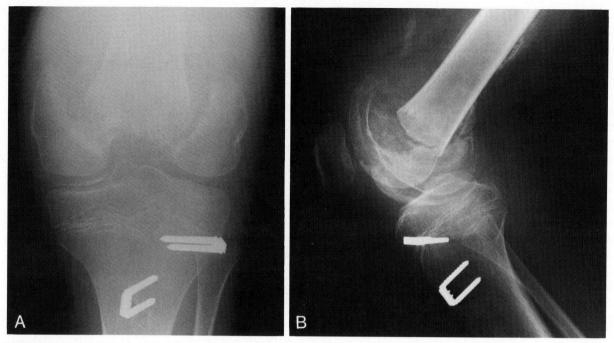

FIGURE 21–13

A and *B,* This patient underwent an anterior-lateral extra-articular reconstruction in which the iliotibial band was passed beneath the fibulocollateral ligament. During the postoperative rehabilitation program, excessive stress was applied to restore motion. Motion occurred at the distal femoral physeal plate rather than at the joint.

defect completely to restore lateral stability. If this extra-articular reconstruction stretches out over time, an intra-articular procedure can be done at a later date when physeal plate closure is complete.

In a knee with chronic marked pathologic anterior laxity (defined as grade III Lachman or a score of 8 mm or more [manual maximum] on KT-1000 arthrometry), an extra-articular reconstruction alone may not provide stability for the knee. In this situation, some authors advocate placing small (6 to 8 mm) drill holes across the tibial physeal plate and inserting tendon grafts (semitendinosus or gracilis) through these drill holes, drawing them over the top of the femur. It is believed that such small holes filled with soft tissue (tendon), especially if placed centrally in the growth plate, will not cause physeal arrest and growth abnormality. However, until a series of such patients with significant growth remaining is presented, I consider this procedure potentially quite risky. In this situation, I prefer to perform a modified intra-articular reconstruction, possibly with an extra-articular back-up. The tomato stake reconstruction described by Bergfeld (see Fig. 21–10) and its modification described by Drez (see Fig. 21–11) are methods of intra-articular reconstruction that I favor because they do not violate the surrounding physes [8, 32]. The remnants of the ACL are exposed surgically. These remnants proximally and distally are carefully teased away from the scar tissue and left intact. The ACL remnants are augmented with a hamstring tendon. I prefer to save the

patellar tendon for use later if this modified procedure fails. The semitendinosus or gracilis is detached proximally and left attached distally. The graft is passed over a groove in the anterior border of the tibia and then drawn to the over-the-top position on the femoral condyle. The remainder of the scar tissue or fat pad is sutured around the graft. The sutures in the graft are brought out through two drill holes in the femoral epiphysis (Fig. 21–11). This procedure produces a reconstruction that is not isometric at the sites of attachment on either the femur or the tibia. This may lead to failure of the graft owing to loss of motion or recurrent instability. Grooving the anterior tibia produces a more isometric tibial graft position than the procedure as Bergfeld described it. However, care must be taken to avoid the tibial physeal plate when the groove is made. Depending on the degree of laxity, an extra-articular reconstruction may be added. Following the tomato stake or modified reconstruction, the patient is placed in a brace, and knee motion from −20 to 90 degrees of flexion is allowed for 2 weeks. Mobilization and rehabilitation are then instituted in much the same way as in an adult who has undergone an intra-articular reconstruction.

One must be extremely careful in selecting patients for this tomato stake type of repair. Although it does accomplish reconstruction of the central pivot ligament (ACL), it has two drawbacks. First, the tibial origin is too anterior, and the femoral insertion is too posterior. These abnormal insertions result in a nonisometric reconstruction and, according to current theory, are certain to result in stretching of the reconstruction with the passage of time. This may result in recurrence of the instability. Second, use of the patellar tendon or semitendinosus in this nonisometric repair leaves the surgeon with a limited selection of autogenous tissue if a repeat reconstruction is necessary. For these reasons, it is best, if the clinical situation allows, to delay intra-articular reconstruction until the danger of sequelae of physeal plate damage has passed and an isometric reconstruction can be performed.

POSTERIOR CRUCIATE LIGAMENT

Disruption of the posterior cruciate ligament (PCL) is a rare injury in adults and is even less common in children [88, 103, 115]. Ringer and Fay [112] recently reviewed reports of PCL injuries in children. Their extensive review of the literature yielded 21 cases of PCL injury in children 15 years of age or younger [9, 18, 23, 43, 52, 68, 69, 86, 89, 95, 102, 110, 115, 125, 126, 132, 133]. The authors reviewed two additional cases of their own in children aged 5 and 12 years. In addition to the rarity of this injury, follow-up of reported cases has been extremely short. Therefore, at present, the functional effect of loss of the PCL in the skeletally immature knee is not known.

The PCL arises from a wide origin on the posterior aspect of the lateral surface of the medial femoral condyle [48] and inserts into a depression behind the articular surface of the tibia [48]. It courses from the posterior surface of the intercondylar area of the tibia in an anterior, superior, and medial direction to attach on the lateral surface of the medial femoral condyle. The tibial attachment passes distally over the posterior aspect of the tibia and blends into the periosteum, giving it a wide base. Anatomically, the PCL has been divided into two portions, a larger anterior bundle and a smaller posterior portion that attaches lower on the posterior tibia. The anterior bundle is tight in flexion whereas the smaller posterior bundle is tight in extension [3, 48]. Two meniscofemoral ligaments may be present either singularly or together with the PCL. When present, both arise from the posterior horn of the lateral meniscus and pass anterior (Humphrey's ligament) and posterior (Wrisberg's ligament) to the PCL. Heller and Langeman [63] report that the ligaments of Wrisberg and Humphrey are found with equal frequency in approximately 70% of knees. They also noted that the ligament of Wrisberg is at least half the diameter of the PCL whereas the ligament of Humphrey is only about one-third the size of the posterior cruciate ligament [63]. The PCL receives its blood supply from the synovium because few anastomoses exist between the endosteum and the ligament at its origin or attachment [1, 37].

The PCL controls posterior translation of the tibia on the femur and helps to stabilize the flexed knee [48]. According to Grood and colleagues [57], the PCL supplies 95% of the restraint to a posterior drawer force. The accessory ligaments of Wrisberg posteriorly and the ligament of Humphrey anteriorly also help to stabilize the knee against posterior displacement [17]. Clancy and associates [17] noted that posterior drawer test results are significantly diminished in patients with intact ligaments of Wrisberg or Humphrey. This decrease in posterior laxity is most apparent when the tibia is internally rotated, a position that causes the ligaments of Wrisberg and Humphrey to become taut. Kennedy and colleagues [82] demonstrated that the PCL is twice as strong as the ACL. This helps to explain why it is infrequently injured.

Mechanism of Injury

According to Kennedy and Grainger [80], the posterior cruciate can be injured by one of two separate mechanisms: first, forceful posterior displacement of the fixed tibia on the femur with the knee in 90 degrees of flexion (Fig. 21–14A), and second, a hyperextension injury of the knee. During hyperextension, the femoral condyles slide posteriorly on the tibia, and the medial femoral condyle abuts against the posterior cruciate ligament, which is stretched. The PCL prevents further backward displacement of the femur, but if the hyperextension force continues past 30 degrees, in-substance failure or avulsion of the PCL will occur (Fig. 21–14B). A third mechanism of injury was reported by Donovan and colleagues [31]. These authors presented three case reports of football players who had documented PCL injuries caused by falling on the proximal tibial crest with the knee flexed at 90 degrees and the foot plantarflexed (Fig. 21–14C). Clancy and associates [17] confirmed this mechanism of injury and reported 10 patients with posterior cruciate injuries that occurred following falls on a flexed knee with the foot plantarflexed. However, according to Fowler [41], the position of the foot is *not* responsible for the PCL injury in this mechanism. Fowler showed that it is the hyperflexion of the knee, *not* the blow to the proximal tibial crest, that produces the PCL lesion (Fig. 21–14D). He also demonstrated that this lesion frequently produces an avulsion of the PCL off the femur, often with some surrounding periosteum or perichondrium, a situation that may allow successful primary repair.

Diagnosis

It must be remembered that a patient with a seemingly isolated PCL injury may have a spontaneously reduced

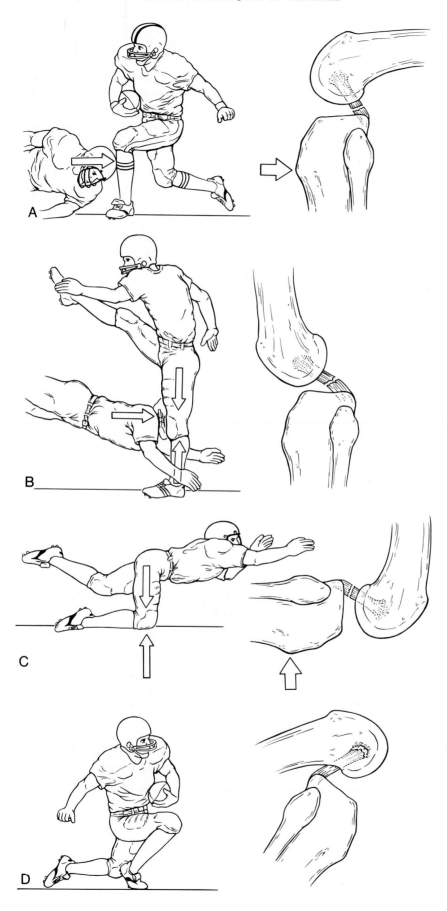

FIGURE 21–14

A, Direct blow to front of fixed tibia with knee in 90 degrees of flexion may produce a midsubstance PCL tear. *B,* Direct blow to front of fixed tibia with knee in 0 degrees of flexion may produce hyperextension and a midsubstance PCL tear. *C,* Direct blow to front of tibial crest secondary to a fall on the proximal tibia with the knee flexed 90 degrees and the foot plantarflexed may produce a force posteriorly on the proximal tibia and a midsubstance PCL tear. *D,* Hyperflexion of the knee with *no* force on the front of the tibia produces an avulsion of the PCL (often with surrounding periosteum or perichondrium) off the femur.

FIGURE 21–15
A and *B,* Quadriceps active drawer test. The knee is flexed to 90 degrees. Slight resistance is applied to the foot. The patient then contracts the quadriceps muscle. The quadriceps contraction pulls the tibia anteriorly from its resting, posteriorly subluxed position, to a neutral, not an anteriorly displaced position.

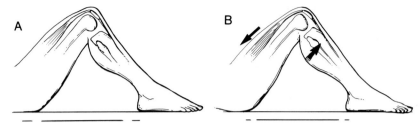

knee dislocation. For this reason, initial and serial vascular and neurologic examinations are essential. An effusion is usually not present with a PCL disruption because of its intrasynovial but extra-capsular location. The involved knee may demonstrate a decreased or painful range of motion [86, 102, 125], and the patient may be unwilling to bear his full weight on the limb [102]. The posterior calf and joint line may be tender and swollen and may show signs of ecchymosis due to a dissecting hematoma. Careful neural and vascular examinations are essential. The knee is initially painful, and motion is limited. In 2 to 3 days the pain subsides and motion returns. The classic "posterior sag" or posterior drawer sign may be absent initially owing to the stability provided by the posterior capsule and the ligaments of Wrisberg and Humphrey [17]. On drawer testing, an unaware examiner may mistakenly believe that a positive anterior drawer test is present if the examination begins with the tibia subluxed posteriorly rather than in its neutral position [118].

The most accurate test for acute PCL disruption is the "quadriceps" active drawer test (Fig. 21–15) [26]. The end-point noted with the posterior Lachman (Lachman-Trillat) test (Fig. 21–16) is also helpful in evaluating the PCL. The quadriceps active drawer test is performed by placing the knee in 70 degrees of flexion with the foot flat on the examination table. The patient then contracts the quadriceps muscle, which pulls the tibial plateau anteriorly [26, 118]. The Lachman-Trillat test is accomplished by placing the knee in 15 to 20 degrees of flexion and stabilizing the distal femur in one hand and the proximal tibia in the other. The examiner must be certain that the tibia is in neutral alignment with the femur and is not anteriorly or posteriorly subluxed to begin the examination. The tibia is then displaced posteriorly by the examiner against the stabilized femur. If a definite end-point is not felt or if there is significant displacement of the tibia posteriorly, the test is positive for a posterior cruciate injury (see Fig. 21–16). Palpation of the loss of the normal tibial plateau step-off when the knee is in 90 degrees of flexion is also a reliable sign of a PCL injury (Fig. 21–17).

Radiographs also play an important role in the diagnosis. Plain radiographs may detect avulsion fractures of the femoral or tibial attachments of the PCL [11, 52, 86, 88, 89, 110]. Ringer and Fay [112] stress the importance

of close scrutiny of routine radiographs to detect slight irregularity at the femoral or tibial origin of the PCL. Stress films are taken to rule out an occult physeal plate injury [18, 22, 28, 29] (Fig. 21–18*A*). The most accurate determination of the site of a PCL injury is obtained by MRI. MRI is used to detect in-substance PCL disruption, PCL avulsion off the femur with a chondral or osseous fragment, and meniscal pathology [73].

The location of the PCL injury is critical in planning treatment. Injuries that result in avulsion of the origin or insertion of the PCL are surgically reparable with an

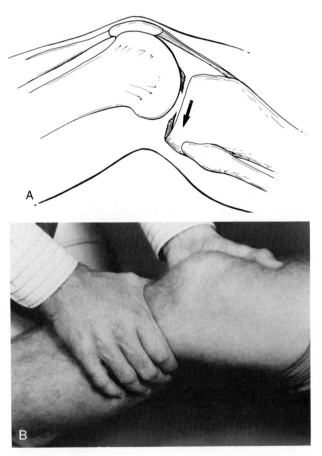

FIGURE 21–16
A and *B,* Posterior or reverse Lachman (Lachman-Trillat) test. The Lachman-Trillat test is performed with the knee in 15 to 20 degrees of flexion. The distal femur is stabilized with one hand while the proximal tibia is displaced posteriorly with the other. Posterior displacement (indicating a PCL injury) is confirmed if a definite end-point is not felt or if significant displacement of the tibia occurs posteriorly.

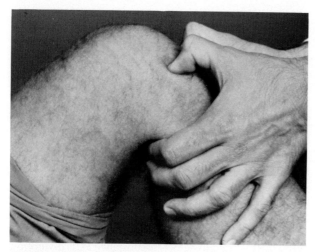

FIGURE 21–17
There is normally a palpable ledge representing the tibial plateau when the knee is flexed 90 degrees. If the PCL is absent, the tibia subluxes posteriorly and the ledge is absent.

expectation of reasonable stability [16], whereas midsubstance tears of the PCL fare no better after primary repair than does the ACL [9, 112]. Ringer and Fay [112] report that of the 23 children with PCL injury described to date, 15 were avulsions (eight were avulsions off the femur [18, 43, 86, 115, 125] and seven off the tibia [52, 89, 102, 110, 132]), and only one was a documented midsubstance tear. In six cases [9, 23, 68, 69, 95, 126] the location of the tear was not noted, and in one case the ligament was "attenuated." In view of this preponderance of avulsion and the improved results of repair of avulsions, the exact location of the PCL injury should be determined by MRI or arthroscopy.

Treatment

Once an acute PCL injury is diagnosed, treatment is directed at associated meniscal pathology and repair of the PCL if it is avulsed from the femur or tibia [11, 52, 86, 88, 89, 110]. As mentioned earlier, if the mechanism of injury is hyperflexion, a repairable PCL avulsion should be suspected.

Arthroscopy is used to confirm the location of the PCL injury, to evaluate meniscal pathology, and to visualize the chondral surfaces. Associated meniscal injury is managed as outlined in the earlier section on ACL injury; meniscal salvage is attempted if at all possible.

If the PCL is avulsed from the femur or tibia, it is repaired with intraepiphyseal sutures [11, 52, 80, 86] (Fig. 21–19A, B) or screw fixation of bony avulsions (Fig. 21–19C) [11, 52, 80, 86, 110]. Ringer and Fay [112] prefer suture fixation of these avulsions. Although replacement of an osteochondral avulsion is expected to restore preinjury stability to the knee, this is not always the result. Hughston and colleagues [69] report persistent laxity and instability of the knee after anatomic replacement of PCL avulsions in adults. Kennedy and associates [82] and Hughston and colleagues [69] report that the laxity is due to the interstitial deformity of the ligament preceding the avulsion. This interstitial tearing results in an increase in resting ligament length and residual laxity.

Isolated midsubstance tears are not repaired because repair in children has proved to be no better than that in adults [18]. Nonoperative treatment of PCL injuries in adults have been advocated by several authors. Dandy

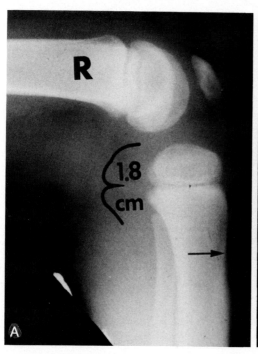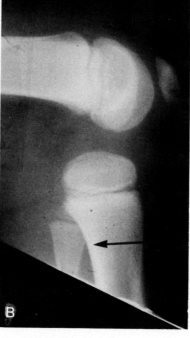

FIGURE 21–18
A and B, Posterior drawer stress test indicating injury to the posterior cruciate ligament.

FIGURE 21-19

A, PCL avulsion off femur repaired with a Bunnell suture through the femoral epiphyses. *B,* PCL avulsion off tibia repaired with a Bunnell suture through the tibial epiphyses. *C,* PCL bony avulsion repaired with an intraepiphyseal screw.

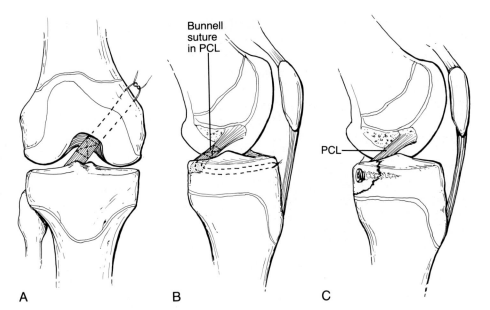

and Pusey [25] reported on 20 patients followed for 7.2 years after PCL injury. Eighteen of the twenty did not have enough instability or discomfort to justify reconstruction. Parolie and Bergfeld [103], describing 25 athletes with untreated PCL injuries who were followed for 6.2 years, reported that 80% of patients were satisfied with their knees without surgical treatment. The authors were unable to demonstrate that instability, as determined by KT-1000 arthrometry, played any role in the patient's activity level. On the other hand, Clancy and colleagues [17] reported in their study that untreated PCL injury leads to medial compartment degenerative joint disease secondary to the instability in a small number of adult patients with limited follow-up and no previous activity modification. For these reasons, these authors favor PCL reconstruction.

Despite these two opposing views, the difficulty with isometry in PCL reconstruction and the fact that some instability usually persists after PCL reconstruction, non-operative treatment of the acute midsubstance PCL injury seems indicated. It must be remembered, however, that there are no reports of the long-term effect of PCL insufficiency on the chondral surfaces or on knee growth in children with PCL insufficiency. Adults with chronic PCL laxity usually do not complain of instability unless there is laxity of the secondary restraints [103]. Clancy and colleagues [17] reported that aching in the knee is the main symptom in the adult with an absent PCL. Children with chronic PCL laxity also do not usually exhibit significant functional disability. In patients with PCL disruption in conjunction with associated complete disruption of either collateral ligament system or the ACL, conservative treatment is not successful [77]. Repair of the PCL, ACL, *and* the collateral ligaments is recommended. If the PCL injury is a midsubstance tear,

a technique similar to that described for the ACL by Marshall and colleagues is utilized, realizing that some persistent posterior laxity is a certainty. If this laxity is symptomatic, PCL reconstruction can be performed when physeal plate closure is complete. It must be emphasized again that due to the small number of skeletally immature patients with PCL injury that have been reported and the extremely short follow-up available, the consequences of loss of PCL function in skeletally immature patients (with and without treatment) is unknown at this time.

Author's Preferred Method of Treatment

In patients with a PCL injury, my primary goal is to determine the exact site of injury. A repairable femoral avulsion is suspected if the history reveals hyperflexion as the mechanism of injury. An MRI is obtained to determine the location of the PCL lesion, any associated bone injury [42] (which may portend a bad prognosis), and meniscal pathology. The patient is then examined under anesthesia, and arthroscopy is done to confirm the location of PCL injury. Avulsions from the femur or tibia are repaired primarily. I prefer to use intra-epiphyseal sutures for these avulsions unless there is a large fragment of bone associated with the avulsion and the patient is near completion of growth. In this situation, I use lag screw fixation. I make no attempt to "countersink" these avulsions as has been recommended to avoid the laxity seen after repair of the avulsion. I have not been impressed by the success of this technique. All meniscal lesions are repaired when technically feasible. Excision is reserved for small unstable fragments.

If the patient is found to have a midsubstance tear of the PCL, conservative treatment, including restoration of range of motion and quadriceps and hamstring strength, is the treatment of choice. The patients are followed annually. If functional instability or pain occur, or if radiographs detect early signs of arthritic changes, consideration of reconstruction of the PCL after growth has ceased is recommended.

If the patient has a complete lesion of either collateral ligament system in conjunction with a PCL injury, the collateral ligament system is repaired surgically, and the meniscal pathology managed as above. The PCL is repaired if it is avulsed from the femur or tibia. If the PCL has a midsubstance tear and there is significant growth remaining, the ligament is repaired primarily using a method similar to that described by Marshall and associates for the ACL [85]. Posterior laxity may result, and if it is clinically significant, a PCL reconstruction can be performed later when the physeal plates are closed. If the patient has less than 1 cm of growth remaining at the time of injury, an acute PCL reconstruction using the patellar tendon is performed in conjunction with repair of the collateral ligaments and menisci.

References

1. Aim, A., and Stromberg, B. Vascular anatomy of the patellar and cruciate ligaments: A microangiopathic and histologic investigation. *Acta Chir Scand* 445:25–35, 1974.
2. Angel, K. R., and Hall, D. J. Anterior cruciate ligament injury in children and adolescents. *J Arthroscop Rel Surg* 5(3):197–200, 1989.
3. Arms, S. W., Johnson R. J., and Pope, M. H. Strain measurement in the human posterior cruciate ligament. *Trans Orthop Med Soc* 9:355, 1984.
4. Arnoczky, S. P., and Warren, R. F. Anatomy of the cruciate ligaments. *In* Fedgin, J. A., Jr. (Ed.), *The Cruciate Ligaments.* New York, Churchill Livingstone, 1988, pp. 179–195.
5. Arnoczky, S. P., and Warren, A. F. Microvasculature of the human meniscus. *Am J Sports Med* 10:90–95, 1982.
6. Baxter, M. P., and Wiley, J. J. Fractures of the tibial spine in children. *J Bone Joint Surg* 70B(2):228–230, 1988.
7. Blokker, C., and Fowler, P. J. Review of tibial eminence fractures. Presented at 17th Annual Clinical Seminar in Orthopaedic Surgery. University of Western Ontario, April, 1989.
8. Bergfeld, J. Personal communication.
9. Bianchi, M. Acute tears of the posterior cruciate ligament: Clinical study and results of operative treatment in 27 cases. *Am J Sports Med* 11:308–314, 1983.
10. Bradley, G. W., Shives, T. C., and Samuelson, K. M. Ligament injuries in the knees of children. *J Bone Joint Surg* 61A(4):588–591, 1979.
11. Brennan, J. Avulsion injuries of the posterior cruciate ligaments. *Clin Orthop* 18:157–162, 1960.
12. Bright, R. W. Physeal injury. *In* Rockwood, C. A., Wilkins, K. E., and King, R. (Eds.), *Fractures in Children.* Philadelphia, J. B. Lippincott, 1984, pp. 87–172.
13. Bright, R. W., Burstein, A. H., and Elmore, S. M. Epiphyseal-plate cartilage: A biomechanical and histological analysis of failure modes. *J Bone Joint Surg* 56A(4):688–703, 1974.
14. Butler, D. L., Noyes, F. R., and Grood, E. S. Ligamentous restraints to anterior-posterior drawer in the human knee. *J Bone Joint Surg* 62A:259–270, 1980.
15. Capra, S., and Fowler, P. J. Personal communication.
16. Chick, R. R., and Jackson, D. W. Tears of the anterior cruciate ligament in young athletes. *J Bone Joint Surg* 60A(7):970–973, 1978.
17. Clancy, W. G., Shelbourne, K. D., Zoellner, G. B., et al., Treatment of knee joint instability secondary to rupture of the posterior cruciate ligament. *J Bone Joint Surg* 65A(3):310–322, 1983.
18. Clanton, T. O., DeLee, J. C., Sanders, B. et al. Knee ligament injuries in children. *J Bone Joint Surg* 61A(8):1195–1200, 1979.
19. Clark, C. R., and Ogden, J. A. Development of the menisci in the human knee joint. *J Bone Joint Surg* 65A:538–547, 1983.
20. Cochran, G. V. *A Primer of Orthopaedic Biomechanics.* New York, Churchill Livingstone, 1982.
21. Committee on the Medical Aspects of Sports. *Standard Nomenclature of Athletic Injuries.* Chicago, American Medical Association, 1968, pp. 99–101.
22. Crawford, A. H. Fractures about the knee in children. *Orthop Clin North Am* 7(3):639–656, 1976.
23. Cross, M. J., and Powell, J. L. Long-term followup of posterior cruciate ligament rupture: A study of 116 cases. *Am J Sports Med* 12:292–297, 1984.
24. Curtis, B. H., and Fisher, R. L. Congenital hyperextension with anterior subluxation of the knee. *J Bone Joint Surg* 51A(2):255–269, 1969.
25. Dandy, D. J., and Pusey, R. J. Long term result of unrepaired tears of the PCL. *J Bone Joint Surg* 64B:92–94, 1982.
26. Daniel, D. M., Stone, M. L., Barnett, P., et al. The quadriceps active drawer. Paper presented at the 52nd Annual Meeting of the American Academy of Orthopaedic Surgeons, Las Vegas, Nevada, January, 1985.
27. DeHaven, K. E., and Wascher, D. C. Management of meniscal problems in the young athlete. *In* Grana, W. A. (Ed.), *Advances in Sports Medicine and Fitness,* Vol. 3. Chicago, Year Book, 1990, pp. 197–213.
28. DeLee, J. C. ACL insufficiency in children. *In* Feagin, J. A., Jr. (Ed.), *The Crucial Ligaments.* New York, Churchill Livingstone, 1988, pp. 439–447.
29. DeLee, J. C., and Curtis, R. Anterior cruciate ligament insufficiency in children. *Clin Orthop* 172:112–118, 1983.
30. Donegan, K. M., DeLee, J. C., Evans, J. A., et al. Comparison of Lysholm and international knee documentation committee scale using extra-articular ACL reconstruction as a model. *Am J Sports Med* May, 1991.
31. Donovan, T. L., Benling, F., and Nagel, D. A. Posterior cruciate injury on artificial turf. *Orthop Trans* 1:20, 1977.
32. Drez, D. J. Personal communication.
33. Eady, J. L., Cardenas, C. D., and Sopa, D. Avulsion of the femoral attachment of the anterior cruciate ligament in a seven year-old child. *J Bone Joint Surg* 64A(9):1376–1378, 1982.
34. Ehrlich, M. G., and Strain, R. E. Epiphyseal injuries about the knee. *Orthop Clin North Am* 10(1):91–103, 1979.
35. Eilert, R. E. Arthroscopy of the knee joint in children. *Orthop Rev* 5(9):61–65, 1976.
36. Engebretsen, S., and Benum, P. Poor results of anterior cruciate ligament repair in adolescence. *Acta Orthop Scand* 59(6):684–686, 1988.
37. Feagin, J. A. (Ed.). *The Crucial Ligaments.* New York, Churchill Livingstone, 1988, pp. 188–194.
38. Feagin, J. A., and Curl, W. W. Isolated tear of the anterior cruciate ligament: Five year followup study. *Am J Sports Med* 4(3):95–100, 1976.
39. Fetto, J. F., and Marshall, J. L. Medial collateral ligament injuries of the knee. *Clin Orthop* 132:206–218, 1978.
40. Fowler, P. J. The classification and early diagnosis of knee of joint instability. *Clin Orthop* 147:15–20, 1980.
41. Fowler, P. J. Personal communication, 1989.
42. Fowler, P. J. Bone injury associated with acute ACL tear. Presented at Herodicus Meeting, Sun Valley, Utah, July, 1990.
43. Frank, S., and Strother, R. Isolated posterior cruciate ligament injury in a child: Literature review and a case report. *Can J Surg* 32:373–374, 1989.
44. Furman, W., Marshall, J. L., and Girgis, F. G. The anterior cruciate ligament. *J Bone Joint Surg* 58A(2):179–185, 1976.

45. Gallagher, S. S., Finison, K., and Gvyer, B. The incidence of injuries among 87,000 Massachusetts children and adolescents. Results of the 1980–1981 statewide Childhood Injury Prevention Program Surveillance System. *Am J Public Health* 74:1340–1347, 1984.

46. Garcia, A., and Neer, C. S. Isolated fractures of the intercondylar eminence of the tibia. *Am J Surg* 95:593–598, 1958.

47. Giorgi, B. Morphologic variations of the intercondylar eminence of the knee. *Clin Orthop* 8:209–217, 1956.

48. Girgis, F. G., Marshall, J. L., and Monajem, A. R. S. The cruciate ligaments of the knee joint. *Clin Orthop* 106:216–231, 1975.

49. Glancy, G. L. The injured knee in the adolescent. *J Musculo Med* 14–27, 1986.

50. Goldberg, B. Pediatric sports medicine. *In* Scott, Nisserson and Nicholas (Eds.); *Principles of Sports Medicine.* Baltimore, Williams & Wilkins, 1984.

51. Gollehon, D. L., Torzilli, P. A., and Warren, R. F. The role of the posterolateral and cruciate ligaments in the stability of the human knee. *J Bone Joint Surg* 69A(2):233–242, 1987.

52. Goodrich, A., and Ballard, A. Posterior cruciate ligament avulsion associated with ipsilateral femur fracture in a 10-year-old child. *J Trauma* 28(9):1393–1396, 1988.

53. Graf, B. K., Fujisaki, K. C., Lange, R. H., et al. Anterior cruciate tears in the skeletally immature athlete. Presented at Arthroscopy Association of North America Annual Meeting, Orlando, Florida, April 1990.

54. Grana, W. A., and Moretz, J. A. Ligamentous laxity in secondary school athletes. *JAMA* 240(18):1975–1976, 1978.

55. Green, W. T., and Anderson, M. Experiences with epiphyseal arrest in correcting discrepancies in length of the lower extremities in infantile paralysis. *J Bone Joint Surg* 29:659–675, July, 1947.

56. Gronkvist, H., Hirsch, G., and Johansson, L. Fracture of the anterior tibial spine in children. *J Pediatr Orthop* 4:465–468, 1984.

57. Grood, A., Stowers, E. S., and Noyes, F. R. Limits of movement in the human knee—effects of sectioning the posterior cruciate ligament and posterolateral structures. *J Bone Joint Surg* 70A:88–97, 1988.

58. Grossman, R. B., and Nicholas, J. Common disorders of the knee. *Orthop Clin North Am* 8:619, 1977.

59. Greulich, W. W., and Pyle, S. I. *Radiographic Atlas of Skeletal Development of the Hand and Wrist* (2nd ed.). Stanford, Stanford University Press, 1959.

60. Halpern, B., Thompson, N., Curl, W. W., et al. High school football injuries: Identifying the risk factors. *Am J Sports Med* 15(4):113–117, 1987.

61. Hargreaves, D. J., and Seedhom, B. B. On the "bucket handle" tear: Partial or total meniscectomy? A quantitative study. *J Bone Joint Surg* 61B:381, 1979.

62. Harris, W. R. The endocrine basis for slipping of the upper femoral epiphysis. An experimental study. *J Bone Joint Surg* 32B:5–11, 1950.

63. Heller, L., and Langeman, J. The menisco-femoral ligaments of the human knee. *J Bone Joint Surg* 46B(2):307–313, 1964.

64. Houseworth, S. W., Mauro, V. J., Mellon, B. A., et al. The intercondylar notch in acute tears of the anterior cruciate ligament: A computer graphics study. *Am J Sports Med* 15(3):221–224, 1987.

65. Hsieh, H., and Walker, P. S. Stabilizing mechanisms of the loaded and unloaded knee joint. *J Bone Joint Surg* 58A(1):87–93, 1976.

66. Hughston, J. C., Andrews, J. R., Cross, M. J., et al. Classification of knee ligament instabilities, Part I. The medial compartment and cruciate ligaments. *J Bone Joint Surg* 58A(2):159–172, 1976.

67. Hughston, J. C., Andrews, J. R., Cross, M. J., et al. Classification of knee ligament instabilities, Part II. The lateral compartment. *J Bone Joint Surg* 58A(2):173–179, 1976.

68. Hughston, J. C., and Degenhavdt, T. C. Reconstruction of the posterior cruciate ligament. *Clin Orthop* 164:59–77, 1982.

69. Hughston, J. C., Bowden, J. A., Andrews, J. A., et al. Acute tears of the posterior cruciate ligament. *J Bone Joint Surg* 62A:438–450, 1980.

70. Hughston, J. C., and Norwood, L. A. The posterolateral drawer test and external rotational recurvatum test for posterolateral rotatory instability of the knee. *Clin Orthop* 147:82–87, 1980.

71. Hyndman, J. C., and Brown, D. G. Major ligament injuries of the knee in children. Read at the annual meeting of the Canadian Orthopaedic Association, British Columbia, June, 1978.

72. Indelicato, P. A. Non-operative treatment of complete tears of the medial collateral ligament of the knee. *J Bone Joint Surg* 65A(3):323–329, 1983.

73. Jackson, D. W., Jennings, L. D., Maywood, R. M., et al. Magnetic resonance imaging of the knee. *Am J Sports Med* 16(1):29–38, 1988.

74. Johansson, E., and Aparisi, T. Congenital absence of the cruciate ligaments. *Clin Orthop* 162:108–111, 1982.

75. Jones, R. E., Henley, M. B., and Francis, P. Nonoperative management of isolated grade III collateral ligament injury in high school football players. *Clin Orthop* 213:137–140, 1986.

76. Joseph, K. N., and Pogrund, H. Traumatic rupture of the medial ligament of the knee in a four year-old boy. *J Bone Joint Surg* 60A(3):402–403, 1978.

77. Kannus, P., and Jarvinen, M. Knee ligament injuries in adolescents. *J Bone Joint Surg* 70B(5):772–776, 1988.

78. Kannus, P. Long term results of conservatively treated medial collateral ligament injuries of the knee joint. *Clin Orthop* 226:103–112, 1988.

79. Kennedy, J. C. *The Injured Adolescent Knee.* Baltimore, Williams & Wilkins, 1979.

80. Kennedy, J. C., and Grainger, R. W. The posterior cruciate ligament. *J Trauma* 7(3):367–377, 1967.

81. Kennedy, J. C., Weinberg, H. W., and Wilson, A. S. The anatomy and function of the anterior cruciate ligament. *J Bone Joint Surg* 56A(2):223–235, 1974.

82. Kennedy, J. C., Hawkins, R. J., Willis, R. B., et al. Tension studies of human knee ligaments. *J Bone Joint Surg* 58A(3):350–355, 1976.

83. Krause, W. R., Pope, M. H., Johnson, R. J., Mechanical changes in the knee after meniscectomy. *J Bone Joint Surg* 58A(5):599–604, 1976.

84. Lipscomb, A. B., and Anderson, A. F. Tears of the anterior cruciate ligament in adolescents. *J Bone Joint Surg* 68A(1):19–28, 1986.

85. Marshall, J. L., Warren, R. F., Wickiewicz, T. L., et al. The anterior cruciate ligament: A technique of repair and reconstruction. *Clin Orthop* 143:98–106, 1979.

86. Mayer, P. J., and Michell, L. J. Avulsion of the femoral attachment of the posterior cruciate ligament in an eleven year-old boy. *J Bone Joint Surg* 16A(3):431–432, 1979.

87. McCarroll, J. R., Rettig, A. C., and Shelbourne, K. D. Anterior cruciate ligament injuries in the young athlete with open physes. *Am J Sports Med* 16(1):44–47, 1988.

88. McMaster, W. C. Isolated posterior cruciate ligament injury: Literature review and case reports. *J Trauma* 15(11):1025–1029, 1975.

89. Meyers, M. H. Isolated avulsion of the tibial attachment of the posterior cruciate ligament of the knee. *J Bone Joint Surg* 57A(5):669–672, 1975.

90. Meyers, H. H., and McKeever, F. M. Fracture of the intercondylar eminence of the tibia. *J Bone Joint Surg* 52A(8):1677–1684, 1970.

91. Meyers, M. H., and McKeever, F. M. Fracture of the intercondylar eminence of the tibia. *J Bone Joint Surg* 41A(2):209–222, 1959.

92. Micheli, L. J. Pediatric and adolescent sports injuries: Recent trends. *Exerc Sport Sci Rev* 14:359–374, 1986.

93. Mirbey, J. Besancenot, J., Chambers, R. T., et al. Avulsion fractures of the tibial tuberosity in the adolescent athlete. *Am J Sports Med* 16(4):336–340, 1988.

94. Molander, M. L., Watkin, G., and Wikstnd, I. Fracture of the intercondylar eminence of the tibia: A review of 35 patients. *J Bone Joint Surg* 63B:89–91, 1981.

95. Moore, H. A., and Larson, R. L. Posterior cruciate ligament injuries: Result of early surgical repair. *Am J Sports Med* 8:68–78, 1980.

96. Morrissy, R. T., Eubanks, R. G., Park, J. P., et al. Arthroscopy of the knee in children. *Clin Orthop* 162:103–107, 1982.

97. Nichols, P. J. R. Short-Leg syndrome. *Br Med J* 1:1863–1865, 1960.

98. Norwood, L. A., and Hughston, J. C. Combined anterolateral-anteromedial rotatory instability of the knee. *Clin Orthop* 147:62–67, 1980.

99. Noyes, F. R., DeLucas, J. L., and Torvik, P. J. Biomechanics of anterior cruciate ligament failure: An analysis of strain-rate sensitivity and mechanisms of failure in primates. *J Bone Joint Surg* 56A(2):236–253, 1974.

100. O'Donoghue, D. H. An analysis of end results of surgical treatment of major injuries to the ligaments of the knee. *J Bone Joint Surg* 37A(1):1–13, 1955.

101. Ogden, J. A., Tross, R. B., and Murphy, M. J. Fractures of the tibial tuberosity in adolescents. *J Bone Joint Surg* 62A(2):205–222, 1980.

102. Palmer, I. On injuries to the ligaments of the knee joint: A clinical study. *Acta Chir Scand* 53:134–135, 1938.

103. Parolie, J. M., and Bergfeld, J. A. Long term results of nonoperative treatment of isolated posterior cruciate ligament injuries in the athlete. *Am J Sports Med* 14(1):35–38, 1986.

104. Price, C. T., and Allen, W. C. Ligament repair in the knee with preservation of the meniscus. *J Bone Joint Surg* 60A(1):61–65, 1978.

105. Rang, M. *Children's Fractures*. Philadelphia, J. B. Lippincott, 1974.

106. Rang, M. *Children's Fractures* (2nd ed.)., Philadelphia, J. B. Lippincott, 1983.

107. Rinaldi, E., and Mazzarella, F. Isolated fracture avulsions of the tibial insertions of the cruciate ligaments of the knee. *Ital J Orthop Traumatol* 6:77–83, 1980.

108. Roberts, J. M. Fractures and dislocations of the knee. *In* Rockwood, C. A., Wilkins, K. E., and King, R. (Eds.), *Fractures in Children*. Philadelphia, J.B. Lippincott, 1984, pp. 891–945.

109. Robinson, S. C., and Driscoll, S. E. Simultaneous osteochondral avulsion of the femoral and tibial insertions of the anterior cruciate ligament. *J Bone Joint Surg* 63A(8):1342–1343, 1981.

110. Ross, A. C., and Chesterman, P. J. Isolated avulsion of the tibial attachment of the posterior cruciate ligament in childhood. *J Bone Joint Surg* 68B(5):747, 1986.

111. Roth, P. B. Fracture of the spine of the tibia. British Orthopaedic Association, Bristol, October 21, 1927.

112. Ringer, J. L., and Fay, M. J. Acute posterior cruciate ligament insufficiency in children. *Am J Knee Surg* 3:192–203, 1990.

113. Rush, W. A., and Steiner, H. A. A study of lower extremity length inequality. *Am J Roentgenol* 56:616–623, 1946.

114. Salter, R. B. *Textbook of Disorders and Injuries of the Musculoskeletal System.* Baltimore, William & Wilkins, 1970.

115. Sanders, W. E., Wilkins, K. E., and Neidre, A. Acute insufficiency of the posterior cruciate ligament in children. *J Bone Joint Surg* 62A(1):129–130, 1980.

116. Shin, S., and Leung, G. Blood supply of the knee joint. *Clin Orthop* 208:119–125, 1986.

117. Singer, I. J. Sports related knee injuries in the pediatric and adolescent athlete. *RI Med J* 70:255–263, 1987.

118. Sisk, T. D. Knee injuries. *In* Crenshaw, A. H. (Ed.), *Campbell's Operative Orthopaedics* (7th ed.). St. Louis, C. V. Mosby, 1987, pp. 2283–2496.

119. Skak, S. V., Jensen, T. T., Poulsen, T. D., et al. Epidemiology of knee injuries in children. *Acta Orthop Scand* 58:78–81, 1987.

120. Smith, J. B. Knee instability after fractures of the intercondylar eminence of the tibia. *J Pediatr Orthop* 4(4):462–464, 1984.

121. Stanitski, C. L., Harvell, J. C., and Fu, F. Observations on acute hemarthrosis in children and adolescents. *J Pediatr Orthop* 13(4):506–510, 1993.

122. Stanitski, C. L. Anterior cruciate ligament injuries in the young athlete with open physes (letter to the editor). *Am J Sports Med* 16(4):424, 1988.

123. Steingard, M., Morrison, D., Schildberg, W., et al. A followup study on adolescent knee injuries. *J AOA,* 87:(12):807–816, 1987.

124. Stoddard, A. *A Manual of Osteopathic Technique.* London, Hutchinson, 1959, pp. 212–213.

125. Strand, T., Molster, A. O., Engesaeter, L. B., et al. Primary repair of the posterior cruciate ligament. *Acta Orthop Scand* 55:545–549, 1984.

126. Suprock, M. D., and Rogers, V. P. Posterior cruciate avulsion in a 4-year-old boy. *Orthopaedics* 13:659–662, 1990.

127. Tanner, J. M. *Foetus Into Man.* Cambridge, Harvard University Press, 1990, p. 218.

128. Thompson, N., Halpern, B., Curl, W. W., et al. High school football injuries: Evaluation. *Am J Sports Med* 15(2):97–117, 1987.

129. Tipton, C. M., Matthes, R. D., and Martin, R. K. Influence of age and sex on the strength of bone-ligament junctions in knee joints of rats. *J Bone Joint Surg* 60A(2):230–234, 1978.

130. Tolo, V. T. Congenital absence of the menisci and cruciate ligaments of the knee. *J Bone Joint Surg* 63A(6):1022–1023, 1981.

131. Torg, J. S., Pavlov, H., and Morris, V. B. Salter-Harris type III fracture of the medial femoral condyle occurring in the adolescent athlete. *J Bone Joint Surg* 63A(4):586–591, 1981.

132. Torisu, T. Isolated avulsion fracture of the tibial attachment of the posterior cruciate ligament. *J Bone Joint Surg* 59A:68–72, 1977.

133. Torisu, T., and Masumi, S. Midsubstance tear of the posterior cruciate ligament: A case report. *Am J Knee Surg* 2:50–52, 1989.

134. Weiss, C. B., Lindberg, M., Hamberg, P., et al. Nonoperative treatment of meniscal tears. *J Bone Joint Surg* 71A:811–822, 1989.

135. Zaricznyj, B. Avulsion fracture of the tibial eminence: treatment by open reduction and pinning. *J Bone Joint Surg* 59A:1111–1115, 1977.

KNEE ARTHROSCOPY IN CHILDREN

Carl L. Stanitski, M.D.

The first arthroscopic procedure was attempted in Tokyo by Takagi in a human cadaver knee in 1918 [27] but was not a successful venture. Eugene Burcher of Switzerland, using a Jacobeus laparoscope, attempted to view the knees endoscopically in 1921; this was the first publication on the topic [5]. Burman [6] in 1931 gave credit to Burcher, who, after a few trials on cadavers, performed knee arthroscopy in 35 clinical cases, noting a range of diagnoses including medial meniscal tears, osteochondritis dissecans, tuberculosis, and other conditions. Burcher used oxygen or nitrogen gas to provide joint distention. At various times he referred to this technique as "endoscopy of the knee joint," "arthroendoscopy," or "arthroscopy." In 1931, Takagi [53] reported limited success in the use of endoscopy of the human knee in a clinical setting. Wiberg [60] commented on arthroscopy in the mid 1930s, noting that "it did not seem to have any potential clinical value but would be more of a research tool."

Pioneers in the United States in the late 1920s and early 1930s gained experience in both cadaveric and clinical trials of arthroscopy of multiple joints. In 1934, in a report on the clinical use of arthroscopy in 30 cases [7] Burman and his colleagues specifically suggested that general anesthesia be used in children under the age of 12. He discussed two cases in 8-year-old children suffering from chronic synovitis of the knee. In that paper he noted that "arthroscopy involves only a minimal risk, and in some cases has actually had a beneficial therapeutic result."

As early as 1925, Kreuscher [28] and others [31] championed the use of the arthroscope to aid early diagnosis of meniscal lesions. In 1931, Finkelstein and Meyer [18] described three cases that were diagnosed arthroscopically as chronic inflammation of the knee secondary to tuberculosis.

After a significant period of quiescence, Watanabe [58, 59], Takagi's pupil, continued further experimentation with the arthroscope. Using an improved lens system, he developed the No. 21 arthroscope, which became the state-of-the-art tool for arthroscopy in the 1950s and 1960s. His arthroscope was often derisively referred to as "the professor's toy."

Interest in arthroscopic techniques burgeoned in the United States in the mid to late 1970s, stimulated and simplified by fiberoptic technology and courses on arthroscopy presented by the American Academy of Orthopaedic Surgeons. Advances in optics, fiberoptic technology, and electronics led to the development of high-quality arthroscopic lens systems and cameras. These provided improved operating ease and accuracy. Courses in diagnostic techniques initially and later in arthroscopically guided surgical procedures heralded an explosion in the use of arthroscopic techniques by orthopedic surgeons. Spurred by commercial profit potential in an expanding market, many companies now offer a myriad of instruments designed to assist the surgeon in procedures dealing with almost all intra-articular structures.

Diagnostic and surgical arthroscopy is now a significant part of the curriculum of all orthopedic residencies. During the past decade and a half, practicing orthopedists have educated themselves by a multitude of courses, hands-on motor skill laboratories, tutorials, and other means of gaining arthroscopic proficiency. Many arthroscopists with limited arthroscopic diagnostic abilities and experience have nonetheless pressed forward trying to develop surgical arthroscopic skills, often to the detriment of the articular surface (Fig. 22–1). As arthroscopic skills and electronics systems have improved, demands for an enhanced visualization technique have increased, and the horizons of procedures capable of being done under arthroscopic control have expanded. An almost insatiable appetite exists for equip-

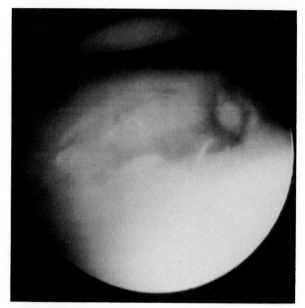

FIGURE 22–1
Iatrogenic osteochondral injury of femoral sulcus seen at time of repeat arthroscopy.

ment (either manually operated or powered by gas or electricity) for surgical probing, trimming, and mending. One must remember that tools do not always make the surgeon. The basic principles of arthroscopic surgery must always be followed. One must be expert in diagnostic arthroscopy, i.e., capable of mastering the stereotaxic demands for triangulation technique before embarking on surgical forays for loose body removal, meniscectomy, and so on. This is especially true with the smaller volume of the child's knee [20].

KNEE ARTHROSCOPY IN CHILDREN

Previous teaching held that knee intra-articular injuries in children were uncommon and that surgery for such disorders was even less common. In the United States, because of the increased numbers of children and adolescents involved in sports and in vehicular trauma (motorcycles, all-terrain vehicles, automobiles, bicycles), the frequency of knee injuries in children and adolescents has risen dramatically during the past dec-

ade. This is certainly in marked contrast to Fairbank's [17] review of 63 cases of "internal derangements of the knee" in children and adolescents a half century ago. Fourteen of his patients had osteochondritis dissecans and 32 had meniscal lesions—20 medial and 12 lateral (discoid type). Although the patient population and the etiology of injury have changed, the caveat expressed by Fairbank in 1937 still holds true: "The diagnosis of a knee case in the child is by no means an easy matter."

Arthroscopy should not be considered a substitute for a careful history and physical examination. However, adequate historical and physical findings are often difficult to elicit and are commonly nonspecific in the pediatric age group. The burden of providing clinical information is often laid on the parents, who may be unaware of the specific details in regard to a particular injury. Following acute knee trauma, children are commonly unwilling to cooperate with a thorough knee examination, and one's clinical diagnostic acumen may not be allowed full expression. Unfortunately, the outmoded attitude of the rarity of intra-articular injuries in children still persists. Delay in diagnosis and treatment results in loss of motion, muscle strength, and flexibility attendant on the injury itself.

Most reports on arthroscopy deal with adult disorders. Few reports have focused on the results of knee arthroscopy for a variety of conditions specifically in children and adolescents [15, 22, 24, 35, 50, 62]. Reports in the 1960s and 1970s on arthroscopy in the United States and Canada [27] did not mention any significant age differentiation in the patients reviewed.

Correlation with Preoperative Clinical Assessment

Because of these factors, most authors of papers on knee arthroscopy in children have noted a major discrepancy between the clinical preoperative diagnoses and the intra-articular findings noted at the time of arthroscopy. In these series, incorrect diagnoses in children less than 13 years old ranged from 36% to 73% (Table 22–1). In the first report that looked specifically at the preadolescent arthroscopy patient, Morrissy and associates [35] found only a 25% correlation between the preoperative clinical diagnosis and the arthroscopic findings. A 61%

TABLE 22–1
Literature Review of the Accuracy of Clinical vs. Arthroscopic Diagnoses

	Morrissey [75]	Ziv [113]	Bergstrom [17]	Juhl [59]	Suman [97]	Angel [7]	Harvell [48]
Number (total)	32	156	71	76	72	205	310
Number of preadolescents	11	43	20	12	20	49	29
Number of adolescents	21	113	51	64	48	156	71
Correct preadolescent diagnoses (%)	27			37.3	42		55
Correct adolescent diagnoses (%)	61			45.4	55	56	70
Additional findings (%)							35/25

correlation was noted in adolescents, i.e., those over 13 years of age in that series. Angel and Hall [1] studied 212 knees in 192 patients and noted a 56% overall accuracy rate for clinical assessments versus a 99% accuracy rate for arthroscopic diagnosis. Harvell and colleagues [22] noted similar limitations in preoperative clinical assessments compared with arthroscopic findings.

In addition to lack of correlation with preoperative clinical assessment, arthroscopic findings revealed a significant amount of unsuspected additional intra-articular pathology. In the largest series reported to date, Harvell and associates [22] studied 310 knees in 285 children. The preoperative clinical diagnoses were correlated with arthroscopic findings. Eighty-three patients (29% of the total) were preadolescents, and two-thirds were between 9 and 12 years of age. Thirty-seven of the patients' injuries occurred during a sport activity. An additional 13% of injuries involved direct knee trauma related to a vehicular accident (Fig. 22–2).

In their preadolescent group, 55% of the preoperative clinical diagnoses were confirmed at surgery. At arthroscopy, an additional 35% of the patients were found to have intra-articular pathology not anticipated on the preoperative clinical examination. In the adolescent group there was improved correlation between the preoperative clinical assessment and intraoperative findings. In children 13 to 18 years old, 70% of preoperative clinical diagnoses were confirmed at arthroscopy. However, additional evidence of intra-articular injury was found at the time of surgery in 25% of this group (Fig. 22–3).

A striking finding in all series was the high frequency of meniscal injuries noted in the preoperative clinical diagnoses. At arthroscopy, no such injury was usually found. In many series, the most common preoperative diagnosis was chondromalacia patella, whereas pristine

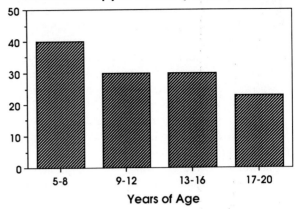

Additional Pathology in the Knee Found at Arthroscopy not Anticipated Clinically

FIGURE 22–3
Children's Hospital of Pittsburgh knee arthroscopy data. Again, note correlation between accuracy and age.

articular surfaces were found on the patella at arthroscopy. Suman and colleagues [52], Bergstrom and co-workers [4], Angel and Hall [1], Morrissy and associates [35], and Harvell and associates [22] all cautioned about the hazards of routine overdiagnosis of meniscal tears in children.

The versatility of arthroscopy in the diagnosis and treatment of a range of intra-articular knee disorders in children is beginning to be appreciated. In acute trauma, accuracy of reduction and enhancement of fixation of tibial eminence fractures has been reported by McLennan [34]. A significant proportion of chondral fractures following acute patellar dislocation was found by Angel and Hall [1] and by Harvell and colleagues [22].

ARTHROSCOPY IN MANAGEMENT

The use of arthroscopy in the management and treatment of various arthritides in children has recently been reported [40]. Synovial biopsy, synovectomy, and objective evaluation of articular surfaces are easily accomplished arthroscopically. The authors emphasize the value of direct observation of the articular surface versus the less accurate radiographic means of assessing arthritic effects on the articular cartilage.

Chondromalacia patella, a nonspecific state of anterior knee pain, is commonly reported as a diagnosis at arthroscopy [24], particularly in females. The opportunity for overzealous arthroscopy exists in patients with this condition and should be resisted in the management of such nonspecific anterior knee pain in children and adolescents, which commonly responds extremely well to nonoperative treatment. Mild patellar instabilities have been successfully managed using arthroscopically guided lateral retinacular release [29, 41].

Meniscal repair has been highlighted in recent years

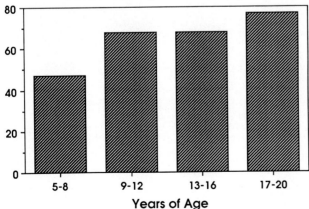

Clinical Diagnosis in the Knee
Confirmed by Arthroscopy

FIGURE 22–2
Children's Hospital of Pittsburgh knee arthroscopy data. Note direct correlation between accuracy and age.

[2, 3, 10, 14, 21, 25, 51]. Although no series has been specifically reported in children, case illustrations in skeletally immature patients have been noted in reported papers on meniscal repair (Fig. 22–4). The current recommended treatment for non-Wrisberg-type discoid lateral menisci is sculpturing of the abnormally shaped meniscus into a more anatomically normal-appearing one with sparing of the remaining meniscus to prevent long-term degenerative disease (Fig. 22–5) [19, 20, 23, 26, 42, 46, 57]. A recent report described a Wrisberg-type unstable discoid meniscus that was stabilized by arthroscopic means [39].

In adolescents who are almost skeletally mature, arthroscopic guidance of anterior cruciate ligament reconstructions has been reported with limited follow-up [32].

The use of the arthroscope in management of acute septic joints in children has been reported by Skyhar and Mubarik [43], Stanitski and associates [49], and others [55], who recommend arthroscopy for the management of acute septic knee in children. These authors believe that the arthroscope provides improved visualization of the joint, enhanced irrigation ability, improved joint distention, and lower morbidity postoperatively than do previous arthrotomy techniques. These authors have reported excellent results following combined arthroscopy and parenteral antibiotic use in the management of acute septic knees. Stanitski and his associates [49] also were able to remove foreign bodies in the knee that were found in one-fourth of the patients in their septic knee series.

DIAGNOSTIC ARTHROSCOPY

Arthroscopy is extremely helpful in diagnosing and staging osteochondritis dissecans [16]. The state of the

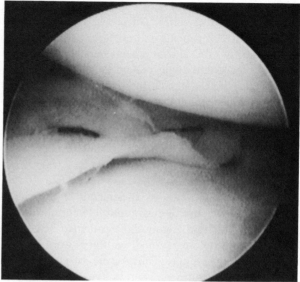

FIGURE 22–4
Medial meniscal repair in a 12-year-old basketball player.

articular surface and the stability of the chondritic fragment are easily assessed and documented arthroscopically (Fig. 22–6). In most cases, there is poor correlation with preoperative roentgenograms of the stability of the osteochondritic defect unless an obvious loose fragment is noted radiographically. In Harvell and colleagues' [22] series of arthroscopies in children and adolescents, osteochondritis dissecans was the most common diagnosis in preadolescent boys. The use of arthroscopy in staging the stability of these osteochondritic lesions will provide further information about the natural course of this disorder and its effective treatment.

Diagnostic arthroscopy of joints other than the knee, particularly the shoulder and ankle, has become more

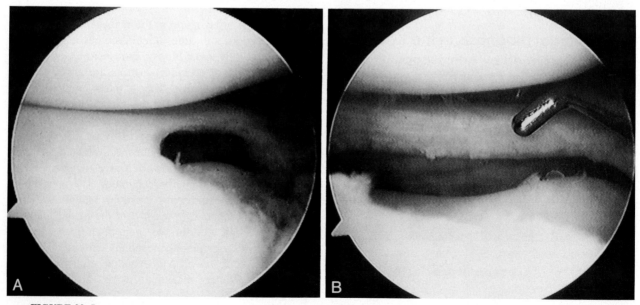

FIGURE 22–5
A, Symptomatic lateral discoid meniscus in a 13-year-old volleyball player. *B,* Following sculpting. (Courtesy of Dr. James Bradley.)

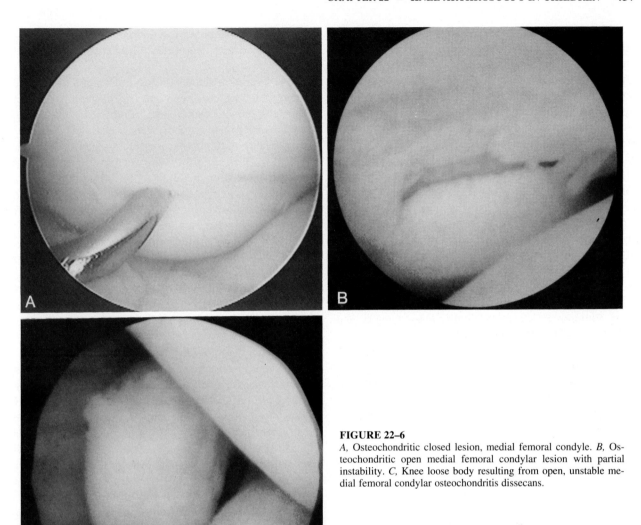

FIGURE 22–6
A, Osteochondritic closed lesion, medial femoral condyle. *B,* Osteochondritic open medial femoral condylar lesion with partial instability. *C,* Knee loose body resulting from open, unstable medial femoral condylar osteochondritis dissecans.

common, and as techniques improve, surgical advances in these areas also can be expected to occur.

Because of the widespread use of arthroscopy, especially in athletic celebrities, patients commonly have an unrealistic view of the procedure and its benefits. Many patients remember the dramatic return of Joan Benoit-Samuelson to the marathon trials 3 weeks after arthroscopic surgery. Commonly, the patient may mention that he has had a "scope" done, not understanding in the least what actually was done. Patients also equate "arthroscopy" with unanimity of procedure for all (Fig. 22–7).

Patients need to understand that arthroscopy is but one technique of surgery of the knee and that it has two phases, diagnostic and surgical. The surgical part of arthroscopy is specific to a particular knee and depends on the preoperative condition of the leg and the knee pathology noted therein. Patients must understand that their

injury and their knee are unique and that comparisons with other patients who have had the procedure performed are unrealistic because the latter may have had a "scope" during which no pathology was discovered or created.

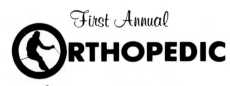

First Annual
ORTHOPEDIC
Invitational Ski Race

A unique race designed specifically for those that have had Orthopedic Surgery.*   *Sorry - Scopes Don't Count!

FIGURE 22–7
Notice "Scopes Don't Count"!—testimony to the public's attitude toward "scopes" vs. "real" surgery. (Courtesy of Dr. John Feagin.)

Arthroscopy provides improved visualization of all knee compartments and increases diagnostic accuracy. As clinicians' index of suspicion and diagnostic skills improve, a surprising number of intra-articular knee injuries in children are being discovered. One of the injuries now frequently seen in children and adolescents is a partial or complete anterior cruciate ligament (ACL) tear [11, 50]. This ligamentous injury without epiphyseal change is seen with increasing frequency in athletic populations, particularly among adolescents. In all reported series of patients with acute knee hemarthroses [9, 13, 36, 50], the authors reinforce the finding that hemarthrosis is a herald of a major intra-articular insult to the knee, most commonly associated with either an ACL tear or a meniscal or osteochondral injury. A high degree of associated injuries, particularly meniscal injuries, also are noted in children with anterior cruciate injuries [9, 50].

At Children's Hospital of Pittsburgh, Stanitski and colleagues [50] evaluated arthroscopically 70 pediatric patients with acute traumatic hemarthroses. In preadolescent patients (less than 12 years old), 47% had a meniscal tear and 47% had an ACL tear in combination with a medial meniscal tear. In adolescents (13 to 18 years old), ACL tears occurred in 70%, 40% of whom had an associated meniscal injury (Table 22–2).

In addition to providing increased diagnostic accuracy, arthroscopy allows precision surgery to be performed. Meniscal injuries that would once have precipitated removal of the entire meniscus can now be repaired, sparing the knee from undue wear and premature degenerative change [8, 30, 33, 38, 48, 54, 56]. By eliminating the extirpation of normal menisci for nefarious diagnoses such as "hypermobility," children's and adolescents' knees are spared the onset of premature joint senescence.

Arthroscopy enhances the diagnosis and allows early formulation of specific treatment and rehabilitation plans, resulting in rapid restoration of function. Intra-articular lesions causing asperities at the articular surfaces are eliminated, thus reducing the subsequent risk of degenerative joint disease. Accurate intra-articular assessment also allows one to make a diagnosis of normalcy. Reinforcement of symptoms of psychic genesis is eliminated and appropriate alternative therapy instituted.

Few long-term studies of postarthroscopic procedures in children have been reported. It is difficult to translate adult results to children and adolescents, but arthroscopic partial meniscectomy versus complete meniscectomy results in adults have certainly been encouraging [33, 54]. The results of meniscectomy in children, in general, have been reported to be only slightly better than those in adults, but much of the data consists of short-term follow-up and all of it was compiled in the prearthroscopic era, a time of almost ritualistic total meniscectomy by formal arthrotomy [8, 30, 38, 48]. Many series also included unstable knees with medial collateral ligament or ACL deficits that were made more unstable by total meniscectomy.

COMPLICATIONS

Although the morbidity associated with arthroscopy is small, complications can and do occur. Such reported complications include septic arthritis, compartment syndrome, neural and vascular damage, reflex sympathetic dystrophy, iatrogenic articular cartilage damage, broken instruments, and others [12, 44], even in experienced hands [45]. In those series that specifically reported diagnostic arthroscopy in children and adolescents, the complication rate is almost nonexistent. Whether these data will hold true when increased numbers of children are reported over a longer time span with closer scrutiny remains to be seen. An especially high incidence of complications is reported with surgery on the quadriceps mechanism, especially lateral retinacular release [46]. Neurologic and muscular damage and infections have been reduced with arthroscopically guided meniscal repair by newer techniques, but these are still potential problems. Knee stiffness, infection, and epiphyseal damage are all potential complications of ACL reconstruction in the skeletally immature patient. Arthroscopy is, after all, a surgical procedure with all the attendant risks of surgery, and it should not be considered cavalierly as a "no-problem, band-aid" type of surgery.

Arthroscopy is a surgical technique that has risen rapidly to the forefront of orthopedics in the recent past. It provides accuracy of diagnosis and a potential for precise surgical correction of a myriad of intra-articular disorders. Arthroscopy in children and adolescents requires perhaps more skill than in adults because of the child's limited articular cavity size despite relative knee laxity. The portals and techniques used in children are similar to those used in adults. Most standard arthroscope sizes are satisfactory for use in the child's knee. Arthroscopic surgical instruments of smaller sizes also are well adapted to pediatric-sized knees. The use of a leg holder in children has not been specifically ad-

TABLE 22–2
Knee Hemarthrosis[a]

	Meniscal Tear	Isolated ACL Tear	Meniscal Plus ACL Tear
Preadolescent (<12 years old)	47%	47%	6%
Adolescent (13 to 18 years old)	45%	70%	40%

[a]Children's Hospital of Pittsburgh data on acute knee hemarthrosis evaluated arthroscopically. Note the significant incidence of ACL tears in the preadolescent group.

dressed, but hypothetically, epiphyseal injury could occur as the counterpart in children of collateral ligament injury due to excessive force during attempted visualization maneuvers.

A careful history and physical examination are still necessary so that non-intra-articular pathology is recognized and premature arthroscopy is not embarked on as the treatment of course. The adage "knee pain is hip pain in children until proven otherwise" will prevent such premature arthroscopic procedures on the knee when pain is referred from hip pathology due to Perthes disease or slipped capital femoral epiphysis. Yaw and colleagues [61] reported on injudicious use of arthroscopy in patients with benign and malignant tumors about the knee that were apparent radiographically but were unrecognized, and an incorrect diagnosis was made preoperatively prior to arthroscopy. In some cases, knee roentgenograms were not taken. As they advise in their paper, "Caveat Arthroscopos," radiologic imaging continues to be part of the standard assessment in patients with knee complaints (Fig. 22–8).

Magnetic resonance imaging (MRI) is a noninvasive and accurate means of assessing intra-articular pathology, especially with the newer, higher strength magnets [37], but its availability, cost, and need for patient cooperation may limit its use in the pediatric population. It unfortunately does not provide a technique for evaluating the stability of meniscal or articular cartilage lesions. No specific data are available about the accuracy of MRI in children's knee disorders.

Arthroscopy has dramatically enhanced our knowledge of intra-articular knee lesions in children and necessitates a rethinking of the old attitude that such injuries are uncommon in children. With improved arthroscopic techniques, children's and adolescents' knees have benefited in many ways.

Arthroscopy allows a precise diagnosis including the diagnosis of a normal knee. Such a diagnosis leads to sparing of normal menisci, which were often removed in the past because they were considered, even though normal, to be the source of knee complaints and were removed for fear of missing a lesion in the posterior horn that could not be well visualized at arthrotomy. Meniscal preservation by repair or by sculpturing of the discoid menisci with preservation of as much tissue as possible allows more physiologic knee function and hopefully prevents premature senescence of the articular cartilage.

Arthroscopy allows an accurate diagnosis with less delay in providing proper treatment. Arthroscopic techniques have significantly reduced the morbidity associated with the variety of intra-articular procedures available (compared with formal arthrotomy) and allow rapid restoration of motion, strength, and function, goals that have often been difficult to achieve in children with lesions requiring arthrotomy.

The indications for arthroscopic surgery on the knee

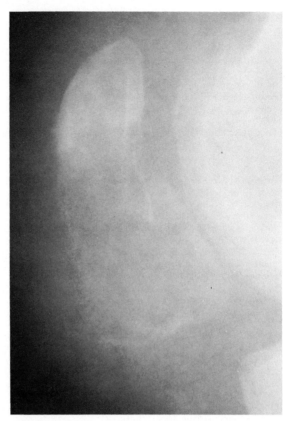

FIGURE 22–8
Patellar cystic lesion in an 11-year-old girl who had recently undergone arthroscopy and plica release for anterior knee symptoms.

in children and adolescents are similar to those used in adults. Surgery should be performed on a problem knee for which no accurate clinical or imaging diagnosis can be made for any of a variety of reasons, the most common of which may be pain limiting the accuracy of the examination. Arthroscopy should be strongly considered in all patients with hemarthrosis because of the high incidence of associated ligament, meniscal, and articular surface involvement in such patients.

Arthroscopy should not be looked upon as a panacea for all knee problems, whether in adults or in skeletally immature patients. Appropriate preoperative clinical evaluation and postoperative rehabilitation are still essential for restoration of function. Patients must understand the uniqueness of their knee problem and the need for their own involvement in the course of rehabilitation to gain maximum return to normalcy. Burman [6], in 1931, said it well when he noted ". . . it is to be expected that arthroscopy will not be used indiscriminately or to satisfy curiosity. Arthroscopy is contraindicated when there is no definite indication for it. It should be used discriminately in collaboration with a good history and physical examination and well-taken roentgenograms." It is certainly difficult to argue with any of those statements, and they should serve as guidelines for current arthroscopists.

References

1. Angel, K. R., and Hall, D. J. The role of arthroscopy in children and adolescents. *Arthroscopy* 5(3):192–196, 1989.
2. Arnoczky, S. P., Warren, R. F., and Spivak, J. M. Meniscal repair using an exogenous fibrin clot. *J Bone Joint Surg* 70A:1209, 1988.
3. Arnoczky, S. P., Warren, R. F., and McDevitt, C. A. Meniscal replacement using a cryopreserved allograft. *Clin Orthop* 252:121, 1990.
4. Bergstrom, R., Gilquist, J., Lysholm, J., et al. Arthroscopy of the knee in children. *J Pediatr Orthop* 4:542–545, 1984.
5. Burcher, E. Die arthroendoscopie. *Z Chir* 48:1460–1461, 1921.
6. Burman, M. S. Arthroscopy or the direct visualization of joints. An experimental cadaver study. *J Bone Joint Surg* 13:669–695, 1931.
7. Burman, M. S., Finkelstein, H., and Meyer, L. Arthroscopy of the knee joint. *J Bone Joint Surg* 13:255–268, 1934.
8. Busch, M. T. Meniscal injuries in children and adolescents. *Clin Sports Med* 9(3):661–680, 1990.
9. Butler, J. C., and Andrews, J. R. The role of arthroscopic surgery in the evaluation of acute traumatic hemarthrosis of the knee. *Clin Orthop* 228:150–152, 1988.
10. Cassidy, R. E., and Shaffer, A. J. Repair of peripheral meniscus tears: A preliminary report. *Am J Sports Med* 9:209, 1981.
11. Clanton, T. O., DeLee, J. C., Sanders, B., et al. Knee ligament injuries in children. *J Bone Joint Surg* 61A:1195, 1979.
12. Committee on Complications of Arthroscopy Association of North America. DeLee, J. D., Chairman. Complications of arthroscopy and arthroscopic surgery: Results in a national survey. *Arthroscopy* 1(4):214–220, 1985.
13. DeHaven, K. E. Diagnosis of acute septic knee injuries with hemarthrosis. *Am J Sports Med* 8:9–14, 1980.
14. DeHaven, K. E. Peripheral meniscus repair. An alternative to meniscectomy. *Orthop Trans* 5:399, 1981.
15. Eilert, R. E. Arthroscopy of the knee joint in children. *Orthop Rev* 9:61, 1976.
16. Ewing, J. W., and Voto, S. J. Arthroscopic surgical management of osteochondritis dissecans of the knee. *Arthroscopy* 4(1):37–40, 1988.
17. Fairbank, H. A. T. Internal derangement of the knee in children and adolescents. *Proc R Soc Med* 30:427, 1934.
18. Finkelstein, H., and Meyer, L. The arthroscope. A new method of examining joints. *J Bone Joint Surg* 13:583–588, 1931.
19. Fujikawa, K., Iseki, F., and Mikura, Y. Partial resection of the discoid meniscus of the child's knee. *J Bone Joint Surg* 63B:391–395, 1981.
20. Fulkerson, J. P., and Winters, T. F., Jr. Articular cartilage response to arthroscopic surgery: A review of current knowledge. *Arthroscopy* 2(3):184–189, 1986.
21. Ghadially, F. N., Wedge, J. H., and Lalonde, J.-M. A. Experimental methods of repairing injured menisci. *J Bone Joint Surg* 68B:106, 1986.
22. Harvell, J. C., Fu, F. H., and Stanitski, C. L. Diagnostic arthroscopy of the knee in children and adolescents. *Orthopaedics* 12(12):1555–1560, 1989.
23. Hayashi, L. K., Yamaga, H., Ida, K., et al.: Arthroscopic meniscectomy for discoid lateral meniscus in children. *J Bone Joint Surg* 70A(10):1495–1500, 1988.
24. Hayes, A. G., and Nageswar, M. The adolescent painful knee: The value of arthroscopy in diagnosis. *J Bone Joint Surg* 59B:499, 1977.
25. Henning, C. E., Lynch, M. A., and Clark, J. R. Vascularity for healing of meniscus repairs. *Arthroscopy* 3:13–18, 1987.
26. Ikeuchi, H. Arthroscopic treatment of the discoid lateral meniscus: Technique and long-term results. *Clin Orthop* 167:19–28, 1982.
27. Jackson, R. W. Current concepts review, arthroscopic surgery. *J Bone Joint Surg* 65A(3):416–420, 1983.
28. Kreuscher, P. H. Semilunar cartilage disease. A plea for the early recognition by means of the arthroscope and the early treatment of this condition. *Illinois Med J* 47:290–292, 1925.
29. Lankenner, P. A., Micheli, L. J., Clancy, R., et al. Arthroscopic percutaneous lateral patellar retinacular release. *Am J Sports Med* 14(4):267–269, 1986.
30. Manzione, M., Pizzutillo, P. A., Peoples, A. B., et al. Meniscectomy in children: A long-term follow-up study. *Am J Sports Med* 11:111, 1983.
31. Mayer, L., and Burman, M. S. Arthroscopy in the diagnosis of meniscal lesions in the knee joint. *Am J Surg* 43:501–511, 1939.
32. McCarroll, J. R., Rettig, A. C., and Shelbourne, K. D. Anterior cruciate ligament injuries in the young athlete with open physes. *Am J Sports Med* 16:44–50, 1988.
33. McGinty, J. B., Geuss, L. F., and Marvin, R. A. Partial or total meniscectomy. A comparative analysis. *J Bone Joint Surg* 59A:763, 1977.
34. McLennan, J. G. The role of arthroscopic surgery in the treatment of fractures of the intercondylar eminence of the tibia. *J Bone Joint Surg* 64B:477–480, 1982.
35. Morrissy, R. T., Eubanks, R. G., Park, J. P., et al. Arthroscopy of the knee in children. *Clin Orthop* 162:103–107, 1982.
36. Noyes, F. R., and Bassett, R. W. Arthroscopy in acute traumatic hemarthrosis of the knee. *J Bone Joint Surg* 62A:687–696, 1980.
37. Polly, D. W., Callaghan, J. J., Sikes, R. A., et al. The accuracy of selective magnetic resonance imaging compared with the findings of arthroscopy of the knee. *J Bone Joint Surg* 70A:192–198, 1988.
38. Ritchie, D. M. Meniscectomy in children. *Aust NZ J Surg* 35:239–241, 1965.
39. Rosenberg, T. D., Paulos, L. E., Parker, R. D., et al. Discoid lateral meniscus: Case report of arthroscopic attachment of a symptomatic Wrisberg-ligament type. *J Arthros Rel Surg* 3:277, 1987.
40. Rydholm, U. Arthroscopy of the knee in juvenile chronic arthritis. *Scand J Rheumatol* 15:109–112, 1986.
41. Schonholtz, G. J., Zahn, M. G., and Magee, C. M. Lateral retinacular release of the patella. *Arthroscopy* 3(4):269–272, 1987.
42. Seger, B. M., and Woods, G. W. Arthroscopic management of lateral meniscal cysts. *Am J Sports Med* 4:105, 1986.
43. Skyhar, M. J., and Mubarik, S. J. Arthroscopic treatment of septic knees in children. *J Pediatr Orthop* 7(6):647–651, 1987.
44. Small, N. C. Complications in arthroscopy: The knee and other joints. *Arthroscopy* 2(4):253–258, 1986.
45. Small, N. C. Complications in arthroscopic surgery performed by experienced arthroscopists. *Arthroscopy* 4(3):215–221, 1988.
46. Small, N. C. An analysis of complications in lateral retinacular release procedures. *Arthroscopy* 5(4):282–286, 1989.
47. Smillie, I. S. The congenital discoid meniscus. *J Bone Joint Surg* 30B:671, 1948.
48. Smillie, I. S. Injuries of the knee joint (4th ed.). Edinburgh, Churchill Livingstone, 1970.
49. Stanitski, C. L., Harvell, J. C., and Fu, F. Arthroscopy in acute septic knees: The pediatric years. *Clin Orthop* 247:66–71, 1989.
50. Stanitski, C. L., Harvell, J. C., and Fu, F. H. Observations on acute knee hemarthroses in children and adolescents. *J Pediatr Orthop* 13(4):506–510, 1993.
51. Stone, K. R., Rodkey, W. G., Webber, R. J., et al. Future directions. Collagen-based prostheses for meniscal regeneration. *Clin Orthop* 252:129, 1990.
52. Suman, R. K., Stother, I. G., and Illingworth, G. Diagnostic arthroscopy of the knee in children. *J Bone Joint Surg* 66B:535–537, 1984.
53. Takagi, K. Practical experience using Takagi's arthroscope. *J Jap Orthop Assoc* 8:132, 1933.
54. Tapper, E. M., and Hoover, N. W. Late results after meniscectomy. *J Bone Joint Surg* 51A:517, 1969.
55. Thiery, J. A. Arthroscopic drainage in septic arthritides of the knee: A multicenter study. *Arthroscopy* 5:65–69, 1989.
56. Thompson, W. O., Theate, F. L., Fu, F. H., et al. Tibial meniscal dynamics using 3D reconstruction of MR images. Personal communication. In press, 1993.
57. Vandermeer, R. D., and Cunningham, F. K. Arthroscopic treatment of the discoid lateral meniscus: Results of long-term follow-up. *Arthroscopy* 5(2):101–109, 1989.
58. Watanabe, M., and Takeda, S. The number 21 arthroscope. *J Jap Orthop Assoc* 34:1041, 1960.
59. Watanabe, M., Takeda, S., and Ikeuchi, H. *Atlas of Arthroscopy* (3rd ed.). Tokyo, Igaku Shoin, 1978.
60. Wiberg, G. Roentgenographic and anatomic studies on the femoropatellar joint: With special references to chondromalacia patellae. *Acta Orthop Scand* 12:319, 1941.
61. Yaw, J., Mankin, H., and McGinty, J. Caveat arthroscopos. *J Bone Joint Surg* 70A:1575, 1988.
62. Ziv, I., and Carroll, N. C. The role of arthroscopy in children. *J Pediatr Orthop* 2:243–247, 1982.

ANKLE AND FOOT INJURIES IN THE PEDIATRIC ATHLETE

J. Andy Sullivan, M.D.

Most of the injuries that occur in the ankle and foot in the pediatric athlete are not unique to athletic participation but occur normally during childhood. Some occur with greater frequency in the athlete. The conditions covered in this chapter occur in childhood and may present in the athlete, raising the question of whether he or she should be allowed to participate.

VARIATIONS OF NORMAL ANATOMY

Tarsal Coalition

Tarsal coalition is a bony or fibrocartilaginous connection of two or more of the tarsal bones. The cause is unknown, but it has been established that the condition results from a failure of differentiation and segmentation of the primitive mesenchyme [15]. The incidence is 1% to 3% [9, 20]. The most common coalitions are the calcaneonavicular and the talocalcaneal. The first is bilateral in about 60% of cases, and the second is bilateral in about 50% [9, 16, 20]. More than one type of coalition can exist in one foot, and coalition may be more common than previously appreciated, as discussed later. The exact mode of inheritance is unknown, but it is postulated to be autosomal dominant with variable penetrance [20].

Most patients present during early adolescence at a time when the coalition is ossifying. The pain is vague in nature and insidious in onset. There may be a history of precipitating trauma. Sports participation or running over uneven ground may accentuate the pain. Physical findings include pain on palpation over the subtalar joint, limited subtalar motion, and at times pes planus and ankle valgus. The peroneal muscles may be tight and resist inversion, but true muscle spasm occurs rarely. Any condition that injures the subtalar joint can produce the same picture.

The clinical diagnosis can be confirmed by radiographic imaging. Plain radiographs, especially the 45-degree oblique view, usually demonstrate the calcaneonavicular coalition. Talocalcaneal coalition is difficult to visualize on plain radiographs, but there may be secondary changes suggesting the need for other studies. These include beaking and shortening of the talar neck, failure to see the middle subtalar facet, elongation of the lateral process of the calcaneus, and ball and socket ankle joint. Special views (e.g., Harris-Beath view), scintigraphy, plain tomography, and arthrography have all been used to demonstrate these coalitions. Computed tomography (CT) is now the method of choice for the diagnosis of tarsal coalitions not identified on plain films [14]. It is comparable in cost and radiation dosage to the other studies. It is technically simple to perform, noninvasive, and accurate. CT provides precise delineation of the anatomy if surgical resection is contemplated. It may also demonstrate the presence of more than one coalition, which is important in planning treatment (Fig. 23–1).

The initial treatment of these conditions should be conservative measures aimed at relieving the pain. These measures are empiric and include casting, various shoe inserts, and orthotics. The main indication for surgical resection is persistent pain. For calcaneonavicular coalition, resection of the bar with interposition of the extensor digitorum brevis is usually associated with good results. Cowell and Jayakumar and Cowell indicated that

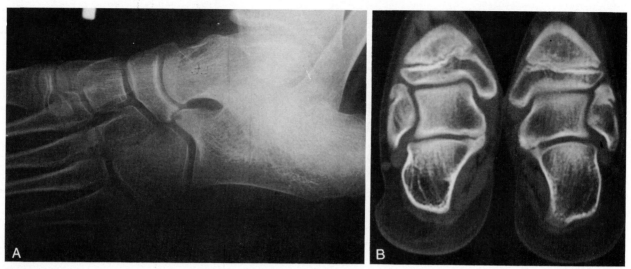

FIGURE 23–1
Plain radiograph *(A)* and CT scan *(B)* showing calcaneonavicular and talocalcaneal coalitions, which occurred bilaterally in this patient. The patient presented with a painful, rigid foot and was having difficulty playing tennis.

23 of 26 feet treated in this manner became symptom-free [9, 16].

Talocalcaneal coalition is harder to recognize and its surgical management less certain. Prior to the use of CT the diagnosis was often confirmed at the time of surgery. Jayakumar and Cowell [16] reported that up to one-third of their patients responded to conservative treatment and believed that there were few indications for resection. This conclusion was based on evidence showing that family studies indicated that many adults with tarsal coalition were asymptomatic. The surgical alternatives are resection of the bar and triple arthrodesis.

Scranton reviewed 14 patients with 23 symptomatic talocalcaneal coalitions [26]. Five feet (three patients) were treated successfully with casts. Four feet were treated by triple arthrodesis. Eight patients with 13 coalitions resected had a good result. The review was done at a mean of 3.9 years after surgery. The size of talocalcaneal bar that can be successfully removed is still unanswered. In Scranton's series approximately one-half the joint surface was removed in some patients. In the series of Swintkowski and colleagues [30] 10 patients were treated for talocalcaneal coalition, four by resection of the bar and the remainder by some type of arthrodesis. This article stressed that the talar beak is not a true degenerative sign and therefore is not a contraindication to resection of the bar. Olney and Asher [21] evaluated nine patients with persistent pain from a middle facet talocalcaneal coalition who were treated by resection of the bar and autogenous fat graft. At an average follow-up of 42 months the results in five were rated excellent, three good, one fair, and one poor. In one patient who underwent reoperation the fat graft had been replaced by fibrous tissue.

The management of these coalitions is still controversial and awaits larger series with longer follow-up. Patients with persistent symptoms who do not have degenerative findings have the option of continued conservative care, resection of the coalition, or arthrodesis. Talar beaking is not necessarily a degenerative sign. Severe malalignment of the foot is a contraindication to resection alone. The size of coalition that can be resected is unknown, and the question of whether interpositional material is beneficial is unanswered.

Adolescent Bunion

The etiology of adolescent bunion is unknown. Fifty to sixty percent of patients have a positive family history [8, 27]. Patients with this condition have an increased intermetatarsal angle (the angle between the first and second metatarsals, normally 10 degrees) and an increased first metatarsal-phalangeal angle (normally 20 degrees). Many also have a relaxed flatfoot and a long first metatarsal ray. None of these conditions is known to be the cause of adolescent bunion. Shoewear has been implicated, but because bunions occur in cultures where shoes are not worn, this theory seems unlikely.

These patients complain of pain, prominence, and difficulty with shoewear. On examination deviation of the toe laterally is found with a prominence medially and a wide forefoot. The bursa that is a prominent part of the adult deformity may be present but is usually less impressive. Arthritis and decreased range of motion are also less common. The patient should be evaluated with anteroposterior (AP) and lateral weight-bearing radiographs. The joint space is usually maintained. The sesamoids may be laterally displaced in advanced cases. The medial eminence of the metatarsal head is prominent, and a sagittal groove may be present medially.

Children should be treated nonsurgically whenever possible. Alteration or stretching of shoewear may alleviate the symptoms. Surgical procedures performed prior to physeal closure are associated with a high recurrence rate [8, 27]. Although some series have claimed a success rate of 80% to 95%, this high rate of success has not been the universal experience. The series of Scranton [27] and of Bonney and McNab [5] both had a high complication rate. Factors implicated in these complications included failure to correct the abnormal deviation of the first metatarsal, failure to correct the soft tissues, too early weight bearing, inadequate immobilization, and osteotomy performed distal to the open physis. Patients with a hypermobile flatfoot or a long first ray also seemed more prone to recurrence.

Indications for surgery include pain that is not responsive to conservative measures and severe deformity. The goals of surgery should include realignment of the first ray and of the metatarsophalangeal joint, cosmesis, and prevention of arthritis. Discussion of the types of surgical procedures used is beyond the scope of this chapter but is found in the reference by Coughlin and Mann [8].

In general, the most common procedures are a distal osteotomy such as the Mitchell procedure or a proximal realignment osteotomy combined with soft tissue procedures. Arthrodesis and resection arthroplasty have no place in surgery in children.

Accessory Navicular

Numerous accessory ossicles can occur in the foot, and one needs to be aware of them to avoid confusion with acute fracture. The most common are the os trigonum posterior to the talus and the os vesalium at the base of the fifth metatarsal. The accessory navicular is a separate ossification center of the navicular. It may be completely separate or joined by a synchondrosis. It may also present as a large or cornuate prominence on the medial side of the navicular (Fig. 23–2). Since the work of Kidner [18] the accessory navicular has been implicated in the genesis of a flatfoot. It was postulated that the posterior tibial tendon inserted into this accessory ossicle, resulting in loss of the normal support of the longitudinal arch. Kidner advocated resection of the bone and plication or reinsertion of the posterior tibial tendon inferior to the navicular. We now know that only a small slip of the tendon inserts into this ossicle and

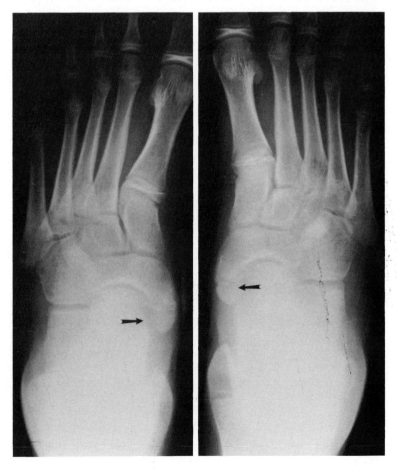

FIGURE 23–2
Large bilateral cornuate of prominent accessory naviculars. These are joined by a synchondrosis to the navicular.

that these patients are no more likely to have a flatfoot than those with a normal navicular [29].

Many of these patients are asymptomatic. Symptomatic patients experience pain directly over the prominence, usually from shoewear over the bump. If the shoes are stretched or altered over this prominence, symptoms may be relieved. Other patients seem to experience pain when the posterior tibial tendon is stretched or put under tension. In those with persistent pain, simple excision of the ossicle without rerouting of the tendon is usually successful [3, 29].

Cavus Foot

Cavus is defined as an increase in the height of the longitudinal arch of the foot. A variety of other modifiers are used to further describe the position of the heel such as cavovarus and calcaneocavus. Often the patient has clawtoes or hammertoes and metatarsal head calluses. The presenting complaint can be pain or abnormal wear of the shoe. A cavus foot is usually the result of muscle imbalance resulting from an underlying neurologic disorder. The patient should undergo a meticulous neurologic examination looking for evidence of disorders such as Charcot-Marie-Tooth disease, spinal dysraphism, or a spinal tumor. Initial radiographic evaluation should in-

clude weight-bearing views of the feet and at least an AP view of the entire spine looking for an occult spinal anomaly.

Miscellaneous Foot Abnormalities

A variety of other bony variations may produce pain. ''Pump bumps'' are soft tissue bursae that are associated with prominent calcaneal tuberosities. They are irritated by the heel counter of some shoes. Treatment consists of altering the shoewear or padding the heel. Bunionettes are similar bursae that occur over the lateral aspect of the fifth metatarsal head. Stretching the shoe is usually curative. Only rarely is removal of the bony prominence or osteotomy of the fifth ray necessary. A dorsal bunion can occur over the first metatarsal head. In most instances it is a result of weakness or loss of function in the peroneus longus, which is responsible for depressing the first metatarsal. Treatment must be individualized to balance the overpull of the dorsiflexors of the first ray and may require tendon transfer, osteotomy, or arthrodesis.

SOFT TISSUE INJURIES

The ligaments of the ankle insert on the epiphyses distal to the physeal line (Fig. 23–3). Because the physis

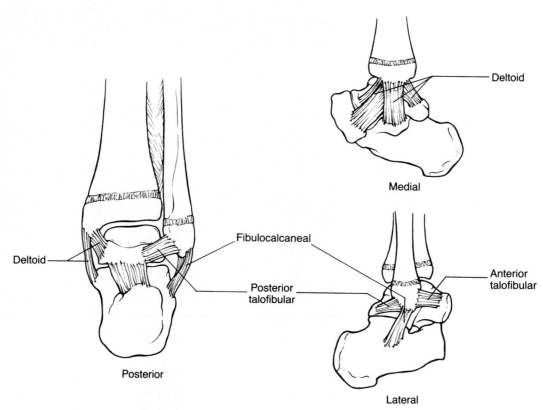

FIGURE 23–3
The ligaments of the ankle in posterior, medial, and lateral views.

is the weakest link in this bone-tendon-bone interface it is usually the part that gives way when significant force is applied to the ankle. Serious ankle sprains are unusual in the skeletally immature athlete. Physeal fractures that do occur are covered in the next section. Minor ankle sprains do occur and are diagnosed by a history of inversion or eversion strain with findings of tenderness over the anterior talofibular or deltoid ligament. Treatment is accomplished by the usual conservative means of ice, compression, elevation, and immobilization. Rehabilitation is rarely necessary. Continued pain or disability should provoke a search for other, more serious injury.

Recurrent subluxation of peroneal tendons can occur in the adolescent athlete. There is usually a history of injury followed by recurrent episodes of a snapping sensation and pain. The subluxation can be provoked by forceful dorsiflexion with the foot everted. In patients whose symptoms are sufficiently severe, surgical correction may be indicated. Surgical alternatives include deepening the groove on the fibula, creating a bony block, or reconstructing the superior peroneal retinaculum. The first two are rarely useful in the pediatric athlete because the physis is still open. Poll reviewed nine patients aged 15 to 45 (average age 25) who had reconstruction using the posterior calcaneofibular ligament attached to a bone block [24]. Results were said to be good.

Contusions on the foot are treated in the same way as any other contusion. Blisters are a frequent problem and require alleviation of the stress, which is usually a new shoe, and protection until healing occurs. Tinea pedis (athlete's foot) usually responds to a regimen of antifungal medication and education about the need to change socks frequently and use antifungal powders.

FRACTURES ABOUT THE ANKLE

Multiple systems have been proposed to classify ankle injuries. Dias proposed using the systems that are applied to adult ankle fractures [10]. All these classification systems take into account the position of the foot at the time of injury and the force applied. The Salter-Harris classification is based on the mechanism of injury and the pathoanatomy of the fracture pattern through the physis [25] (Fig. 23–4).

Dias and Giergerich [10] proposed a modification of the Lauge-Hanson system by combining it with the Salter-Harris classification, suggesting that it is of benefit in planning the closed reduction of these injuries. Although these other systems may be important in the adult, the Salter-Harris classification is the most important system in the child for planning treatment and predicting outcome. In the skeletally immature patient the tibiotalar joint surface is rarely disturbed. The outcome of the injury depends on the type of physeal injury and its

management. Tension injuries usually produce Salter-Harris type I and II injuries of the physis. Compression forces can produce Salter-Harris type III and IV injuries.

Salter-Harris type V injuries are severe crush injuries. A type VI injury in which the perichondrial ring is injured has been described [25]. These injuries do not occur during usual sport activities.

Clinical Evaluation. The mechanism of injury and the time elapsed since the accident should be noted. The neurovascular status of the foot should be carefully documented. The amount of swelling and the status of the skin are important. Gentle examination should be carried out to seek areas of point tenderness, especially over the physis. This examination may be more useful in the diagnosis of Salter-Harris type I injuries than radiographs.

Radiographs should always include three views of the ankle. Only in this manner will the physician be able to see some fractures, and radiography is of benefit in determining the Salter-Harris classification of the fracture. Plain tomography and CT may be indicated in the juvenile fracture of Tillaux and in triplane fractures, which are discussed below. Because treatment and prognosis depend on the Salter-Harris classification, the fractures will be discussed by fracture type.

Salter-Harris Type I

Salter-Harris type I injuries of the tibia occur in very young children and are not a consideration in the athlete. Salter-Harris type I fractures of the fibula are common and may be missed entirely or misdiagnosed as a sprain. The characteristic history of an external rotation force in a patient who presents with localized tenderness and swelling directly over the distal fibular physis is diagnostic. The radiograph shows only localized swelling and widening of the fibular physis. Many of these injuries probably go unrecognized and untreated. They respond quite well to 2 to 3 weeks of immobilization in a short-leg walking cast.

Salter-Harris Type II

This injury is uncommon or infrequently recognized in the fibula. Salter-Harris type II injury of the distal tibia combined with a fracture of the distal fibula is one of the most common injuries about the ankle, accounting for 47.3% of cases in the series compiled by Peterson and Cass [22]. In most instances this injury can be reduced closed under sedation. Periosteum or other soft tissue can block the reduction if it is inverted into the fracture site. Traditional treatment consists of a long-leg bent knee cast for 2 to 3 weeks followed by a short-leg walking cast for 4 weeks. Dugan and Herndon [11] re-

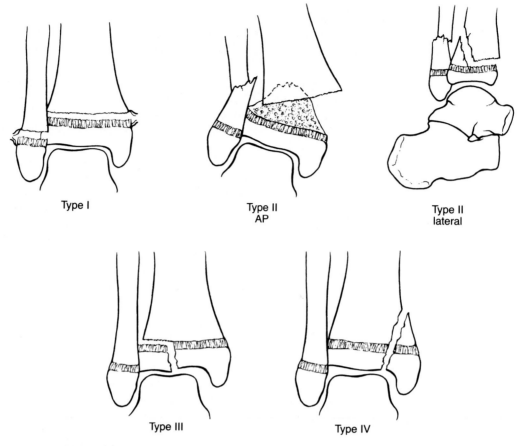

Type I   Type II
               AP   Type II
                           lateral

Type III   Type IV

FIGURE 23–4
Fracture patterns of the distal tibial and fibular physes classified by the Salter-Harris system.

viewed 56 patients with this injury who were treated with a long-leg weight-bearing cast for 4 weeks. There were no nonunions and no angular deformities. There was one case of clinically insignificant premature closure of the growth plate. This seems to be the treatment of choice because it allows early healing, low morbidity, and rapid rehabilitation.

Salter-Harris Type III

This injury is also known as the juvenile fracture of Tillaux. The distal tibial physis closes first in the central region and then from the medial side toward the fibula. An external rotation force applied to the partially closed physis applies traction on the physis through the anterior talofibular ligament. This avulses a fragment of the lateral physis, which remains attached to the ligament (see Fig. 23–5). Closed reduction under anesthesia should be attempted. The injury can be treated closed if the fragment is not displaced more than 2 mm. Most of these injuries require open reduction and fixation of the fragment with a pin or cancellous screw.

Fractures of the medial malleolus can be either type III or IV injuries. If displaced less than 2 mm they may be treated closed. This treatment should consist initially of a long-leg nonweight-bearing cast for 3 weeks followed by a short-leg walking cast for 3 weeks. These injuries are the most unpredictable of ankle epiphyseal injuries. Near-anatomic reduction must be obtained.

Salter-Harris Type IV

This group includes some of the medial malleolar fractures and the triplane fractures. The triplane fracture, first described by Marmour, is so named because the fracture lines extend from the physis into the transverse, sagittal, and coronal planes [7, 12, 28] (see Fig. 23–5). This may be mistaken for a Salter-Harris type II injury if the radiographs are not carefully scrutinized.

Many authors have described this fracture and have argued over the number of fragments involved [7, 10, 12, 25, 28]. Rang [25] depicted this as a three-part fracture. Cooperman and colleagues [7] studied 15 triplane fractures (average age 13 years). This number represented 6% of 237 consecutive physeal fractures of the tibia and fibula. Average follow-up was 26 months.

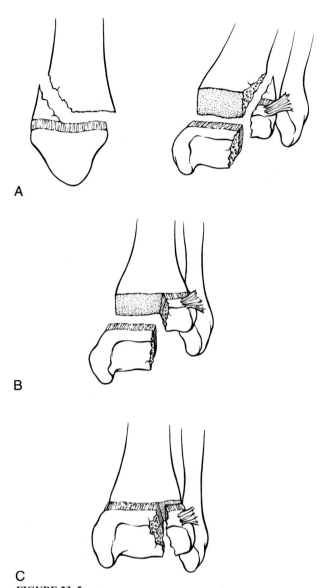

FIGURE 23–5
A and *B*, The triplane fracture can consist of two or more fragments. *C*, The juvenile fracture of Tillaux.

Figure 23–5 illustrates the possibilities. In the two-part fracture the main fragment is the tibial shaft including the medial malleolus and a portion of the medial epiphysis. The second fragment is the remaining epiphysis, which is attached to the fibula. In the three-part injury the third fragment is usually an anterior free epiphyseal fragment.

If this injury can be reduced to within 2 mm it may be treated closed. In Cooperman and colleagues' series [7] 13 of 15 fractures were treated closed, and in the series of Dias and Giergerich [10] five of eight were treated in this way. In the series by Ertl and co-workers [12] residual displacement of more than 2 mm was associated with a high incidence of late symptoms. Obtaining a reduction of less than 2 mm by either closed or open means did not ensure an excellent result. Poor results may be related to damage done to the articular surface or to the amount of displacement. Fractures outside the weight-bearing area did not show this tendency toward poor results.

Evaluation of the adequacy of reduction in this injury is very difficult, and because most authors recommend manipulation under general anesthesia the only radiographic means of diagnosis available is plain radiography. The author's preferred method is manipulation by internal rotation of the foot under sedation, usually in the emergency room. If there is any question about the adequacy of reduction on plain radiographs, CT or plain tomography is used to evaluate the articular surface and the reduction (Fig. 23–6). If there is displacement of more than 2 mm, open reduction and internal fixation are carried out. This may require two incisions. The first is an anterolateral incision and allows identification of the anterolateral fragment. Usually it is first necessary to reduce and fix the posterior fragment. If this cannot be done closed or percutaneously, a second incision is required. These injuries require 6 weeks in a cast.

Prediction of Outcome

The prognosis for an ankle fracture in a skeletally immature patient depends on the following factors:

1. Salter-Harris classification
2. Quality of reduction
3. State of skeletal maturity
4. Amount of displacement
5. Miscellaneous modifiers (open fracture, vascular injury, infection, systemic illness, and so on)

Thirteen fractures had been treated closed, and two had been treated by open reduction and internal fixation. In this series plain tomographic studies supported the opinion that this was a two-part fracture. Dias and Giergerich [10] reviewed a series of fractures that included eight triplane fractures, which included both two-part and three-part fractures. Three patients were treated by open reduction, at which time it was confirmed that these were three-part fractures. In two patients studies confirmed that it was a two-part injury, and they were treated in long-leg cast for 6 weeks. Ertl and associates [12] reviewed 23 patients with this injury. Eleven of fifteen had a three-part fracture. In these patients plain radiographs did not accurately demonstrate the configuration of the fracture and were unreliable in distinguishing two-part from three-part fractures.

Spiegel and colleagues [28] retrospectively studied a series of closed distal tibial physeal injuries. One hundred and eighty-four patients (of 237) were followed for an average of 28 months. The authors looked specifically at the complications of angular deformity of

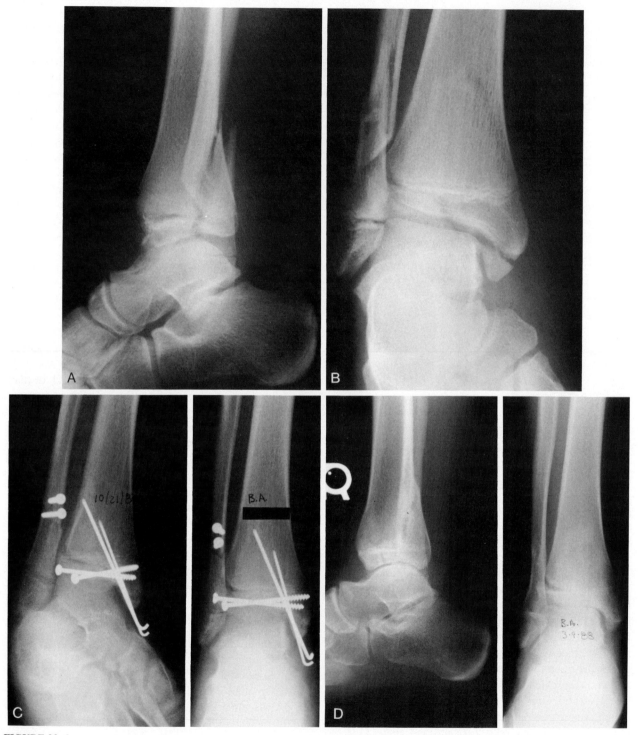

FIGURE 23–6

A and *B*, The position obtained after manipulation of a severely displaced triplane fracture. The position was not acceptable, so further imaging was not necessary. *C*, The position obtained by open reduction. *D*, The position present after hardware removal.

greater than 5 degrees and shortening of more than 1 cm, joint incongruity, or asymmetrical closure of the physis. These complications seemed to correlate with the Salter-Harris grade, the amount of displacement or comminution, and the adequacy of reduction. The patients were divided into the groups shown in Table 23–1.

The overall complication rate was 14.1% for 184 patients. Salter-Harris type II injuries of the tibia seemed to be the least predictable because the incidence of complications remained approximately the same regardless of the amount of displacement. Displacement is not always mentioned as one of the factors involved in prediction of outcome, but it is intuitive that greater displacement implies greater force with more likely damage to the articular cartilage, the circulation, and the soft tissues important in healing. The result may be that more displacement has a greater tendency to lead to a poor result.

Anatomic reduction of type II injuries of the tibia seems necessary. These injuries are easy to reduce and often benign but must be followed until the patient attains skeletal maturity or a normal growth pattern is ensured because some will go on to premature closure and angular deformity.

The juvenile fracture of Tillaux and the triplane fracture result from incomplete closure of the physis. Because growth is nearing an end, angular deformity and shortening are uncommon. In these patients the tibiotalar joint surface is disturbed and must be restored to as near normal as possible to prevent incongruity and subsequent traumatic arthritis. In Cooperman and colleagues' series [7] triplane fractures were reduced under general anesthesia by internally rotating the foot. The adequacy of reduction was determined by plain tomography. Dias and Giergerich [10] had nine Tillaux and triplane fractures that were followed for an average of 18 months and all did well.

Peterson and Cass [22] reviewed all Salter-Harris type IV distal tibial injuries seen at the Mayo Clinic, paying particular attention to injuries of the medial malleolus.

Nine of eighteen of these injuries went on to premature physeal closure sufficient to require additional surgery for physeal bar resection, angular deformity, or leg length discrepancy. Thirteen of these patients received their care at the Mayo Clinic, and of these, 11 were closed injuries. Six were treated by closed reduction and a short-leg cast. Five had open reduction and internal fixation. Five additional patients in the study had been referred to the clinic because of complications of a closed injury that had been treated closed. Peterson and Cass concluded that oblique radiographs may be necessary to make an accurate diagnosis. Some injuries that resemble type III injuries are actually type IV. The authors also found that partial arrest that results in angular deformity was more common than complete arrest. They concluded that there are three patterns of medial malleolar injury and that type IV injuries comprise the most common and most dangerous pattern because they usually occur in a patient who has remaining growth potential (Fig. 23–7). They also concluded that the medial malleolus requires anatomic reduction, which often necessitates open reduction and internal fixation.

In any patient with an open physis, it is preferable to avoid crossing the physis with any fixation device. This goal can usually be achieved by placing smooth pins from metaphysis to metaphysis or from epiphysis to epiphysis. At times crossing the physis cannot be avoided. In these instances smooth pins can be used. The patients need to be followed to skeletal maturity or until one is certain that a normal growth pattern is occurring. An asymmetrical Harris growth arrest line may be the earliest clue to an abnormal growth pattern (Fig. 23–7).

FRACTURES IN THE FOOT

Fractures about the foot resulting from sports are unusual in children. Fractures of the metatarsals can result from direct trauma (Fig. 23–8). These can be treated by immobilization in a short-leg walking cast. The most controversial fracture about the foot may be an avulsion injury at the base of the fifth metatarsal.

Fractures of the fifth metatarsal in children can be divided into distal physeal fractures, fractures of the proximal diaphysis, and avulsion fractures of the apophysis. The fifth metatarsal has its epiphysis distally and an apophysis proximally. The tendon of the peroneus brevis is inserted into the apophysis. With inversion stress the apophysis can be avulsed. The findings include tenderness at the base of the fifth metatarsal and radiographic confirmation of widening of the apophysis. Treatment should be symptomatic with compression and partial weight bearing until the pain subsides. Crutches and an elastic bandage may be sufficient. Two to three weeks in a short-leg cast also yield good results.

TABLE 23–1
Complications of Ankle Fractures

Group	Complication Rate (%)	Salter-Harris Group and Bone Involved
Low risk (89 patients)	6.7	Type I and II of fibula, I of tibia, III and IV with displacement of less than 2 mm, epiphyseal avulsion injuries
High risk (28 patients)	32	Types III, IV, and V of tibia
		Tillaux and triplane
Unpredictable (66 patients)	16.7	Type II of the tibia

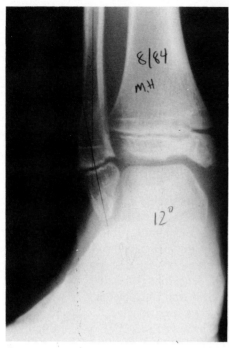
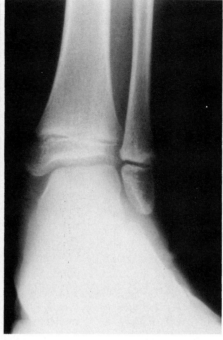

FIGURE 23–7
This patient sustained a Salter-Harris type IV medial malleolar fracture, which was treated closed. The patient was referred 6 months after injury, at which time she had trouble remembering which ankle had been injured. These radiographs were taken 18 months after the injury. Resection of a bony bridge and interposition were required. She resumed growth, and the fibular angular deformity has been corrected. Note the irregular Harris growth arrest lines.

Fractures of the proximal diaphysis of the fifth metatarsal (the Jones fracture) are less common in skeletally immature patients and usually occur in the 15- to 20-year-old age range [17]. When such fractures do occur a trial of immobilization in a short-leg walking cast is indicated because many acute fractures will heal. Even fractures with delayed union may heal if they are treated conservatively [1]. Early operative intervention in highly competitive athletes has been advocated by some, but others have shown that each patient needs to be treated individually because some of these fractures will heal if treated conservatively allowing early return to athletics [1, 17, 19]. Early operative intervention in the pediatric athlete is rarely if ever indicated. Patients with established nonunion require operative treatment that includes reopening of the medullary canal, bone grafting, and internal fixation.

Fractures of the toes are unusual in sports. Most phalangeal fractures can be treated by ''buddy-taping'' them to the adjacent toe, wearing appropriate shoes for a few weeks, and avoiding sports until the toe is asymptomatic. Articular fractures are even more rare. The only one that may merit consideration of operative management is an interarticular physeal fracture of the great toe. These should be reduced to as near anatomic alignment as possible by whatever means necessary.

Stress fractures are less common in children than in adults but cannot be entirely dismissed. Some children participate in marathons and other sporting events that can result in stress fractures. Basketball, soccer, and other team sports have tournaments that can require considerable running. The stress fracture shown in Figure 23–9 resulted from a tournament and was thought to be a sprain.

Yngve found 131 pediatric stress fractures in 23 references in the literature [32]. There were only two reports of metatarsal fracture, two of the tarsal navicular, and one of the medial sesamoid. The primary training error was too much too soon. Other factors that should be considered are a change in training surface, equipment (shoes), or a sudden change in intensity of training (tournaments). The diagnosis depends on an appropriate history, a high index of suspicion, and the presence of localized tenderness. The differential diagnosis includes contusion, tendinitis, and sprains.

The initial radiograph may be normal but should be diagnostic in half the cases. One should look for cortical thickening or a translucent fracture line. A bone scan may be diagnostic at this stage and may be particularly helpful if the diagnosis is in question and one wishes to avoid immobilization. On the other hand, immobilization for 2 weeks in a cast is usually diagnostic in that the pain is relieved and repeat radiographs are then positive, making a bone scan unnecessary. Although some of these fractures heal without a cast, the athlete should be immobilized for protection from himself or herself as well as from well-meaning parents and coaches.

OSTEOCHONDRAL LESIONS OF THE TALUS

The term *osteochondritis dissecans* has been used to describe lesions in the dome of the talus. These lesions

FIGURE 23–8
A, This patient sustained fractures of the lateral four metatarsal necks when he caught his foot on a base while sliding. *B*, This patient fractured his first metatarsal when he was stepped on during a football game.

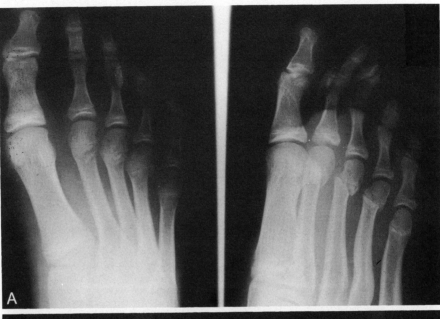

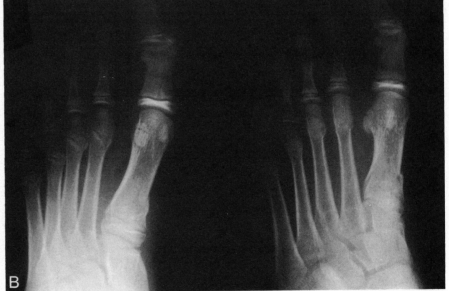

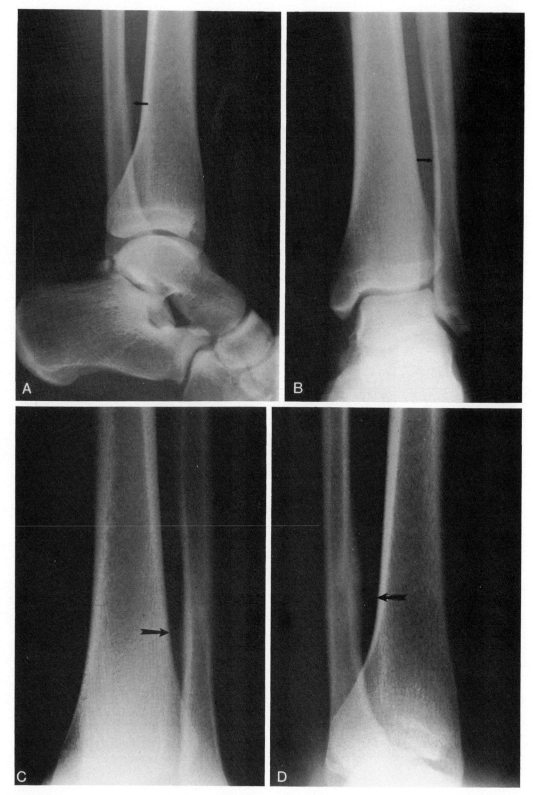

FIGURE 23–9

This patient presented with localized tenderness just above the ankle. After being injured in a basketball tournament she had continued to play with a presumptive diagnosis of a sprained ankle. The initial radiographs (*A* and *B*) showed periosteal elevation. Follow-up radiographs (*C* and *D*) taken after two weeks of short-leg walking cast treatment illustrate new bone formation.

have been attributed to a vascular insult, but most authors now attribute them to previous trauma to the ankle, most often inversion stress [2, 4, 6]. Berndt and Hart [4] thought that both the medial and lateral lesions were the sequelae of trauma and developed a four-stage classification system based on the amount of damage and the degree of displacement. This system, modified slightly, is still in use [2].

Stage I: Localized trabecular compression
Stage II: Incompletely separated fragment
Stage IIA: Formation of a subchondral cyst
Stage III: Undetached, undisplaced fragment
Stage IV: Displaced or inverted fragment

Most series consist predominantly of adults; however, 21 of 29 patients studied by Canale and Belding [6] experienced onset of symptoms in the second decade. Newer diagnostic methods may reveal that these lesions, which are often hard to see on plain radiographs, are more common in adolescents than previously suspected. Proper treatment depends on identification of the lesion and accurate staging.

Anderson and colleagues [2] have recommended scintigraphy as a screening procedure for patients in whom this diagnosis is suspected but in whom radiographs are normal. They recommended that patients with positive scintigraphy be further evaluated by magnetic resonance imaging (MRI). Patients with positive plain radiographs do not need either of these two studies. CT in these patients allows staging of the lesion and selection of the proper treatment.

Canale and Belding [6] recommended that nonoperative treatment by immobilization of all stage I, stage II, and medial stage III (Berndt and Harty classification) lesions would result in a high percentage of good clinical results and delayed development of arthrosis. Persistent symptoms after conservative treatment were an indication for operative treatment by excision and curettage. They further recommended that all stage III lateral lesions and all stage IV lesions be treated by immediate excision and curettage of the lesion. Anderson and colleagues [2] recommended immobilization for 6 weeks for patients with stage I and II fractures but cautioned that these patients need to be followed for a prolonged period of time to detect the delayed development of arthrosis. Operative treatment was recommended for stage IIA, III, and IV lesions. Arthroscopic treatment is now gaining favor, but follow-up in reported cases is brief.

OSTEOCHONDROSES IN THE FOOT

The osteochondroses are a group of conditions of unknown etiology. Suggested causes have included endo-crinopathies, vascular phenomena, infection, and trauma [23]. Many of these conditions are now known to represent radiographic variations of normal ossification of the epiphysis. Most are named by the person or persons who originally described them. They all include a pattern of clinical symptoms coupled with a radiograph that suggests that the epiphysis or apophysis is undergoing necrosis. In the foot the most commonly described conditions are Kohler's syndrome and Freiberg's infarction.

Kohler's syndrome is a clinical syndrome comprising pain in the midfoot coupled with a finding of localized tenderness over the navicular. Radiographs demonstrate increased density and narrowing of the tarsal navicular. Irregular ossification in this bone may be the rule rather than the exception, so that the existence of this condition is in question (Fig. 23–10). Thirty percent of males and 20% of females have irregular ossification in the tarsal navicular [31]. Most patients seem to respond to 6 weeks of immobilization in a cast. In the series of Williams and Cowell [31], all 23 patients eventually became asymptomatic, and the navicular became normal. The authors believed that patients treated in a cast became asymptomatic sooner than those treated with shoe inserts. There are no long-term problems from this condition, again raising the question of whether it is a distinct pathologic condition.

Freiberg's infarction is a condition of condensation and collapse of the metatarsal head and articular surface. It commonly occurs in the second decade of life while the epiphysis is still present [13]. It is of unknown cause and is more common in females. Many causes have been proposed, but repetitive trauma probably plays a role. The lesion occurs most commonly in the second or third metatarsal [23]. These are the longest and least mobile of the metatarsals. The patient presents with pain on weight bearing and has localized tenderness over the metatarsal head. Radiographs reveal collapse of the articular surface. Conservative treatment with a cast or orthotic device that minimizes weight bearing over the involved head is often successful in relieving the pain. Surgical treatment consisting of removal of loose bodies or bone grafting has been reported for persistent symptoms. A dorsiflexion osteotomy to relieve weight bearing has also been reported to work well. Removal of the metatarsal head should be avoided because this will result in transfer of weight bearing to the adjacent metatarsal heads. Prosthetic replacement has also been tried but is not indicated in children. In most instances the disease runs its course, and the head reossifies in 2 to 3 years.

Sever's disease is a term used to refer to a nonarticular osteochondrosis or a traction apophysitis. The real question is whether a distinct syndrome exists and, if it does, whether the apophysis has anything to do with it. The calcaneal apophysis appears and develops in the 5- to

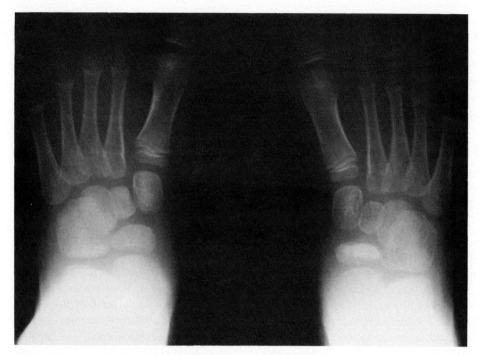

FIGURE 23–10
This patient presented with undisplaced fractures of the metatarsals. The condensed narrowed appearance of the navicular is the same as that seen in patients with Kohler's syndrome but was an incidental finding in this patient.

12-year-old age range and is typically irregular. Often a child with heel pain and an irregular apophysis has the same radiographic finding in the opposite asymptomatic heel. These children are usually in the 9- to 12-year-old age range and are active in sports. They may have a tight heel cord. The calcaneus serves as the insertion of the powerful gastrocnemius-soleus muscle and the origin of the plantar fascia. Traction or overuse can strain these structures, producing pain. Stretching may be beneficial. Symptomatic treatment by avoidance of the offending exercise is usually curative. Shock-absorbing insoles may be advantageous. A heel lift to relieve some of the pull of the gastrocnemius-soleus or at times an arch support for a child with a high arch may give symptomatic relief as well. Heel cord stretching exercises may be tried. One must carefully search for the point of maximum tenderness and seek its cause rather than implicating an irregular apophysis, which is probably not a part of the problem. The exact time frame for resolution of symptoms in children with heel pain is unknown and at times can be vexing. If I feel that the child has followed the above conservative measures and is no better after 6 to 8 weeks, I then proceed with a further workup such as a bone scan and other studies to seek more occult sources of the pain.

SYSTEMIC ILLNESS

Systemic illness can present with foot pain and must be remembered in the athlete as well as in other children. Rheumatoid arthritis can involve the subtalar joint. Os-teomyelitis can involve the foot but is unusual unless there is a history of a puncture wound. Acute lympho-cytic leukemia is a great masquerader and can infiltrate the bones of the foot. Although they are very rare, these sorts of diseases must be considered. One cannot develop tunnel vision and believe that all pain in an athlete is of traumatic origin.

SHOES AND ORTHOTICS

The athletic shoe business is a lucrative one as shown by the intense marketing and competition for the introduction of new technology and an edge in the marketplace. There is very little scientific evidence to support the hype associated with shoe sales. More often the advertisements depict current sports heroes wearing shoewear on the high end of the price scale and tell us little about the shoes themselves. The models and range of widths available are more limited for children. Athletic shoes should fit adequately in both width and length. The material should be reasonably soft. Too often children's athletic shoes are made of stiff, unyielding synthetic material and are poorly padded around the heel counter. Multisport shoes with small-diameter, evenly spaced cleats that distribute weight bearing more evenly are preferable to cleated or studded shoes. Padding over the heel counter and ankle may increase comfort. Most shoes now come with a built-in arch support that has very little scientific basis but may give some support to children with a well-developed arch. Those with a flatter foot may actually find it necessary to remove the pad.

Orthotics are another area of controversy. An asymptomatic flexible flatfoot should be left alone. There is no evidence to support the idea that an orthotic will bring about any structural change in such a foot. A painful flatfoot should prompt a thorough search for its cause such as a tarsal coalition. Orthotics may be tried in a patient with aching feet or shins and a flexible flatfoot. Heel cups may be beneficial in the symptomatic treatment of heel pain. There is little if any scientific information available about the use of sports orthotics in children.

References

1. Acker, J. H., and Drez, D., Jr. Non-operative treatment of stress fractures of the proximal shaft of the fifth metatarsal (Jones' fracture). *Foot Ankle* 7:152–155, 1986.
2. Anderson, I. F., Crichton, K. J., Gratton-Smith, T., et al. Osteochondral fractures of the dome of the talus. *J Bone Joint Surg* 71A:1143–1152, 1989.
3. Bennet, G. L., Weiner, D. S., and Leighley, B. Surgical treatment of symptomatic accessory tarsal navicular. *J Pediatr Orthop* (In press, 1993).
4. Berndt, A. L., and Harty, M. Transchondral fractures (osteochondritis dissecans) of the talus. *J Bone Joint Surg* 41A:988–1020, 1959.
5. Bonney, G., and McNab, I. Hallux valgus and hallux rigidus. A critical appraisal of operative results. *J Bone Joint Surg* 34B:366–385, 1952.
6. Canale, S. T., and Belding, R. H. Osteochondral lesions of the talus. *J Bone Joint Surg* 62A:97–102, 1980.
7. Cooperman, D. R., Spiegel, P. G., and Laros, G. R. Tibial fractures involving the ankle in children: The so-called triplane epiphyseal fracture. *J Bone Joint Surg* 60A:1040–1046, 1978.
8. Coughlin, M. J., and Mann, R. A. The pathophysiology of juvenile bunion. *Instr Course Lect* 36:123–136, 1987.
9. Cowell, H. R. Diagnosis and management of peroneal spastic flatfoot. *Instr Course Lect* 24:94–103, 1975.
10. Dias, L. S., and Giergerich, C. R. Fractures of the distal tibial epiphysis in adolescence. *J Bone Joint Surg* 65A:438–444, 1983.
11. Dugan, G., Herndon, W. H., and McGuire, R. Distal tibial physeal injuries in children: A different treatment concept. *J Orthop Trauma* 1:63–67, 1987.
12. Ertl, J. P., Barrack, R. L., Alexander, A. H., et al. Triplane fracture of the distal tibial epiphysis. *J Bone Joint Surg* 70A:967–976, 1989.
13. Gauthier, G., and Elbaz, R. Freiberg's infarction: A subchondral bone fatigue fracture. *Clin Orthop* 142:93–95, 1979.
14. Gerzenberg, J. E., Goldner, J. L., Martinez, S., et al. Computerized tomography of talocalcaneal tarsal coalition: A clinical and anatomic study. *Foot Ankle* 6:273–288, 1986.
15. Harris, B. J. Anomalous structures in the developing human foot. (Abstract) *Anat Rec* 121:399, 1955.
16. Jayakumar, S., and Cowell, H. R. Rigid flatfoot. *Clin Orthop* 122:77–84, 1977.
17. Kavanaugh, J. H., Brower, T. D., and Mann, R. V. The Jones fracture revisited. *J Bone Joint Surg* 60A:776–782, 1978.
18. Kidner, F. C. The pre-hallux in relation to flatfoot. *JAMA* 101:1539, 1933.
19. Lehman, R. C., Torg, J. S., Pavlov, H., et al. Fractures of the base of the fifth metatarsal distal to the tuberosity: A review. *Foot Ankle* 7:245–252, 1987.
20. Olney, B. W., and Asher, M. A. Tarsal coalition and peroneal spastic flatfoot: A review. *J Bone Joint Surg* 66A:976–984, 1984.
21. Olney, B. W., and Asher, M. A. Excision of symptomatic coalition of the middle facet of the talocalcaneal joint. *J Bone Joint Surg* 69A:539–544, 1987.
22. Peterson, H., and Cass, J. R. Salter-Harris IV injuries of the distal tibial epiphysis. *J Bone Joint Surg* 65A:1059, 1983.
23. Pizzutillo, P. The osteochondroses. *In* Sullivan, J. A., and Grana, W. A. (Eds.), *The Pediatric Athlete: Guidelines to Participation.* Park Ridge, IL, American Academy of Orthopedic Surgeons, 1990.
24. Poll, R. G. The treatment of recurrent dislocation of the peroneal tendons. *J Bone Joint Surg* 66B:98–100, 1984.
25. Rang, M. *Children's Fractures* (2nd ed.). Philadelphia, J. B. Lippincott, 1983.
26. Scranton, P. E., Jr. Treatment of symptomatic talocalcaneal coalition. *J Bone Joint Surg* 69A:533–539, 1987.
27. Scranton, P. E., Jr., and Zuckerman, J. D. Bunion surgery in adolescents: The results of treatment. *J Pediatr Orthop* 4:39–43, 1984.
28. Spiegel, P. G., Cooperman, D. R., and Laros, G. S. Epiphyseal fractures of the distal end of the tibia and fibula. *J Bone Joint Surg* 60A:1096, 1978.
29. Sullivan, J. A., and Miller, W. A. The relationship of the accessory navicular to the development of the flatfoot. *Clin Orthop* 144:233–237, 1979.
30. Swintkowski, M. F., Scranton, P. E., Jr., and Hansen, S. Tarsal coalitions: Long-term results of surgical treatment. *J Pediatr Orthop* 3:287–292, 1983.
31. Williams, G. A., and Cowell, H. R. Kohler's disease of the tarsal navicular. *Clin Orthop* 158:53–58, 1981.
32. Yngve, D. A. Stress fractures in children. *In* Sullivan, J. A., and Grana, W. A. (Eds.), *The Pediatric Athlete: Guidelines to Participation.* Park Ridge, IL, American Academy of Orthopedic Surgeons, 1990.

IMAGING

George W. Gross, M.D.

Although less prone to injury than adults, children and adolescents are subject to a wide variety of sports-related musculoskeletal injuries [1–4, 6, 11, 12, 18, 27, 28, 30, 32, 39, 46, 48, 54, 64, 66, 70, 95, 97, 103, 106, 107, 109, 126, 132, 137, 139, 141, 143, 146–148, 152–155, 157, 160, 166–168]. These injuries are of two types: acute, following episodes of macrotrauma, and overuse injuries resulting from repetitive unrepaired microtrauma [74, 100, 148]. This chapter focuses on the applicability and limitations of various imaging techniques to the identification and assessment of sports-related musculoskeletal injuries in the child and adolescent.

Strains and sprains account for almost two-thirds of sports-related injuries [47]. The pattern of injury often reflects the nature of the athletic activity involved. For example, cranial and facial trauma occurs with a higher frequency in ice hockey, whereas gymnastics and figure skating, which are associated with significant repetitive low back stress, are associated with a prevalence of lower back injuries [54, 110]. In girls' high school athletics, injury rates and the need for radiographic evaluation are greatest for softball, cross-country running, and gymnastics [47].

Bone injury in children can differ from that in adults in several ways: The growing ends of long bones are commonly affected, carrying the potential for subsequent growth damage and deformity; the capacity for anatomic correction, with growth and remodeling, is considerable in the child; and slight overlap of fragment ends on reduction may be preferable to end-to-end apposition because of increased growth in fractured bone [59]. Compared to the adult, the child's bone is more flexible, predisposing it to plastic deformation (bending) with trauma [118]. As a consequence, traumatic forces that in the adult might produce gross fracture may result in a bowing or torus fracture in the child [118].

Unique to the immature skeleton are fractures involving the physis or growth plate [74, 125]. The Salter-Harris classification of physeal injuries, the most widely used classification, divides such fractures into five basic types depending on the pattern of involvement of the adjacent ossified bone: type I (physis involved alone, 6%); type II (physis and metaphysis, 75%); type III (physis and epiphysis, 8%); type IV (vertical fracture through a portion of the metaphysis, the physis, and the epiphysis, 10%); and type V (crush injury to physis, 1%) [74, 125, 130, 149].

The most common locations of fractures in children are the clavicle, proximal end of the humerus, supracondylar portion of the humerus, midshaft and distal third of the radius and ulna (the most common fracture of childhood), fracture separation of the distal radial epiphysis (the most common growth plate injury), midshaft of the femur, and tibial shaft [59].

Children and adolescents are at risk for overuse injuries resulting from a wide range of athletic activities [99]. These injuries include stress fractures, tendinitides of the shoulder, ankle, elbow, or hips, and the patellofemoral stress syndrome of the knee [99]. All of the major structural components of the extremities and torso (muscle-tendon units, ligaments, bone, and articular cartilage) are potential sites of overuse injury in children and adolescents [99]. Stress fractures most commonly involve the tibia and fibula but occur at numerous additional sites [99, 161]. Tendinitis usually occurs at the site of tendon insertion, the apophysis, which usually becomes symptomatic before the tendon itself does [99].

ANATOMIC DIFFERENCES BETWEEN THE MATURE AND IMMATURE SKELETON

All skeletal components initially form as mesenchymal cellular condensations in utero [84, 110]. The appendicular and axial skeleton derives from the initial transformation of the mesenchymal model to cartilage, which is subsequently changed to bone by two discrete processes: (1) the formation of an osseous collar around the midshaft of the cartilaginous anlage with associated vascular invasion forming the primary ossification center; and (2) a later osseous transformation of the cartilaginous epiphysis forming the secondary or epiphyseal ossification center at the bone end, a process termed "endochondral ossification" [74, 84, 110].

Subsequent growth of any particular bone after this initial differentiation may involve discrete, juxtaposed, or interspersed areas of both basic patterns within the same bone [86, 110]. Endochondral-derived bones generally undergo intramembranous ossification by appositional bone growth from the periosteum [110]. Membranous bone may subsequently grow and elongate by means of a modified endochondral process (e.g., the clavicle) [110].

The diaphysis develops primarily by endosteal and periosteal remodeling and bone formation [110]. During childhood, increasingly complex Haversian systems and increased intercellular matrix develop, which increases the hardness of cortical bone [110]. Compared to the mature (adult) bone, the periosteum in childhood is much thicker, more vascular, more loosely attached to the underlying diaphysis, and capable of more rigid callus formation in response to a similar degree of injury [110]. The periosteum serves as the origin for most muscle fibers along the metaphysis and diaphysis, permitting coordinated growth of bone and muscle units [110].

The metaphyses in childhood are characterized by variably contoured flaring, decreased thickness of the cortical bone and increased amounts of trabecular bone comprising both primary and secondary spongiosa [110]. The metaphysis is the site of greatest metabolic activity and bone turnover during childhood [110]. The metaphyseal region does not develop significant Haversian systems until skeletal maturity approaches [110]. In contrast to the diaphysis, the periosteum is more firmly fixed to the metaphysis [110]. As in the diaphysis, there are no significant direct muscle attachments into the metaphyseal bone; instead, muscle fibers blend primarily into the periosteum [110].

At birth, each epiphysis is a completely cartilaginous structure at both ends of each long bone (with the exception of the distal femur) [110]. At a time characteristic for each cartilaginous epiphysis, a secondary center of ossification gradually enlarges until, at skeletal maturity, virtually the entire cartilage model has been replaced by bone, leaving only articular cartilage unossified [110]. The pattern of development of the secondary ossification center is thought to affect its susceptibility to certain injury, including fracture patterns [110]. As the osseous tissue expands, the ossification center imparts increasing rigidity to the more resilient epiphyseal cartilage [110].

The physis is the essential mechanism of endochondral ossification both prenatally and postnatally [110]. Although most physes maintain their basic structural contour throughout development, a few undergo major changes [110]. Among the latter are the proximal humerus and the proximal femur, which change from initially transverse to highly contoured structures with growth [110].

There are two basic types of growth plates: discoid and spherical [110]. Most primary growth plates of the major long bones are discoid and are characterized by a relatively planar area of rapidly differentiating and maturing cartilage that grades imperceptibly from the epiphyseal hyaline cartilage [110]. As they respond to subsequent growth and biomechanical stresses, most discoid physes assume a characteristic contour while retaining their basic planar nature [110]. The spherical growth plate, which is the major growth mechanism of the epiphyseal ossification center, gradually assumes the contours of the particular bone or physis by means of progressive centrifugal expansion [110].

RADIOLOGIC DIFFERENCES BETWEEN THE MATURE AND IMMATURE SKELETON

The presence of skeletal immaturity and the associated variable degree of incomplete ossification of the child's skeleton introduces several unique and potentially confusing aspects to musculoskeletal imaging in children.

The imaging appearance of various musculoskeletal structures in the child reflects the mode of imaging employed and the histologic and chemical nature of the specific anatomic part. Conventional radiography and tomography cannot differentiate between various water-density soft tissue structures such as tendons, ligaments, muscles, and unossified cartilage but can differentiate between calcium, fat, air, and water-density tissues. Computed tomography (CT) is more sensitive in identifying calcium but has limited ability to differentiate between different soft tissue structures. Magnetic resonance imaging (MRI) can differentiate between different types of cartilage and has proved to be excellent at identifying a variety of soft tissue abnormalities. However, MRI is inferior to CT and plain film radiography in defining the finer anatomic details of the calcified osseous structures. Radionuclide examination depends on the incorporation of radioactive isotopes into tissues of differing metabolic activity. Although they are highly sensitive in identifying certain musculoskeletal traumatic abnormalities, bone scanning and other radionuclide procedures have poor spatial resolution and therefore provide limited anatomic detail. The pediatric skeleton, owing to the normal increase in activity at the growth plates, presents a unique scintigraphic appearance on bone scans.

The normal growth plate appears as a radiolucent zone between the epiphysis and the metaphysis of a long bone on radiographs and CT scans but is dark on MRI images due to limited signal emission [84]. The radiolucent portion of the growth plate consists of the resting, proliferating, and hypertrophic zones, all made up of nonmineralized cartilage [84]. A fourth, or calcifying, zone is partially radiodense due to matrix calcification [84].

Trauma can produce a variety of abnormal radiographic appearances of the growth plate [149]. Growth plate injuries account for 30% of fractures in children [93]. Widening can result from Salter-Harris epiphyseal-metaphyseal fractures; the fracture line characteristically passes through the hypertrophic zone, the weakest point in the growth plate [84, 86]. Narrowing can result from Salter-Harris type V compression fractures, which are notoriously difficult to identify even when comparison radiographs of the contralateral normal bone are available [84]. An irregular contour of the growth plate can result from Salter-Harris fractures types I to IV as well as from many nontraumatic disorders [84, 86, 149].

APPROACH TO IMAGING OF PEDIATRIC AND ADOLESCENT SPORTS INJURIES

Selection of Patients for Imaging

Patient history can be a significant factor in the determination of whether or not an imaging procedure needs to be done, what anatomic areas require imaging, what imaging procedure should be done, and how the patient should be handled. For example, the acute onset of localized pain in a case of documented trauma would merit imaging as part of patient evaluation. More chronic symptoms of lesser severity often require imaging for proper evaluation as well.

The type of athletic activity producing a certain degree and location of symptoms (i.e., back pain) may influence the need for imaging studies; for example, radiographic evaluation of the back in a runner with lower back pain would be less likely to demonstrate positive findings than images in a gymnast with similar symptoms.

Additionally, a history of symptoms and athletic activity can be significant in determining whether supplemental imaging procedures are warranted when the initial radiographic examination is normal (e.g., should a bone scan be obtained for foot pain in a runner with normal foot radiographs?).

Positive physical findings (e.g., soft tissue swelling, deformities) and localization of pain are obviously of paramount importance in defining the scope of any imaging procedure in children and adolescents with athletic injuries. However, referred pain can be misleading about the site of primary abnormality (e.g., a hip abnormality in a child may produce pain referred to the knee).

A falling hematocrit in a patient subjected to acute trauma could signify extensive bleeding within soft tissues (including muscles) or contained areas such as the peritoneal cavity and may warrant more extensive imaging with CT or MRI. An elevated sedimentation rate in the appropriate setting might suggest infection and might warrant a three-phase bone scan to assess for possible septic arthritis or osteomyelitis.

Because clothing can produce a variety of artifactual shadows in various imaging procedures, it is advisable to remove as much of the patient's clothing overlying the area being imaged as possible. Special considerations for MRI include removal of any external metallic objects, which can accelerate to high speed in the magnetic field and present a hazard to the patient.

In the usual situation involving imaging of the injured athlete, sufficient voluntary cooperation is present so that patient restraints are not required. Occasionally, gentle positional stabilization of the extremity or patient restraint may be required. The nature and severity of some injuries may necessitate passive patient movement. Occasionally, patients sustaining acute trauma may be dazed or confused and are therefore unable to remain immobile during imaging procedures. A technical assistant in attendance during the procedure will permit patient monitoring and stabilization.

RADIATION PROTECTION AND REDUCTION

Although radiation exposure is important regardless of patient age, greater consideration should be given to minimizing exposure when imaging the pediatric or adolescent patient, including but not limited to imaging in circumstances of musculoskeletal trauma.

Staff. Anyone required to aid in patient positioning must be given appropriate radiation protection. When a child or adolescent must be restrained during imaging, it is often best to enlist the aid of the parent or other person not normally engaged in radiographic work [9]. Parents especially may be best able to calm and reassure an injured child [9]. Assistants should wear lead aprons and (depending on the proximity of hands to the irradiated field) lead gloves in the radiographic room [9].

Patient. Many factors contribute to minimizing patient radiation exposure. Proper positioning aids (restraints, sandbags, sponges) and exposure factors (MAS, kV) help to reduce the need for radiographic retakes [9]. Proper collimation decreases exposure and increases image quality; through collimation, only the area(s) of clinical interest should be radiographed [9]. Gonadal shielding with lead aprons should be used routinely, especially when the gonads lie within 5 cm of the primary beam (assuming that critical anatomic information will not be obscured by use of a gonadal shield) [9].

To ensure that a patient with an unknown pregnancy is not irradiated, all postmenarchal teenage girls should be interviewed for the date of their last menstrual period. Radiographic procedures on potentially pregnant girls should be postponed, if clinically possible, to satisfy the 10-day rule, which states that radiographic examinations should be performed only during the first 10 days following the onset of menstruation, when a potential pregnancy can be reliably excluded.

All imaging studies must be performed by a properly trained and licensed radiologic technician. For many types of imaging procedures (e.g., CT, MRI, nuclear medicine), more specialized technical training with the specific imaging modality is preferred in order to optimize imaging quality.

IMAGING OPTIONS (Table 24–1)

Plain Film Radiography

Conventional plain film radiography remains the mainstay for the diagnostic imaging evaluation of most orthopedic problems [9]. Only in very limited circumstances is a single projection adequate for evaluation of a possible musculoskeletal abnormality. More typically, two projections, preferably taken at a 90-degree orientation

to each other, constitute the minimum acceptable radiographic examination [8, 130] (Fig. 24–1). Depending on the clinical circumstances and specific needs, additional supplemental radiographic projections may be obtained [8, 130] (Fig. 24–2). There are a large number of specialized radiographic projections related to specific anatomic areas [59, 96].

Magnification and high-resolution radiography is a variation of conventional radiography that employs a small focal spot x-ray tube and a high-resolution x-ray film system to improve anatomic detail and reveal subtle signs of fracture in sports-related injuries [8, 56].

Stress Views

In some circumstances, a ligamentous injury to a joint will not be apparent on conventional radiographs unless ''stress views'' are obtained to demonstrate the excess motion at the site of injury [8]. Application of graded stress to the affected joint by a physician or assistant is usually required. Patient discomfort may dictate the amount of stress that can be applied. Joint instability secondary to ligamentous injury may occur with (Fig. 24–3) or without (Fig. 24–4) an associated fracture.

Fluoroscopy

Fluoroscopic imaging, which provides continuous monitoring of a site of interest, is only infrequently used

TABLE 24–1
Selection of Imaging Modality in Pediatric Athletes

Imaging Modality	Advantages	Disadvantages
Conventional radiography	Universal availability Variation in projection Lower cost (relative) Highest anatomic resolution	Radiation exposure Poor differentiation of soft tissue structures
Ultrasonography	Widely available Variation in projection Lower cost No radiation	Cannot image bone or through air Application to soft tissue structures only
CT	Excellent bone–soft tissue differentiation Good anatomic detail Three-dimensional capability	Limited imaging planes Radiation exposure (relatively higher) Cost (moderate)
Conventional tomography	High resolution Imaging in predetermined planes	Radiation exposure (relatively high) Longer examination time
MRI	Excellent soft-tissue differentiation Unique soft tissue evaluation No radiation exposure	Not universally available Higher cost Longer examination time
Nuclear medicine	Physiologic information Lower radiation dosage Unique imaging features	Cost (moderate) Long examination time Poor anatomic detail

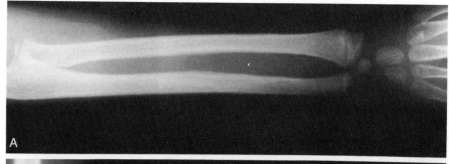

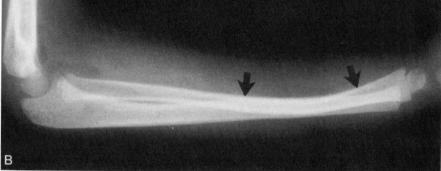

FIGURE 24–1

Plastic or bowing fracture of forearm. This 5-year-old boy sustained a laterally directed blow to his left forearm when a playmate fell on him. The AP view *(A)* demonstrates no abnormality. A plastic or bowing fracture of the radius is demonstrated (arrows) only on the lateral projection *(B)*. The ulna is intact. This case illustrates the importance of obtaining at least two radiographic views, preferably at right angles to each other, in all cases of trauma to the extremities.

in orthopedic radiology outside of the operating room, where it can be invaluable in assisting in fracture fragment positioning and in assessing the position of orthopedic devices during their internal placement. Fluoroscopy may also show the degree of angulation of fracture fragments, demonstrate abnormal motion through a fracture, and identify ligamentous injury [8]. Fluoroscopy can result in significant supplemental patient radiation exposure and should be used judiciously.

Conventional Tomography

Conventional tomography (laminography, planography, body section radiography) provides an image of a selected plane in the body while blurring structures above and below that plane [9]. Compared to CT, conventional tomography has greater resolution and therefore may be able to define subtle fracture lines not seen on radiographs or CT scans [8] (Fig. 24–5). Tomographic motions can be simple (linear) or complex (circular, hypocycloidal, elliptical, or trispiral) [9]. For evaluating skeletal structures (which have inherent high contrast) wide angle tomography using an arc of 30 to 50 degrees is usually preferred [9].

Potential orthopedic indications for tomography include better evaluation of metallic fixation devices and acute trauma (using linear motion) and evaluation of subtle fractures, stress fractures, and fracture healing (with more complex motion tomography) [9] (Fig. 24–6). The primary limitations of tomography are the ability

of the patient to remain immobile during the exposure and restrictions on patient positioning [9].

Xeroradiography

Introduced in 1952, xeroradiography was formerly used in mammography and for evaluation of bone and soft tissue disorders of the extremities, but it is rarely if ever utilized at present in orthopedic disorders. Xeroradiography was useful in the past for detecting subtle fractures and providing better bone detail through cast material [9].

Ultrasonography

The advantages of ultrasonography in general are the absence of radiation exposure, lack of known adverse biologic effects, and ability to show on image in a wide variety of planes [9]. Ultrasonography cannot show calcified (e.g., bone) or air-containing (e.g., bowel) structures.

Applications of ultrasonography to orthopedics are limited to the evaluation of soft tissue structures [8, 9]. Ultrasonography can easily distinguish fluid collections (which are echo-free) from solid tissues (which are echogenic due to internal tissue plane interfaces) [9]. The evaluation of the popliteal fossa is an important musculoskeletal application of ultrasonography because it permits differentiation of popliteal artery aneurysms, poplit-

Text continued on page 465

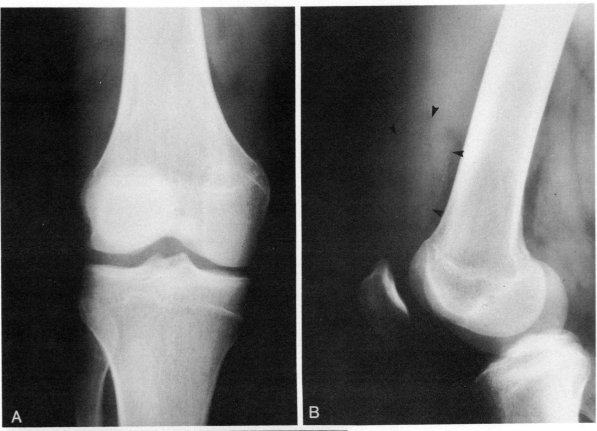

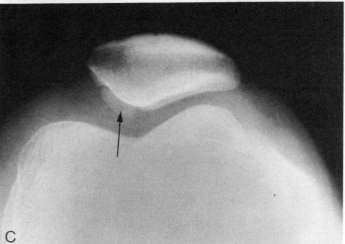

FIGURE 24–2

Post-traumatic osteochondral fracture. This 17-year-old football player had persistent left knee pain following a direct blow. Radiographic evaluation 4 weeks after injury consisted of AP *(A),* lateral *(B),* and skyline *(C)* views. The AP view is unremarkable. The lateral view demonstrates a large suprapatellar bursal effusion (arrowheads) but no fracture. The skyline view alone identifies a nonunited osteochondral fracture of the posterior patellar margin (arrow).

The lateral projection of the knee is best for identifying joint fluid, which tends to localize in the suprapatellar bursa. Nonroutine views (oblique, tunnel, skyline) may be required to identify atypical or subtle fractures, as in this patient.

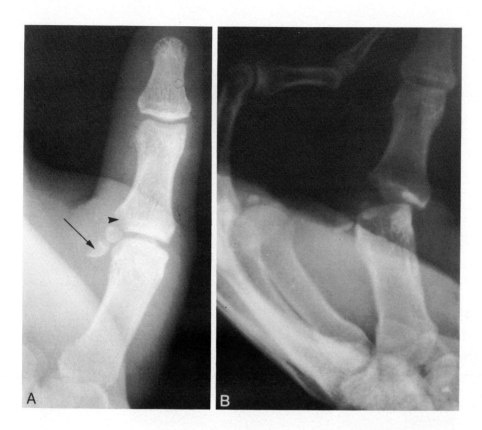

FIGURE 24–3
Game-keeper's thumb. This 16-year-old basketball player sustained an injury to the left thumb while going up for a rebound. The initial AP view *(A)* demonstrates an avulsion fracture (arrow) displaced from its site of origin at the base of the proximal phalanx (arrowhead). The first metacarpal-phalangeal joint appears grossly normal. A stress view *(B)* demonstrates subluxation of the thumb and marked widening of the medial joint space due to associated ligamentous injury and secondary joint instability. Stress views may be required to fully evaluate post-traumatic joint damage.

FIGURE 24–4
Stress views for ligamentous injury. This 14-year-old basketball player had a prior ankle injury but without fracture. Persistence of ankle discomfort led to additional stress views of both ankles being made. The inversion stress AP view of the symptomatic ankle *(A)* demonstrates excessive widening of the lateral portion of the ankle joint space, reflecting lateral ligamentous injury. The inversion stress AP view of the opposite ankle *(B),* made for comparison, is normal.

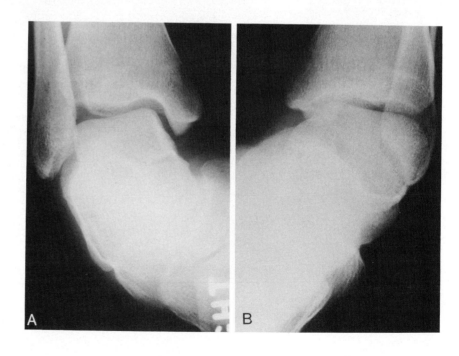

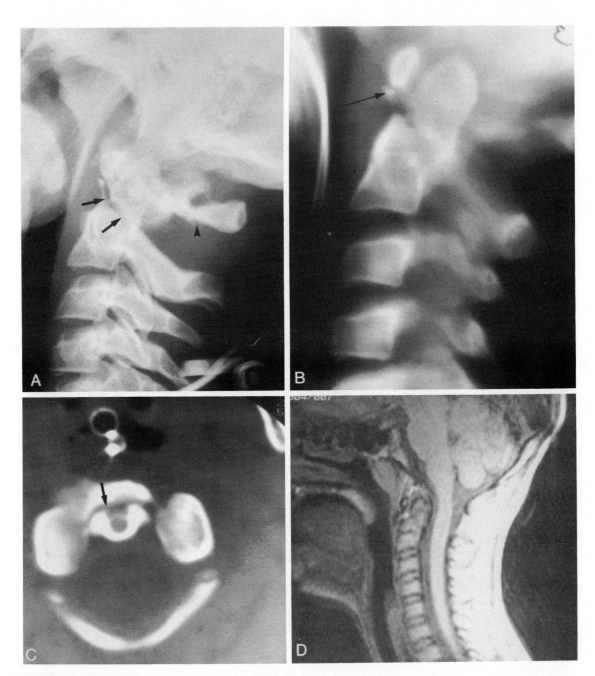

FIGURE 24–5

Fractures of C1 and C2. This 14-year-old diver struck the bottom of the pool and was pulled from the water unconscious. Lateral radiograph of the cervical spine with halo immobilization device in place *(A)* demonstrates an oblique radiolucent line at the base of the odontoid process of C2, representing a fracture (arrows). A second fracture of the neural arch of C1 is suggested (arrowhead). Lateral tomogram of the cervical spine *(B)* confirms the C2 fracture and also identifies a small fracture fragment from C2 displaced beneath the anterior margin of C1 (arrow). The fracture of the neural arch of C1 is not in the plane of tomography and therefore cannot be identified here. Axial CT through C2 *(C)* confirms the odontoid fracture (arrow). Midsagittal plane MRI of the cervical region *(D)* shows slight posterior displacement of the C2 fracture with minimal compression of the upper cervical cord. The cervical cord itself appears intrinsically normal. The patient suffered no permanent neurologic damage.

Although most vertebral fractures are definable by conventional radiographs, improved fracture definition is usually provided by thin-section, complex motion tomography or CT. Conventional tomography should be performed, in most cases, in both the AP and lateral planes of imaging to optimize the definition of fracture or subluxation. CT is optimal for identifying neural arch fractures and any fracture extension into the neural canal but may miss a vertebral fracture when it is aligned primarily with the axial imaging plane employed with CT. MRI demonstrates vertebral fractures and any fragment displacement, although not as well as either conventional tomography or CT, and it is unsurpassed at identifying encroachment on or damage to the spinal cord.

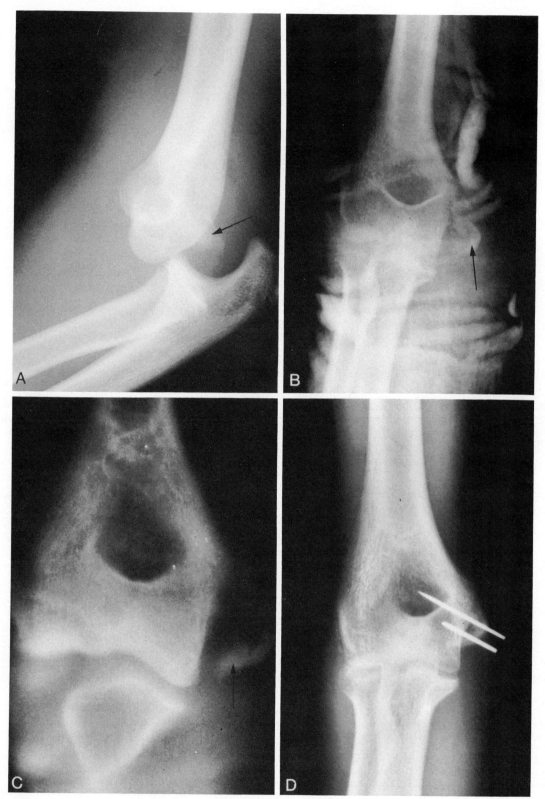

FIGURE 24–6

Avulsion fracture of medial humeral epicondyle. This 14-year-old ice hockey player fell hard onto the ice and experienced a sharp pain in his elbow. Lateral projection *(A)* demonstrates complete posterior dislocation at the elbow with an associated avulsion fracture of the medial humeral epicondyle (arrow) displaced into the joint space. Following closed reduction and immobilization in a cast, an AP radiograph *(B)* shows satisfactory reduction of the dislocation. The medial epicondylar fracture fragment is partially obscured by overlying cast density but appears to be separated from its site of origin by up to 10 mm (arrow). Subsequent tomogram of the casted elbow in the AP projection *(C)* confirms the separation (arrow shows the medial epicondylar fragment). Open reduction with pinning was required to obtain acceptable and stable fragment reduction *(D)*.

eal cysts, abscesses, hematomas, and malignant tumors [8, 9]. Additionally, patients with acute calf pain can be evaluated for suspected thrombophlebitis [9]. Although it is used to some degree in the evaluation of possible rotator cuff tears of the shoulder, ultrasonography is less sensitive and specific than arthrography and MRI [8, 23].

Ultrasonography can contribute to the assessment of sports injuries, including hematomas and muscle tears [62]. Hematomas usually present as anechoic fluid collections [62]. A torn or ruptured muscle may have a different echogenic pattern than an intact uninjured muscle [62].

Computed Tomography

Modern CT scanners produce images with superior image contrast but less spatial resolution than routine radiographs [9]. CT provides better differentiation of soft tissue planes than conventional radiographs, and the transverse (axial) orientation of CT images is frequently an important supplement to conventional radiographic examination of skeletal structures [9].

Spine CT scans should consist of a set of axial-plane images that completely cover the area of suspected pathology [133] (see Fig. 24–5). CT images are typically photographed twice, once to display soft tissue and the other to show bony detail [133]. Reformatted images in the sagittal and coronal planes may be added [133].

CT is particularly useful in defining bone structure in areas of complex anatomy such as the pelvis, hips, sacrum, spine, shoulders, and face [8, 9, 87, 109] (Fig. 24–

7). In addition, areas such as the sternoclavicular joints that are not easily displayed on routine radiographs may be well demonstrated on the cross-sectional images of CT [9]. Occult fractures, especially in the spine, that are not visible on plain films or tomography are often identified on CT [9]. CT is particularly valuable for evaluating the spine following trauma; in addition to fractures, CT can demonstrate bone, disc material, blood, or foreign bodies in the spinal canal [8, 9, 63, 109] (Fig. 24–8). CT can accurately detect soft tissue injuries and is particularly valuable in evaluating the abdomen after trauma [9]. CT is effective at imaging a variety of appendicular skeletal injuries and other abnormalities including fractures, osteochondritis dissecans, and dislocations that may be difficult to identify on conventional radiographs [105] (Fig. 24–9).

In general, the radiation dose delivered by CT scanning is greater than that needed for a conventional radiographic study but less than that for conventional tomograms of the same anatomic area [9]. CT doses can vary from less than 1 rad to greater than 10 rads [9]. Limitations of CT, in addition to greater radiation dosage and higher cost, are its lack of ability to define horizontal fractures of the spine, vertebral body compression fractures, and some subluxations [9].

Three-Dimensional Computed Tomography

More recently, computer programs have been developed that permit three-dimensional computed tomo-

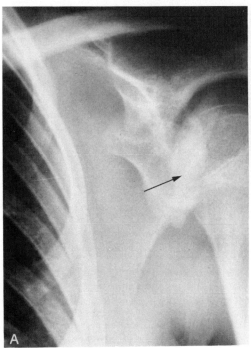

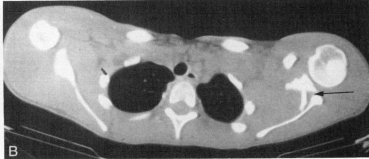

FIGURE 24–7
Comminuted fracture of scapula. This 15-year-old cyclist flipped over the handlebars, sustaining an injury to the left shoulder region. An AP radiograph of the left shoulder *(A)* demonstrates irregular deformity of the subglenoid region of the left scapula (arrow), indicating a probable fracture. However, the exact pattern of fracture as well as the direction and degree of fragment displacement is not well defined. An axial CT image *(B)* better demonstrates the true nature of the comminuted scapular fracture (arrow) and the pattern of fragment displacement. Computed tomography is frequently essential for optimal definition of complex fractures with fragment displacement.

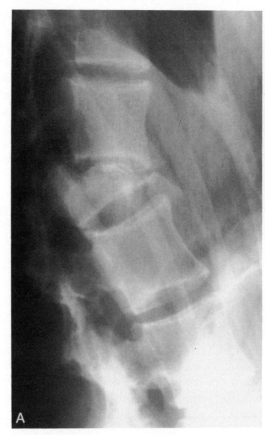

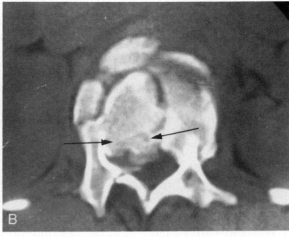

FIGURE 24–8
Comminuted fracture of L1. This 15-year-old equestrian was thrown off her horse while going over a jump. *A*, Lateral radiograph of the thoracolumbar spine demonstrates a severe compression fracture of L1 with both anterior and posterior fragment extension and a secondary gibbus angulation deformity. *B*, Axial plane CT image without intrathecal contrast nicely demonstrates the severe vertebral compression fracture as well as the marked fragment extension into the neural canal (arrows).

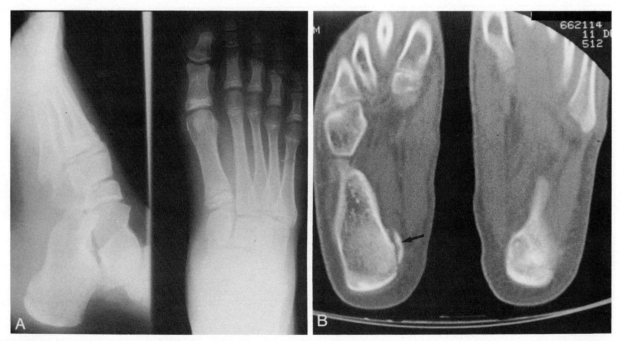

FIGURE 24–9
Calcaneal fracture demonstrated with CT. Fourteen-year-old youth with severe pain in left hindfoot following trauma. AP and lateral views of the foot *(A)* are normal. Noncontrast coronal plane CT of the foot *(B)* demonstrates an avulsion fracture of the medial aspect of the posterior portion of the right calcaneus (arrow). CT is excellent for demonstrating subtle fractures that may not be adequately depicted on plain radiographs.

graphic reconstruction and display of anatomic abnormalities. These have particular applicability to certain complex fractures (e.g., craniofacial, shoulder, and pelvic fractures) [41, 42, 82, 86]. The advantages of three-dimensional CT need to be weighed against the additional expense and procedure time needed for the examination. The addition of two- and three-dimensional CT imaging to conventional radiography can alter patient management and performance of surgery in 20% to 30% of orthopedic patients [42].

Magnetic Resonance Imaging

The primary advantages of MRI in musculoskeletal imaging are its high soft tissue contrast, which allows good differentiation between various soft tissue structures; absence of bone artifact (in contrast to CT); availability of a variety of pulse sequences to improve definition of abnormal processes; and absence of any known adverse biologic effects [9, 61, 75]. The use of limited flip-angle, gradient-recalled pulse sequences such as GRASS and fast low-angle shots (FLASH) have proved highly valuable in pediatric patients [80]. The disadvantages of MRI include its lack of cortical bone detail (compared to conventional radiographs and CT) and its relatively high cost [9]. Ferromagnetic contrast agents are increasingly used in MRI, further improving the differentiation of pathologic processes from normal structures [9]. With technical improvements in MRI, the previous long scanning time required is being significantly reduced.

Contraindications to the use of MRI at present are limited to the presence of cardiac pacemakers (which may revert to the asynchronous mode) or cerebral aneurysm clips (which could potentially change orientation or position within a magnetic field and perhaps induce hemorrhage). Neither is of practical concern in the child or adolescent with a sports-related injury. Orthopedic appliances composed of stainless steel or Vitallium (prosthetic joint replacements, metal plates and screws, and vascular clips) are not magnetic and are not associated with heating when placed in a magnetic field. Claustrophobia associated with placement in the MRI unit is a significant practical problem and may result in studies that are incomplete or not performable.

MRI has many applications in spinal cord imaging in children and adolescents, including those with spinal cord injury [35, 55, 83, 101] (see Fig. 24–5). Both acute and chronic spinal cord changes can be readily demonstrated with MRI [83, 101]. MRI has to date had limited application in the patient with an acute spine injury owing to the common presence of ferromagnetic stabilization devices [101]. However, early use of MRI in patients with a neurologic deficit following conventional radiography has been advocated [55]. In the subacute stage, vertebral body fractures show morphologic changes and increased signal intensity on both T1- and T2-weighted images, presumably owing to hemorrhage [101]. In the chronic phase, fractures are decreased or isointense on T1-weighted images and increased or isointense on T2-weighted images [101]. The advantage of MRI in the evaluation of spinal trauma is its ability to image not only extradural defects but also intramedullary sequelae of trauma such as cord atrophy, hematoma, necrosis, and syringomyelia [65, 101].

MRI is of limited use in imaging acute trauma to the appendicular skeleton [37] (Fig. 24–10). It is capable of identifying stress fractures and differentiating them from bone neoplasms but is not superior to radiographs or bone scanning in this regard [37, 144]. MRI can also show initial and evolving growth plate abnormalities following trauma [21, 73, 102]. Joint effusions are readily identified on MRI (Fig. 24–11). MRI provides excellent definition of the soft tissue component of trauma and is superior to plain films and CT at demonstrating edema and hemorrhage [21, 34, 37, 38, 44] (Fig. 24–12). Various compartment syndromes can be imaged with MRI [37]. MRI is comparable to arthrography and arthroscopy in defining tears of the menisci of the knee joint as well as other intra-articular pathology following trauma [8, 29, 38, 45, 75, 165] (Fig. 24–13). In complex intra-articular fractures and unstable fractures after closed reduction, MRI is an excellent method of assessing fragment alignment [102]. MRI is effective at staging the abnormality associated with osteochondritis dissecans [75, 102] and at defining rotator cuff tears and other shoulder disorders [60, 104, 158].

Dynamic or real-time MRI has been used primarily in evaluation of the cardiovascular and central nervous systems but has to date been little used with musculoskeletal abnormalities [108]. Three-dimensional MRI display has significant potential value in evaluation of musculoskeletal disorders but has been little used so far.

Arthrography

Arthrography is an invasive but generally benign procedure with a very low complication rate [9]. After sterile preparation of the skin surface, water-soluble contrast material, air, or a combination of contrast agent and air (double-contrast technique) is injected into the specified joint space, and fluoroscopic spot or overhead radiographs are exposed [9].

Arthrography has been used most frequently to evaluate internal knee joint anatomy, specifically, in patients with cruciate ligament tears and disrupted menisci [8, 9].

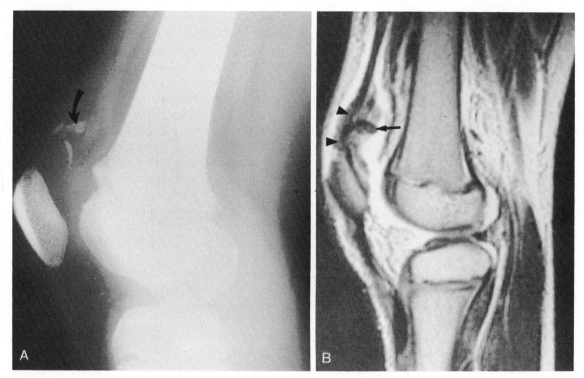

FIGURE 24–10
Patellar avulsion fracture with quadriceps tendon disruption. This 7-year-old child jumped from a tree limb and sustained a right knee injury with severe pain and swelling. A lateral knee radiograph *(A)* demonstrates avulsion fracture fragments originating from the superior patellar margin and displaced cephalad (arrows). There is associated soft tissue swelling. *B,* Improved definition of patellar and quadriceps mechanism injuries demonstrated by MRI scan. A midsagittal T2-weighted MRI of the right knee *(B)* also demonstrates an avulsion fracture of the patella (arrows). In addition, there is inhomogeneous signal intensity (arrowheads) in the distal quadriceps tendon that is compatible with a tendon disruption or tear. The full extent of soft tissue injury is often demonstrated only with MRI.

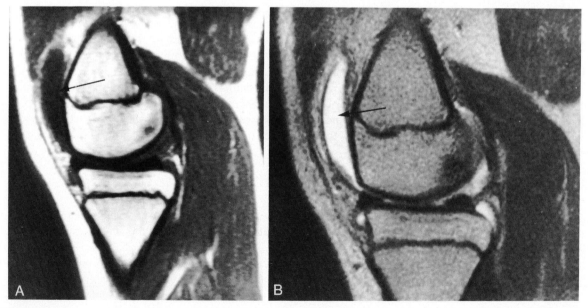

FIGURE 24–11
Joint effusion. This 13-year-old field hockey player had chronic knee pain following an injury. Physical examination revealed a knee effusion. MRI study of the knee was normal except for a large suprapatellar bursal effusion, which has low signal intensity (dark) on T1-weighted images *(A)* and high signal intensity (white) on T2-weighted images *(B)* (arrows). MRI is optimal, and in many instances unique, at demonstrating a variety of sports-related soft tissue injuries, including ligamentous and tendon disruptions, meniscal tears, and abnormal fluid collections.

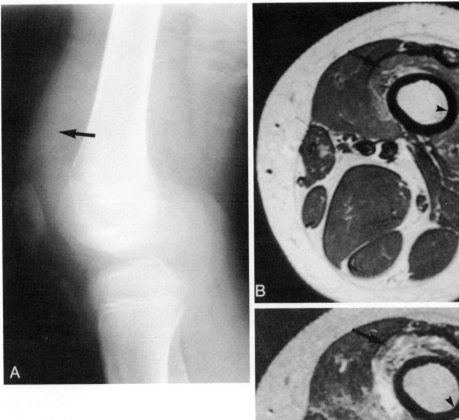

FIGURE 24–12
Soft tissue injury. A 10-year-old football player had chronic pain in the left knee region. A lateral radiograph of the left knee *(A)* demonstrates ill-defined soft tissue swelling in the suprapatellar region (arrows). Axial plane MRI with first *(B)* and second *(C)* echo T2-weighted images demonstrates increased signal intensity in the vasti muscles (arrows) compatible with post-traumatic edema. The intact adjacent femoral cortex (arrowheads) appears a homogeneous black (absence of signal).

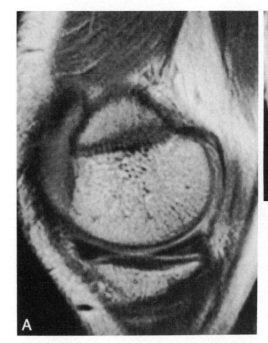

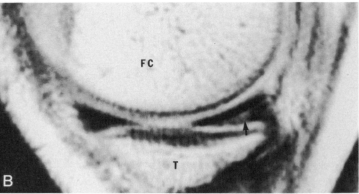

FIGURE 24–13
Complex meniscal tear. This 15-year-old halfback had acute onset of knee pain after a tackle. Sagittal MRI of knee (*A* and *B*) demonstrates a zone of high signal intensity (arrow) in the posterior horn of the medial meniscus extending to the articular surface that reflects a meniscal tear. FC = femoral condyle; T = tibia.

In the shoulder, arthrography is most typically used to evaluate rotator cuff tears [8, 9, 14, 104] (Fig. 24–14). Arthrography of the wrist can demonstrate abnormal intercompartmental communication, tears of the triangular fibrocartilage, post-traumatic synovitis, and secondary degenerative arthritis [85] (Fig. 24–15). At present, MRI is an alternative and perhaps superior method of identifying many of these abnormalities [85].

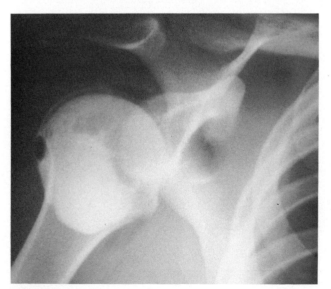

FIGURE 24–14
Normal double-contrast shoulder arthrogram. This 17-year-old rower presented with right shoulder pain. Plain radiographs of the shoulder (not shown) were normal. Double contrast shoulder arthrography was performed to exclude a rotator cuff tear. The AP view with internal rotation of the arm demonstrates a normal appearance of the shoulder joint, and there is no cephalad extension of either contrast or air to indicate a rotator cuff tear.

Computed Arthrography

Computed arthrography (a combination of arthrography and computed tomography) has been used primarily in adults and older adolescents [33, 52, 53, 79, 121, 140, 142]. Single- or, preferably, double-contrast arthrography is performed initially, followed by thin-section computed tomography of the affected joint [111, 121] (Fig. 24–16). The procedure is less invasive than arthroscopy [121]. Combining CT scanning with arthrography provides three-dimensional definition of joint structures, including definition of nonossified cartilaginous structures and capsular tears [29].

Shoulder instability, unexplained shoulder pain, and osteochondritis dissecans with sequestra are among the main indications for the use of this technique [13, 80, 111]. In evaluating disorders of the shoulder CT arthrography is less effective than conventional arthrography in detecting bony glenoid margin fractures but more reliable in identifying Hill-Sachs fractures and rotator cuff tears [164]. In general, computed arthrography should be reserved for cases in which conventional arthrography has not provided adequate anatomic information [13].

Angiography and Digital Subtraction Angiography

Angiography in pediatric orthopedics is limited to assessment of the vascularity of tumors and the diagnosis and treatment of vascular injuries following blunt, penetrating, or operative trauma [8, 9]. Vascular trauma may

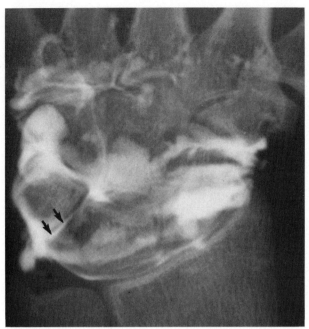

FIGURE 24–15
Torn left triquetrolunate ligament. This 14-year-old tennis player presented with persistent left wrist pain. Plain radiographs of the wrist (not shown) were normal. The AP view of the wrist after injection of water-soluble contrast material into the radiocarpal joint shows contrast extending into the intercarpal and carpal-metacarpal joints through a tear in the triquetrolunate ligament (arrows). Conventional wrist arthrography is satisfactory at demonstrating intra-articular ligamentous and cartilage tears.

be asymptomatic or may result in hemorrhage, pulse defects, expanding masses, bruits, or signs of distal ischemia [9].

Angiography as a therapeutic modality has almost no applicability in pediatric orthopedic trauma except in occasional cases of post-traumatic pelvic arterial hemorrhage [9]. Bleeding arteries can be accurately localized and occluded through the catheter, resulting in cessation of hemorrhage in most cases [9].

Nuclear Medicine Procedures

Nuclear medicine (scintigraphic) imaging of the pediatric musculoskeletal system relies on the three-phase bone scan [9, 22, 135]. The bone imaging isotope used is typically technetium-99m compounded to a diphosphonate [94, 135]. A gamma camera and a display monitor with photographic hard-copy recording capability are required [9, 59]. In conjunction with the bolus intravenous injection of a predetermined quantity of ^{99m}Tc-diphosphonate, a rapid series of images are initially obtained (phase 1, angiographic phase) to determine relative blood flow [9, 22]. Almost immediately afterward, high-count static images are obtained (phase 2, blood-pool segment) [9, 22]. After an interval of ap-

proximately 3 hours to allow the incorporation of the isotope-diphosphonate into the osseous structures in a pattern reflecting regional bone perfusion and metabolism, the entire musculoskeletal system or a portion thereof is imaged in the third or bone imaging phase [9, 22]. Occasionally, a delayed phase is obtained up to 24 hours after isotope injection when soft tissue background activity is minimal [22]. The various patterns of isotope localization permit differentiation between neoplastic, infectious, and traumatic abnormalities [9, 22].

Bone scintigraphy has become an important imaging procedure in sports medicine because it identifies the site of focal metabolic changes secondary to the chronic repeated stress characteristic of physical activity [51, 109, 131, 134, 135, 163]. Although routine radiographs usually demonstrate the site and nature of any fracture, bone scintigraphy can identify subtle fractures when initial radiographs are normal [9, 22, 94]. Fractures on bone scintiscans are seen as focal areas of increased uptake early, with 80% visible in 24 hours and 95% in 72 hours [9, 94]. Bone scintigraphy can detect stress fractures earlier than is possible with conventional radiography [9, 72, 94, 109, 131, 135].

Bone scintigraphy is occasionally specific for the type of injury; for example, stress injuries of the proximal tibia and "shin splints" in runners [22, 135]. In adolescent athletes with chronic localized pain suggestive of a stress injury, a radionuclide bone scan is recommended as the initial imaging study, supplemented by radiographs of regions with abnormal isotope activity [131].

Whereas the major advantage of bone scintigraphy is its high sensitivity to various abnormal bone processes, its major disadvantage is poor anatomic detail and typical lack of specificity [9, 94]. A positive bone scintiscan

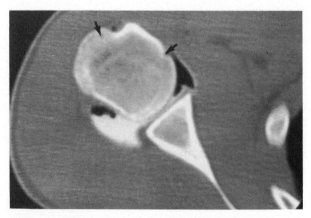

FIGURE 24–16
CT arthrography of shoulder. This 17-year-old pitcher had intermittent pain in the right shoulder. Axial plane CT of the right shoulder following intra-articular injection of air and water-soluble contrast material demonstrates a normal relationship between the humeral head and the glenoid fossa. Slight cortical irregularity and cystic change (arrows) reflect early rotator cuff degenerative change. There was no actual rotator cuff tear.

usually requires supplemental conventional radiographs or other imaging studies (e.g., CT) for actual definition of the abnormality [9]. A positive bone scintigram is not necessarily specific for trauma because it may mimic infection or tumor [113]. In addition, bone scintigraphy may impart a higher absorbed radiation dose than conventional radiographs [50].

Myelography

There are two basic techniques for performing myelography: conventional film myelography with fluoroscopy, and CT imaging of the spine following intrathecal injection of contrast medium [7, 9, 124] (Fig. 24–17). Currently, both techniques use nonionic water-soluble contrast agents (e.g., metrizamide) injected into the lumbar subarachnoid space [7, 9, 124]. CT of the spine, with or without intrathecal injection of metrizamide, is preferred over conventional myelography in the patient with post-traumatic spinal injury [9]. Either procedure can be used to evaluate the patient for nerve root compression due to disc herniation [9].

SPECIFIC ANATOMIC SITES OF INJURY

Neck and Cervical Spine

Trauma to the child's spine can be classified into a three basic groups: (1) cord injury without fracture, (2) cord injury with fracture or dislocation, and (3) fracture or dislocation alone, without neurologic injury [110]. Owing to the relatively greater strength of the posterior neck muscles and the restriction on the potential degree of neck flexion by the chin hitting the sternum, extension injuries of the cervical spine are potentially more serious for an equivalent amount of force than are flexion injuries [17]. Flexion injury to the cervical spine tends to result in vertebral body anterior wedge fractures, chip fractures, and anterior dislocations as well as ruptures of the posterior longitudinal, interspinal, and supraspinal ligaments [17]. With an extension (whiplash) spine injury, the anterior elements are disrupted and the posterior elements compressed, resulting in rupture of the anterior longitudinal ligament and injury to the spinous processes, facets, and neural arch [17]. Vertical loading of the spine from a blow to the vertex with the neck flexed predisposes to a compression or burst injury [17, 116, 162]. This is a major mechanism of cervical fracture-dislocation and quadriplegia in many athletes sustaining diving, football, or ice hockey neck injuries [17, 116, 162]. A combined flexion-rotation injury is more likely

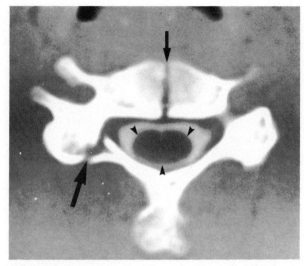

FIGURE 24–17
CT myelography. This 16-year-old cyclist struck a tree, sustaining brief loss of consciousness and upper extremity weakness. Axial CT image of the fifth cervical vertebral body after intrathecal injection of water-soluble contrast medium (CT myelography) demonstrates a mid-sagittal vertebral body fracture (small arrow) and a second fracture through the junction of the right lamina and pedicle (large arrow). Myelographic contrast material outlines the adjacent cervical cord (arrowheads). The axial CT image accurately demonstrates the fractures as well as the absence of fragment extension into the neural canal or enlargement of the adjacent spinal cord.

to result in a flexion injury accompanied by anterior subluxation [17].

The patterns of cervical spine injury in children are in part related to the changes in their anatomy with age [110]. Compared to other body proportions, the head of the developing child is relatively large at birth [110]. With increasing age and development, the head-to-body ratio decreases so that less relative mass or potential angular momentum is presented to the cervical spine following trauma to the head [110].

The risk of sustaining a sports-related cervical spine injury varies with the sport; both serious and minor spine injuries are associated with diving, football, gymnastics, horseback riding, rugby, ice hockey, and wrestling [17, 116, 156, 162].

The natural history of spinal fractures in children may differ significantly from that in adults owing to the child's inherent ability to withstand trauma and the potential for growth and development subsequent to the injury [110]. The principal differences observed in children are the relatively benign clinical course, the gradual restoration of vertebral body height when the vertebrae are anteriorly wedged, and the development of progressive spinal deformity when there is either end-plate injury or paralysis [110]. Fractures, dislocations, and fracture-dislocations of the spine in children and adolescents are much less common than in adults [110].

Fractures of the cervical spine in children under the age of 7 tend to involve the atlas and axis and consist of distraction of the osseous ring [36]. The pediatric cervical spine attains an adult form by approximately 8 years of age [36]. In older children and adolescents cervical fractures tend to be more evenly distributed throughout the cervical spine and are compressive in nature [36]. The decreased incidence of spinal cord injuries in children is thought to reflect, at least in part, the greater flexibility of the child's spine, which causes force to be more easily dissipated over a greater number of segments [110]. Dislocation of the spine is rare in children because the ligaments are generally stronger than the bone [110].

Vertebral or spinal cord damage should be suspected in the unconscious child with an injury that can cause flexion or rotation of the spine, in the awake child who complains of loss of sensation or motor power below a transverse level of the body, and in the injured child who complains of localized vertebral pain or tenderness or pain radiating along a radicular distribution [110]. A possible spinal injury should not be overlooked in a child or adolescent whose primary site of injury is the head [110].

Radiographic evaluation of the cervical spine must be accomplished with regard for potentially severe and unstable injuries and must include prior adequate immobilization of the spine [110, 116]. One of the most frequent errors made in evaluating suspected injury of the cervical spine is failure to obtain good visualization of the C7–T1 vertebral bodies and posterior elements [110, 116].

In a patient with acute neck trauma, a cross-table lateral projection of the cervical spine with the neck immobilized in a protective collar or brace is obtained initially, followed by anteroposterior (AP) and odontoid views taken without moving the patient [8, 17, 110, 116, 156]. If no obvious fracture or subluxation is present, additional views are obtained as needed clinically. A minimum cervical spine study should consist of AP, lateral, both oblique, and open-mouth atlantoaxial views [9, 20, 116, 156]. The oblique views require limited patient repositioning and can be deleted if CT of the cervical spine is to follow. Lateral flexion and hyperextension views may be required to assess the stability of the cervical spine [47, 156]. Pleuridirectional (complex motion) tomography is superior for defining fractures and other injuries of the vertebral facets, whereas CT adds the most additional information in patients with laminar and posterior element fractures and C1 fractures [20]. Tomography is preferred over CT for defining fractures of the odontoid process of C2 [91]. Both conventional and computed tomography can define rotary subluxation of C1 and C2 (Fig. 24–18). A more detailed

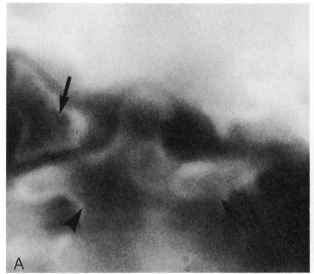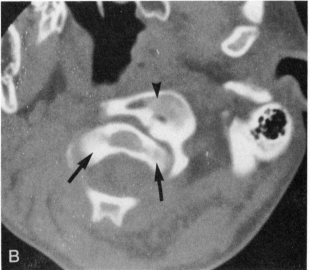

FIGURE 24–18
Rotatory subluxation of C1 on C2. This 10-year-old fell off a bicycle, striking her head on the pavement and twisting her neck. A persistent torticollis prompted radiologic evaluation. Standard cervical spine views (not shown) suggested a rotatory subluxation of C1 on C2, which was confirmed by conventional tomography. A true anteroposterior tomographic projection *(A)* demonstrates an intact C2 (arrowheads). Note that the right lateral mass of C1 (arrow) is in the plane of imaging, while the left is not, indicating rotatory subluxation. Axial CT *(B)* was confirmatory (arrowhead = C1; arrows = C2). There was no associated fracture.

Although rotatory subluxation of the cervical spine can be demonstrated by conventional radiographs and radiographic tomography, CT is superior at demonstrating the actual direction and degree of rotation and subluxation. CT also more reliably excludes any associated neural arch fracture.

discussion of specific injuries of the cervical spine is beyond the scope of this chapter but can be found elsewhere [110].

When spinal cord injury is documented on neurologic examination, only a cross-table lateral view of the cervical spine (with the neck in protective immobilization) is taken; oblique and other supplemental projections are deferred to prevent risk of further cord injury [17, 116]. Instead, a CT scan of the spine is obtained to define the extent of trauma and the presence of spinal cord compression by bone, disc, or hematoma [17]. MRI of the spine is an alternative method of defining post-traumatic intraspinal pathology [17].

Thoracic Spine

Injury to the vertebral elements in the thoracic region is uncommon in childhood [110]. The intrinsic elasticity of the region, coupled with the protective effect of the rib cage to prevent excessive translational movements, minimizes the abnormal stresses necessary to cause fracture or dislocation [110]. In the thoracic region, especially in younger children, injury to the spinal cord occurs more often without associated vertebral fracture. [110].

Wedge fractures of the vertebral bodies, usually of minor degree, are more common in older children and adolescents [110]. Unlike the situation in adults, the intrinsic elasticity of children's bones allows these injuries to occur without major damage to the posterior elements, resulting in an intrinsically more stable injury [110]. The posterior and anterior longitudinal ligaments usually remain intact [110].

Scheuermann's disease is an irregularity of three or more contiguous vertebral end plates with anterior wedging and resultant kyphosis [16]. Repetitive microtrauma caused by jumping with axial loading and forced hyperextension and hyperflexion may account for many cases [16].

Radiographic evaluation of the thoracic spine usually consists of AP and lateral projections [8, 110]. A "coned-down" lateral projection centering on the level of primary concern is frequently performed as a supplemental view. CT of the spine is best for identifying more complex fractures, particularly fractures of the posterior elements, as well as for detecting extension of fracture fragments into the neural canal [110].

Thoracic Cage (Ribs, Sternum, Sternoclavicular Joints)

Injuries of the thoracic cage are common occurrences in sport-related trauma [9]. Blunt chest trauma may result in acute rib fractures, almost always involving the middle and lower ribs [57]. Acute fractures of the upper ribs are much less common and are not associated with an increased incidence of great vessel or airway injury, as previously thought [57]. Noncontact sports (e.g., golf, rowing, tennis) can result in stress fractures of the ribs owing to repetitive application of submaximal stress on the ribs [57]. Displaced rib fractures from blunt trauma are easily recognized on radiographs of the ribs [57]. Associated complications such as pneumothorax, hemothorax, and lung contusion may be readily evident on rib and chest radiographs, although damage to the spleen, kidneys, and liver will require additional imaging by ultrasound or CT for proper definition [57]. Acute stress fractures of the ribs are typically not definable radiographically until sufficient healing has occurred, usually in 10 to 14 days. Costochondritis produces no specific findings on imaging and remains essentially a clinical diagnosis [57]. Sternoclavicular dislocations are usually anterior (three times more frequent than posterior dislocations) and are usually easily reduced [104].

Radiographic evaluation of the ribs should include an AP view of the thorax optimized for rib detail as well as oblique projections of the ribs, either unilaterally or bilaterally, according to clinical indications [9]. An AP view of the thorax optimized for lung definition should be considered to exclude pneumothorax.

Radiographic examination of the sternum should consist of right and left posteroanterior (PA) oblique projections with the patient prone as well as an erect or recumbent lateral view [96]. Examination of the sternoclavicular joints should consist of PA oblique views as well as a straight PA view [96]. In patients with more severe trauma, in whom movement must be minimized, AP rather than PA views are appropriate.

CT is also good for assessing the sternoclavicular joints and the medial ends of the clavicles, areas that are frequently difficult to image well with conventional radiographs [9, 57, 104].

Lumbosacral Spine and Lower Back

The lumbar region is infrequently involved in significant injury until the adolescent period, when the developing spine assumes more of the biomechanical characteristics of the adult spine [110]. Acute wedge fractures may occur at all levels [110]. Fracture-dislocation injuries are more common in adolescent athletes, thereby increasing the likelihood of significant spinal cord or cauda equina injury [110] (see Fig. 24–8).

Vertebral end plate fractures resulting from intervertebral disc material being forced into the vertebral body may occur; these fragments are usually stable because the posterior elements remain intact [110]. The resultant Schmorl's node is identified radiographically as a corticated notch in the superior or inferior vertebral end plate [114].

Herniated nucleus pulposus in adolescents usually has no specific findings on plain radiographs, although occasionally narrowing of the affected intervertebral disc space may be demonstrated; this is best seen on the lateral projection. CT and especially MRI are optimal for defining disc herniation and are increasingly being used to replace myelography in the diagnosis of this disorder.

Fractures of the vertebral apophyseal rings in older children and adolescents usually require fragment displacement for diagnosis on plain radiographs. Both conventional tomography and CT can identify apophyseal ring fractures, although the former is generally more reliable because of its greater anatomic resolution and the availability of multiple imaging planes.

Traumatic spondylolysis representing a stress fracture through the pars interarticularis of the neural arch, usually at the L5 level, is a recognized consequence of adolescent trauma, especially in young gymnasts [43, 54, 114] (Figs. 24–19 and 24–20). A baseline radiographic assessment of the lumbosacral spine in a child or adoles-

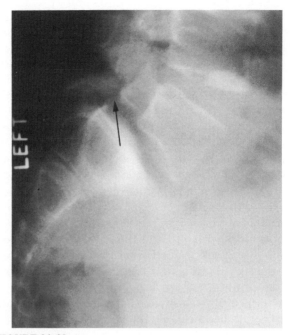

FIGURE 24–20
Spondylolisthesis. A 15-year-old weight-lifter had chronic lower back pain. A lateral spine radiograph coned down to the lumbosacral junction demonstrates 15-mm anterior subluxation of L5 on the sacrum in association with an L5 neural arch defect (spondylolisthesis) (arrow). Characteristic posterior wedging of the L5 vertebral body is also present. This view is best for assessing the degree of vertebral slippage associated with spondylolysis.

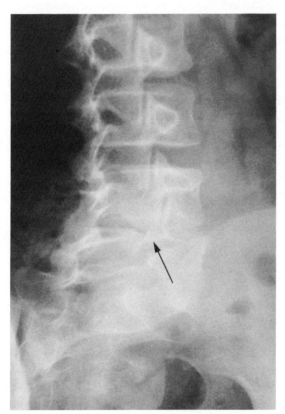

FIGURE 24–19
L5 spondylolisthesis. A 10-year-old gymnast presented with chronic lower back pain. Standard views (not shown) of the lumbar spine demonstrated first-degree L5 spondylolisthesis. The actual pars interarticularis defect (arrow) is usually best depicted on oblique views. If conventional radiographs fail to identify a neural arch defect and clinical suspicion is high, a radionuclide bone scan should be obtained. Focally increased isotope localization within the neural arch would be highly suggestive. A spinal CT scan would optimize demonstration of a subtle neural arch defect with or without associated subluxation.

cent with back pain or a back injury consists of a minimum of AP and lateral projections [156]. Especially if the symptoms are recurrent or chronic, supplemental oblique as well as "coned-down" lateral views of the L5–S1 region are generally recommended [16, 110, 156]. However, the addition of routine oblique projections to the pediatric lumbar spine examination increases the diagnostic accuracy by only 5% but more than doubles the gonadal radiation dose [129]. Angling the tube 30 degrees cephalad on the AP view of the lumbosacral junction (Ferguson view) may assist in demonstrating a pars interarticularis defect, a transitional vertebra, or sacroiliac joint disease [9]. Instability of the lumbar spine, as with spondylolysis, can be suggested by obtaining Knuttsen bending (forward and backward) lateral projections [16, 156]. In many instances of stress reaction or fracture of the pars interarticularis (isthmus) of the lumbar vertebrae, the bone scan is positive when conventional radiographs are normal [71].

Routine radiographic examination of the sacrum and coccyx consists of AP and lateral projections [9]. To focus on the sacrum in the AP view, the x-ray tube is angled 15 degrees cephalad [96]. To focus on the coccyx, the tube should be angled 10 degrees caudad [96]. Defects of the pars interarticularis vertebral segment are readily identified on axial spine CT, as are less common transverse process and facet fractures [133].

MRI should be used as the primary screening study for the detection of a herniated disc and or spinal cord compression resulting from vertebral fractures [16, 114].

Shoulder Girdle and Upper Arm

A variety of injuries to the shoulder region, including fractures, subluxations, and acromioclavicular joint separations, occur in the adolescent athlete [67, 104] (Fig. 24–21). Fractures and dislocations resulting from macrotrauma are common in football, wrestling, and ice hockey [67]. Fractures of the proximal humeral epiphysis are either Salter-Harris type I or II [130]. Type I injuries are frequent in 10- to 12-year-olds, an exception to the general rule that type I injuries occur in younger individuals [130] (Fig. 24–22). Shoulder injury related to throwing is usually an anterior subluxation, although epiphyseal avulsion and proximal humeral growth plate fractures can occur [11, 67, 104]. Chronic overuse of the shoulder ("pitcher's shoulder") is associated with widening of the proximal humeral physeal plate and meta-

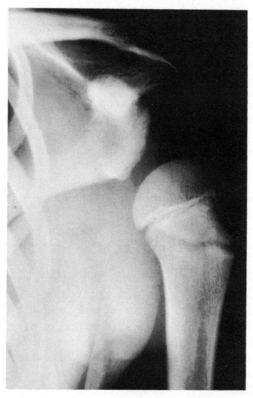

FIGURE 24–21
Subluxable right shoulder secondary to rotator cuff tear. This 11-year-old boy developed chronic recurrent right shoulder pain following repeated soccer injuries. The AP view demonstrates caudad displacement of the intact humeral head, reflecting subluxability of the right shoulder. No fracture is present, and the acromioclavicular joint is intact. A rotator cuff tear was subsequently identified by shoulder arthrography.

physeal cystic changes [104]. Excessive external rotation and extension can lead to relaxation of the anterior ligaments, and degenerative changes may develop on the posterior surface of the humeral head [11,104].

The most commonly dislocated joint in the young athlete is the glenohumeral joint, which accounts for 85% of all shoulder area dislocations [104]. Ninety-five percent of all glenohumeral dislocations are anterior, with the humeral head coming to rest under the coracoid process [78, 104]. Recurrent glenohumeral dislocation is common (occurring in up to 80% to 90% of patients) if the first dislocation occurs when the patient is under age 20. Most anterior dislocations are definable on the AP shoulder radiograph, the scapular Y view being most helpful [104] (Fig. 24–23). Any resultant compression fracture of the posterior and lateral aspects of the humeral head (Hill-Sachs lesion) is recognizable on AP films of the shoulder if the arm is maximally internally rotated [104]. A fracture of the anterior-inferior glenoid rim or avulsion of the fibrocartilaginous attachments (the Bankart lesion) is best evaluated on the West Point view [104].

Rotator cuff strains and tears may result from throwing a baseball, other overhead sports, and direct contact blows [67]. Injuries to the rotator cuff are not as common in young, skeletally immature athletes as they are in older athletes [67].

Defined as a painful arc of motion when the arm is actively abducted between 40 and 120 degrees, the impingement syndrome can occur in younger athletes involved in overhead throwing sports, such as baseball, swimming, and tennis [104]. Radiographic findings vary from normal to subacromial bony spurs, degenerative changes in the humeral tuberosities and acromioclavicular joints, and narrowing of the acromial humeral distance [104].

Uncommon injuries include long thoracic nerve palsy and subluxation of the biceps tendon with tendinitis [67].

Acromioclavicular joint sprains occur with and without fractures of the clavicle [67]. Grade I and grade II sprains are more common than complete grade III dislocations [67]. Following acromioclavicular separation, heterotopic ossification can develop in the coracoclavicular ligament [104].

The standard radiographic examination of the shoulder consists of AP external and internal rotation and axillary views [9, 59, 67, 104, 117]. Supplemental projections are the posterior oblique view (with the patient rotated 40 degrees to the affected side, allowing better visualization of the glenohumeral joint space), the West Point view (to assess the anterior inferior glenoid), the apical oblique view, and the Stryker notch view (to assess the posterior inferior glenoid) [9, 67, 81, 104, 117]. The transthoracic lateral projection requires little or no movement of the injured shoulder and upper arm but

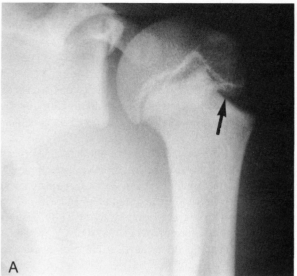

FIGURE 24–22
Proximal humeral Salter-Harris type I fracture. This 12-year-old pitcher developed chronic shoulder pain aggravated by throwing a baseball. An AP view of the shoulder *(A)* demonstrates widening of the proximal humeral growth plate (arrow) that is most severe in the lateral portion and represents a Salter-Harris type I growth plate fracture. A normal shoulder is shown in *B* for comparison.

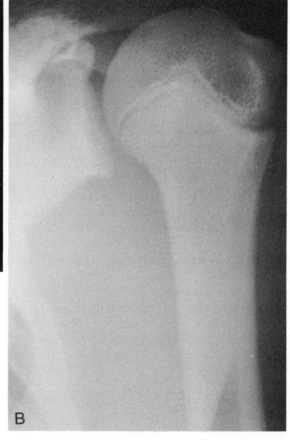

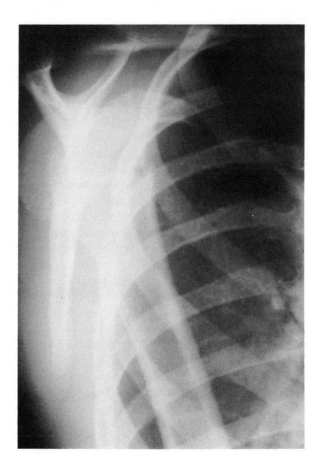

FIGURE 24–23
The scapular Y view assists in identifying fractures of the scapula and dislocation of the humeral head.

superimposes numerous skeletal structures, resulting in an often confusing radiographic appearance (Fig. 24–24). Standard projections of the humerus and upper arm include recumbent AP and lateral views [9, 59].

Standard projections of the scapula include AP and lateral views [9, 104]. The scapular 4 view (with the patient rotated 60 degrees toward the cassette) allows best visualization of the anterior and posterior surfaces of the scapula [9, 104]. CT has proved to be especially useful for better definition of glenoid fractures of the scapula and more complex scapular fractures as well [9] (see Fig. 24–7).

The acromioclavicular joint is seen on AP, posterior oblique, and axillary views of the shoulder [9]. In patients with potential injury to the acromioclavicular joint, stress views with 8 to 10 pounds of weight hung from both wrists are recommended [9, 67]. Because the radiographic findings may be subtle, comparison views of both shoulders are mandatory [104]. When comparing the two acromioclavicular joints, asymmetry is significant [104]. Of particular importance is the alignment of the lower end of the clavicle with the acromion and the distance between the coracoid and the undersurface of the clavicle [104]. Osteolysis of the distal clavicle can

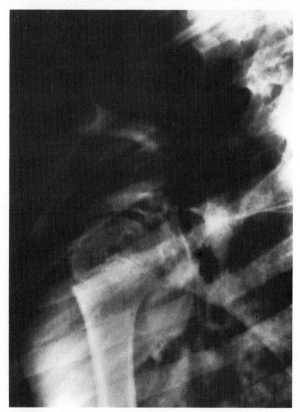

FIGURE 24–24
The transthoracic lateral view has the disadvantage of superimposing multiple osseous structures (e.g., humerus, scapula, ribs), resulting in a confusing radiographic appearance that may preclude identification of a fracture or dislocation.

develop in weight lifters and other athletes in conjunction with grade I and grade II acromioclavicular joint sprains [9, 67, 104]. Radiographic findings include osteoporosis of the distal clavicle, loss of subchondral bone, cystic changes, or bone resorption [9]. When the radiographic findings are minimal, a bone scan may corroborate the clinically suspected abnormality by demonstrating increased uptake at the acromioclavicular joint [9].

Rotator cuff tears, which are not definable on conventional radiographs, have traditionally been imaged with shoulder arthrography [9]. In general, ultrasonography is less sensitive than arthrography in identifying rotator cuff tears unless they are large. MRI is effective in identifying rotator cuff tears [9, 14, 75, 158] and structural changes secondary to recurrent shoulder dislocation [78, 158].

Double-contrast CT arthrography is a highly accurate technique for investigating glenohumeral joint derangement, including labral, capsular, and rotator cuff tears, but is less reliable in evaluating rotator cuff tears and impingement syndromes of the extracapsular structures [33, 80, 120, 121, 140]. Compared to conventional radiographs, CT arthrography is superior at defining rotator cuff and glenoid labrum tears but is less effective at detecting fractures of the bony glenoid labrum [164].

Elbow and Forearm

Elbow injuries are most common in athletes participating in throwing or overhead sports, especially baseball, although fractures, dislocations, ligamentous injuries, and post-traumatic myositis ossificans do occur in the adolescent athlete [67]. A variety of fractures and dislocations of the forearm have been described [25] (Fig. 24–25).

Synovitis and compression and traction injuries to the distal humeral epiphyses, especially the medial ulnar aspect of the elbow, occur in teenage gymnasts [54]. Tennis elbow may appear radiographically as soft tissue calcification adjacent to the lateral humeral epicondyle [104]. Little Leaguer's elbow is caused by repetitive and excessive stress on the origin of the flexor-pronator muscle group at the medial epicondylar apophysis [104, 147]. Radiographically, there is separation of the medial epicondyle with associated soft tissue swelling [104, 147] (Fig. 24–26). The more serious injury of isolated entrapment of the medial epicondyle into the elbow joint may be easily overlooked on elbow radiographs [104] (see Fig. 24–6). An intra-articular location of the medial epicondyle and its absence from the expected normal location are the keys to the radiographic diagnosis [104, 130]. Comparison views of the opposite elbow can be invaluable in making the diagnosis [104, 130] (see Fig.

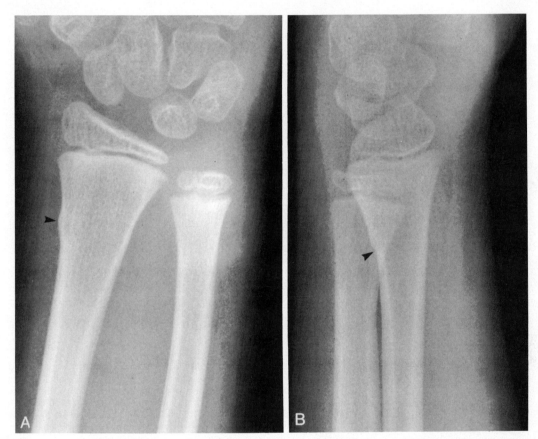

FIGURE 24–25

Torus fracture of distal forearm. This 9-year-old boy tripped while running and fell forward on his outstretched arms. He subsequently had pain in the distal left forearm region. Anteroposterior *(A)* and lateral *(B)* views of the distal forearm and wrist demonstrate a mild torus fracture of the distal radial shaft (arrowheads). Distal radial and ulnar fractures are among the most common pediatric fractures and can be very subtle and difficult to diagnose. Any alteration (e.g., localized bulge or angulation deformity) of the normally straight or slightly curved radial or ulnar cortex must be considered a fracture in the appropriate clinical setting of trauma.

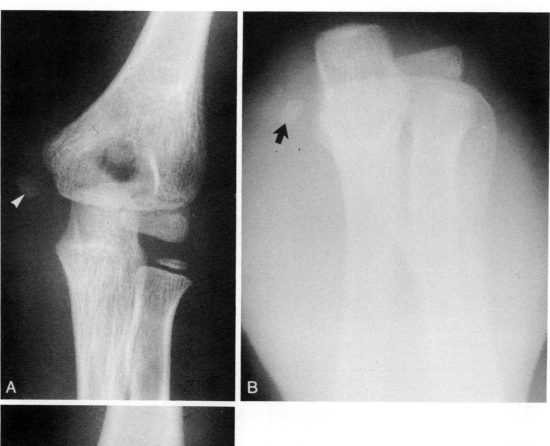

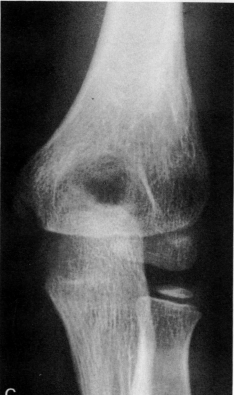

FIGURE 24–26

Avulsion fracture of medial epicondyle. This 8-year-old football player presented with sudden onset of right elbow pain after being tackled. A lateral elbow radiograph (not shown) demonstrated distal humeral fat pad displacement reflecting an elbow joint effusion. The standard AP view *(A)* shows an avulsion fracture of the medial (ulnar) epicondylar ossific nucleus (arrowhead) with mild lateral displacement. A supplemental tangential view *(B)* with maximal elbow flexion confirms the fracture (arrow). An AP view of the opposite elbow, shown for purposes of comparison, demonstrates the normal and medial epicondyle position *(C)*.

The immature elbow is a potentially confusing area of imaging evaluation because of the various ages of appearance of the secondary or epiphyseal ossification centers. The sequence and mean age of development are: capitellum (4 to 5 months); radial head (4 to 5 years); medial epicondyle (5 to 7 years); trochlea (8 to 9 years); olecranon process of ulna (8 to 10 years); and lateral epicondyle (11 to 12 years). Comparison views of the opposite elbow are frequently necessary to optimize assessment of possible elbow region injury.

24–26). Chronic separation of the olecranon epiphysis can occur in adolescent baseball pitchers and is best identified on the lateral elbow radiograph [104].

Osteochondritis dissecans, a potential component of Little Leaguer's elbow, typically involves the capitellum [104, 147] (Fig. 24–27). Radiographic findings may include flattening of the capitellum, areas of fragmentation of the capitellum, or an ill-defined lucency within the capitellum [104]. Routine radiographic evaluation includes AP, lateral, and both oblique views [104]. Conventional multidirectional tomography, noncontrast CT, and arthrography of the elbow have been used for identifying associated loose joint bodies and other structural changes [104].

Radiographic examination of the elbow region must include, as a minimum, AP and lateral views [9, 59, 67, 118]. For the AP projection, the elbow is extended, and for the lateral view the elbow is flexed to 90 degrees [9, 118]. A true lateral projection is essential for the definition of elbow joint fluid (Fig. 24–28). In trauma patients, oblique views with 45 degrees of internal and external rotation are also recommended [9, 118]. In addition, radial head projections can identify subtle fractures of the radial head or tendon calcifications in athletes with tendinitis [9]. The olecranon process is best demonstrated on the lateral and axial projections taken with the elbow completely flexed [9, 67]. To assess the status of the ulnar collateral ligament, stress views may be required [67].

Radiographic examination of the forearm consists of AP and lateral projections with inclusion of both the elbow and wrist joints [9]. For the AP projection the elbow is extended; for the lateral projection, the elbow is flexed to 90 degrees [9].

Although infrequently performed, elbow arthrography is indicated for evaluation of loose bodies or subtle synovial or articular changes that can result from osteochondritis dissecans, osteochondromatosis, acute trauma, and injuries to the ulnar collateral ligament that are not apparent on conventional and stress radiographic views [9, 67, 80]. Single- or double-contrast may be used, but the latter is generally preferred [9]. Linear or complex motion tomography is usually employed [9]. Double-contrast elbow arthrography combined with CT (CT arthrography) enhances the detection and characterization of a variety of pathologic processes, including fractures,

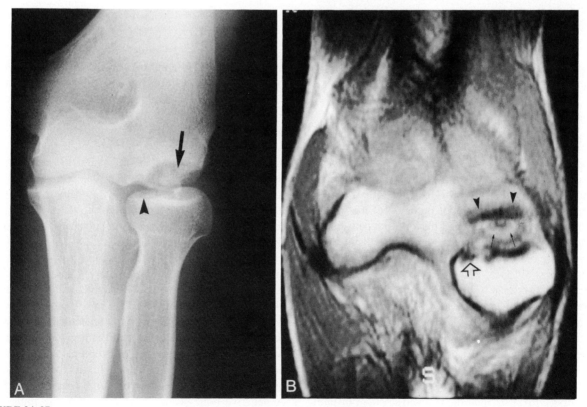

FIGURE 24–27
Osteochondritis dissecans of the capitellum. This 15-year-old baseball pitcher had chronic elbow pain. An AP radiograph of the elbow *(A)* demonstrates a large zone of lucency with a faintly sclerotic proximal margin and a central zone of ossification in the capitellum (arrow), which is highly suggestive of osteochondritis dissecans. There is focal irregularity of the adjacent radial head cortex (arrowhead). Coronal plane proton density MRI *(B)* demonstrates a zone of inhomogeneous low signal intensity in the capitellum (arrowheads), representing the marginal sclerosis seen on the radiograph. Fluid (high signal intensity; arrows) surrounds the central low signal focus of osteochondritis and indicates fragment loosening or instability. The adjacent radial head cortical irregularity is also demonstrated (open arrow).

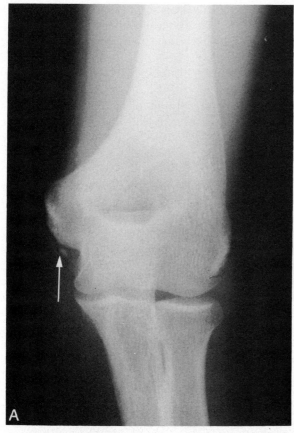

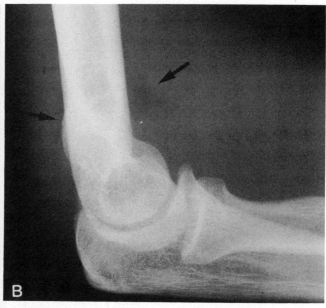

FIGURE 24–28

Avulsion fracture of medial epicondyle with associated elbow effusion. This 16-year-old quarterback was hit while throwing a football. The AP view of the right elbow *(A)* demonstrates two ossifications adjacent to the medial epicondyle (arrow) reflecting avulsion fractures. Displacement of the distal humeral fat pads (arrows) on the lateral view *(B)* reflects an associated elbow fluid collection. The presence of a sizable elbow joint effusion in association with trauma is strong presumptive evidence of an occult intracapsular elbow fracture even if a fracture is not definable on standard radiographic views.

osteochondral and cartilaginous bodies, and articular surface abnormalities [142].

Wrist and Hand

Wrist and hand injuries are common in athletes [122]. The most common carpal fracture is a fracture of the navicular, which accounts for 70% to 80% of all carpal fractures and is especially prevalent in football players [122] (Fig. 24–29). Fractures of the hook of the hamate are common in golfers, baseball players, and participants in racquet sports [122]. Separations of the distal radial epiphysis are most common in athletes over age 10 years [130]. Almost all distal radial growth plate fractures are of the Salter II type [130]. Gymnasts with stress injuries of the distal radial growth plate tend to have delayed skeletal maturation, thereby prolonging the period of risk [18a].

The most common wrist dislocations are rotary subluxation of the navicular, perilunate dislocations, and lunate dislocations [122]. Dorsal intercalated segment instability (DISI) and volar intercalated segment instability (VISI) are the two most common post-traumatic carpal instability patterns [122]. Ligamentous and fibrocartilaginous injuries about the wrist can result from athletic stress and trauma (Fig. 24–30).

Athletic injuries of the hand include tendon injuries,

ligamentous injuries, and fractures [122]. The three most common tendon injuries are avulsion of the terminal extensor tendon, injury of the central slip of the extensor tendon over the PIP joint, and avulsion of the flexor profundus from the base of the distal phalanx [122]. Ligamentous injuries of the hand include injuries of the ulnar collateral ligament of the thumb (''gamekeeper's thumb'') and rupture of the volar plate at the base of the middle phalanx [122]. Phalangeal and metacarpal fractures usually involve a crush injury to the distal phalanx or fractures of the first and fifth metacarpals (''boxer's fracture'') [122] (Fig. 24–31).

Routine evaluation of the wrist and hand requires PA, lateral, and oblique (approximately 45 degrees) views [9, 122]. A scaphoid view is supplemented if there is clinical concern about a fracture of the navicular carpal bone [9, 122]. Obliteration of the navicular fat stripe and tissue swelling over the dorsum of the wrist are present with navicular fractures [122]. If clinical suspicion of a navicular fracture is high and radiographs do not demonstrate a fracture, a bone scan can be performed [122]. A negative bone scan 3 days after an acute injury virtually excludes a navicular fracture [122]. In patients with a navicular fracture, periodic radiographic follow-up is required because possible long-term complications such as delayed union, nonunion, or avascular necrosis of the proximal portion may occur [122].

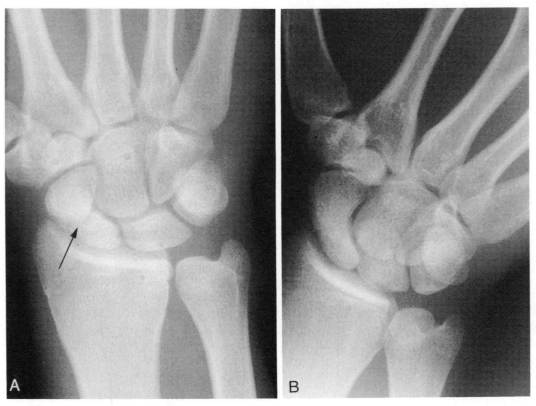

FIGURE 24–29
Navicular carpal fracture. This 17-year-old sustained a direct blow to the wrist. The AP view *(A)* demonstrates a fracture through the middle third of the navicular carpal (arrow) and is adequate for diagnosis in this case. However, navicular fractures may not be apparent on standard views of the wrist. If clinical suspicion is high, a supplemental oblique navicular view *(B)* should be obtained to improve diagnostic accuracy.

FIGURE 24–30
Tear of the triangular fibrocartilage of the wrist. This 14-year-old gymnast presented with recurrent right wrist pain. Coronal plane T2-weighted MRI of the right wrist demonstrates high signal intensity fluid in the triangular fibrocartilage (arrow), representing a cartilage tear. Fluid extends into the distal radioulnar joint (arrowhead). Of incidental note is a small bone island of the proximal scaphoid (small arrowhead).

MRI can provide excellent noninvasive evaluation of internal derangement of the joints.

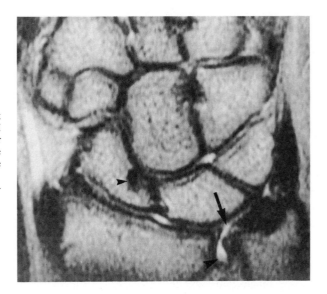

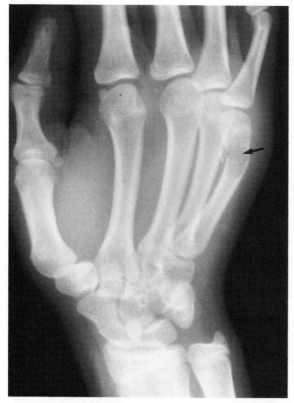

FIGURE 24–31
Boxer's fracture through a bone cyst. This 14-year-old football player slammed his right hand against an opponent's helmet. An acute fracture of the distal portion of the fifth metacarpal is present. There is a mild resultant volar angulation deformity. An associated area of lucency (arrow) within the fifth metacarpal reflects a pre-existing cyst and means that this is a pathologic fracture.

If a fracture of the hook of the hamate is suspected clinically and standard views of the wrist are negative, specialized projections (carpal tunnel), lateral tomography, or CT of the wrist can be utilized [122]. Rotary subluxation of the navicular carpal appears as widening (greater than 4 mm) of the navicular lunate distance (Terry Thomas sign) and foreshortening of the navicular on the PA view [122]. On wrist arthrography, contrast injected into the radiocarpal joint enters the midcarpal row between the navicular and lunate [122]. Perilunate and lunate dislocations are best evaluated on the lateral view [122]. In dorsal perilunate dislocations, the capitate is positioned dorsal to the lunate and radius, whereas in a lunate dislocation the lunate is visually displaced in a volar direction relative to the capitate and radius [122].

With DISI, the lateral view shows dorsal tilting of the distal articulating surface of the lunate, and the navicular angle exceeds 80 degrees [122]. The PA view shows widening of the navicular lunate distance and an overlap of the lunate and capitate bones [122]. With VISI, the lateral view shows volar tilting of the distal articulating surface of the lunate and a capitolunate angle of greater than 30 degrees [122]. The PA view shows overlap of the capitate and lunate [122].

With avulsion of the terminal extensor tendon, the lateral view is optimal and shows a flexion deformity of the DIP joint and (in 25% of cases) an avulsion fracture from the dorsal surface of the base of the distal phalanx [122]. Disruption of the central slip of the extensor tendon can produce the boutonniere deformity; radiographs may be negative except for soft tissue swelling or a small avulsion fracture from the dorsum of the middle phalanx [122]. With avulsion of the flexor profundus tendon soft tissue swelling is usually the only radiographic abnormality [122].

Injury of the ulnar collateral ligament may show an avulsion fracture at the base of the proximal phalanx, or there may be no associated radiographic findings [122]. Rotation of any avulsed fragment should be identified because surgical intervention is then required [122]. When plain radiographs are negative, stress views may show more than 10 degrees difference in abduction between the injured and normal thumb [122]. Rupture of the volar plate at the PIP joint may produce soft tissue swelling only, an avulsion fracture at the base of the middle phalanx, or dorsal dislocation of the PIP joint [122]. The majority of avulsed fragments are seen on the lateral view, but the oblique view provides the best or only visualization of the bony fragment in one-third of cases [122]. Phalangeal and metacarpal fractures are well demonstrated on standard radiographic projections [122].

Arthrography of the wrist is occasionally performed to assess the integrity of the ligaments, triangular cartilage, and joint compartments of the wrist in patients who have post-traumatic wrist pain [9]. Wrist arthrography usually employs single-contrast injection into the radiocarpal joint [9].

Pelvis and Hips

Avulsion injuries to the pubic symphysis occur in young athletes involved in soccer, rugby, ice hockey, karate, and cycling [77, 114]. A variety of other pelvic apophyseal avulsion injuries (ischial tuberosity, anterior inferior and anterior superior iliac spines, iliac crest apophysis, lesser femoral trochanter) occur in adolescent sprinters, hurdlers, long jumpers, weight lifters, and cheerleaders [40, 77, 114, 115] (Figs. 24–32 and 24–33). The discontinuity of the anterior part of the iliac apophysis noted on radiographs of adolescent athletes suffering a "hip-pointer" injury is probably an anatomic anomaly rather than a stress fracture as previously thought [92].

Hip joint pathology secondary to sports activity is rare [114] (Fig. 24–34). Idiopathic avascular necrosis of the femoral head (Legg-Calvé-Perthes disease) may occa-

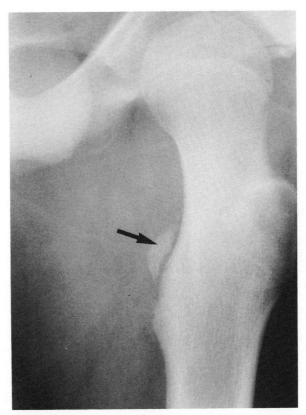

FIGURE 24–32
Avulsion fracture of lesser trochanter of femur. This 13-year-old ice hockey player experienced a sudden onset of pain in the left groin region after tripping and falling hard. An avulsion fracture of the lesser trochanter apophysis of the left femur (arrow) with mild cephalad displacement is present. Apophyseal avulsion injuries are a relatively common occurrence in adolescent sports injuries and can usually be diagnosed by plain radiographs alone because sufficient ossification of the apophysis is present at the time of injury.

sionally be attributable to athletic activity in children 4 to 8 years of age [114] (Fig. 24–35). Degenerative osteoarthritis secondary to chronic, athletically related hip trauma is rarely evident in adolescents and children.

Although newer imaging modalities, especially CT and MRI, have significantly influenced the radiographic approach to diagnostic problems of the pelvis and hips in children and adolescents, routine radiography remains the primary technique for initial evaluation [9]. In most cases, more than one radiographic projection is necessary to allow adequate evaluation [9]. The AP view of the pelvis and hips should be the initial film taken in patients with suspected trauma [9, 59]. The AP view is obtained with the patient in the supine position, with 15 degrees of internal rotation of the feet to optimize definition of the greater trochanters and femoral necks [9]. Gonadal shielding should not be used during the initial projection to avoid obscuring potentially significant bony and soft tissue structures [9]. The AP view of the pelvis provides, in most cases, excellent overall assess-

ment of the bony pelvis and hip regions and may be the only view required [9].

Clarification of findings on the AP view may be accomplished by using inlet and tangential projections [9]. The inlet projection, obtained with the patient in the supine position and the tube angled 40 degrees caudad, aids in evaluating the pelvic ring and more easily assesses displaced fracture fragments [9]. The tangential view allows better evaluation of the anterior pelvis, ventral foramina, and margins of the sacrum [9]. Individual hip regions can be evaluated with lateral, AP, Judet, and oblique views [9].

Radiographic findings associated with injuries of the pubic symphysis include loss of cortical definition, widening of the symphysis, marginal erosions and sclerosis, periosteal reaction, and hypertrophic changes [114]. The changes usually occur on only one side of the symphysis [114].

An apophyseal avulsion injury usually presents radiographically as a curvilinear, corticated osseous fragment displaced less than 1 cm from its site of origin [40, 114]

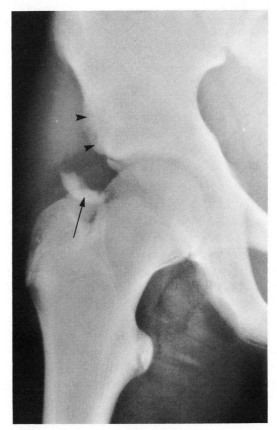

FIGURE 24–33
Avulsion fracture of anterior-inferior iliac spine. This 15-year-old male football player sustained a sudden onset of pain in the right hip region after being tackled. An AP view of the right hip demonstrates a large avulsion fracture fragment (arrow) arising from the anterior inferior iliac spine (arrowheads), the site of origin of the rectus femoris muscle.

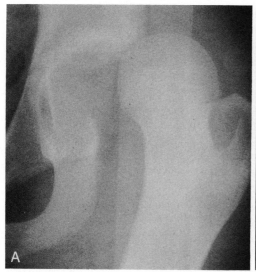

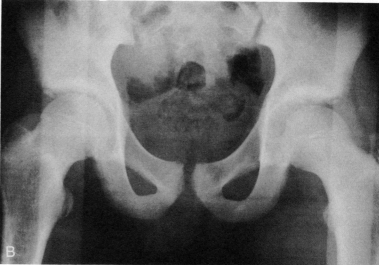

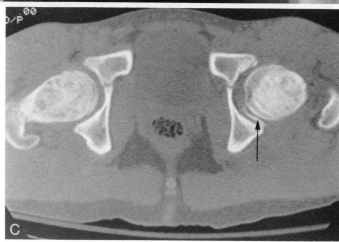

FIGURE 24–34
Dislocated hip with intra-articular fracture. This 18-year-old half-back experienced sudden onset of severe left hip pain following a tackle. An AP radiograph of the left hip *(A)* demonstrates lateral dislocation but no apparent fracture. Following hip reduction, there is residual widening of the left hip joint space, suggesting post-traumatic intra-articular fluid *(B)*. Because of persistent left hip pain, CT of the hips was performed. The axial CT image *(C)* demonstrates an intra-articular fracture fragment (arrow) arising from the posterior acetabular margin. CT is excellent at demonstrating subtle intra- or periarticular fractures that may not be definable on conventional radiographs.

(see Figs. 24–32 and 24–33). During the healing phase, a mixed pattern of increased and decreased density that can simulate a neoplastic process may be seen [40, 114]. Later stages of healing may include extensive heterotopic ossification or an exostosis [114]. Conventional radiographs are almost always sufficient for the identification of avulsion injuries [40].

MRI of the hips is very valuable in the diagnosis of several pediatric hip disorders [75]. MRI is as sensitive as bone scintigraphy in the early identification of avascular necrosis of the femoral head, but it also provides superior anatomic detail, especially of joint cartilage and regional soft tissue structures [75]. Fluid or hemorrhage in the hip joint secondary to hip trauma as well as cartilaginous fragments within the joint space are readily definable on MRI [75].

Thigh and Femur

Injuries to the femur are uncommon in adolescent athletes. Macrotrauma (e.g., due to football) can produce femoral shaft fractures. Stress fractures, such as those occurring in runners, usually involve the medial cortex proximal to the lesser trochanter but may also involve the superior lateral aspect of the femoral neck or the subtrochanteric medial femoral cortex [114]. Myositis ossificans of the thigh can develop secondary to trauma-related hematomas [114].

Baseline radiographic evaluation of the femur consists of AP and lateral projections, with inclusion of the hip and knee joints [9, 59]. The AP view is obtained with the patient supine, the legs extended, and the foot internally rotated 15 degrees in order to position the patella anteriorly and to minimize anteversion of the femoral neck [9]. Except in situations of acute trauma, the lateral view is obtained with the patient turned onto the affected side and the dependent knee slightly flexed [9]. Evaluation of the proximal femur is usually done using lateral hip views [9].

Fractures of the femoral shaft secondary to macrotrauma are readily demonstrated on standard radiographic views [114]. In the early stages of a femoral

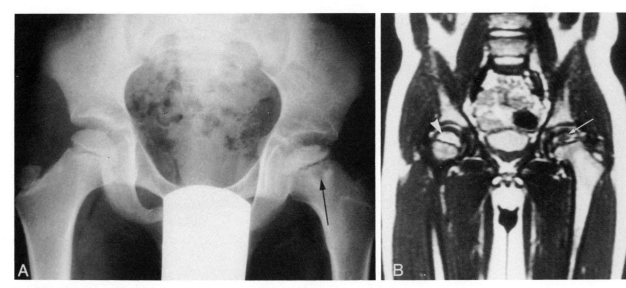

FIGURE 24–35

Legg-Calvé-Perthes disease. This 7-year-old soccer player presented with a 5-month history of persistent pain in his left hip unrelated to any specific injury. An AP radiograph of the pelvis and hips *(A)* demonstrates partial collapse of the left femoral epiphysis, with relative flattening and an increase in density of the epiphysis. There are associated cystic changes in the adjacent femoral metaphysis (arrow). The right hip is normal.

At the time of initial presentation 5 months earlier, radiographs of the pelvis and hips were normal. However, MRI *(B)* demonstrated low signal intensity in the left femoral epiphysis (arrow), which is characteristic of avascular necrosis. The proximal right femoral epiphysis (arrowhead) demonstrates the expected normal high signal intensity of marrow fat.

In the acute phase, avascular necrosis of the femoral head (or elsewhere) may produce no positive plain radiographic findings. Previously, in this situation, diagnosing or excluding avascular necrosis depended on demonstrating a photopenic area corresponding to the affected femoral epiphysis on radionuclide bone scanning. MRI is more sensitive than either plain radiographs or bone scanning for the earliest possible diagnosis of avascular necrosis and is the preferred imaging study in the appropriate clinical situation when plain radiographs are normal.

neck stress fracture, radiographs may be normal, and the abnormality is only definable as an area of increased activity on the bone scan [114]. After 2 weeks, a stress fracture appears as a linear area of increased density [114]. Conventional tomography may be necessary to identify the lucent fracture line within the area of sclerosis [114]. Radiographic definition of a post-traumatic hematoma usually requires 2 months [114]. An ossific mass oriented along the longitudinal axis of the involved muscle with a central area of relative lucency and maximal density peripherally is characteristic [114].

Knee

Athletically derived injuries to the adolescent's knee include collateral and cruciate ligament tears, meniscal injuries, osteochondral fractures, osteochondritis dissecans, injuries to the quadriceps mechanism, and stress fractures [76] (Figs. 24–36 and 24–37). Knee effusions are frequently a sign of an intra-articular knee fracture and are often subtle and difficult to diagnose [19, 76] (see Fig. 24–2). Acute tears of the medial collateral ligament may be associated with anterior cruciate ligament injuries and medial meniscal tears (O'Donahue's triad) [76]. Anterior cruciate ligament tears occur more frequently than posterior cruciate ligament tears [76]. Osteochondritis dissecans may present as an osteochon-

dral fracture and tends to occur at three main sites within the knee: the medial condyle near the intercondylar notch, the lateral femoral condyle near the notch, and the posterior aspect of the patella [76]. Osteochondral fragments may become detached and form loose bodies within the joint [76]. Injuries of the quadriceps mechanism may comprise one or more of four types: ruptures of the quadriceps or patellar tendons, transverse fractures of the patella, and chronic avulsion of the tibial tubercle (Osgood-Schlatter disease) [76, 147] (Fig. 24–38). Acute avulsion fracture of the tibial tuberosity may occur in high jumpers [5]. Stress fractures are usually located along the posterior aspect of the proximal tibia [76].

Chondromalacia of the patella and traction osteochondrosis of the patella ligament (seen in patients with both Osgood-Schlatter disease and Sinding-Larsen-Johansson syndrome) occur in a variety of sports, including gymnastics [54]. Chondromalacia patella is a term used to describe vague anterior knee complaints [147]. Arthroscopic examination may be normal, and there are no specific plain radiographic findings [147]. Identification of any cartilage defect will depend on the results of arthrography, CT, or MRI [115] (Fig. 24–39).

Routine radiographic examination of the knee following trauma requires AP, lateral, and both oblique projections. The lateral view is obtained with the involved knee dependent and flexed about 30 degrees [9]. Joint

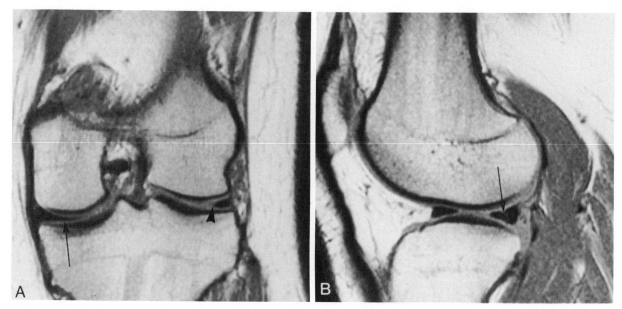

FIGURE 24–36
Lateral meniscal tear. This 16-year-old figure skater had recurrent knee pain and intermittent locking of the knee. Knee radiographs were normal. Proton density T2-weighted coronal and sagittal plane MRI of the knee was performed. The coronal image *(A)* demonstrates a normally sharply pointed medial meniscus of homogeneous low signal intensity (arrow). The medial edge of the lateral meniscus is blunted (arrowhead), reflecting a meniscal tear with fragment separation. The sagittal image *(B)* demonstrates a linear higher signal intensity change (arrow) in the posterior horn of the lateral meniscus, representing an additional segment of tear.

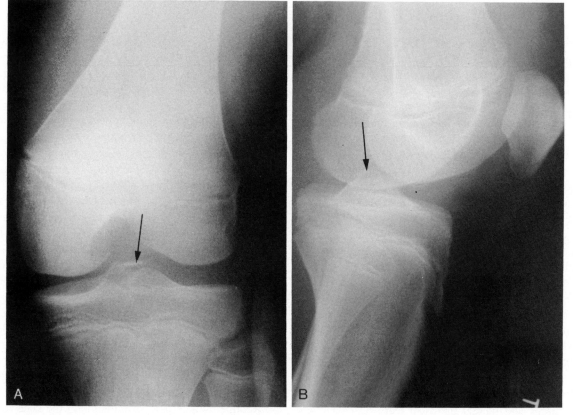

FIGURE 24–37
Fracture of tibial spine. This 14-year-old soccer player sustained a blow to his right knee. Anteroposterior *(A)* and lateral *(B)* views demonstrate an avulsion fracture of the tibial spine (arrows). Conventional radiographic projections usually suffice for defining articular fractures, although at least two projections, preferably at right angles, are considered a minimum study.

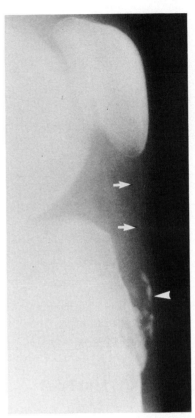

FIGURE 24–38
Osgood-Schlatter disease. This 16-year-old baseball catcher repeatedly and intentionally fell on his knees. Tenderness and soft tissue swelling in each pretibial region resulted in a clinical diagnosis of Osgood-Schlatter disease, which was confirmed on a lateral knee radiograph. Radiographic findings characteristic of Osgood-Schlatter disease are loss of sharp definition of the posterior margin of the lower infrapatellar tendon (arrows), pretibial soft tissue swelling, and fragmentation and irregularity of the anterior tibial tubercle (arrowhead). In cases of clinically suspected Osgood-Schlatter disease, lateral knee radiographs are recommended to exclude a possible osteosarcoma or even osteomyelitis.

Assessment of suspected medial collateral ligamentous injury can be accomplished with stress views, although pain and swelling may make it difficult to perform this technique in patients with an acutely injured knee [9, 151]. The examination is usually performed manually by fixing the extremity with a bolster or strap and applying force in the opposite direction. AP views are obtained with the leg extended, lateral views with the knee flexed 90 degrees [9]. Measured differences of more than 3 mm between the normal and abnormal knees suggest ligamentous injury [9]. Heterotopic new bone formation adjacent to the medial femoral condyle (Pellegrini-Stieda lesion) may occur when a medial collateral ligamentous injury is old [76].

An anterior or posterior cruciate ligamentous tear may present as a post-traumatic hemarthrosis, appearing as fluid within the suprapatellar bursa on lateral radiographs [76]. Avulsion fracture fragments may also be evident on radiographs [76]. Graded stress radiographs employing lateral projections and variable stress can distinguish partial from complete tears of the anterior cruciate ligament [128].

Double-contrast arthrography of the knee had been a

effusions are best detected on the lateral view and appear as increased soft tissue density within the suprapatellar pouch [76]. A cross-table lateral view may be substituted in patients who cannot be moved [9]. In a patient with a fracture within the knee joint compartment, the cross-table lateral view may permit visualization of a fat-fluid level within the joint space, indicating a lipohemarthrosis [9, 76]. Additional projections that may be important in specific instances of trauma are the notch and patella projections [9]. Radiographic findings in Osgood-Schlatter disease are loss of sharp definition of the posterior margin of the infrapatellar tendon due to edema, swelling of the soft tissue anterior to the tibial tubercle, and irregularity and fragmentation of the tibial tubercle [76].

Injury to the medial collateral ligament may appear as soft tissue swelling adjacent to the medial femoral condyle on the AP view, a finding that is nonspecific [76].

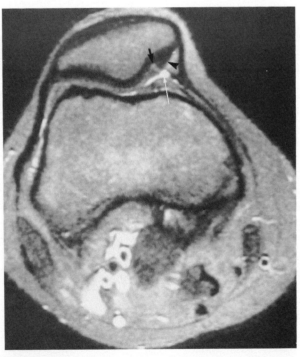

FIGURE 24–39
Chondromalacia patellae. This 15-year-old figure skater had left knee pain but no history of specific injury. Radiographs of the knee were normal. Axial plane fast-spin echo (T2-weighted) MRI demonstrates a focal area of linear increased signal intensity (arrow) within the articular cartilage of the medial patellar facet adjacent to an area of low signal intensity (arrowhead); these findings together are indicative of chondromalacia. There is a small amount of high signal intensity fluid (white arrow) in the adjacent joint space. MRI is the only imaging modality presently available that can diagnose chondromalacia.

widely employed technique that permits evaluation of the menisci, cruciate ligaments, articular cartilage, synovial diseases, loose bodies, intra-articular fractures, and patellar alignment [9]. Accuracy of arthrography is greater than 90% in experienced hands [9, 76]. The most common indication for knee arthrography is evaluation of the menisci [9]. High-resolution CT following double-contrast arthrography permits improved definition of intra-articular structures and meniscal tears [52]. MRI has replaced most knee arthroscopy.

MRI is well suited for evaluation of many pathologic conditions of the knee, including post-traumatic changes [15, 45, 75, 123, 137, 138, 159]. Tears of the menisci, patellar tendon, and anterior and posterior cruciate ligaments are readily identified by MRI [15, 45, 58, 75, 89, 102, 123, 150, 159, 165] (Figs. 24–40 and 24–41). MRI findings consistent with a cruciate ligament tear include frank disruption of the ligament, waviness of the margin of the ligament, and an area of heterogeneous high signal within the ligament [15, 58, 89, 123, 159]. Occult intraosseous fractures of the knee have been identified by MRI when conventional radiographs were normal [88]. MRI is excellent for excluding significant intra-articular pathology of the knee [123].

Ultrasonography has had limited use in evaluating the

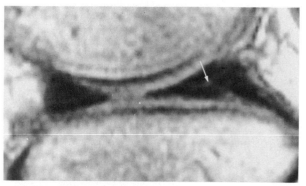

FIGURE 24–41
Meniscal tear. This 16-year-old football player had left knee pain. Proton density sagittal MRI demonstrates a high signal intensity linear change (arrow) in the posterior horn of the lateral meniscus, representing a complex meniscal tear. MRI is rapidly replacing arthrography for the diagnosis of internal joint derangement, including meniscal tears.

soft tissue component of osteochondrosis of the tibial tuberosity (Osgood-Schlatter disease) and of the patella (Sinding-Larsen-Johansson disease) [31].

Lower Leg, Ankle, and Foot

Injuries of the lower leg, ankle, and foot include acute fractures, soft tissue injuries, and dislocations, chondral fractures, stress fractures, and tenosynovitis [127] (Fig. 24–42). Contusions and ankle sprains are the most common athletic injuries [147]. Nondisplaced Salter-Harris type I fractures of the distal fibular physis are common and present a diagnostic challenge in the pediatric and adolescent athlete [127, 130, 147]. Other common ankle fractures in the child and adolescent are Salter-Harris II, triplane, and Tillaux fractures [26, 90, 130]. Chronic foot pain in the young athlete may be due to osteochondritis of the metatarsal head (Freiberg's disease) [127]. Stress fractures of the foot are less common in adolescent athletes; when present, they usually involve the second and third metatarsals [127]. Osteochondritis dissecans of the dome of the talus may produce pain in the ankle [147]. Sever's disease is calcaneal apophysitis occurring in the preadolescent athlete [147].

Standard AP and lateral views of the tibia and fibula should include the adjacent knee and ankle joints [9]. Oblique projections can give additional information about fracture rotation and alignment [9]. Because the distal tibial growth plate closes in a medial-to-lateral direction, fractures of the lateral plafond of the tibia may be obscured by the overlying fibula on the AP view and only appreciated on the oblique view [90].

Radiographic examination of the ankle following trauma requires AP, lateral, mortise (internal oblique), and external oblique views [26]. The AP view best demonstrates the tibiotalar joint and medial joint mortise, the

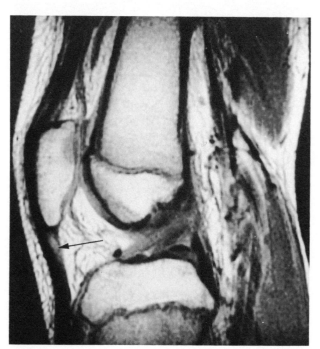

FIGURE 24–40
Chronic tendinitis of the infrapatellar tendon. This 15-year-old basketball player had chronic pain in the infrapatellar region of the left knee. Midsagittal plane, proton density spin echo MRI demonstrates an area of increased signal intensity (arrow) within the infrapatellar tendon, which is suggestive of infrapatellar tendinitis. The normal infrapatellar tendon should appear homogeneously dark. In addition, the infrapatellar tendon is thickened, suggesting that the process is chronic, and the patella is inferiorly displaced by at least 5 mm.

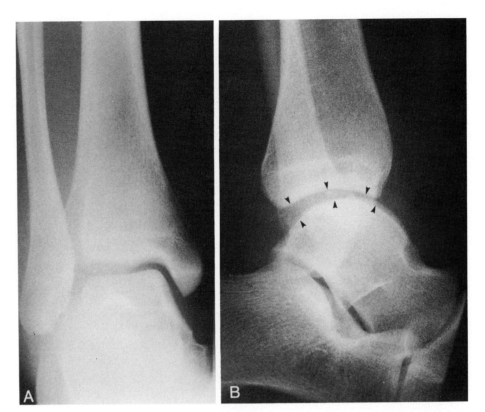

FIGURE 24–42
Post-traumatic ankle joint instability. This 17-year-old basketball player landed hard on his right ankle and experienced subsequent severe pain and soft tissue swelling. The AP view *(A)* shows prominent lateral soft tissue swelling and slight asymmetry of the ankle mortise. The lateral view *(B)* demonstrates mild anterior subluxation of the talus relative to the distal tibia (arrowheads). Although plain radiographs can exclude a fracture and suggest ligamentous injury, stress views may be necessary to identify post-traumatic joint instability adequately.

lateral view demonstrates the AP dimensions of the tibiotalar and the posterior subtalar joint, and the mortise view allows visualization of the entire ankle mortise [9].

Varus and valgus stress views of the ankle are obtained to evaluate ligamentous injury following ankle sprains [26]. A difference of 3 mm between the injured and uninjured sides indicates ligamentous injury.

AP, lateral, and oblique views are routinely obtained in patients with foot trauma [9]. The AP view best demonstrates the articular relationship of the tarsal-metatarsal and phalangeal joints, and the medial oblique view improves definition of the third through fifth tarsal-metatarsal joints, which overlap on the AP view [9]. More specialized additional views include axial calcaneal, subtalar, and sesamoid views. The axial calcaneal view more clearly demonstrates the trochlear process, sustentaculum tali, and calcaneocuboid articulation [9]. The subtalar view demonstrates the subtalar joint and sinus tarsi region [9]. The sesamoid view projects the sesamoid bones away from the first metatarsal, allowing sesamoid fractures to be more readily identified [9].

Radiographic evaluation for possible tarsal coalition as a cause of chronic hindfoot pain should begin with AP, lateral, and 45-degree oblique projections [127]. Tarsal beaking, widening of the lateral process, and talocalcaneal midfacet coalitions may indicate the presence of a hindfoot coalition [127]. A coronal plane CT scan of the foot and ankle is the optimal way to evaluate a patient for a hindfoot coalition, however [127].

Stress-related injuries of the tibia, as demonstrated by radionuclide bone scanning, may be one of three types: stress fractures, shin splints, and "indeterminate bone stress" [135]. The posterior tibial cortex is the most common site of involvement [135].

Ankle arthrography is most frequently performed to evaluate suspected ligamentous tears [9]. Both routine and stress views are usually obtained [9].

SPECIAL PROBLEMS AND SITUATIONS

Slipped Capital Femoral Epiphysis

Slipped capital femoral epiphysis (SCFE) is the most common disorder of the hips in adolescents and has an incidence of 2 cases per 100,000 [24, 125] (Fig. 24–43). The goals of treatment of SCFE are stabilization and prevention of additional slipping, stimulation of early physeal closure, and prevention of avascular necrosis, chondrolysis, and osteoarthritis as complications of treatment [24].

Radiographic evaluation for SCFE must include both AP and frog-leg lateral projections of the pelvis and both hips [24]. Because slippage always involves a posterior but not necessarily a medial component, milder degrees of SCFE may be apparent only on the lateral view and may be overlooked or not diagnosable on the AP projec-

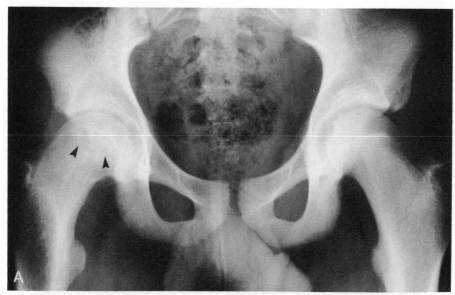

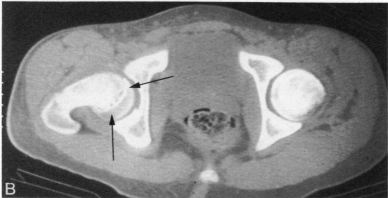

FIGURE 24–43
Slipped capital femoral epiphysis (SCFE). This 14-year-old male football player complained for 2 months of persistent right hip pain but continued to play football. The initial AP view of the pelvis *(A)* demonstrates narrowing of the width of the right femoral capital epiphysis compared to the normal left side and lucency on the metaphyseal side of the right femoral physis or growth plate (arrowheads). The proximal right femur is relatively osteopenic, reflecting a voluntary decrease in usage and stress placed on the right leg. These findings suggest a slipped right capital femoral epiphysis, which was confirmed on a lateral view. The lateral view of the proximal femur is considerably more sensitive than the AP view in defining epiphyseal slippage and should be included in any hip radiographic study when SCFE is suspected.

An axial CT image of the hips *(B)* demonstrates the posteriorly rotated, slipped right femoral epiphysis (arrows). CT is excellent at demonstrating the epiphyseal slip, any associated metaphyseal cystic change, and secondary deformity of the acetabulum. In this case, the acetabulum is normal.

tion alone [125]. Radiographic classification of SCFE, based on the amount of movement of the femoral head on the neck of the femur, is as follows: minimum, less than one-third of the femoral neck diameter; moderate, between one-third and two-thirds; and severe, more than two-thirds [24].

If treatment of SCFE involves pinning, fluoroscopy is employed to confirm satisfactory position of the pins, which traverse the physis and end in the epiphysis but do not extend into the joint space. Two projections taken at 90 degrees are usually sufficient to confirm satisfactory position [24].

Subsequent imaging of patients with SCFE is essential to assess for the following potential complications: varus deformity with a short and broad femoral neck, osteonecrosis, chondrolysis, and early degenerative joint disease [125].

Low Back Pain in Athletes

Low back pain in children and adolescents is usually due to organic disease; possible causes include biome-chanical factors, infection, metabolic and developmental disorders, neoplasms, trauma, and spondylolysis or spondylolisthesis [64, 98, 112, 145, 156]. Sports-related injuries to the spine are seen with increasing frequency in young persons participating in a wide variety of sports activities [39, 54, 68–70, 112]. When low back pain is acute in onset and follows a clearly defined episode of trauma, conventional radiographic examination of the lumbosacral spine consisting of AP, lateral, and both oblique projections is recommended [145]. If the low back pain is chronic or recurrent, thereby indicating the possibility of an overuse or stress injury, both conventional lumbosacral spine radiographs and bone scintiscans using ^{99m}Tc methylene diphosphonate (MDP) are recommended [112]. Whereas radiography is anatomically superior and more specific, bone scintigraphy is a very sensitive indicator of bone remodeling and therefore permits detection of abnormalities when conventional radiographs are normal [64, 65, 112]. CT or conventional tomography of the lumbosacral spine is recommended only if the bone scan demonstrates a focal abnormality and conventional radiographs fail to adequately categorize the nature of the lesion.

Single photon emission computed tomography (SPECT) is more sensitive than conventional radiography and CT in identifying structural abnormalities of the lumbosacral spine in patients with chronic low back pain [10, 49, 136]. SPECT can also provide improved anatomic localization compared to radiography and CT [136].

Vertebral body apophyseal fractures (representing localized injuries to the vertebral growth plate) and spondylolysis with or without spondylolisthesis are usually detectable on conventional spine radiographs [50, 64, 112]. The pars defect of spondylolysis is best detected radiographically on the lateral view by a break in the "neck of the Scottie dog" sign or on the oblique views [64, 114] (see Figs. 24–19 and 24–20). In cases of isthmic stress fracture, bone scintigraphy can be positive when conventional radiographs are normal [50, 112, 114, 147]. Subsequent radiographs may or may not be abnormal depending on the pattern of healing of the initial injury [112]. Osteoid osteomas causing low back pain are best defined anatomically by CT; bone scintigraphy reliably identifies the presence and site of abnormality but is seldom specific for the type of abnormality present.

MRI currently provides the most accurate morphologic evaluation of the intervertebral disc, including nerve root compression secondary to disc herniation, and without using ionizing radiation [64].

The major contribution of imaging studies to the evaluation of low back pain in young patients is their ability to diagnose spondylolysis or focal stress reaction and to exclude infection or neoplasm as the cause of the pain [112]. A recommended imaging algorithm in young patients with low back pain is shown in Figure 24–44.

Stress Fractures

Stress fractures in children and adolescents are most commonly secondary to repetitive microtrauma that eventually overcomes the ability of normal bone to resist fracturing [125]. The proximal tibia is most commonly affected in children [77, 125].

In its early stages a stress fracture may not be definable on conventional radiographs [77, 125]. Abnormal isotope localization on a bone scan can often achieve the earliest diagnosis by imaging when radiographs are nor-

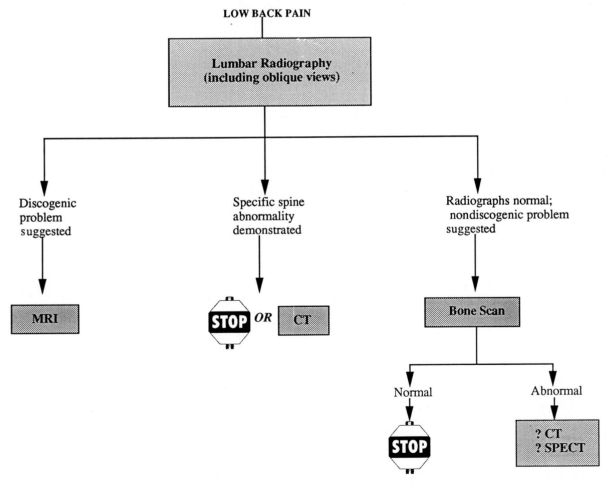

FIGURE 24–44
Imaging algorithm in adolescents with low back pain.

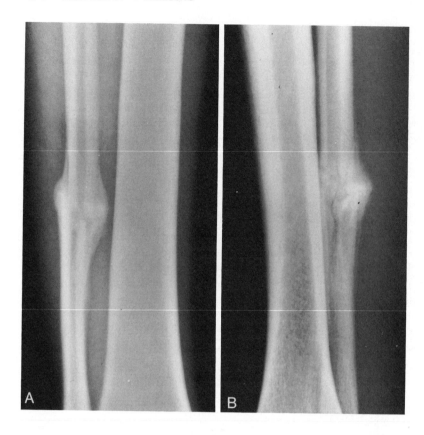

FIGURE 24–45

Healing stress fracture. This 15-year-old high school cross-country runner experienced 3 months of chronic pain in the outer aspect of the left lower leg that was aggravated by running and walking. A localized associated bump in the region of pain had developed. AP *(A)* and lateral *(B)* radiographs of the left lower leg demonstrate extensive localized callus around a distal fibular stress fracture. A bone scan showed increased isotope localization in the same area.

Acute stress fractures are commonly not visible radiographically. A radionuclide bone scan is usually positive when the radiograph is negative and is the best way to diagnose an acute stress fracture. Within a week or two, sufficient healing and callus formation has normally occurred to permit a radiographic diagnosis.

mal [77, 125]. MRI may show increased cortical signal intensity and decreased medullary signal intensity as early abnormal signs of stress fractures [125].

Depending on the location of a stress fracture, the radiographic findings will vary; a metaphyseal stress fracture may appear as a transverse intraosseous band of sclerosis, representing traumatic condensation of trabeculae, whereas a diaphyseal stress fracture may be indicated by a linear cortical radiolucency accompanied by periosteal and endosteal cortical thickening [77, 125] (Fig. 24–45).

References

1. Abel, M.S. Jogger's fracture and other stress fractures of the lumbosacral spine. *Skel Radiol* 13(3):221–227, 1985.
2. Adams, J.E. Injury to the throwing arm. A study of traumatic changes in the elbow joints of boy baseball players. *Calif Med* 102:127–132, 1965.
3. Adams, J.E. Little League shoulder: Osteochondrosis of the proximal humeral epiphysis in boy baseball players. *Calif Med* 105:22–25, 1966.
4. Alley, R.H., Jr. Head and neck injuries in high school football. *JAMA* 188:418–422, 1964.
5. Balmat, P., Vichard, P., and Pem, R. Treatment of avulsion fractures of the tibial tuberosity in adolescent athletes. *Sports Med* 9(5):311–316, 1990.
6. Barone, G.W., and Rodgers, B.M. Pediatric equestrian injuries: A 14-year review. *J Trauma* 29(2):245–247, 1989.
7. Barry, J.F., Harwood-Nash, D.C., Fitz, C.R., et al. Metrizamide in pediatric myelography. *Radiology* 124:409–418, 1977.
8. Becker, E., and Griffiths, H.J.L. Radiologic diagnosis of pain in the athlete. *Clin Sports Med* 6(4):699–711, 1987.
9. Berquist, T.H. *Imaging of Orthopedic Trauma and Surgery.* Philadelphia, W.B. Saunders, 1986.
10. Bodner, R.J., Heyman, S., Drummond, D.S., et al. The use of single photon emission computed tomography (SPECT) in the diagnosis of low back pain in young patients. *Spine* 13:1155–1160, 1988.
11. Bowerman, J.W., and McDonnell, E.J. Radiology of athletic injuries: Baseball. *Radiology* 116:611–615, 1975.
12. Bowerman, J.W., and McDonnell, E.J. Radiology of athletic injuries: Football. *Radiology* 117:33–36, 1975.
13. Brody, A.S., Ball, W.S., and Towbin, R.B. Computed arthrotomography as an adjunct to pediatric arthrography. *Radiology* 170:99–102, 1989.
14. Burk, D.L., Jr., Karasick, D., Mitchell, D.G., et al. MR imaging of the shoulder: Correlation with plain radiology. *AJR* 154:549–553, 1990.
15. Burk, D.L., Jr., Mitchell, D.G., Rifkin, M.D., et al. Recent advances in magnetic resonance imaging of the knee. *Radiol Clin North Am* 28(1):379–393, 1990.
16. Cacayorin, E.D., Hochhauser, L., and Petro, G.R. Lumbar and thoracic spine pain in the athlete: Radiographic evaluation. *Clin Sports Med* 6(4):767–783, 1987.
17. Cantu, R.C. Head and spine injuries in the young athlete. *Clin Sports Med* 7(3):459–472, 1988.
18. Carter, S.R., Aldridge, M.J., Fitzgerald, R., et al. Stress changes of the wrist in adolescent gymnasts. *Br J Radiol* 61(722):109–112, 1988.
18a. Carter, S. R., and Aldridge, M. J.: Stress injury of the distal radial growth plate. *J Bone Joint Surg* 70B:834–836, 1988.
19. Clanton, T., et al. Knee ligament injuries in children. *J Bone Joint Surg* 61A:1195, 1979.
20. Clark, C.R., Igram, C.M., El-Khoury, G.Y., et al. Radiographic evaluation of cervical spine injuries. *Spine* 13(7):742–747, 1988.
21. Cohen, M.D. MRI of the gastrointestinal and musculoskeletal systems in children. *Appl Radiol*, July, 1987.
22. Conway, J.J. Radionuclide bone scintigraphy in pediatric orthopedics. *Pediatr Clin North Am* 33(6):1313–1334, 1986.
23. Crass, J.R., Craig, E.V., Cretzke, C., et al. Ultrasonography of the rotator cuff. *RadioGraphics* 5:941–953, 1985.

24. Crawford, A.H. Current concept review: Slipped capital femoral epiphysis. *J Bone Joint Surg* 70A(9):1422–1427, 1988.

25. Curtis, R.J., Jr., and Corley, F.G., Jr. Fractures and dislocation of the forearm. *Clin Sports Med* 5(4):663–680, 1986.

26. Daffner, R.H. Ankle trauma. *Radiol Clin North Am* 28(2):395–421, 1990.

27. Daffner, R.H., Martinez, S., and Gehweiler, J.A. Stress fractures in runners. *JAMA* 247(7):1037–1041, 1982.

28. Daffner, R.H., Martinez, S., Gehweiler, J.A., Jr., et al. Stress fractures of the proximal tibia in runners. *Radiology* 142:63–65, 1982.

29. Daffner, R.N., Riemer, B.L., Lupetin, A.R., et al. Magnetic resonance imaging in acute tendon ruptures. *Skel Radiol* 15:619–621, 1986.

30. Daly, P.J., Sim, F.H., and Simonet, W.T. Ice hockey injuries: A review. *Sports Med* 10(3):122–131, 1990.

31. DeFlaviis, L., Nessi, R., Scaglione, P., et al. Ultrasonic diagnosis of Osgood-Schlatter and Sinding-Larsen-Johansson diseases of the knee. *Skel Radiol* 18:193–197, 1989.

32. DeHaven, K.E., and Lintner, D.M. Athletic injuries: Comparison by age, sport and gender. *Am J Sports Med* 14:218–224, 1986.

33. Deutch, A.L., Resnick, D., Mink, J.H., et al. Computed and conventional arthrotomography of the glenohumeral joint: Normal anatomy and clinical experience. *Radiology* 153:603, 1984.

34. Dooms, G.C., Fisher, M.R., Hricak, H., et al. MR imaging of intramuscular hemorrhage. *J Compu Assis Tomogr* 9:908–913, 1985.

35. Duthoy, M.J., and Lund, G. MR imaging of the spine in children. *Eur J Radiol* 8:188–195, 1988.

36. Ehara, S., El-Khoury, G.Y., and Soto, Y. Cervical spine injury in children: Radiologic manifestations. *AJR* 151:1175–1178, 1988.

37. Ehman, R.L., and Berguist, J.H. Magnetic resonance imaging of musculoskeletal trauma. *Radiol Clin North Am* 24:291–319, 1986.

38. Ehman, R.L., Berguist, T.H., and McLeod, R.A. MR imaging of the musculoskeletal system: A 5-year appraisal. *Radiology* 166:313–320, 1988.

39. Ferguson, R.H., McMaster, J.H., and Stanitski, C.L. Low back pain in college football linemen. *Am J Sports Med* 2:63–69, 1974.

40. Fernbach, S.K., and Wilkinson, R.H. Avulsion injuries of the pelvis and proximal femur. *AJR* 137(3):581–584, 1981.

41. Fishman, E.K., Magid, D., Ney, D.R., et al. Three dimensional imaging in orthopedics: State of the art 1988. *Orthopedics* 11(7):1021–1026, 1988.

42. Fishman, E.K., Magid, D., Ney, D.R., et al. Three-dimensional imaging. *Radiology* 181:321–337, 1991.

43. Fitz, C.R. Diagnostic imaging in children with spinal disorders. *Pediatr Clin North Am* 32(6):1537, 1985.

44. Fleckenstein, J.L., Weatherall, P.T., Parker, R.W., et al. Sports-related muscle injuries: Evaluation with MR imaging. *Radiology* 172:793–798, 1989.

45. Gallimore, G.W., and Harris, S.E. Knee injuries: High resolution MR imaging. *Radiology* 160:457–461, 1986.

46. Garrick, J.G., and Requa, R.H. Injury patterns in children and adolescent skiers. *Am J Sports Med* 7:245, 1979.

47. Garrick, J.G., and Requa, R.K. Girls sports injuries in high school athletics. *JAMA* 239(21):2245–2248, 1978.

48. Garrick, J.G., and Requa, R.H. Injuries in high school sports. *Pediatrics* 61:465–469, 1978.

49. Gates, G.F. SPECT imaging of the lumbosacral spine and pelvis. *Clin Nucl Med* 13:907–914, 1988.

50. Gelfand, M.J., Strife, J.L., and Kereiakes, J.G. Radionuclide bone imaging in spondylolysis of the lumbar spine in children. *Radiology* 140:191–195, 1981.

51. Geslieu, G.E., Thrall, J.H., Espinosa, J.L., et al. Early detection of stress fractures using ^{99m}Tc-polyphosphate. *Radiology* 121:683–687, 1976.

52. Ghelman, B. Meniscal tears of the knee: Evaluation by high resolution CT combined with arthrography. *Radiology* 157:23, 1985.

53. Glynn, T.P., Jr., Kreipke, D.L., and DeRosa, G.P. Computed tomography arthrography in traumatic hip dislocation. *Skel Radiol* 18:29–31, 1989.

54. Goldberg, M.J. Gymnastics injuries. *Orthop Clin North Am* 11:717, 1980.

55. Goldberg, L., Rothfus, W.E., Deeb, Z.L., et al. The impact of magnetic resonance on diagnostic evaluation of acute cervicothoracic spinal trauma. *Skel Radiol* 17:89–95, 1988.

56. Griffiths, H.J., and DeHaven, K.E. Magnification and high resolution radiography in sports-related injuries. *Am J Sports Med* 9(6):394–399, 1981.

57. Groskin, S. The radiologic evaluation of chest pain in the athlete. *Clin Sports Med* 6(4):845–871, 1987.

58. Grover, J.S., Bassett, L.W., Gross, M.L., et al. Posterior cruciate ligament: MR imaging. *Radiology* 174:527–530, 1990.

59. Gyll, C., and Blake, N.S. *Paediatric Diagnostic Imaging.* London, W. Heineman, 1986.

60. Habibian, A., Stauffer, A., Resnick, D., et al. Comparison of conventional and computed arthrotomography with MR imaging in the evaluation of the shoulder. *J Compu Assis Tomogr* 13(6):968–975, 1989.

61. Hall, T.R., and Kangarloo, H. Magnetic resonance imaging of the musculoskeletal system in children. *Clin Orthop* 244:119–130, 1989.

62. Harcke, H.T., Grissom, L.E., and Finkelstein, M.S. Evaluation of the musculoskeletal system with sonography. *AJR* 150:1253–1261, 1988.

63. Harris, J.H. Radiologic evaluation of spinal trauma. *Orthop Clin North Am* 17:75–86, 1986.

64. Harvey, J., and Tanner, S. Low back pain in young athletes. A practical approach. *Sports Med* 12(6):394–406, 1991.

65. Haughton, V.M. MR imaging of the spine. *Radiology* 166:297–301, 1988.

66. Ireland, D. Common hand injuries in sport. *Austr Fam Phys* 13(11):797–800, 1984.

67. Ireland, M.L., and Andrews, J.R. Shoulder and elbow injuries in the young athlete. *Clin Sports Med* 7(3):473–494, 1988.

68. Jackson, D.W. Low back pain in young athletes: Evaluation of stress reaction and discogenic problems. *Am J Sports Med* 4:364–366, 1979.

69. Jackson, D.W., and Wiltse, L.L. Low back pain in young athletes. *Physician Sportsmed* 2:53–60, 1974.

70. Jackson, D.W., Wiltse, L.L., and Cirincione, R.J. Spondylolysis in the female gymnast. *Clin Orthop* 117:68–73, 1976.

71. Jackson, D.W., Wiltse, L.L., and Dingeman, R.D. Stress reactions involving the pars interarticularis in young athletes. *Am J Sports Med* 9:304–312, 1981.

72. Jackson, D.W., Wiltse, L.L., Dingeman, R.D., et al. Stress reactions involving the pars interarticularis in young athletes. *Am J Sports Med* 9:304–312, 1981.

73. Jaramillo, D., Hoffer, F.A., Shapiro, F., et al. MR imaging of fractures of the growth plate. *AJR* 155:1261–1265, 1990.

74. Jokl, P., and Lynch, J.K. Epiphyseal growth plate: Physiology and effects of sports. *Ann Sports Med* 2(2):55–58, 1985.

75. Kanal, E., Burk, D.L., Jr., Brunberg, J.A., et al. Pediatric musculoskeletal magnetic resonance imaging. *Radiol Clin North Am* 26(2):211–239, 1988.

76. Kaye, J.J., Nance, E.P., Jr. Pain in the athlete's knee. *Clin Sports Med* 6(4):873–883, 1987.

77. Keats, T.E. The spectrum of musculoskeletal stress injury. *Curr Prob Diagn Radiol* 13(2):7–51, 1984.

78. Kieft, G.J., Sartoris, D.J., Bloem, J.L., et al. Magnetic resonance imaging of glenohumeral joint diseases. *Skel Radiol* 16:285–290, 1987.

79. Klein, A., Sumner, T.E., Volberg, F.M., et al. Combined CT-arthrography in recurrent traumatic hip dislocation. *AJR* 138:963, 1982.

80. Kleinman, P.K., and Spevak, M.R. Advanced pediatric joint imaging. *Radiol Clin North Am* 28(5):1073–1109, 1990.

81. Kornguth, P.J., and Salazar, A.M. The apical oblique view of the shoulder: Its usefulness in acute trauma. *AJR* 149:113–116, 1987.

82. Kuhlman, J.E., Fishman, E.K., Ney, D.R., et al. Complex shoulder trauma: Three-dimensional CT imaging. *Orthopedics* 11:1561–1563, 199.

83. Kulkarni, M.V., McArdle, C.B., Kopanicky, D., et al. Acute spinal cord injury: MR imaging at 1.5T. *Radiology* 164:837–843, 1987.

84. Kumar, R., Madewell, J.E., Swischuk, L.E. The normal and abnormal growth plates. *Radiol Clin North Am* 25(6):1133–1153, 1987.

85. Kursunoglu-Brahme, S., Gundry, C.R., and Resnick, D. Advanced imaging of the wrist. *Radiol Clin North Am* 28(2):307–320, 1990.

86. Ledesma-Medina, J., Newman, B., and Oh, K.S. Disturbances of bone growth and development. *Radiol Clin North Am* 26(2):441–463, 1988.

87. Lee, B.C.P., Kazam, E., and Newman, A.D. Computed tomography of the spine and spinal cord. *Radiology* 128:95–102, 1978.

88. Lee, J.K., and Yao, L. Occult intraosseous fracture: Magnetic resonance appearance versus age of injury. *Amer J Sports Med* 17(5):620–623, 1989.

89. Lee, J.K., Yao, L., and Wirth, C.R. Magnetic resonance imaging of major ligamentous knee injuries. *Physician Sportsmed* 18(4), 1990.

90. Letts, R.M. The hidden adolescent fracture. *J Pediatr Orthop* 2(2):161–164, 1982.

91. Levine, A.M., and Edwards, C.C. Traumatic lesions of the occipitoatlantoaxial complex. *Clin Orthop* 239:53–68, 1989.

92. Lombardo, S.J., Retting, A.C., and Kerlan, R.K. Radiographic abnormalities of the iliac apophysis in adolescent athletes. *J Bone Joint Surg* 65(4)A:444–446, 1983.

93. Mann, D.C., and Rajmaira, S. Distribution of physeal and non-physeal fractures in 2,650 long-bone fractures in children aged 0–16 years. *J Pediatr Orthop* 10:713–716, 1990.

94. Martire, J.R. The role of nuclear medicine bone scans in evaluating pain in athletic injuries. *Clin Sports Med* 6(4):713–737, 1987.

95. McCauley, E., Hudash, G., Shields, K., et al. Injuries in women's gymnastics—the state of the art. *Am J Sports Med* 15:558–565, 1987.

96. *Merrill's Atlas of Radiographic Positions and Radiologic Procedures* (5th ed.). Ballinger, P.W. (Ed.). St. Louis, C.V. Mosby, 1982.

97. Meyers, M.C., Elledge, J.R., Sterling, J.C., et al. Injuries in intercollegiate rodeo athletes. *Am J Sports Med* 18(1):87–91, 1990.

98. Micheli, L.J. Low back pain in the adolescent: Differential diagnosis. *Am J Sports Med* 7:362–364, 1979.

99. Micheli, L.J. Overuse injuries in children's sports: The growth factor. *Orthop Clin North Am* 14:337–360, 1983.

100. Micheli, L.J. Common painful sports injuries: Assessment and treatment. *Clin J Pain* 5(2):551–560, 1989.

101. Modic, M.T., Masaryk, T., and Paushter, D. Magnetic resonance imaging of the spine. *Radiol Clin North Am* 24(2):229–245, 1986.

102. Moore, S.G., Bisset, G.S., III, Siegel, M.J., et al. Pediatric musculoskeletal MR imaging. *Radiology* 179:345–360, 1991.

103. Moskwa, C.A., Jr., and Nicholas, J.A. Musculoskeletal risk factors in the young athlete. *Phys Sportsmed* 17(11), 1989.

104. Newberg, A.H. The radiographic evaluation of shoulder and elbow pain in the athlete. *Clin Sports Med* 6(4):785–809, 1987.

105. Newberg, A.H. Computed tomography of joint injuries. *Radiol Clin North Am* 28(2):445–460, 1990.

106. Nielsen, A.B., and Yde, J. Epidemiology and traumatology of injuries in soccer. *Am J Sports Med* 17(6):803–807, 1989.

107. Nielsen, A.B., and Yde, J. An epidemiologic and traumatologic study of injuries in handball. *Int J Sport Med* 9:341–344, 1988.

108. Niitsu, M., Anno, I., Fukubayashi, T., et al. Tears of cruciate ligaments and menisci: Evaluation with cine MR imaging. *Radiology* 178:859, 1991.

109. Nussbaum, A.R., Treves, S.T., and Micheli, L. Bone stress lesions in ballet dancers: Scintigraphic assessment. *AJR* 150:851–855, 1988.

110. Ogden, J.A. *Skeletal Injury in the Child.* Philadelphia, Lea & Febiger, 1982.

111. Paille, P., Quesnel, C., Baunin, C., et al. Computed arthrography: Its role in the screening of joint diseases in pediatric radiology. *Pediatr Radiol* 18:386–390, 1988.

112. Papanicolaou, N., Wilkinson, R.H., Evans, J.B., et al. Bone scintigraphy and radiography in young athletes with low back pain. *AJR* 145:1039–1044, 1985.

113. Park, H.M., Rothschild, P.A., and Kernek, C.B. Scintigraphic evaluation of extremity pain in children: Efficacy and pitfalls. *AJR* 145:1079–1084, 1985.

114. Pavlov, H. Roentgen examination of groin and hip pain in the athlete. *Clin Sports Med* 6(4):829–843, 1987.

115. Pavlov, H. Athletic injuries. *Radiol Clin North Am* 28(2):435–443, 1990.

116. Pavlov, H., and Torg, J.S., Roentgen examination of cervical spine injuries in the athlete. *Clin Sports Med* 6(4):751–766, 1987.

117. Pavlov, H., Warren, R.F., Weiss, C.B., Jr., et al. The roentgenographic evaluation of anterior shoulder instability. *Clin Orthop* 194:153–158, 1985.

118. Pitt, M.J., and Speer, D.P. Imaging of the elbow with the emphysis on trauma. *Radiol Clin North Am* 28(2):293–305, 1990.

119. Post, M.J.D., and Green, B.A. The use of computed tomography in spinal trauma. *Radiol Clin North Am* 21:327–375, 1983.

120. Rafii, M., Firooznia, H., Bonamo, J.J., et al. Athlete shoulder injuries: CT arthrographic findings. *Radiology* 162(2):559–564, 1987.

121. Rafii, M., Minkoff, J., Bonamo, J., et al. Computed tomography (CT) arthrography of shoulder instabilities in athletes. *Am J Sports Med* 16(4):352–361, 1988.

122. Recht, M.P., Burk, D.L., Jr., and Dalinka, M.K. Radiology of wrist and hand injuries in athletes. *Clin Sports Med* 6(4):811–828, 1987.

123. Reicher, M.A., Hartzman, S., Bassett, L.W., et al. MR imaging of the knee. Part I. Traumatic disorders. *Radiology* 162:547–551, 1987.

124. Resjo, M., Harwood-Nash, D.C., Fitz, C.R., et al. Normal cord in infant and children examined with computed tomographic metrizamide myelography. *Radiology* 130:691–696, 1979.

125. Resnik, C.S. Diagnostic imaging of pediatric skeletal trauma. *Radiol Clin North Am* 27(5):1013–1022, 1989.

126. Retsky, J., Jaffe, D., and Christoffel, K. Skateboarding injuries in children: A second wave. *Am J Dis Child* 145:188–192, 1991.

127. Rettig, A.C., Shelbourne, K.D., Beltz, H.F., et al. Radiographic evaluation of foot and ankle injuries in the athlete. *Clin Sports Med* 6(4):905–919, 1987.

128. Rijke, A.M., Goitz, H.T., McCue, F.C., III, et al. Graded stress radiography of injured anterior cruciate ligaments. *Invest Radiol* 26:926–933, 1991.

129. Roberts, F.F., Kishore, P.R.S., and Cunningham, M.E. Routine oblique radiography of the pediatric lumbar spine: Is it necessary? *AJR* 131:287–298, 1978.

130. Rogers, L.F. The radiography of epiphyseal injuries. *Radiology* 96:289–299, 1970.

131. Rosen, P.R., Micheli, L.J., and Treves, S. Early scintigraphic diagnosis of bone stress and fractures in athletic adolescents. *Pediatrics* 70:11–15, 1982.

132. Roser, L.A., and Clauson, D. Football injuries in the very young athlete. *Clin Orthop* 69:212, 1970.

133. Rothman, S.L. Computed tomography of the spine in older children and teenagers. *Clin Sports Med* 5(2):247–270, 1986.

134. Roub, L.W., Gumerman, L.W., Hanley, EN., et al. Bone stress: A radionuclide imaging perspective. *Radiology* 132:431–438, 1979.

135. Rupani, H.D., Holder, L.E., Espinola, D.A., et al. Three-phase radionuclide bone imaging in sports medicine. *Radiology* 156:187–196, 1985.

136. Ryan, P.J., Evans, P.A., Gibson, T., et al. Chronic low back pain: Comparison of bone SPECT with radiography and CT. *Radiology* 182:849–854, 1992.

137. Shellock, F.G., Foo, T.K.F., Deutsch, A.L., et al. Patellofemoral joint: Evaluation during active flexion with ultrafast spoiled GRASS MR imaging. *Radiology* 180:581–585, 1991.

138. Shellock, F.G., Mink, J.H., Deutsch, A.L., et al. Patellar tracking abnormalities: Clinical experience with kinematic MR imaging in 130 patients. *Radiology* 172:799–804, 1989.

139. Sherry, E. Radiology of skiing injuries. *Austr Radiol* 29(4):359–369, 1985.

140. Shuman, W.P., Kilcoyne, R.F., Matson, F.A., et al. Double contrast computed tomography of the glenoid labrum. *AJR* 141:581, 1983.

141. Siffert, R.S., and Levy, R.N. Athletic injuries in children. *Pediatr Clin North Am* 12:1027–1037, 1965.

142. Singson, R.D., Feldman, F., and Rosenberg, Z.S. Elbow joint: Assessment with double contrast CT arthrography. *Radiology* 160:167, 1986.

143. Smith, A.D. Foot and ankle injuries in figure skaters. *Physician Sportsmed* 18(3), 1990.

144. Stafford, S.A., Rosenthal, D.I., Gebhardt, M.C., et al. MRI in stress fracture. *AJR* 147:553–556, 1986.

145. Stanitski, C.L. Low back pain in athletes. *Physician Sportsmed* 10:77–91, 1982.

146. Stanitski, C.L. Pediatric sports injuries. *Adv Orthop Surg* 9:53–57, 1985.

147. Stanitski, C.L. Management of sports injuries in children and adolescents. *Orthop Clin North Am* 19(4):689–698, 1988.

148. Stanitski, C.L. Common injuries in preadolescent and adolescent athletes: Recommendations for prevention. *Sports Med* 7:32–41, 1989.

149. Stiffert, R.S. The effect of trauma to the epiphysis and growth plate. *Skel Radiol* 2:21–30, 1977.

150. Stoller, D.W., Martin, C., Cruse, J.V., et al. Meniscal tears: Pathologic correlation with MR imaging. *Radiology* 163:731–735, 1987.

151. Sullivan, J.A. Ligamentous injuries of the knee in children. *Clin Orthop Pediatr Res* 255:44–50, 1990.

152. Sullivan, J.A., et al. Evaluation of injuries in youth soccer. *Am J Sports Med* 8:325, 1980.

153. Sullivan, J.A., et al. Outdoor and indoor soccer: Injuries among youth players. *Am J Sports Med* 14:231–233, 1986.

154. Tator, C.H., Ekong, C.E., Rowed, D.W., et al. Spinal injuries due to hockey. *Can J Neurol Sci* 11(1):34–41, 1984.

155. Tertti, M., Paajanen, H., Kujala, U.M., et al. Disc degeneration in young gymnasts: A magnetic resonance imaging study. *Am J Sports Med* 18(2):206–208, 1990.

156. Thomas, J.C., Jr. Plain roentgenograms of the spine in the injured athlete. *Clin Sports Med* 5(2):353–371, 1986.

157. Thompson, N., Halpern, B., Curl, W.W., et al. High school football injuries: Evaluation. *Am J Sports Med* 15:117–124, 1987.

158. Tsai, J.C., and Zlatkin, M.B. Magnetic resonance imaging of the shoulder. *Radiol Clin North Am* 28(2):279–291, 1990.

159. Turner, D.A., Prodromos, C.C., Petasnick, J.P., et al. Acute injury of the ligaments of the knee: Magnetic resonance evaluation. *Radiology* 154:717–722, 1985.

160. Tursz, A., and Crost, M. Sports-related injuries in children. A study of their characteristics, frequency, and severity, with comparison to other types of accidental injuries. *Am J Sports Med* 14:294–299, 1986.

161. Walter, M., and Wolf, M. Stress fractures in young athletes. *Am J Sports Med* 5:165, 1977.

162. Wilberger, J.E., and Maroon, J.C. Cervical spine injuries in athletes. *Physician Sportsmed* 18(3):000, 1990.

163. Wilcox, J.R., Moniot, A.L., and Green, J.P. Bone scanning in the evaluation of exercise-related stress injuries. *Radiology* 123:699–703, 1977.

164. Wilson, A.J., Totty, W.G., Murphy, W.A., et al. Shoulder joint: Arthrographic CT and long-term follow-up, with surgical correlation. *Radiology* 173:329–333, 1989.

165. Wirtz, C.R., Yao, L., and Lee, J.K. Magnetic resonance imaging of meniscal tears. *Physician Sportsmed* 18(3), 1990.

166. Wroble, R.R., Mysnyk, M.C., Foster, D.T., et al. Patterns of knee injuries in wrestling: A 6-year study. *Am J Sports Med* 14:55–66, 1986.

167. Yde, J., and Nielsen, A.B. Sports injuries in adolescents' ball games: Soccer, handball, and basketball. *Br J Sports Med* 24:51–54, 1990.

168. Zaricznyj, B., et al. Sports-related injuries in school-aged children. *Am J Sports Med* 8:318, 1980.

REHABILITATION FOR CHILDHOOD AND ADOLESCENT ORTHOPAEDIC SPORTS-RELATED INJURIES

James J. Irrgang, M.S., P.T., A.T.C.
Rajiv Sawhney, M.S., P.T.

A striking number of young girls and boys enter organized and unorganized sports yearly. Are these young children ready for sports? From a physiologic point of view, the muscle strength and endurance capacity of children and adolescents is more than adequate for sports [44]. Participation in sports for many children is a positive experience in normal development. Sports involvement provides an opportunity for children to have fun, socialize, and be physically active while acquiring new skills.

Despite the many positive benefits of sports participation for children, negative experiences may occur. In addition to the possibility of incurring physical injury from sports participation, another plausible negative feature may be the problem of development of low self-esteem, depression, and excessive anxiety related to involvement in sports [31].

To ensure the safe conduct of sports and to minimize sports injuries in the young, the American Academy of Pediatrics and the American Academy of Sports Medicine have issued guidelines for participation in sports [22]. The importance of proper coaching is stressed in the guidelines.

Following an injury, rehabilitation is necessary before an athlete can return safely to sport or activity participation. This concept is readily identifiable in the adolescent and adult population, but little information is available on the rehabilitation of the pediatric athlete. The rehabilitation of musculoskeletal injuries in pediatric and adolescent athletes is discussed in this chapter with special emphasis on physiologic and psychological considerations.

DEFINITIONS OF REHABILITATION

Rehabilitation is defined as any measure used to restore the injured athlete to normal activity as quickly and safely as possible. The overall goal of rehabilitation is restoration of the prior level of function. In athletics, time is of the essence when an athlete is recovering from an injury; however, complete resolution of the injury and prevention of recurrence should not be sacrificed to allow an early return to sport.

The primary concern following an injury is to reduce the pain and swelling associated with acute inflammation. As the reparative process begins, one should focus on techniques that enhance tissue healing. These include restoration of joint motion, musculotendinous flexibility, muscular strength, power, and endurance, cardiovascular endurance, proprioception, coordination, and agility.

Restoration of the prior level of function, including a safe return to athletic activities, should be the final outcome of the rehabilitation process. The return to athletics should be a gradual process. It should include a period of reconditioning that allows a transition from rehabilitation to full participation. Often this transition period is overlooked, resulting in reinjury. If return to the prior level of function is not possible, the health care team must counsel the athlete and parents on realistic expectations, which may include modified sports participation. When necessary, alternative sports and activities should be recommended. At all times the long-term welfare of the child should be considered. A long active lifestyle should not be sacrificed for a few moments of glory for the child or parent.

Rehabilitation includes the application of physical modalities and therapeutic exercises to promote healing and restore function. Modalities include a variety of physical agents such as various forms of heat, cold, sound, electricity, and massage to effect healing, reduce pain, swelling, and spasm, and control blood flow. Therapeutic exercise includes movements prescribed to restore or favorably alter factors such as range of motion, flexibility, strength, and endurance.

Several concerns need to be addressed when one is developing a rehabilitation program for children. These concerns include the effects of physical modalities and therapeutic exercise on the open epiphysis, the length of the musculotendinous unit relative to the length of bone during growth, and the lack of androgenic hormones in the prepubescent child, which are necessary for increasing muscle mass and strength. These factors are addressed throughout the remainder of the chapter as they pertain to rehabilitation of sports-related injuries.

Psychological factors such as emotional maturity, motivation, and level of understanding of the injury should also be considered. These factors dictate that the rationale for treatment and instructions be given in terms that are easily understood by both the child and the parent. When possible, activities and games should be incorporated into the rehabilitation program to improve compliance and prevent boredom.

INFLAMMATION AND REPAIR

Acute Inflammation

Acute inflammation includes a series of reactions of vascularized tissue in response to injury. The purpose of inflammation is to control the effects of the injurious agent and prepare the area for the subsequent repair process. The basic inflammatory response is nonspecific in that it is the same whether the injurious agent is trauma, bacteria, heat, or cold. Acute inflammation is characterized by swelling, redness, warmth, pain, and loss of function. It is an immediate response to injury and lasts for up to 72 hours. The events of acute inflammation include transient vasoconstriction followed by

vasodilation, exudation, consolidation, and finally neutralization of the noxious stimuli.

A period of transient vasoconstriction occurs immediately after the injury and lasts for 5 to 10 minutes. This transient vasoconstriction is followed by active vasodilation of the blood vessels in the injured area. This vasodilation is associated with increased permeability of the capillary membranes. Clinically, this results in swelling of the involved area. Pain results from chemical irritation and pressure on free nerve endings. Pain results in atrophy, loss of motion, and impaired function.

Migration of leukocytes into the area is mediated by chemotactic agents that have yet to be identified but are called leukotoxins [11]. The proteolytic enzymes released from the neutrophils include protease and collagenase, which solubilize connective tissue and interfere with formation of ground substance and collagen in the process of fibroplasia. The presence of the proteolytic enzymes released from neutrophils can delay or prevent the process of repair.

Monocytes are predominant in the later stages of inflammation. They merge to form macrophages, which further ingest and digest debris. Successful macrophage function with neutralization of the area marks the end of the acute inflammatory phase.

Repair

Repair includes the process of fibroplasia as well as maturation and remodeling of the scar. Fibroplasia begins as the noxious stimuli are neutralized. Fibroblasts migrate into the area along the fibrin network.

Fibroblasts begin to produce collagen by the fourth to fifth day following injury and continue to produce collagen for 2 to 4 weeks.

During fibroplasia the tensile strength of the scar increases significantly in relation to the amount of collagen produced. Molecular cross-linking between the fibrils lends further strength to the scar at this time. Once sufficient collagen has been produced, the number of fibroblasts in the area decreases. The end result of fibroblasia is a large disorganized dense scar. The fibers are randomly oriented, and the tissue is very fragile.

Maturation and remodeling of the scar result in pronounced changes in the form, bulk, and strength of the scar. During this period the collagen fibers become more regularly oriented. The tensile strength of the scar increases in relation to increased intra- and intermolecular cross-linking. Stresses placed on the scar directly affect the remodeling and maturation process, which may continue for many years.

Soft tissue wounds including defects in muscle, ligament, and tendon heal by formation of scar tissue through the processes of acute inflammation, fibroplasia, and maturation and remodeling. Unfortunately, the scar is never as strong as the tissue it replaces. It is important to remember that healing is a continuum, so that the stages of the process overlap. Fibroplasia overlaps with acute inflammation, and maturation and remodeling begin during the process of fibroplasia.

An understanding of the soft tissue healing process is imperative in establishing an appropriate rehabilitation program. The clinical signs and symptoms associated with each stage of healing can be used to mark the progress of the rehabilitation program so that it produces the desired outcome within the shortest period of time without exceeding the limits of the healing tissue. The rehabilitation program must be individually designed to account for the nature, severity, and current state of healing of the injury.

PHYSICAL MODALITIES

Physics of Heat and Cold

Heat flows from one body to another only when one body is at a higher temperature; heat flows from the hotter to the cooler body. In this sense, application of a cold pack to the body results in heat flow from the body to the cold pack with a lowering of tissue temperature. Classification of body temperatures is shown in Table 25–1 [30].

Heat can be transferred by conduction, convection, conversion, and radiation. Transfer of heat by conduction is the result of direct molecular impact between two bodies in contact with each other. An example of heating by conduction is the application of a hot pack to the body.

Heating by convection occurs in fluids and gases and is the result of currents created from unequal temperature densities. As liquids or gases are heated, they expand and become less dense and are forced upward. Cooler portions of the liquid or gas are more dense and move downward. Temperature gradients set up convection currents within the liquid or gas and act to transfer heat. The process of convection continues until all por-

tions of the liquid or gas are heated to the same temperature. A whirlpool is an example of heating by convection.

Heating by conversion involves the application of one form of energy to the body that acts to increase the molecular motion of body tissues. Ultrasound is an example of heating by conversion.

Radiation involves transference of heat through intervening spaces between two bodies not in actual contact. The kinetic energy of a given body is constantly being converted and emitted as radiant energy. When radiant energy strikes another body, it can be reflected, transmitted, or absorbed. Radiant energy that is absorbed imparts kinetic energy or heat to the body. Examples of heating by radiation include microwave and shortwave diathermy.

Cold is defined as the absence of kinetic energy or heat. Cooling can occur by conduction or evaporation. Cooling by conduction is similar to heating by conduction in that heat transfer occurs through direct molecular impact. Energy is transferred from the faster moving molecules of the hotter body to the slower moving molecules of the cooler body.

Cooling by evaporation occurs as heat is lost through evaporation of liquids from the surface of an object. The quicker the rate of evaporation, the greater the rate of heat loss. The use of vapocoolant sprays such as fluoromethane is an example of cooling by evaporation.

The magnitude of temperature change that occurs when heating or cooling an object by conduction depends on the temperature difference between the two objects, the time of exposure, the thermal conductivity of tissues, and the type of agent used to produce the heating or cooling [53]. The rate of heat transfer can be summarized by the equation:

$$D = \frac{Area \times K \times (T1 - T2)}{Thickness \ of \ tissue}$$

where D is the rate of heat transfer in calories/second, K is the thermal conductivity of the tissues, and T1 − T2 is the temperature difference between warm and cool objects. Area is the amount of body surface that is exposed to the heating or cooling agent. An increase in the area being heated or cooled results in a greater rate of heat exchange. Thermal conductivity (K) is the measure of a material's ability to conduct heat. Generally, tissues higher in water content are better conductors of heat. For this reason, muscle, which has a higher water content than fat, is a better conductor of heat than fat. Adipose tissue acts as an insulator of heat transfer. The greater the temperature gradient between the body surface and the heating or cooling agent, the greater the rate of heat exchange. The thickness of tissue refers to the depth of the structure targeted for heating or cooling beneath the

TABLE 25–1
Classification of Temperature with Respect to the Human Body

32–55°F	Very cold
55–65°F	Cold
65–80°F	Cool
80–92°F	Neutral
92–98°F	Warm
98–104°F	Hot
>104°F	Very hot

surface of the body. Structures that lie far beneath the surface of the body have a slower rate of heat exchange. All these factors must be considered when conductive forms of heat or cold are applied to the body in order to regulate the dose and extent of the physiologic reactions produced.

Therapeutic Application of Cold

Cryotherapy is the local application of cold for therapeutic purposes. It involves producing relatively low tissue temperatures for a short period of time. The reduction in temperature is localized to the area being cooled.

Physiologic Responses to the Application of Cold

The local application of cold results in vasoconstriction of blood vessels in the area exposed to cold with a resultant decrease in blood flow. Vasoconstriction is the body's attempt to conserve heat. It is caused by direct and reflex nervous responses of the blood vessels to cold. The application of cold stimulates thermal receptors in the skin that reflexively excite sympathetic nerves, resulting in contraction of smooth muscle in the wall of the blood vessel. Cooling can also result in generalized cutaneous vasoconstriction. As the cooled blood returns to the central circulation, it stimulates the anterior hypothalamus, which can result in generalized vasoconstriction [53].

Vasodilation can develop in response to prolonged application of cold. This was described as the "hunting response" by Lewis [42]. Secondary vasodilation in response to cold results in increased blood flow to the area and is a protective response to prevent injury of the tissues due to prolonged exposure to cold. Continued cooling results in alternate periods of vasoconstriction followed by vasodilation. The mechanism of secondary vasodilation in response to prolonged application of cold is not clearly understood but may be related to an axon reflex with release of a neurotransmitter similar to histamine [42] or to a slowing of nerve conduction velocity with subsequent paralysis of smooth muscle within the blood vessel wall [15, 47].

Cold also reduces blood flow by increasing the viscosity of blood. As blood is cooled, its viscosity increases. Increased resistance to flow of the cooled blood results in slowing of blood flow.

Cold inhibits the action of histamine, thereby limiting its ability to produce vasodilation and increase capillary permeability. This further decreases blood flow in the cooled area and restricts formation of exudate.

Cold reduces the metabolic activity of cells in the cooled area, resulting in decreased requirements for oxygen and other nutrients.

Stiffness reflects the ability of tissues to lengthen in response to stress. Plasticity is the tissue's ability to lengthen permanently. Cold increases stiffness and decreases plasticity of connective tissue. Application of cold makes it more difficult for connective tissue to stretch and to maintain its new length.

Cold is an effective analgesic, particularly for acute throbbing pain, lowering the excitability of free nerve endings and peripheral nerve fibers. Cold slows nerve conduction velocity, leading to eventual conduction failure with extreme cooling. Slowing of nerve conduction velocity results in decreased perception of pain. Additionally, application of cold following injury minimizes edema formation, which in turn results in less pressure on free nerve endings, limiting the development of pain. Histamine is a strong pain-producing substance whose action is inhibited by the application of cold.

Muscle spasm is reduced by cold. Spasm is a sustained contraction of the muscle that often accompanies injury to protect the injured area. Spasm occurs reflexly in response to pain as well as to chemical or mechanical irritation of the nerve or muscle. Cold decreases spasm by lowering the sensitivity of the muscle spindle to stretch, allowing the muscle to relax [54].

Indications for Uses of Cold

The physiologic actions of cold make cryotherapy an effective anti-inflammatory agent. Cold can be used to limit acute inflammatory reactions following traumatic injuries such as contusions, sprains, and strains. Cold can also be effective in limiting acute inflammation associated with surgery. As an anti-inflammatory agent, cold reduces pain, limits hemorrhage and swelling, and limits secondary tissue damage related to hypoxia. Application of cold following therapeutic exercise helps to control pain and swelling and limits inflammation caused by the exercise. When cold is applied to treat acute traumatic conditions, it should be coupled with compression and elevation (Fig. 25–1). Cold can be used as an analgesic for painful conditions and is particularly useful for treatment of acute throbbing pain.

Cryokinetics combines exercise with the use of cold. Application of cold desensitizes the area to allow pain-free range of motion exercise. Cryokinetics has been found to be an effective means of treatment for acute musculoskeletal injuries [25, 29]. Cold can be used with stretching exercises to reduce muscle spasm [57].

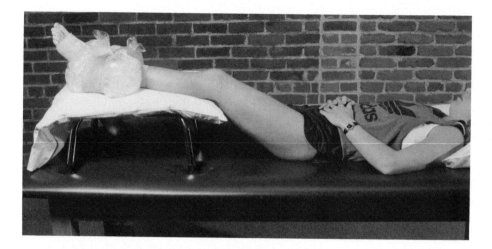

FIGURE 25–1
Cold combined with compression and elevation.

Contraindications and Precautions for the Use of Cold

Prolonged use of cold may cause tissue damage. Drez and colleagues [21] reported neurapraxia and axonotmesis following prolonged application of cold over superficial nerves. Additionally, prolonged application of cold may elicit the hunting reaction, alternately increasing and decreasing blood flow. This may increase hemorrhage and edema formation following acute injury. Cold should not be used in areas of compromised blood flow. Cooling an ischemic area may further compromise blood flow, increasing the potential for ischemic necrosis. Areas of decreased sensation should be treated with caution. Insensitive areas may be inadvertently exposed to toxic amounts of cold because the individual is unable to perceive the danger.

Application of cold should be avoided in individuals who have cold sensitivity symptoms, including those who experience cold urticaria, which is an allergic reaction to cold. Urticaria may result in the development of hives and joint pain. Systemically, cold urticaria may result in flushing of the face, a drop in blood pressure, increased pulse rate, and syncope [54].

Individuals with Raynaud's phenomenon experience abnormal extreme vasoconstriction in response to cold, resulting in inadequate blood flow to maintain metabolism of the tissues. Pain develops in response to the ischemia. Hyperemia follows the period of ischemia. An individual with Raynaud's phenomenon will report pain and blanching of the skin when it is exposed to cold. This is followed by reddening of the area. Raynaud's phenomenon is common in those with rheumatic disease, particularly lupus erythematosus and scleroderma.

Other conditions for which cold is contraindicated include cryoglobinemia and paroxysmal cold hemoglobinuria [54]. Cryoglobinemia is characterized by abnormal protein that forms a gel or precipitate at low temper-

atures. Precipitate or gel formation can result in ischemia or gangrene of the involved area. Paroxysmal cold hemoglobinuria results in lysis of red blood cells with release of hemoglobin that appears in the urine.

The application of cold to healing wounds may delay the normal healing process. This may be related to decreased blood flow to the wound in response to cooling. Some individuals do not respond well psychologically to the application of cold. Those with an aversion to cold should not be treated with cold. Hypertensive patients should be treated with caution because cold may increase systolic and diastolic blood pressure. Caution should be used to avoid treating a large surface area for a prolonged period of time in hypertensive individuals.

In athletes, caution must be exercised when using cold as an analgesic to mask protective pain. Cold used as an analgesic to allow continued participation may cause further injury. Additionally, the use of cold prior to intense physical exercise may increase stiffness of connective tissue and predispose the athlete to injury.

When cold is used to treat athletic injuries in the child or adolescent, care must be taken to avoid the problems identified earlier. Often children are unreliable judges of temperature and may be exposed to toxic doses of cold. Also, the child's thermoregulatory mechanisms are not well developed, and prolonged application of cold may result in hypothermia. The use of cold by a child should be closely supervised by an adult to avoid problems and to ensure compliance with the recommendations.

Methods of Application of Cold

Many methods of cold application are available. The method of choice is dependent on the part to be treated and the specific aims of the treatment. Generally, the time needed for the use of cold is 10 to 30 minutes. Treatment time should be shorter for more localized superficial conditions. Treatment time should be extended for treatment of more deep-seated lesions, particularly if they are covered by an insulating layer of fat. Prolonged continuous treatment with cold should be avoided. Applications of cold can be reapplied every 2 to 4 hours as needed. Once the acute symptoms following injury have subsided, the use of ice should be discontinued because cold can delay healing [30].

Ice Packs

Ice packs can be created by placing ice in a plastic bag or a towel. Crushed or shaved ice is preferred to cubes or blocks of ice because it can be shaped to fit the treatment area. Ice packs are the preferred method of treatment if prolonged cooling to low temperatures is desired. They are also more economical than commercial cold packs. A moist towel should be placed between the plastic bag and the athlete's skin to modify cold transfer, making treatment more comfortable.

Commercial Cold Packs

Commercial cold packs consist of a plastic cover surrounding a hydrated silica gel that is kept in a freezer or cooling unit at 0° to 10°F. Commercial cold packs are neat and conform well to the body part being treated. They can maintain a low temperature for a relatively long period of time but do not lower skin temperature as much as an ice pack. Commercial cold packs are used to produce a less intense and more prolonged cooling. Commercial cold packs probably do not lower temperatures enough to produce an analgesic effect.

Ice Massage

Ice massage is the use of a block of ice over the area to be cooled (Fig. 25–2). The ice block is made by freezing water in a paper or Styrofoam cup after inserting a tongue depressor in the water to provide a handle for use when massaging the area. Ice massage is indicated for treatment of small areas of pain or localized inflammation. The block of ice should be massaged over the area to be treated using a rhythmic motion at moderate speed. Treatment time is 5 to 10 minutes or until anesthesia is produced when treating pain. When the goal of treatment is to limit inflammation, the length of treatment should be extended to 10 to 20 minutes.

Therapeutic Applications of Heat

Physiologic Responses to the Application of Heat

The physiologic effects of heat are essentially the opposite of those described for cold. The vascular response to the local application of heat is vasodilation of blood vessels in the warmed area. This results in increased blood flow to the area accompanied by delivery of oxygen and nutrients and removal of waste products. Following acute injury, application of heat encourages hemorrhage and edema formation and will delay the healing process. Vasodilation is the body's attempt to dissipate the excess build-up of heat. Increased blood flow produced by vasodilation helps to remove heat from the area, preventing damage to the tissues. Vasodilation in response to application of heat may be the result of axon or local spinal cord reflexes, release of a chemical mediator, or stimulation of the anterior hypothalamus [53].

Heat stimulates cutaneous thermoreceptors, resulting in activation of sensory nerves. A portion of this sensory nerve activity is carried antidromically to blood vessels lying in the skin, resulting in vasodilation. Local spinal cord reflexes are initiated by sensory input originating from the cutaneous thermal receptors and result in de-

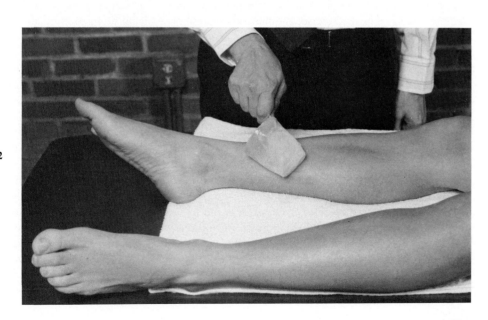

FIGURE 25–2
Ice massage.

creased postganglionic sympathetic nerve activity and vasodilation of the heated area. Additionally, these reflexes can produce vasodilation in areas remote from the application of heat and can be used to increase blood flow safely in areas of peripheral vascular disease. For example, application of heat to the back may be used to increase cutaneous blood flow to the lower extremities.

Afferent stimulation produced by activation of thermal receptors in response to heat can also travel to the higher levels of the central nervous system to stimulate the vasomotor center of the anterior hypothalamus. This results in cutaneous vasodilation in an attempt to remove the excess build-up of heat from the body.

Application of heat causes the release of chemical mediators associated with inflammation including histamine and prostaglandins. These substances produce a mild inflammatory reaction in response to heat. This reaction includes vasodilation, which results in increased capillary membrane permeability and thus in mild edema. The application of heat primarily affects blood flow through the skin. Redness of the skin following application of heat is evidence that blood flow through the cutaneous vessels has increased. Application of heat produces a sharp increase in skin temperature during the first 4 minutes of application. A more gradual increase in temperature occurs until the maximum temperature is reached by the seventh to eighth minute. During the remaining 20 minutes of treatment time, skin temperature remains the same or slowly declines [1, 41]. These effects are explained by the fact that after the seventh to eighth minute of heating, cutaneous blood flow has increased and is able to remove excess heat from the area.

The effect of blood flow through skeletal muscles is primarily regulated by the metabolic activity of the muscle and can be increased by exercise of the muscle. Blood flow through muscle is unaffected or minimally increased by application of heat. Greenberg [26] evaluated the effects of heat, exercise, and the combination of heat and exercise on blood flow. One minute of exercise alone produced a ninefold increase in blood flow over the resting level. Blood flow quickly returned to resting level after exercise was terminated. The application of heat for 20 minutes produced a gradual and longer lasting increase in blood flow. Twenty minutes of heat increased blood flow twofold over the resting level, and blood flow remained elevated for at least 15 minutes after termination of the heat. The increase in blood flow occurred primarily through the skin as evidenced by redness. The increase in blood flow due to exercise was produced in the active muscles. Exercise was the treatment of choice to improve blood flow to the muscle. The combination of heat and exercise together produced an additive effect on blood flow and resulted in the greatest increase in total blood flow.

The effects of application of heat on joint temperature and blood flow are not clear. Horvath and Hollander [33] reported a decrease in intra-articular temperature following the application of superficial heat. They postulated that application of heat caused a reflexive decrease in joint temperature as blood flow was shunted from the joint to the skin. Cobbold and Lewis [16] demonstrated an increase in blood flow to the knee joint following application of radiant heat. Borrell and colleagues [9] demonstrated increased joint temperature of the foot and hand following 20 minutes of dry heat. A 5°C increase in joint temperature was associated with a fourfold increase in enzymaticolysis of articular cartilage collagen [28]. This may accelerate degeneration of articular cartilage.

Application of heat increases tissue metabolism. Increased tissue metabolism increases the demands for oxygen and nutrients and can stimulate blood flow to the area. Following acute injury, heat will increase secondary hypoxic injury in tissues that survived the initial trauma.

The application of heat also increases the acute inflammatory response following injury. Vasodilation caused by heating enhances edema and hemorrhage formation, resulting in a longer time necessary for resolution.

Once exudation and consolidation are complete, application of heat during the subacute phase of inflammation may aid in neutralizing the noxious stimuli through removal of waste and debris as a result of increased blood flow in the heated area. Repair during the fibroblastic stage may be enhanced by increased delivery of nutrients and oxygen.

The application of heat enhances plasticity, or permanent deformation, of connective tissue. Lehman and associates [40] studied the effects of heat and stretching on the extensibility of rat tail tendons. The results indicated that heating alone produced no elongation and that stretching alone produced no residual elongation. Significant elongation occurred if heat and stretch were combined. A greater increase in length was found if the stretch was applied during the period of heating rather than after the application of heat. A greater increase in length was maintained if the stretch was maintained during the period of cooling. Overall, the most effective method of producing a residual increase in length of connective tissue was to apply a sustained stretch during the application of heat and to maintain the stretch during the period of cooling.

Application of heat increases the pain associated with acute inflammation. This is related to enhanced vasodilation and blood flow through the heated area, which produces increased edema and hemorrhage with increased pressure on free nerve endings. Additionally, heat enhances the action of histamine, which is a strong pain-producing agent.

Subacute and chronic pain described as soreness,

aches, or stiffness may be decreased by the local application of heat. Heat affects the free nerve endings and peripheral nerves, increasing the threshold for pain perception. Lehman and colleagues [38] demonstrated increased pain threshold measurements over the heated area and fifth finger following application of heat to the ulnar nerve at the medial aspect of the elbow. Pain produced by the accumulation of metabolites and waste products such as lactic acid may be decreased by application of heat. Joint stiffness is relieved following application of heat. This may be related to alteration of the viscous flow properties of collagen with heating.

The application of heat can reduce muscle spasm. This may be related to the clearance of waste products such as lactic acid, which acts as a chemical irritant to the muscle. Elimination of chemical irritation to the muscle allows the muscle to relax. Additionally, heat can reduce muscle spasm by decreasing the muscle spindle's sensitivity to stretch. Mease [51] reported decreased activity of the group II afferents from the muscle spindle and increased activity of group I fibers from the Golgi tendon organ (GTO) in response to increased muscle temperature. These changes could decrease alpha motor neuron activity and reduce muscle spasm.

Systemic effects of heating occur away from the site of application of heat. They are produced by stimulation of thermoreceptors in the skin that provide input to the anterior hypothalamus. The systemic effects of heating are less pronounced than the local effects and are dependent on the size of the area heated. Systemic responses to heat reflect the body's attempt to prevent elevation of the core temperature. The body strives to maintain homeostasis by distal vasodilation to aid in the removal of heat. Other systemic responses to heat include increased sweat production, increased metabolism, and increased oxygen consumption with an increase in respiratory and heart rates. Heart rate increases 10 beats/minute for every 1°F increase in core temperature. The ability to dissipate heat systematically is reduced in the child, and therefore local application of heat may produce an artificial fever [30].

The extent of the physiologic reactions produced by heat depend on the temperature reached in the tissues, treatment time, rate of temperature change, and size of the area heated. The therapeutic range for the application of heat is 40° to 45°C. Tissue temperatures less than 40°C are not effective in producing physiologic changes. Temperatures greater than 45°C are associated with tissue destruction. The technique of application of heat is important to ensure that the therapeutic range is reached in the desired tissue without exceeding the therapeutic temperature range in adjacent tissues. This is especially important when one is using deep heat modalities such as ultrasound where one cannot rely on the sensation of warmth to regulate dosage.

The minimum effective duration for the application of heat is 3 to 5 minutes. More complete reactions are achieved after heat has been applied for 20 to 30 minutes. Treatment in excess of 30 minutes will not result in further physiologic changes. A more vigorous physiologic response to heat is achieved when the rate of temperature change is rapid. This is explained by the fact that of the total treatment time, only that portion that produces therapeutic temperatures in the tissues will be biologically effective. A greater physiologic response also can be produced by heating a larger surface area.

Indications for the Therapeutic Use of Heat

The indications for the therapeutic use of heat are derived from the physiologic actions of heat. Heat is indicated in traumatic conditions *after* the acute symptoms have subsided. Application of heat increases blood flow to aid in the process of neutralization by removing debris and waste and aid in repair by bringing nutrients and oxygen to the healing area. Heat can be used to increase an athlete's range of motion if it is used in combination with therapeutic exercise. Heat increases the viscous flow properties of connective tissue, allowing greater plasticity. Heat can be used to decrease subacute or chronic pain by increasing the pain threshold of peripheral nerves and free nerve endings and by increasing blood flow to clear metabolites that irritate free nerve endings. Muscle spasm can be reduced by the application of heat by removing chemical irritants to muscles and reducing the sensitivity of the muscle spindle to stretch.

Contraindications and Precautions for the Use of Heat

Heat is contraindicated in patients with acute traumatic conditions. Application of heat to acute injuries will increase both secondary hypoxic injury to the surrounding tissues and edema and hemorrhage formation. Active bleeding may be increased by the application of heat. Malignancies are a contraindication to heat because heat is hypothesized to increase the rate of cell growth and the chance of metastasis [53]. Use of heat is contraindicated in individuals who have a fever. Application of heat in an individual who has a fever may result in a further increase in core temperature and may place additional stress on the cardiorespiratory system. Individuals with cardiac insufficiency may not be able to tolerate the additional stress on the heart produced by generalized exposure to heat.

Special care must be taken during the heating of insensitive or ischemic areas. Application of heat to an area of decreased sensation may result in overheating and tissue damage. Ischemic areas may not be able to dissipate the build-up of heat and may result in tissue injury. Special precautions must be taken when applying heat in children because they are unreliable judges of heat and their thermoregulatory mechanisms for the dissipation of heat are not well developed.

Methods of Heating

All methods of heating produce the same physiologic effects. The only difference between the various methods of heating is the depth at which the effects are produced. The choice of heating modality depends on the depth of the structure to be heated, the accessibility of part, the need for movement, the availability of a therapeutic heating agent, and the patient's, physician's, or therapist's preference.

Superficial vs. Deep Heating Modalities

Superficial heating modalities produce heat that penetrates 1 to 5 mm beneath the surface of the body. They produce a vigorous heating response in the skin and subcutaneous tissues and a mild heating response in the deeper structures. It should be noted that superficial heating modalities can produce a vigorous heating response in superficial joints such as the ankle and knee owing to the minimal soft tissue covering of these areas. Examples of superficial heating modalities include hot packs, whirlpool, paraffin, and infrared lamps.

Deep heating modalities include short wave and microwave diathermy and ultrasound. Deep heating modalities are capable of producing a vigorous heating response. Selection of a deep heating modality is dependent on the temperature distribution produced by the modality and the location of the lesion. Attempts should be made to use the modality that produces the highest temperature in the tissue that is injured. However, for practical reasons, ultrasound is the deep heating modality that is most commonly used.

Hot Packs

Hot packs are canvas bags filled with a silica gel that is capable of absorbing water. They are heated by placing them in a thermostatically controlled tank of hot water that is heated to 170°F (Fig. 25–3). Hot packs deliver heat to the body by conduction. They are capable of retaining heat for approximately one-half hour.

Hot packs are a superficial form of heat; however, they can heat deeper tissues through conduction of heat from the superficial tissues. They can be used effectively to treat a localized area. Since hot packs lose heat during treatment, the risk of burning the skin decreases as treatment progresses. The weight of the hot pack may aggravate tender areas. Contact of the hot pack with the skin or repeated use of unwashed toweling may be a potential avenue for the spread of infection.

Paraffin Bath

A paraffin bath contains a mixture of paraffin wax and mineral oil in a ratio of 5 pounds of paraffin to 1 pint of mineral oil. It is heated in a thermostatically controlled unit to 125° to 127°F (Fig. 25–4). Paraffin is an effective means of delivering heat to the hands and feet, which are difficult to heat unless a liquid medium is used. Paraffin is a superficial form of heating by conduction. Deeper tissues are heated by conduction of heat from the superficial tissues. In addition to the effects of heating,

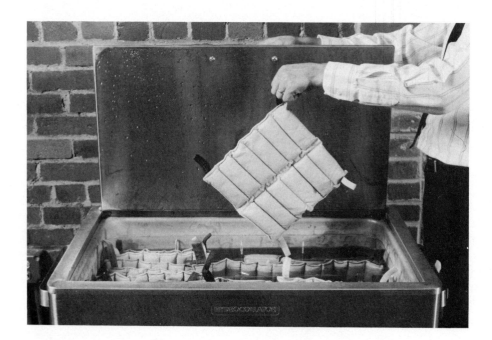

FIGURE 25–3
Hot packs—canvas bags filled with silica gel stored in a thermostatically controlled tank of hot water.

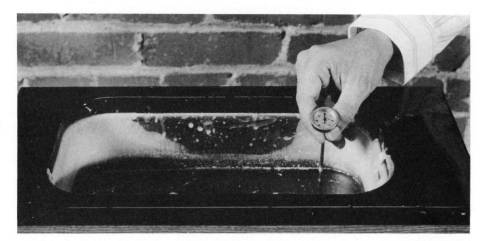

FIGURE 25–4
Paraffin bath.

the wax coating helps to retain perspiration and softens the skin.

Some individuals are unable to tolerate the heat required to keep the paraffin in its molten form. Movement during treatment must be minimized, and there is a potential for messiness, making it a less useful treatment for children. Individuals with open wounds in the area to be heated should not be treated with paraffin to prevent the spread of infection.

Contrast Bath

A contrast bath involves immersion of the affected body part alternately in warm and cold water. Contrast baths provide alternate vasoconstriction and vasodilation, which stimulates peripheral blood flow and promotes healing. Combining the effects of heat and cold makes the adverse effects of each less likely to occur. For example, edema, which might be aggravated by heat, is less likely to occur when alternated with cold. The indications and contraindications for contrast baths are similar to those for the use of heat. Additionally, hypersensitivity to cold is a contraindication for contrast baths.

A contrast bath makes use of two containers of water, one heated to 100° to 110°F, the other cooled to 55° to 65°F. The part to be treated is initially immersed in the hot water for 3 to 5 minutes and then is immersed in cold water for 1 to 2 minutes. The part is alternately immersed in hot and then cold water in this manner for 20 to 30 minutes. Treatment is terminated in either hot or cold water depending on the condition the treatment is being used for. Treatment is terminated in cold water if edema is a concern, and in hot water if stiffness and connective tissue extensibility are a concern.

Whirlpool

Whirlpools use water agitated by an electric turbine (Fig. 25–5). They can be used to provide heat or cooling but are most commonly used as a source of heat. Warm

whirlpools combine the therapeutic effects of heat with exercise in water.

The use of a warm whirlpool heats the body part by means of conduction and convection and produces physiologic changes similar to those produced by other forms of superficial heat. Subcutaneous tissues are heated by conduction of heat from adjacent tissues.

The water also exerts hydrostatic pressure on the im-

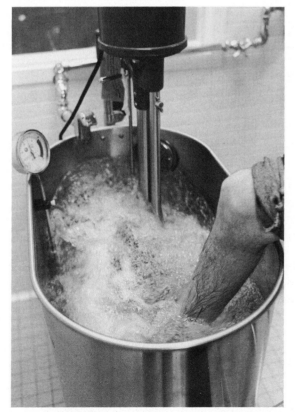

FIGURE 25–5
Whirlpools. Water is agitated by electric turbine.

mersed limb. The hydrostatic pressure increases with increasing depth of immersion and tends to increase the rate of venous and lymphatic flow. Hydrostatic pressure may counteract edema, which would otherwise be produced by heat when the part is in the dependent position.

Agitation of the water increases hydrostatic pressure against the immersed body part and aids venous return. Agitation of the water also provides a means of grading exercise. Movement against the turbulence is resisted while movement in the same direction of the turbulence is assisted. Agitation of the water decreases the thermal gradients in the water, keeping the temperature of the water in the whirlpool consistent throughout. The cleansing action of the whirlpool is enhanced by agitation of the water.

The whirlpool offers several advantages over other forms of superficial heat. Higher tissue temperatures can be created because the part is insulated from evaporative heat loss. The patient can move the part to take advantage of combining tissue temperature changes with exercise. Exercise in the whirlpool is aided by buoyancy and the specific gravity of water to reduce the effects of gravity. Additionally, the viscous properties of water provide resistance to movement of the part in the water. Areas with open wounds can be heated with reduced risk of infection providing proper cleaning procedures are followed.

The disadvantage of a whirlpool is that the part is in a dependent position while it is being treated, which may increase the tendency for edema formation during treatment. However, this tendency toward edema formation is somewhat offset by the hydrostatic pressure exerted on the limb.

Caution must be used when immersing a large portion of the patient in a warm or hot whirlpool. The remaining surface area exposed to the air may not be sufficient to eliminate heat, and the core temperature may rise. If this situation is not recognized the athlete may faint as blood is shunted to the skin in an attempt to dissipate heat. Children should not be completely immersed in a warm or hot whirlpool because their thermoregulatory mechanism is not well developed, making them susceptible to elevated core temperatures and its consequences.

Guidelines for selection of the proper water temperature are listed in Table 25–2 [30]. Small local areas may be treated with warmer temperatures than larger, more generalized areas. Water temperatures for full-body immersion should not exceed 100°F. Water temperatures should never exceed 110°F.

A disinfectant should be added to the water if an open wound is present. Betadine is suggested if the individual is not allergic to iodine.

The duration of the treatment is 15 to 20 minutes. Individuals, particularly children and adolescents, should be supervised at all times to avoid accidents. If the

TABLE 25–2

Guidelines for Selection of Water Temperature for Use in Whirlpools

Condition	Temperature Ranges
Open wounds	Neutral to warm (80–98°F)
Circulatory/cardiac disorders	Neutral to warm (80–98°F)
Chronic conditions	Hot (98–104°F)
Painful conditions with no other contraindications	Hot to very hot (98–110°F)

dependent position is likely to produce increased edema, the athlete should actively move the part during treatment to activate the muscle pump and assist in venous return. Also, the part should be elevated after treatment.

Ultrasound

Ultrasound is a high-frequency mechanical energy that produces deep heating. Ultrasound is not part of the electromagnetic spectrum. It is transmitted as a longitudinal wave that causes the molecules of the medium it is traveling through to vibrate parallel to the direction of the sound wave. As the sound wave passes through a medium, the molecules of the medium are alternately compressed and spread further apart. When sound energy is applied to the body, it is either transmitted or absorbed by the tissues. Ultrasound is transmitted by tissues with a high water content and is absorbed by tissues high in protein content. Therefore, ultrasound is selectively absorbed by muscle, nerve, and connective tissue. When sound energy is absorbed by tissues, its energy is converted to heat.

Absorption of ultrasound is also influenced by the frequency of the sound wave in such a way that absorption increases as the frequency increases [69]. Absorption is in part related to the internal friction of the tissues that must be overcome by the sound wave. As the frequency increases, molecules are forced to move against increased friction. At frequencies greater than 20 megahertz (mHz), superficial absorption becomes so great that less than 1% of the sound energy penetrates beyond the first centimeter [69]. The frequency of 0.8 to 1.0 mHz was selected for the therapeutic use of ultrasound in physical therapy because it offers a good compromise between penetration and absorption.

The power output from the ultrasound unit can be either continuous or interrupted. Interrupted or pulsed ultrasound is created by interrupting the oscillating circuit. Pulsed ultrasound is characterized by specifying the duty cycle, which is the ratio of the duration of the delivery of the sound to the pulse period (time on plus time off). Typical duty cycles for modern ultrasound units are 0.2 (20%) and 0.5 (50%). Use of pulsed ultrasound decreases the thermal effects produced.

The physiologic effects produced by ultrasound are

thermal and nonthermal. The thermal effects produced by ultrasound are similar to those produced by other forms of heat. However, ultrasound elevates tissue temperature at depths of up to 5 cm beneath the surface of the body. Intensities required to elevate tissue temperature to a range of 40° to 45°C vary from 1.0 to 2.0 watts/cm^2 for a duration of 5 to 10 minutes [69]. Tissues high in protein content appear to absorb ultrasound energy selectively. Therefore, structures such as nerve, muscle, tendon, ligaments, and joint capsule may be selectively heated by the use of ultrasound. Very small temperature increases are found in the skin, subcutaneous tissues, and fat. The lack of heat production in the skin, where thermal receptors lie, results in a minimal sensation of heat during ultrasound treatment.

Ultrasound may also produce nonthermal effects. Cavitation is a result of the vibrational effect of ultrasound on small gas bubbles in the tissues and blood stream. Changes in local pressure caused by ultrasound result in expansion and compression of gas bubbles. These pulsations of gas bubbles induced by the ultrasound can cause changes in cellular activity and destruction of tissues. If the pulsation of gas bubbles is not excessive, cavitation can result in altered diffusion across the cell membrane and altered cell activity [39]. Excessive expansion of gas bubbles results in violent collapse of the bubble and damage to the surrounding tissues. Cavitation may result in separation of collagen fibers and may account for increased extensibility of connective tissue. Cavitation may occur at therapeutic levels of ultrasound [69]. As the intensity of ultrasound increases beyond the therapeutic range, the risk of destructive cavitation increases.

Increases in cell membrane and vascular wall permeability have been demonstrated with therapeutic ranges of ultrasound. These changes may be the result of acoustic streaming, which is the movement of fluids along the boundaries of the cell membrane caused by a mechanical wave of pressure that in turn causes a change in ion flux [69]. Increases in fibroblastic activity including increased protein synthesis and increases in calcium flux across smooth muscle membranes of the mouse uterus have been demonstrated using pulsed ultrasound [23].

Ultrasound is commonly used to decrease pain and muscle spasm and to improve connective tissue extensibility and healing. Ultrasound may also be used for phonophoresis, which is a noninvasive technique of delivering medication through the skin.

In addition to the contraindications already mentioned for other forms of heat, ultrasound should not be used around the eyes or over the heart, pregnant uterus, testes, spinal cord, or malignant tissues. Ultrasound at intensities higher than therapeutic range have been demonstrated to retard growth of the long bones and damage the spinal cord and other tissues. Epiphyseal areas in children should be only minimally exposed to ultrasound. Research indicates that therapeutic intensities of ultrasound over open epiphyseal areas are safe, but intensities of greater than 3.0 watts/cm^2 result in demineralization of bone, damage to epiphyseal plates, and retardation of long bone growth [8, 13, 18, 63].

The therapeutic range for ultrasound when using a moving transducer is 0.5 to 3.0 watts/cm^2. Subacute and superficial lesions should be treated with lower power outputs. Higher power outputs should be used for more chronic or deep-seated lesions. An additional 0.5 watt/cm^2 should be used when water is used as the coupling agent.

The treatment time for ultrasound is generally 3 to 10 minutes. Treatment of less than 3 minutes in duration is ineffective, and maximal effects are achieved after 10 minutes. Initial treatments should be shorter. Chronic and deep-seated lesions require longer treatment times. A general rule of thumb for determining treatment time is 5 minutes for every 25 square inches of area being treated [30].

Daily ultrasound treatment is recommended initially. As the condition improves, the frequency of treatment can be decreased. Generally, a series of 10 to 12 treatments is recommended with a 2-week interval before another series of treatments is started. Three to six ultrasound treatments may be required before any noticeable change can be expected. Occasionally patients may feel a slight increase in symptoms after the initial treatment.

When performing an ultrasound treatment, precautions should be taken to prevent concentration of energy that may result in hot spots and pain. The sound head should be kept moving in a slow rhythmic manner throughout the treatment. Even contact with the skin must be maintained. If surface contact decreases without a decrease in output, the intensity of sound energy could be concentrated in the remaining area of contact between the body and the transducer. Air bubbles in the coupling medium should be removed if they develop. The presence of air bubbles may result in uneven distribution of the sound energy. The transducer should be kept off bony prominences to eliminate concentration of sound energy at the periosteum, which may cause a deep aching pain known as periosteal pain. The recommended dosage should not be exceeded.

The sensation of surface heating or an increase in temperature of the transducer indicates inadequate use of coupling medium or loosening of the crystal within the transducer. If superficial heating is not eliminated by the use of additional coupling medium, the unit should be checked by a qualified service technician.

The transducer should not be held in the air while it is emitting sound energy for more than a few seconds. Since air is a relatively poor transmitter of sound energy, energy will be reflected back to and absorbed by the transducer, causing it to overheat and resulting in possible damage to the crystal.

When treating open epiphyseal areas in children and adolescents, the intensity of the ultrasound should not exceed 2 watts/cm². Additionally, the use of pulsed ultrasound is recommended to reduce the risk of injury to the epiphyseal plate.

Phonophoresis

Phonophoresis is the process by which medicinal molecules are driven across the skin and cell membranes by ultrasound. The primary purpose of phonophoresis is to deliver medicine to a localized area without invading the skin. Phonophoresis results from the increased cell membrane permeability produced by ultrasound. Changes in cell membrane permeability appear to be related to both the thermal and nonthermal effects of ultrasound.

Phonophoresis with anti-inflammatory drugs is indicated for treatment of subacute inflammatory conditions. Ten percent hydrocortisone cream is the most common agent used for phonophoresis. Contraindications for phonophoresis are those previously listed for ultrasound as well as those listed for the drug being administered.

The medication is applied directly to the body and is rubbed in to eliminate air bubbles and improve transmission of the ultrasound. The coupling medium is applied to the area, and the ultrasound treatment is performed using the standard technique. Because the increase in cell membrane permeability is thermal as well as nonthermal, elevation of tissue temperature is desirable. Higher intensities of continuous ultrasound should be used if they are appropriate for the acuteness and location of the lesion.

THERAPEUTIC EXERCISE

Rationale for Therapeutic Exercise

Therapeutic exercises must be specific for the condition for which they are prescribed. When prescribing therapeutic exercises one must consider the purpose of the exercise. The exercise must be appropriate to accomplish the desired goals. Contraindications and precautions for exercise must be considered including any existing condition that might alter the individual's response to exercise. The current state of healing and the nature of the injury impose limits on exercise prescription. Generally, the intensity and duration of the exercise must be limited in the early stages of healing. As healing progresses, the intensity and duration of exercise must be increased to make continued progress toward restoration of maximal function. Eventually, rehabilitative exercises must give way to conditioning exercises to make the transition for return to sport.

Soft Tissue Response to Immobilization

A plethora of research exists on connective tissue response to prolonged immobilization. After injury it is extremely important to minimize the effects of prolonged immobilization. Prolonged immobilization can lead to contractures, decrease in the strength of ligamentous structures, muscle atrophy, bone density loss, and loss of range of motion (ROM) [3, 5, 55, 62, 67, 68]. Minimizing the effects of immobilization can be beneficial to the eventual outcome after an injury. The physician determines whether immobilization is necessary after an injury. Many types of devices that limit range of motion are available on the market today. These devices can provide total cessation of movement or allow some limited degree of motion. The physical therapist may be consulted by the physician about the type of devices available.

Flexibility

"Flexibility can be most simply defined as the full range of motion possible at or in a joint or series of joints" [61]. To allow fluid motion and to avoid injuries all athletes need a moderate degree of flexibility for function [61, 65]. For some individuals superior flexibility is a key to performance. A gymnast needs greater intervertebral flexibility, whereas a baseball pitcher needs greater shoulder external rotation. The diver who cannot execute a deep pike position will never gain stardom. Flexibility is dependent on the alignment of bones and joints, the amount of muscle and fat tissue that may restrict movement by approximation, and the length of soft tissue structures, specifically muscle and tendon. The major components that determine an individual's flexibility are the muscles, ligaments, and tendons that join bones together. Flexibility is a necessary component of exercise, practice, competition, and rehabilitation. Flexibility can be improved by stretching, participation in sport, and exercise. Flexibility is very specific to both the individual and the sport or activity an individual pursues.

Research indicates that stretching improves flexibility. Clinical studies conducted on laboratory animals have shown that tissue temperature can significantly influence the extensibility of connective tissue and therefore may affect flexibility [65]. The literature is inconclusive about the theory of warm-up exercises increasing the tissue temperature prior to stretching. Significant improvements in flexibility are noted with static stretching programs in which a position of stretch is held for 30 seconds or longer [65].

Stretching exercises can be performed by the athlete himself or can be therapist-assisted utilizing proprioceptive neuromuscular facilitation (PNF) techniques [56]. The effectiveness of PNF is attributed to neurophysiologic mechanisms involving the stretch reflex. The stretch reflex involves two types of somatosensory receptors. One is the muscle spindle, which is sensitive to a change in length as well as to rate of change in length of the muscle fiber. The second is the Golgi tendon organ, which detects changes in tension.

Two neurophysiologic phenomena may help to explain the effectiveness of stretching in improving flexibility. The first phenomenon is known as autogenic inhibition, which is thought to be mediated by afferent fibers from a stretched muscle acting on the alpha motor neurons supplying the particular muscle, causing it to relax [14]. Motor neurons supplying a stretched muscle receive both excitatory and inhibitory impulses from the receptors. If the stretch is continued for an extended period of time, the inhibitory signals from the Golgi tendon organ override the excitatory impulses, causing relaxation [49]. The muscle spindle transmits excitatory impulses, which initially stimulate contraction of the muscle being stretched. With prolonged stretch, the inhibitory signals transmitted by the Golgi tendon override the weaker excitatory signals, causing relaxation [56].

The second mechanism to explain the effectiveness of stretching is known as reciprocal inhibition and deals with the relationships of the agonist and antagonist muscles. When the motor neurons of the agonist muscle receive excitatory impulses from afferent nerves, the motor neurons supplying the antagonist muscles are inhibited by the afferent impulses [14]. ''Thus contraction of the agonist muscle will elicit relaxation of the antagonist'' [56].

Muscle Strengthening

Strength training in prepubescent children remains controversial. For years, young boys and girls have been discouraged from using weights for fear that they might incur injuries that would impede normal growth. It is unethical to design a study to observe the possible harmful results of heavy strength training on children. To date most research has been performed on animals.

From birth through adolescence there is an increase in the muscle mass of the body that parallels weight gain [66]. Peak development of muscle in boys coincides with puberty, and this is related to the sudden increase in circulating androgens (testosterone) [4, 66]. In girls, there is a decrease in the rate of strength development relative to the increase in body weight at puberty [66]. In girls muscle mass reaches its peak, unless altered by diet, consumption of anabolic steroids, and exercise, by

18 years of age. This peak occurs in males between 18 and 22 years of age.

Sewall and Micheli [60] and Servedio and associates [59] postulated that prepubescent children of both sexes gain muscle strength in response to appropriate resistive exercise programs. Vrijens [64], on the other hand, concludes that strength training has little effect on the prepubescent. Bar-Or [7] states that the effects of puberty on response to exercise are not fully understood, but it is highly likely that major changes in muscle power occur at puberty.

Muscle strength can be increased by utilizing different forms of isometric, isotonic, and isokinetic exercise. Many different muscle strengthening devices are available. The three forms of exercise are described elsewhere in this chapter.

In addition to the effects of puberty on muscle power, the onset of puberty alters anaerobic energy turnover, sweating responses, trainability, and other exercise-related functions. The lactic acid capacity for anaerobic exercise is reduced in children compared to adults. This has a very limited practical significance in daily life but may become important with physical exercise and sports. Reduced lactic acid tolerance in children should not impede the brief, intense exercise episodes in which lactic acid anaerobic metabolism is involved. However, in less intense exercise bouts of 2 to 3 minutes, before aerobic metabolism kicks in, the child may not be capable of doing as well as the adult. By puberty, there should be no difference between children and adults in regard to lactic acid tolerance [44].

Special Considerations

Physicians and other health care providers have long been concerned about heat dissipation in athletes during strenuous exercise, especially in warm humid climates. The thermoregulatory system of prepubescent children is not fully developed, and therefore heat dissipation with prolonged exercise is a major concern in both boys and girls [7]. Females may be more susceptible to the negative effects of heat. In females the body temperature rises two to three degrees higher than it does in males before the cooling process of sweating occurs. Once full maturity is reached females continues to have fewer functioning sweat glands than males [27].

Maximum oxygen uptake (VO_2 max) is regarded by most sport scientists as the single best determinant of cardiovascular fitness [44, 61, 66]. VO_2 max can be defined as the highest oxygen uptake rate attainable in exhaustive exercise and is commonly described in terms of milliliters of oxygen per kilogram of body weight per minute. The higher the VO_2 max the greater the ability or capacity to perform prolonged exercise. Exercise at levels above the VO_2 max requires the support of anaerobic metabolism. Aerobic metabolism that relies on muscle glycogen has a limited capacity as a fuel source. When muscle glycogen is depleted, exercise must be halted; this may occur within minutes during aerobic exercise [2,66].

Maximum oxygen uptake is affected by age, sex, health status, physical training, and heredity. In children, cardiovascular endurance increases in both sexes until the age of 8, but girls may experience a gradual decline in VO_2 max from this point on. The sex difference in VO_2 max is in part a result of the relatively large amount of body fat in females compared to males after puberty [61, 66].

Maximum oxygen uptake declines with advancing age after middle age [66]. This phenomenon was evident in a cross-sectional sample of boys and men ranging from 6 to 91 years of age. VO_2 max attained its peak value at 17 to 20 years of age and then decreased as a linear function of age [66]. Adams and associates [2] found a similar relationship between VO_2 max and age in a large population of adult males.

Improvement in VO_2 max is dependent on the initial level of fitness and the type and amount of exercise an athlete is involved in. Athletes initiating a program to increase cardiovascular endurance may experience a 25% increase in VO_2 max. Athletes who are normally active and have a normally high VO_2 max may experience only a 5% improvement with training [66]. Ekblom [24] stated that pubescent children could gain aerobic capacity in excess of what is considered a normal improvement for their age group. His research supports the concept that pubescence may increase the child's response to aerobic exercise.

The optimal method of exercising to improve VO_2 max involves repetitive movements using the large muscles of the legs. Training sessions should last at least 20 to 30 minutes, 3 to 5 days a week. Most young athletes, even with training, will not attain the levels of VO_2 max achieved by world-class athletes [66]. The upper limits of cardiovascular endurance are determined by heredity and can be improved slightly with training [66].

The limited information available at this time suggests that no measurable physiologic damage results from cardiovascular training in children.

Forms of Therapeutic Exercise

Therapeutic exercise includes passive, active-assisted, active, active-resisted, isometric, and stretching exercises. Each form of exercise can be used to achieve specific objectives in the rehabilitation process. A knowledge of the purpose and effects of each form of exercise is essential to the successful rehabilitation of the injured

athlete. Inappropriate use of therapeutic exercise can cause aggravation of the injury and delay healing.

Passive exercise is movement that is performed by a force external to the athlete with no voluntary effort on his part. Passive exercise is utilized when muscles are paralyzed or weak or when active contraction of muscle is contraindicated. Passive exercise can be used to maintain or increase joint or soft tissue mobility, to increase musculotendinous length, and to maintain or improve kinesthetic sense.

Passive movement of a joint can be either physiologic or accessory. Physiologic joint motion is a result of rotation of the bone about the axis of motion for the joint. An example of physiologic joint motion is flexion and extension of the knee or abduction and adduction of the shoulder. Accessory joint motion involves the gliding or translation of the articular surfaces over each other and is necessary for normal physiologic movement of the joint. An example of accessory joint motion is the inferior gliding of the head of the humerus on the glenoid during abduction of the shoulder. Accessory joint motion is dependent on the configuration of the joint surface that is moving. Convex joint surfaces glide in the opposite direction of the swing of the bone, and concave joint surfaces glide in the same direction as the swing of the bone.

Passive exercise can be graded according to Maitland's classification [45]. Grade I movement is a small-amplitude movement at the beginning of the range of movement. Grade II movement is a large-amplitude movement that does not go to the end of the range of motion. Grade III movement is a large-amplitude movement that goes to the end of the range. Grade IV movement is a small-amplitude movement at the end of the range of motion. Grade I to II movements are useful to decrease pain and increase motion in acute and subacute conditions. Grade III to IV movements are indicated to increase the range of motion in the later phases of healing.

Active assisted exercise is movement performed by the voluntary activity of the injured athlete with assistance from external forces to complete the motion. External assistance may be provided by another individual, the athlete's uninvolved extremity, or gravity. Active assisted exercise may also be performed in water. The buoyant properties of water assist upward movements in water. Active assisted exercises are used to maintain or increase motion when the athlete's muscles are weak and to strengthen weak muscles.

Active exercise is movement performed voluntarily by the athlete's muscles with no external assistance or resistance. Active exercise can be used to maintain or increase joint motion and soft tissue mobility and to strengthen weak muscles. Active exercises can be performed against gravity or with gravity reduced. Active exercise against gravity occurs as an upward movement in the vertical plane. The muscle must generate sufficient force to lift the body part against gravity.

The effects of gravity can be reduced by moving the part in the horizontal plane. Moving the part in the horizontal plane requires less force to move the body part through a full range of motion than attempting to move the part against gravity. When muscles act on a small body segment such as the fingers, the difference in force required to move the part against gravity or in the horizontal plane is small. However, the difference between active motion against gravity and in the horizontal plane is significant for movement of larger body parts such as raising the arm from the shoulder or the leg from the hip.

Active exercise can be undertaken gradually by having the athlete progress from movement in the horizontal plane to movement against gravity. Progression of movement from the horizontal to the vertical plane requires greater muscular force and can increase the strength of muscles that are weak. Generally, the athlete should be able to demonstrate a full range of motion against gravity before external resistance is applied.

Voluntary movement performed against external resistance can be used to increase muscular strength and endurance. The terms strength, work power, and endurance are often misused when applied to exercise and muscular performance. Before further discussion of active resisted exercise these terms require further clarification. *Strength* is defined as the maximum amount of force a muscle can generate for a given type and speed of contraction [34, 36]. *Force* is that which tends to change the state of rest or motion of matter [36, 52]. Force is a linear measure and is the product of mass times acceleration. It is produced by a muscle as it attempts to shorten along its longitudinal axis. Force is measured in Newtons (N); 1 N is the amount of force required to accelerate a 1-kg mass 1 meter per second.

When a muscle exerts its force on the skeleton it produces a rotation about an axis [36, 52]. *Torque* is a rotational measure and is equal to the product of force times the perpendicular distance from the line of action of the force to the axis of rotation. When assessing strength or the force generated by a muscle acting on the bony skeleton, one is actually measuring torque. Torque is expressed in Newton meters (Nm). Torque can be calculated as the product of the measured force times the perpendicular distance between the line of force and the axis of rotation.

Work and *power* are often included in the discussion of strength. Work is force expressed through a distance with no limitation on time [36]. For linear motion, work is the product of force times distance, whereas for rotational movements work is equal to the product of torque times distance. Work is expressed in joules such that 1 joule is the amount of work done by a force of 1 N being expressed a distance of 1 m.

Power is the rate of doing work [36]. Power is work per unit of time. It can also be expressed as the product of force times velocity. Power is measured in watts so that 1 watt is the production of 1 joule of work per second. Power should not be confused with torque generated at high contractile velocities. Maximum power is generated at intermediate contractile speeds [36].

Muscular *endurance* is the ability of a muscle or muscle group to generate force or perform work over time without fatigue. Muscle endurance can be quantified as the length of time that a contraction can be maintained or as the number of repetitions that can be performed at a particular force or power level through a specified range of motion [34]. As endurance improves, the muscle is able to perform a greater number of contractions or hold against a load for a longer period of time.

Active resisted exercises can be performed isotonically or isokinetically. Strictly speaking, isotonic exercises involve movement against resistance with constant muscular tension. However, this condition rarely occurs owing to the length tension curve for muscles and to the fact that a muscle's mechanical advantage changes as the body segment moves through the range of motion. In practical terms isotonic exercise involves moving against a fixed external resistance. No attempt is made to control the speed of isotonic exercise. An example of an isotonic exercise is an arm curl performed against a fixed weight. As the weight is moved through the range of motion, the resistance remains constant. However, tension in the elbow flexors varies as a function of the length of the muscle and the mechanical advantage exerted on the skeletal system. With isotonic exercise the amount of weight that can be lifted is limited by the weakest point in the range of motion. Generally, the muscle can generate the least torque in the fully lengthened or fully shortened position and can generate the greatest torque in the middle of the range of motion that it produces. Therefore, a muscle is not maximally stressed through the entire range of motion with isotonic exercise.

Variable resistance weight machines have been developed in an attempt to provide a mechanical means of changing the resistance as the part is moved through the range of motion. These machines use a cam that changes the length of the lever arm that the resistance is acting upon to match the torque created by the muscle as it moves the part through the range of motion. Generally, the muscle is capable of generating greater torque in the middle of its range of motion. To match this the cam of the variable resistance weight machine is designed to provide a greater lever arm and therefore more resistance in the middle of the range of motion (Fig. 25–6).

Isokinetic exercise makes use of movement at a constant velocity. The resistance provided by isokinetic devices is variable and accommodating. The amount of resistance is directly proportional to the effort provided

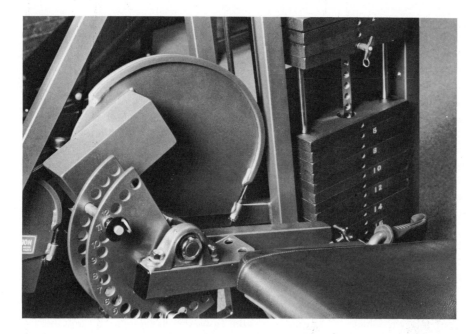

FIGURE 25–6
Variable resistance exercise machine. Cam provides increasing torque in the midportion of the range of motion. A longer lever arm is provided by the cam to provide increased resistance to the muscle in the mid range of motion.

by the athlete. Once the part has been accelerated to the preselected velocity of movement, attempts to contract the muscle with greater force will result in a proportionate increase in resistance by the isokinetic device.

Isotonic and isokinetic exercise can be performed both concentrically and eccentrically. A concentric contraction results in shortening of the muscle as it contracts causing the bony attachments of the muscle to move closer together. An example of a concentric contraction is lifting a weight against gravity. In an eccentric contraction the muscle lengthens as it contracts. During an eccentric contraction, the bony attachments of the muscle are moved further apart by an external force that overcomes the internal force created by the muscle. A controlled lowering of a weight is an example of an eccentric contraction. Both eccentric and concentric contractions are important for normal movement of the body. Concentric contractions result in acceleration of the body whereas eccentric contractions result in deceleration of the body.

The torque generated by a muscle contraction depends upon the speed of contraction [17]. For a concentric contraction, the force generated by the muscle decreases as the speed of contraction increases. However, for an eccentric contraction, the force generated by the muscle increases as the speed of contraction increases. The force-velocity relationship for eccentric contractions is correct only up to certain speeds, after which an increase in speed does not result in greater force generation. McLane and associates [50] demonstrated that peak isokinetic torque of the quadriceps occurs eccentrically at 120 degrees/second. Further increases in the speed of contraction fail to result in a further increase in isokinetic torque. A maximal concentric contraction results in

lower force development than a maximal eccentric contraction at the same speed. The greater force generation with eccentric contraction is the result of stretching of the series elastic component and facilitation of the stretch reflex as the muscle is lengthened [17]. The greater the speed of lengthening the more these factors contribute to the force produced by an eccentric contraction. Because eccentric contractions are important for normal movement and produce greater stress on the musculoskeletal system, it is important to include eccentric exercises in the rehabilitation program; otherwise, the rehabilitation program will not fully prepare the athlete for return to sport.

Isometric exercises result in development of tension within the muscle but produce no joint motion. During an isometric contraction the length of the muscle does not change. An isometric contraction can involve a maximal effort or any percentage thereof. Isometric exercises can be incorporated in the early rehabilitation period to increase strength when motion is contraindicated or limited. Isometric exercises result in increased strength only at the angle at which the exercise was performed. To improve strength throughout the entire range of motion, isometric exercises must be performed every 15 to 20 degrees. Strength gains with isometric exercises have been reported with 10 repetitions daily at two-thirds maximal effort and held for 5 to 6 seconds each [20].

Stretching exercises are used to increase range of motion and flexibility. Flexibility is the ability of the musculotendinous unit to relax and lengthen in response to a stretching force [34]. Passive stretching exercises use an external force, applied either manually or mechanically, to lengthen the shortened tissues. The patient remains relaxed during passive stretching exercises. With active stretching exercises, the patient contracts the antagonistic muscle to lengthen the tight muscle. Active stretching results in reflex inhibition of the tight muscle. Stretching exercises should be performed statically to minimize activation of the stretch reflex. Additionally, static stretching, when coupled with the application of heat, results in a greater residual increase in length than cyclic stretching [40]. Ballistic stretching results in a quick stretch of the muscle, which elicits the stretch reflex and is associated with increased muscle soreness [19, 43]. The use of heat or light exercise to elevate tissue temperatures prior to stretching may be beneficial because heat improves extensibility and plasticity of connective tissue.

REHABILITATION PROGRESSION PROGRAM

Rehabilitation after injury must be goal-oriented with specific outcomes in mind. A team approach is necessary for optimal care. The physical therapist must give consideration to the diagnosis, the results of the physical therapy initial assessment, the child and his or her parents' wishes, the opinions of the referring physician, and the family's ability to bring the child in for care. Rowland [58] stated that children, like adults, must be goal-directed during the exercise regimen. A sense of self-worth, which may serve as a strong motivational force, is observed with the achievement of established goals. "Clearly, exercise programs for children must be designed to provide realistic expectations for improvement and success" [58].

To achieve the established goals, a plan of care is developed after the problems have been identified. The plan of care outlines the therapeutic procedures to be used in the treatment of a patient. The plan of care is continuously reviewed and revised as established goals are met or changed. The rehabilitation program must be individualized to each patient.

The rehabilitation process can be divided into three phases that coincide with the stages of inflammation and repair [10]. The three phases have been described as the acute inflammation, fibroplasia, and maturation and remodeling. Each phase correlates with the normal healing response in the human body and is associated with characteristic signs and symptoms. The stages can be used as guidelines for the progression of treatment within the established plan of care (Table 25–3).

Treatment During Acute Inflammation

Immediate care after an injury can have many positive effects on the length of the total rehabilitation and the time elapsed before return to activity. Immediately after assessment of an injury, the PRICE concept (protection, rest, ice, compression, and elevation) should be instituted. Protection of the injured area may require a cast, brace, splint, strapping, or assistive devices to prevent further injury. Rest, ice, compression, and elevation can help to minimize the edema and its ill effects after an injury. The use and benefits of cold have been discussed earlier in this chapter. Rest is important immediately after an injury to promote healing and decrease the chance for further injury. Compression increases extravascular pressure. External pressure assists in controlling the formation of edema and may help to reduce swelling by promoting reabsorption of fluid [35]. Elevation is beneficial during acute treatment of the injury. Elevation decreases capillary hydrostatic pressure, which decreases capillary filtration pressure. This in turn decreases the amount of edema that develops [35]. Oral anti-inflammatory medications may help to relieve pain and reduce the inflammatory reaction.

The goals of treatment during the acute stage of inflammation are to decrease pain and swelling, retard atrophy, increase patient comfort, provide patient edu-

TABLE 25–3
Phases of Inflammation Correlated with Rehabilitation

Phases of Inflammation	Pain	Range of Motion	Motion Barrier
Acute inflammation	Constant Felt at rest Predominant feature Distal reference zone before motion barrier	Capsular	Muscle guarding
Fibroplasia	Intermittent Felt during movement Synchronous with motion barrier	Capsular	Muscle guarding
Maturation and remodeling	Pain not severe Only felt with forceful movement after motion barrier Proximal extent of reference zone	Capsular	Capsular

Adapted from Bowling, R. W., Rockar, P. A., and Erhard, R. *Physical Therapy* 66 (12):1866–1877, 1986.

cation, and prevent secondary problems associated with immobilization. Exercise, education and physical modalities work in conjunction to meet the treatment goals. An educated patient becomes an active member of the rehabilitation process.

During the acute phase of rehabilitation, passive, active-assisted, and active range of motion exercises should be started in the pain-free range of motion. Passive motion in the pain-free range of motion assists in pain control [46]. It is theorized that pain reduction results from a neuromodulation effect on the mechanoreceptors within the joint [6]. By moving tissues engorged with blood and inflammatory exudate, exercise stimulates circulation and promotes resorption of debris. Exercise should be done at least three times a day for 10 to 15 minutes at a time. Range of motion exercises should be performed in the physiologic range (i.e., motion in the range that is usually achieved actively). Isometric exercises for the antigravity muscles should be started to reduce the negative effects of injury on muscle atrophy. The uninvolved extremities are exercised to maintain cardiopulmonary endurance and prior levels of strength and flexibility. Physical agents or modalities are employed to help reduce pain and inflammation.

Treatment During the Fibroblasia Stage of Healing

The goals of treatment during the fibroblastic phase of inflammation include pain reduction, increasing range of motion, decreasing the ill effects of immobilization, increasing flexibility, increasing functional strength, and improving pain-free function. The patient progresses from the acute to the fibroblastic stage when the pain becomes intermittent in nature. During the fibroblastic phase, pain is felt at the end ranges of passive joint movement [10]. The physical therapist again uses a combination of exercise and physical modalities during the fibroblastic stage to promote pain control and the restoration of motion and strength.

During the fibroblastic phase of treatment protection of the injured area continues to be important to prevent complications. Protective strapping, padding, or bracing may be utilized. A combination of exercise and physical modalities may be used for pain control. Restoration of motion is of great importance at this stage; however, the guidelines relating to healing and limitations in the range of motion must be observed. Range of motion is restricted by the therapist and the physician. It is dependent on the type and severity of the injury, the type of surgery performed, the stage of healing, the stability of the joint involved, and the philosophy of the referring physician. In the literature it is clear that prolonged immobilization can have many ill effects. Early mobiliza-

tion within the limits of the healing tissues may assist the body's natural healing process.

Range of motion exercises can be performed in many ways. Passive, active-assisted, active, and buoyancy-assisted range of motion exercises may be utilized. Passive movements should be performed in the fibroblastic stage to control pain and restore normal arthrokinematics (joint gliding). In this stage, range of motion exercises should be taken to the limit of the available range of motion of the joint or body part being moved. Range of motion exercises should be performed for 20 to 30 repetitions at least three times a day and should be held for 2 to 3 seconds at the end of each movement.

In addition to restoration of joint kinematics, flexibility of tight musculature must be improved. It must be noted that flexibility is specific to each individual and to each sport, and there are no ideal norms that are appropriate for every sport. Stretching exercises must be designed with careful consideration for the sport, the specific muscle to be stretched, the individual, and the need to protect the injured area. Clinical observations of the authors show that stretching is most effective when careful consideration is given to the muscle being stretched and the position used to obtain the most ideal stretch. Stretches should be static and should be prolonged for 30 seconds or more. Stretching exercises should be performed for three to five repetitions three times a day.

Muscle atrophy and strength loss after injury are extensively documented in the literature. The early use of isometric exercises is recommended to retard muscle atrophy and prevent rapid strength loss after injury or surgery. Electrical stimulation and electromyographic (EMG) biofeedback can be used to reeducate weak muscles. Progressive resistive exercises (PRE) can be started in the fibroblastic stage. Isometric exercises started in the acute phase should be progressed to isotonic, weight-bearing functional, and isokinetic exercises. Both concentric and eccentric contractions should be considered. Antigravity muscles such as the quadriceps function eccentrically in weight-bearing positions. The clinician should have a good understanding of sports and their effect on the athlete. Consideration must be given to the strength needs of each sport without predisposing an individual to injury.

In the area of strength building, the future of the child should be considered, and injuries should be avoided to prevent problems later in life. In the pediatric population it is appropriate to take a conservative approach and use low amounts of weight and high numbers of repetitions. For maximum strength gains high repetitions and low weights are preferred. In patients undergoing strength training after injury or surgery it is very important to follow the biomechanical principles of joint mechanics. Special consideration must be given to the joint reaction forces that occur with resisted exercise. Strength training should not be the cause of iatrogenic pain (e.g., patello-femoral pathology with heavy nonweight-bearing isotonic exercise). Weight training should start slowly, using low weights and low repetitions initially, and then slowly progress as tolerated without pain. Clinical experience of the authors shows that sets of 50 to 75 repetitions at a given weight should be used with children. When an individual is able to perform 50 to 75 repetitions comfortably, the weight may be increased and repetitions decreased to 20 to 30. The athlete works with the new weight until 50 to 75 repetitions can be performed with it.

Pain-free improvement of function is a very important part of the fibroblastic stage of rehabilitation. The patient can progress from the use of assistive devices or immobilizers to ambulating and functioning without the use of aids. The extent and type of healing will dictate the functional progression of the individual patient.

Treatment During the Maturation and Remodeling (Late) Stages of Inflammation

During the maturation and remodeling stage of rehabilitation the emphasis of treatment is on restoring a full range of motion, gaining full flexibility, attaining full muscle strength, encouraging proprioceptive training, and restoring full function without limitation so that the athlete is able to return to his or her sport.

The principles of treatment used in the fibroblastic stage are carried into the late stages of rehabilitation. The intensity of the rehabilitation program is increased. At this time the patient should not be experiencing pain at rest; the pain should be intermittent in nature and felt only with forceful movements at the extremes of motion [10]. Range of motion exercises at this time should address any limitations in motion still present. Passive stretching is used with the assistance of a therapist to attain full joint movement. The patient also continues active and active-assisted range of motion exercises. Education of the pediatric patient and his or her family is important for rehabilitation. The concepts of normal range of motion, biomechanics of joint movement, and proper movement required by the joint for return to sport are stressed.

Prior to return to sports the individual must have adequate strength to perform all the functions necessary without limitation. It should be noted that in children isokinetic muscle strengthening may be the ideal mode of strengthening because the resistance is accommodating to the amount of work done by the athlete.

In the area of sports medicine, rehabilitation teams are placing greater emphasis on the etiology and functional rehabilitation of soft tissue injuries and the proprioceptive role of these structures. Because the scope of this discussion is limited, the term postural stability will be used here synonymously with proprioception. Postural stability was defined by Horak as the ability to maintain equilibrium in a gravitational field [32]. To maintain postural stability one needs normal input from the visual, vestibular, and somatosensory systems and an ability to execute coordinated motor responses [32]. Joint receptors (mechanoreceptors) provide information about position and movement. These receptors are found in the ligaments and capsule of the synovial joints [12]. Muscle receptors also play a role in providing proprioceptive input. McClosky [48] reports that in a cat knee joint there are by conservative estimate 4000 myelinated muscle afferents and fewer than 400 myelinated joint afferents. The role of cutaneous receptors in proprioceptive input is not totally clear at this time.

An injury to a joint or to the soft tissues around a joint may lead to proprioceptive deficits, which may lead to further injury with activity [37]. Throughout each stage of rehabilitation, balance and coordination training are incorporated into the treatment regimen. Initially, exercises may be performed in a closed chain position with the patient not exerting more than a few pounds of force through the involved extremity. During the late stages of rehabilitation, proprioceptive training is performed using full weight-bearing functional activities. Proprioceptive training can be implemented into the functional component of the late stages of rehabilitation before return to sport.

Functional training is an integral component of the late phase of the rehabilitation program. Inclusion of functional training can make the difference between success and failure when an athlete returns to competition. During the functional training period the focus shifts from the more traditional treatments already discussed to activities that are specific to the sport or activity an individual performs. Functional activities should be started at low intensities and then progressed slowly to full speed. A patient must be able to perform all activities at 100% of normal prior to discharge and return to full activity. Prior to return to activity protective bracing, padding, or strapping may be used to protect the individual from further injury.

The number of injuries to youth is increasing with the increasing number of children involved in sports. Pediatric injury prevention and rehabilitation programs are also increasing. The clinician who treats pediatric injuries must be cognizant of the motivational factors involved in dealing with this population of athletes. Rowland [58] explained that parent support of the program is of great importance in ensuring the compliance of the child. He also stated that highly structured programs fared much better than unstructured home programs.

References

1. Abramson, D.L., Mitchell, R.E., Tuck, S., et al. Changes in blood flow and oxygen uptake and tissue temperatures produced by the

topical application of wet heat. *Arch Phys Med Rehabil* 42:305–318, 1961.

2. Adams, W.C., McHenry, M.M., and Bernauer, E.M. Multistage treadmill walking performance and associated cardiorespiratory responses of middle aged men. *Clin Sci* 42:355–370, 1972.

3. Akeson, W.H., Amiel, D., Mechanic, G.L., et al. Collagen cross-linking alterations in joint contractures: Changes in the reducible cross–links in periarticular connective tissue collagen after nine weeks of immobilization. *Connect Tissue Res* 5:15–19, 1977.

4. American Academy of Pediatrics. Weight training and weight lifting: Information for the pediatrician. *Physician Sportsmed* 11(3):157–159, 1983.

5. Amiel, D., Woo, S.L., Harwood, F.L., et al. The effect of immobilization on collagen turnover in connective tissue: A biochemical–biomechanical correlation. *Acta Orthop Scand* 53:325–332, 1982.

6. Barak, T., Rosen, E.R., and Sofer, R. Mobility: Passive orthopaedic manual therapy. *In* Gould, J.A., and Davies, G.J. (Eds.), *Orthopaedic and Sports Physical Therapy.* St. Louis, C.V. Mosby, 1985, pp. 212–227.

7. Bar-Or, O. Trainability of the prepubescent child. *Physician Sportsmed* 17(5):65–82, 1989.

8. Bender, L.F., Jones, J.M., and Herrick, J.F. Histologic studies following exposure of bone to ultrasound. *Arch Phys Med Rehabil* 35:555–559, 1954.

9. Borrell, R.M., Parker, R., Henley, E.J., et al. Comparison of in vitro temperatures produce by hydrotherapy, paraffin wax treatment and fluidotherapy. *Phys Ther* 60:1273–1276, 1980.

10. Bowling, R.W., Rockar, P.A., and Erhard, R. *Physical Therapy* 66(12):1866–1877, 1986.

11. Bryant, M.W. Wound healing. *Ciba Clin Symp* 29:1–36, 1977.

12. Carvell, G.E. *Introduction to Neurosciences.* University of Pittsburgh, School of Health Related Professions, 1988–1989.

13. Cerino, L.E., Ackerman, E., and Janes, J.M. Effects of ultrasound on experimental bone tumor. *Surg Forum* 16:466, 1965.

14. Chusid, J.G. *Correlative Neuroanatomy and Functional Neurology.* Los Altos, California, Lange Medical Publications, 1976.

15. Clarke, R.S.J., Hellon, R.F., and Lind, A.R. Vascular reactions of the human forearm to cold. *Clin Sci* 17:165, 1958.

16. Cobbold, A.F., and Lewis, O.J. Blood flow to the knee joint of the dog: Effect of heating, cooling and adrenaline. *J Physiol* 132:379–383, 1956.

17. Curwin, S., and Stanish W.P. *Tendinitis: Its Etiology and Treatment.* Lexington MA, D.E. Heath, 1984.

18. DeForest, R.E., Herrick, J.F., and Janes, J.M. Effects of ultrasound on growing bone: An experimental study. *Arch Phys Med Rehabil* 34:21–31, 1953.

19. deVries, H.A. Evaluation of static stretching procedures for improvement of flexibility. *Res Qu Am Assoc Health Phys Educ Rec* 33:222–229, 1962.

20. deVries, H.A. *Physiology of Exercise for Physical Education and Athletics* (4th ed.). Dubuque, Wm C. Brown, 1986.

21. Drez, D., Faust, D.L., and Evans, J.P. Cryotherapy and nerve palsy. *Am J Sports Med* 9:256–257, 1981.

22. Dyment, P.G. Controversies in pediatric sports medicine. *Physician Sportsmed* 17(7):57–71, 1989.

23. Dyson, M., and terHaar, G.R. The response of smooth muscle to ultrasound. *In* Proceedings from an International Symposium on Therapeutic Ultrasound, Winnipeg, Manitoba, Canada, September 10–12, 1981.

24. Ekblom, B. Effect of physical training in adolescent boys. *J Appl Physiol* 27:350–355, 1962.

25. Grant, A.E. Massage with ice (cryokinetics) in the treatment of painful conditions of the musculoskeletal system. *Arch Phys Med Rehabil* 45:233–238, 1964.

26. Greenberg, R.S. The effects of hot packs and exercise on local blood flow. *Phys Ther* 52:273–278, 1972.

27. Harris, D.V. Women in sports: Some misconceptions. *J Sports Med* 1:15, 1973.

28. Harris, E.D., and McCroskery, P.A. Influence of temperature and fibril stability on degradation of cartilage collagen by rheumatoid synovial collagenase. *N Engl J Med* 290:1–6, 1974.

29. Hayden, C.A. Cryokinetics in an early treatment program. *J Am Phys Ther Assoc* 44:990–993, 1964.

30. Hayes, K.W. *Manual for Physical Agents.* Chicago, Northwestern University, 1984.

31. Hellstedt, J.C. Kids, parents, and sports: Some questions and answers. *Physician Sportsmed* 16(4):59–71, 1988.

32. Horak, F.B. Clinical measurements of postural control in adults. *Phys Ther J* 67(12):1881–1885, 1987.

33. Horvath, S.M., and Hollander, J.L. Intra-articular temperature as a measure of joint reaction. *J Clin Invest* 28:469–473, 1949.

34. Kisner, L., and Colby, L.A. *Therapeutic Exercise: Foundations and Techniques.* Philadelphia, F.A. Davis, 1985.

35. Knight, K.L. *Cryotherapy Theory, Technique and Physiology.* Chattanooga, Chattanooga Corporation, 1985.

36. Knuttgen, H.G., and Kraemer, W.J. Terminology and measurement in exercise performance. *J Appl Sport Sci Res* 1:1–10, 1987.

37. Kotwick, J.E. Biomechanics of the foot and ankle. *Clin Sports Med* 1(1):19–34, 1982.

38. Lehman, J.F., Brunner, L.D., and Stow, R.W. Pain threshold measurements after therapeutic application of ultrasound, microwaves and infrared. *Arch Phys Med Rehabil* 39:560–565, 1958.

39. Lehman, J.F., and Guy, A.W. Ultrasound therapy. *In* Reid, J., and Sikov, M.K. (Eds.), *Interaction of Ultrasound and Biological Tissues.* DHEW Pub. No. (FDA) 73-8008, Session 3:8. Washington, D.C., U.S. Government Printing Office, 1971, pp. 141–172.

40. Lehman, J.F., Masock, A.J., Warren, C.G., et al. Effect of therapeutic temperatures on tendon extensibility. *Arch Phys Med Rehabil* 51:481–487, 1970.

41. Lehman, J.F., Silverman, D.R., Baum, B.A., et al. Temperature distribution in the human thigh produced by infrared hot pack and microwave applications. *Arch Phys Med Rehabil* 47:291–199, 1966.

42. Lewis, T. Observations upon the reactions of the vessels of the human skin to cold. *Heart* 15:177, 1930.

43. Logan, G.A., and Egstrom, G.H. Effects of slow and fast stretching on the sacra-femoral angle. *J Assoc Phys Mental Rehabil* 15:85–89, 1961.

44. Magill, R.A., Ash, M.J., and Smoll, F.L. *Children in Sport.* Illinois, Human Kinetics Publishers, 1982.

45. Maitland, G.D. *Vertebral Manipulation* (5th ed.). Boston, Butterworths, 1986.

46. Maitland, G.D. Treatment of the glenohumeral joint by passive movement. *Physiotherapy* 69:3–7, 1983.

47. Major, T.C., Schwinghammer, J.M., and Winston, S. Cutaneous and skeletal muscle vascular responses to hypothermia. *Am J Physiol* 240 (*Heart Circ Physiol* 9):H868–H873, 1981.

48. McCloskey, D.I. Kinesthetic sensibility. *Phys Rev* 58(4):763–820, 1978.

49. McCough, G., Deery, I., and Stewart, W. Inhibition of knee jerk from tendon spindles and crureus. *J Neurophysiol* 13:343–350, 1950.

50. McLane, T., Dearwater, S., Irrgang, J.J., et al. The relationship of velocity to force and work output during eccentric exercise. Presented at the Annual Conference of the American College of Sports Medicine, Baltimore, MD, May 1989.

51. Mease, S. Effects of temperature on the discharges of muscle spindles and tendon organs. *Pfluegers Arch* 374:159–166, 1978.

52. Meyhew, T.P., and Rothstein, J.M. Measurement of muscle performance with instruments. *In* Rothstein, J.M. (Ed.), *Clinics in Physical Therapy: Measurement in Physical Therapy.* New York, Churchill Livingston, 1985, pp. 57–102.

53. Michlovitz, S.L. Biophysical principles of heating and superficial heat agents. *In* Michlovitz, S.L. (Ed.), *Thermal Agents in Rehabilitation.* Philadelphia, F.A. Davis, 1986, pp. 99–118.

54. Michlovitz, S.L. Cryotherapy: The use of cold as a therapeutic agent. *In* Michlovitz, S.L. (Ed.), *Thermal Agents in Rehabilitation.* Philadelphia, F.A. Davis, 1986, pp. 73–98.

55. Noyes, F.R., Torvik, P.J., Hyde, W.B., et al. Biomechanics of ligament failure. *J Bone Joint Surg* 56A(7):1406–1418, 1974.

56. Prentice, W.E. A comparison of static stretch and proprioceptive neuromuscular facilitation stretching for improving hip joint flexibility. *Athletic Training* Spring, 56–59, 1983.

57. Prentice, W.E. An electromyographic analysis of the effectiveness

of heat or cold and stretching for inducing relaxation in injured muscle. *J Orthop Sports Phys Ther* 3:133–140, 1982.

58. Rowland, T.W. Motivational factors in exercise training programs for children. *Physician Sportsmed* 14(2):122–128, 1986.

59. Servedio, F.J., Bartels, R.L., and Hamlin, R.L. The effects of weight training, using olympic style lifts, on various physiological variables in prepubescent boys (Abstract). *Med Sci Sport Exerc* 17:288, 1985.

60. Sewall, L., and Micheli, L.J. Strength development in children. *J Pediatr Orthop* 6(2):143–146, 1986.

61. Smith, N.J. *Sports Medicine: Health Care for Young Athletes.* Chicago, IL, American Academy of Pediatrics, 1983.

62. Thaxter, T.H., Mann, R.A., and Anderson, C.E. Degeneration of immobilized knee joint in rats. *J Bone Joint Surg* 47A:567–585, 1965.

63. Vaugh, J.L., and Bender, C.F. Effects of ultrasound on growing bone. *Arch Phys Med Rehabil* 40:158–160, 1959.

64. Vrijens, J. Muscle strength development in the pre and post pubescent age. *Med Sport* 11:152–158, 1978.

65. Williford, H.N., East, J.B., Smith, F.H., et al. Evaluation of warm-up for improvement in flexibility. *Am J Sports Med* 14(4):316–319, 1986.

66. Wilmore, J.H. *Training for Sport and Activity: The Physiological Basis of the Conditioning Process* (2nd ed.). Boston, Allyn and Bacon, 1982.

67. Witzmann, F.A., Kim, D.H., and Fitts, R.A. Hind limb immobilization: Length tension and contractile properties of skeletal muscle. *J Appl Physiol* 53(2):335–345, 1982.

68. Woo, S.I., Mathew, J.V., Akeson, W.H., et al. Connective tissue response to immobility. *Arthritis Rheum* 18(3):257–264, 1975.

69. Ziskin, M.C., and Michlovitz, S.L. Therapeutic ultrasound. *In* Michlovitz, S.L. (Ed.), *Thermal Agents in Rehabilitation.* Philadelphia, F.A. Davis, 1986, pp. 141–176.

STRENGTH TRAINING

William A. Grana, M.D.

In 1983 the Committee on Sports Medicine of the American Academy of Pediatrics published a position statement on weight training in the prepubescent that concluded that "maximal benefits are obtained from appropriate weight training in the postpubertal athlete and minimal benefits are obtained from weight training in the prepubertal athlete" [1]. That assessment of strength training for the prepubertal athlete has been a long-standing precept but has been contested recently. In 1985 the American Orthopaedic Society for Sports Medicine sponsored a conference on Strength Training and the Prepubescent Child [2]. The conclusions of that workshop were that weight training in the prepubescent athlete does increase muscle strength, may increase or improve motor skills, protects against injury, increases muscle endurance, and provides positive psychological benefits when conducted in a *carefully structured and monitored* program on an *individual* basis. Although there is lessening controversy about the ability of the prepubescent child to realize strength gains from resistance training, there remain both short- and long-term concerns about the value and safety of such training in the prepubescent and its *safety* in the postpubescent [20]. The purpose of this chapter is to present current knowledge about weight training in the prepubescent and postpubescent athlete.

DEFINITIONS

To begin, the area of exercise evaluated in this chapter is defined. *Strength training* is the use of progressive resistance exercise to increase the ability to exert force or resist force. Other terms that mean the same thing include *resistive training* and *weight training* [2]. Strength training is part of any overall conditioning program, which includes as its other components aerobic and anaerobic endurance training, flexibility, instruction in and accomplishment of physical skills, and instruction in and accomplishment of sports skills [3, 16].

Strength training is distinguished from the terms weight lifting, power lifting, olympic, and competitive lifting. Olympic-type weight lifting is not covered under the definition of strength training because such lifting involves the use of weights to improve appearance or for competition. These body-shaping activities are considered sports rather than training modalities. These sport activities are not appropriate for prepubescent athletes because of the significant risk of injury, especially in unsupervised settings [2, 20].

UNIQUENESS OF THE PREPUBESCENT

The prepubescent is any child considered to be in Tanner stage I [21]. In general, this category includes children up to the age of 12 years. From a musculoskeletal standpoint, certain changes occur following puberty that lead to the occurrence of certain kinds of musculoskeletal problems in the postpubescent that are different from the kinds of problems seen in the prepubescent [3, 8]. These are unique problems for both groups of athletes and are considered in this section.

In the prepubescent child there are unique features in the musculoskeletal system that lead to specific injury patterns. Growing bone tends to bend or deform with microfractures rather than macrofractures, which occur in the postpubescent. The growth centers of the prepubescent athlete's bones are weak owing to the degenerating layer of cartilage cells in the physis. The peak incidence of physeal fractures is the 12- to 13-year-old age group [2]. Finally, the secondary growth centers, the apophyses, are also sites of stress concentration and are vulnerable to the large muscle forces applied through the tendon attachments at these sites. These areas of cartilage can separate or fracture as well. Therefore, these three specific types of injury are seen in the skeletally immature [2]. In addition, disruption of the normal areas of these growing structures may produce permanent deformity or growth arrest when the injury is severe. It is these injury patterns that one expects to see in the prepubescent involved in strength training [24].

PHYSIOLOGIC EFFECTS OF ANAEROBIC TRAINING AND STRENGTH TRAINING

The pediatric athlete is often treated as if he or she were a miniature adult. Faced with a lack of research indicating the appropriate way to train a growing athlete, coaches too often use exercise prescriptions based on experience with more mature athletes. The young athlete is not a scaled-down adult but a special person with age and development-related differences in response to exercise and training. The short-term consequences of treating the prepubescent child as an adult include illness or injury due to overtraining, and the long-term consequences may include serious injury, burnout, and loss of interest. Children are far less able to perform intense anaerobic exercise, but they do recover quickly and therefore are suited physiologically and psychologically to intermittent anaerobic activity [18].

Although the prepubescent compares favorably with the adult and the postpubescent in endurance-related training parameters, his ability to perform anaerobically is less, even when weight-adjusted measures are considered. Children do not utilize glycogen as a metabolite as efficiently as adults. Chemically, this is due to reduced or decreased levels of phosphofructokinase activity, a key enzyme in the glycolytic reaction process [19].

On the other hand, with respect to muscle strength, investigators have routinely found that strength gains parallel growth, with maximum gains occurring sometime in the second decade of life. Strength expressed per unit area of muscle tissue is similar for both adults and children of both sexes. Children's muscle strength increases in response to the same relative overloads that have been found effective for adults [18, 19].

The postpubescent gains strength by means of a combination of neurogenic and myogenic adaptations [18]. Neurogenic changes include improved recruitment of motor units, reduced inhibition, and learned motor skills in the application of force. Myogenic adaptations include increases in contractile proteins, thickening of connective tissue, and increases in short-term energy sources such as creatine phosphate. Although the prepubescent probably experiences neurogenic changes, evidence of myogenic changes occurring in prepubescent athletes is lacking. Recent studies show that children are able to increase strength by means of resistance training but are less likely to increase muscle development in a strength training program. Although there is clear evidence of improvement in strength with resistance training, muscle hypertrophy or increased lean body mass beyond that associated with normal growth is seldom seen, and the training can be viewed as largely neurogenic in nature. It is possible to achieve the neurogenic benefits of resistance training with lighter weights and more repetitions, thereby reducing the risk of injury to the immature skeleton.

The principle of aggressive resistive weight training is well established, and the technique has been used for some time [15]. It now appears that applying this principle to the prepubescent as well as the postpubescent athlete can result in strength gains. Strength training in both prepubescent and postpubescent athletes does increase muscle strength. Until recently there was little scientific information about strength training in the prepubescent, and much of the existing scientific literature stated that it was ineffective [12]. However, a number of recent studies have indicated that strength training in the prepubescent does increase muscle strength when the children are enrolled in a properly designed strength training program. These findings are similar to those reported in the postpubescent athlete [9, 10, 11, 13, 14, 23].

STRENGTH TRAINING AND SAFETY

If one defines strength training as we have in this chapter, there are very few data substantiating the idea that strength training is a cause of large numbers of acute or chronic musculoskeletal injuries in either prepubescent or adolescent participants. On the other hand, it is clear from the literature that in both age groups the use of weights as resistance to increase strength can produce injury in certain circumstances [26, 29, 30, 31]. In particular, competitive weight lifting, which makes use of olympic-type lifting maneuvers, is associated with injury. Strength training, on the other hand, has not been documented to cause acute or chronic injury in musculoskeletal tissues [2]. In this section we will consider occurrence of injury in many forms of resistance training that involves the use of weights.

In 1979 the Consumer Product Safety Commission's National Electronic Injury Surveillance System estimated that over 35,000 weight-lifting injuries that required a visit to the emergency room occur each year. In 1979, half of these were in the 10- to 19-year-old age group and occurred at home. Although most of these injuries were minor sprains and strains, fractures and other serious injuries do occur as well [25]. Moreover, there is little direct evidence to substantiate the safety of strength training as opposed to weight lifting [20]. In addition, most problems tend to occur when competition is added to the strength training program as well as attempts to perform maximum lifts. Competition and maximal lifts are activities that are not recommended by the National Strength and Conditioning Association, the American Orthopaedic Society for Sports Medicine, or the American Academy of Pediatrics [2]. Nonetheless, Brady and colleagues [5] reported on 43 athletes who incurred injury that had a direct causal relationship to a weight-training program. Twenty-nine of these had low back pain, with seven requiring hospitalization, and four of these required surgical treatment. Avulsion of the anterior superior iliac spine occurred in six, meniscal tear in four, and these four required surgery. The conclusion of this paper was that weight-training programs require supervision to permit safe increases in resistance in the use of sophisticated weight-training routines within specific limits. Trainers must recognize the danger of overloading the young athlete in a weight-training program. Athletes in this study were all 13 years old or older and therefore were probably in the postpubescent age group [26].

Further caution is expressed for this age group about olympic-type lifting, in which the spine is not in a stabilized position. This type of lifting creates enormous stress on the lower back and can lead to serious lumbosacral problems [27, 28].

Competitive weight-lifting of any kind is dangerous. It is associated with a high incidence of low back pain due to strained muscles and ligaments as well as acquired spinal defects such as spondylolysis and spondylolisthesis. Both the postpubescent and prepubescent athlete should avoid olympic lifting movements in weight-training programs. Athletes should avoid pressing or jerking overhead any weight exceeding 40% of body weight until 1 year has been spent on basic strength development of the spinal muscles through a full range of movement and full flexion rotation and lateral flexion. Hyperextension exercises of any type should be prohibited [27, 28].

In an evaluation of olympic weight-lifting injuries during a tournament, 80 lifters reported 111 injuries related to the lifting. Most injuries occurred with the clean-and-jerk lift. The shoulder, knee, wrist, and elbow were the most frequently injured anatomic areas. On the basis of this study, Kulund and colleagues [20] developed recommendations for preventing injury. Involvement of a coach is needed who develops appropriate movements to bail out of a lift when it is impossible to complete. Appropriate stretching should be carried out before each work-out to limit the occurrence of shoulder and knee injuries resulting from the rotation of the bar and the press involved in squatting exercises. Safety rack or spotters can help to prevent injuries during maximum lifting activity. Proper breathing techniques can avoid blackouts or excessive increases in blood pressure. If there has been a lay-off, lifters should decrease the weight used. Finally, mats or platforms are useful to

encourage young lifters to drop the weight if it is too heavy [28].

In the prepubescent athlete, the need for supervision is even more important because of the potential risk of growth center injury. Schools and clubs frequently cannot afford a weight coach, or the information an athlete receives may be erroneous. Coaching is often based on the observations and experiences of adults and does not consider the fact that children have a different musculoskeletal physiology and anatomy. The most important guideline for the prepubescent seems to be that competitive lifting, in which the athlete strives for a maximum lift, is never appropriate. Competition in itself may be a healthy motivating factor, but the concern in strength training is about excessive and obsessive competition, which may result in serious musculoskeletal injury [2].

In a controlled study of strength training in prepubescent boys by Cahill [6], no adverse effects on heart rate or blood pressure were reported, and there were no musculoskeletal injuries. In this short-term study, concentric strength training resulted in a low injury rate and did not adversely affect bone, muscle, or physes. Nor did it adversely affect growth development, flexibility, or motor performance, as evidenced by the very well defined guidelines. Nonetheless, the authors concluded that although strength training as defined in this particular study seems to be safe, further research is needed.

The key here seems to lie in the development of safe training regimens and schedules for the prepubescent athlete as well as appropriate supervision to limit the occurrence of injury. There have been reports of distal radial physeal fractures in the prepubescent athlete during military presses [32]. Apart from these occasional case reports of growth center injury in the prepubescent athlete, concern seems to be focused on the potential for injury in training programs that are unsupervised or involve competition [2, 33].

There is at least a theoretical concern about the possibility that strength training may cause acute and chronic injury of bone growth tissue. The studies from the literature that indicate that heavy work or heavy training can result in stunted growth are mainly anecdotal and have not been scientifically referenced; therefore caution is needed [34–37]. In addition, training error can result from improper instruction or insufficient supervision. Either overuse or injudicious training may lead to poor technique, which results in such chronic injury.

Finally, there are some problems that affect both prepubescent and postpubescent athletes. These include the effect of weight training on blood pressure and hemodynamics. Weight lifter's blackout and hypertension can occur in either group of athletes. Weight lifter's blackout is apparently associated with the Valsalva maneuver, which is done during very heavy lifting. Blood pressure falls acutely, and blackout ensues. It is recommended that weight lifters avoid hyperventilation and keep squatting as brief as possible. The weight to be lifted should be raised as rapidly as possible to a position in which it can be supported while normal breathing is resumed. In this way, blackout can be avoided [38, 39]. In the prepubescent athlete, avoiding maximal lifts is the primary way to prevent this complication [2].

FEMALES AND WEIGHT TRAINING

Nothing has been specifically written about weight training in the preadolescent girl, and therefore the following comments are the author's opinion augmented with information gained about adolescent and adult female weight trainers. Without the stimulus provided by added anabolic steroids, females do not develop the muscle hypertrophy and muscle definition characteristic of males. However, this primary difference has been investigated when absolute strength is expressed as a percentage of lean body weight. In this situation there is no strength difference between the sexes. This evidence suggests that neural adaptations are primarily responsible for the increases achieved in muscle strength in females, and therefore the same principles used in male weight training can be applied to weight training in girls. In general, the weights used by women compared to those used by similarly trained and conditioned men are less [11, 39].

A SAMPLE TRAINING PROGRAM

The training regimen recommended for young athletes is a program that requires high repetitions and lower weights that the athlete can handle well to develop good technique safely. A force equivalent to 60% to 80% of a muscle's capacity is required to increase muscular strength. These requirements can be met by selecting a weight that permits approximately ten repetitions before muscle fatigue occurs. One to two sets of 10 to 15 repetitions, with a 2- to 3-minute rest between sets, meets these requirements. Furthermore, these repetitions are high enough to allow the athlete to perfect the lifting technique, improve coordination and motor skills, and allow time for the young body to adapt to the demands of weight training.

Determination of an appropriate resistance weight is to a certain extent a trial and error process and therefore requires intelligent adult supervision. Initially, a light weight should be selected and a lower number of repetitions. Gradually, the repetitions are increased, and then the resistance selected is a weight that can be lifted correctly at least 10 times. This amount of resistance should be used until two complete sets of 15 repetitions can be executed with good form before fatigue. At that time, resistance is increased. After 1 to 3 months of consistent weight training (2 to 3 days a week), the training regimen may be increased to permit two to three sets of 8 to 12 repetitions each to fatigue with a 2- to 3-minute rest interval between sets. Resistance should be increased in increments of 2½ to 5 pounds.

Table 26–1 outlines specific exercises recommended to cover the major muscle groups and to secure balanced increases in strength. By alternating upper and lower extremity exercises, the young athlete can facilitate recovery from fatigue and decrease the potential for injury. If at any time during a set the athlete experiences loss of form or severe fatigue, that set should be terminated and the recovery time increased. As noted in the next section, continuous supervision is required by a knowledgeable adult in a weight-training room in a safe and noncompetitive environment [6,11].

EQUIPMENT AND SUPERVISION FOR STRENGTH TRAINING

Informed coaching and supervision are the most important factors ensuring the safety and effectiveness of weight training in the prepubescent youngster [25]. Often the major emphasis of the coach is on the development of the primary muscles involved in a particular sport, and the synergistic and antagonistic muscle groups are neglected. Injury is the result. For example, overdevelopment of the quadriceps with respect to the hamstrings may lead to problems in the patellofemoral joint. A skilled coach should consider the muscular needs of the injuries common to the sport played. An important part of any weight-training program is the goal of strengthening areas susceptible to injury. High school athletes who participate in a comprehensive weight-

TABLE 26–1
Recommended Specific Exercises

Exercise
1. Leg press
2. Bench press
3. Leg curls (hamstring)
4. Lateral pulls or bent over rows (utilizing a bench for support)
5. Leg extensions (quadriceps)
6. Lateral raises (elbows bent and raise arms to shoulder level)
7. Back extensions (avoid hyperextensions)
8. Tricep extensions
9. Abdominal crunches
10. Bicep curls

Beginners	1–2 sets	10–15 repetitions
Intermediate	2–3 sets	10–15 repetitions
Advanced	2–3 sets	8–12 repetitions

training program may experience 30% fewer injuries and spend half as much time in rehabilitation for injuries related to their sport than athletes who do not undertake weight training.

The risk especially in prepubescent athletes is to allow inadequate supervision or improper instruction to translate into poor technique that results in accidents [2, 40]. Competition, although it may be a healthy motivating factor in sports, can become a driving influence leading to excesses that lead to injury in strength training. In addition to supervision of the use of equipment and the amount of weight used, care must be taken to limit the natural rivalry that forms between youngsters in any athletic endeavor and to individualize the training program.

The prescription for a strength training program in the prepubescent or postpubescent athlete should involve considerations pertaining to the frequency and intensity of the program. The American Orthopaedic Society for Sports Medicine (AOSSM) Workshop on Strength Training recommended two or three training sessions per week with a maximum of four, each session lasting for 20 to 30 minutes including warm-up and cool-down periods as deemed adequate. Increases in weight or resistance should not occur until the participant has achieved proper form. Therefore, initial training requires resistance or weight. The child works on form until the skills are mastered and then begins at a resistance level at which he can perform the lowest number of repetitions. A progressive resistance program should then consist of between 6 and 15 repetitions done in sets of one to three. The child progressively increases the number of repetitions until he can do 15 repetitions with a given weight; weight is then added at 1- to 3-pound increments until the participant can complete six repetitions [2].

Equipment must be appropriate for the size of the child. Most postpubescents involved in strength training will be able to use most of the free weight machine-type equipment that is currently available by making minor adjustments of lever arms and weight. However, for the prepubescent child the so-called isokinetic or variable resistance devices may not be appropriate because such equipment will not be adaptable to his smaller physical dimensions. For this reason, simple free-weight equipment such as barbells and weights are the best devices and can be used safely if the tightness of the fittings is checked routinely as each weight is used. In addition, spotting is necessary with this equipment to prevent loss of control of a weight and resultant injury. If these simple guidelines are followed, strength training in both prepubescent and postpubescent athletes can be safe and effective [40].

SUMMARY

The major benefits of strength training in both prepubescent and postpubescent athletes are improvements in strength and the potential for protection against injury. Although these benefits are not documented in the prepubescents, a number of reports on postpubescent athlete support this concept. The risks of strength training are real. In a short time strength training has the potential to cause acute and chronic musculoskeletal injury, particularly if competitive participation is involved. The long-term effects of strength training are unknown, but in analogous situations chronic injury to bone growth tissue and to joints occurs. A watchword for resistance exercise in the prepubescent athlete is close supervision by knowledgeable adults to decrease the risk to the developing musculoskeletal system.

References

1. American Academy of Pediatrics. Weight training and weight lifting: Information for the pediatrician. *Physician Sportsmed* 11:157–161, 1983.
2. Bar-Or, O. Clinical implications of pediatric exercise physiology. *Ann Clin Res* 34:97–106, 1982.
3. Beckham-Burnett, S., and Grana, W.A. Safe and effective weight training for fitness and sport. *J Musculo Med* 26–46, 1987.
4. Bever, H.G. The influence of exercise on growth. *J Exp Med* 1:546, 1896.
5. Brady, T.A., Cahill, B.R., and Bodnar, L.M. Weight training-related injuries in the high school athlete. *Med Sci Sports Exerc* 18:629–638, 1986.
6. Cahill, B.R. Proceedings of the Conference on Strength Training and the Prepubescent. *Am Orthop Soc Sports Med* 1988.
7. Campton, D., Hill, P.M., and Sinclair, J.D. Weight-lifters' black-out. *Lancet* 1234–1237, 1973.
8. Dangles, C.J., and Bilos, Z.J. Ulnar nerve neuritis in a world champion weightlifter. *Am J Sports Med* 8(6):443–445, 1980.
9. Delmas, M.A. Sur l'entrainement physique intense chez les enfants et les adolescents. *Bull Acad Nat Med* 165:121–126, 1989.
10. Duda, M. Prepubescent strength training gains support. *Physician Sportsmed* 14:157–161, 1986.
11. Fleck, S., and Kraema, W. *Designing Resistance Training Programs.* Champaign, IL, Human Kinetics, 1987, p. 191.
12. Gallagher, R.J., and Delmore, T.L. The use of the technique of progressive-resistance exercise in adolescence. *J Bone Joint Surg* 31A:817–858, 1949.
13. Godin, P. *Growth During School Age* (translated by S.L. Eby). Boston, Gorham Press, 1920.
14. Hagberg, J.M., Ehsani, A.A., Goldring, D., et al. Effect of weight training on blood pressure and hemodynamics in hypertensive adolescents. *J Pediatr* 104:147–151, 1984.
15. Hamilton, H.K. Stress fracture of the diaphysis of the ulna in a body builder. *Am J Sports Med* 12:405–406, 1984.
16. Jesse, J.P. Olympic lifting movements endanger adolescents. *Physician Sportsmed* 61–67, 1977.
17. Jokl, E., Cluver, E.H., Goedvolk, C., et al. *Training and Efficiency.* South African Institute for Medical Research, Reprint No. 303, 1941.
18. Kato, S., and Ishiko, T. Obstructed growth of children's bones due to excessive labor in remote corners. *In* Kato, K. (Ed.), *Proceedings of International Congress of Sport Sciences, 1964.* Tokyo, Japanese Union of Sport Sciences, 1966, p. 479.
19. Kulling, F.A. *Children and Exercise: A Physiological Perspective.*
20. Kulund, D.N., Dewey, J.B., Brubaker, C.E., et al. Olympic weight-lifting injuries. *Physician Sportsmed* 111–117, 1987.
21. Legwold, G. Does lifting weights harm a prepubescent athlete? *Physician Sportsmed* 10:141–144, 1982.
22. Mannis, C.I. Transchondral fracture of the dome of the talus sustained during weight training. *Am J Sports Med* 11:354–356, 1983.

23. O'Neill, D.B., and Micheli, L.J. Overuse injuries in the young athlete. *Clin Sports Med* 7:591–610, 1988.
24. Peterson, C.A., and Peterson, H.A. Analysis of the incidence of injuries to the epiphyseal growth plate. *J Trauma* 12:275–281, 1972.
25. Pfeiffer, R.D., and Rulon, S.F. Effects of Strength Training on muscle development in prepubescent, pubescent, and postpubescent males. *Physician Sportsmed* 14:134–143, 1986.
26. Rians, C.B., Weltman, A., Cahill, B.R., et al. Strength training for prepubescent males: Is it safe? *Am J Sports Med* 15:483–489, 1987.
27. Ryan, J.R., and Sakiicciolsi, G.G. Fracture of the distal radial epiphysis in adolescent weight lifters. *Am J Sports Med* 4:26–27, 1975.
28. Sailors, M., and Berg, K. Comparison of responses to weight training in pubescent boys and men. *J Sports Med* 1987.
29. Servedio, F.J., Bartels, R.L., Hamlin, R.L., et al. The effects of weight training, using Olympic style lifts, on various physiological variables in prepubescent boys. *Med Sci Sports Exerc.*
30. Sewall, L., and Mitcheli, L.J. Strength training for children. *J Pediatr Orthop* 6:143–146, 1986.
31. Sharkey, B.J. Training techniques and issues. *Pediatr Athletics.*
32. Sherman, O.H., Snyder, S.J., and Fox, J.M. Triceps tendon avulsion in a professional body builder. *Am J Sports Med* 12:328–329, 1984.
33. Siegel, J.A., Camaione, D.N., and Manfredi, T.G. Upper body strength and prepubescent children. *Med Sci Sports Exerc*
34. Stover, C.N. Physical conditioning of the immature athlete. *Orthop Clin North Am* 13:525–540, 1982.
35. Tanner, J.M. *Growth at Adolescence* (2nd ed.). Oxford, Blackwell Scientific, 1962.
36. Vrijens, J. Muscle strength development in the pre- and postpubescent age. *Med Sports* 11:152–158, 1978.
37. Weltman, A., Janney, C., Rians, C.B., et al. The effects of hydraulic resistance strength training in pre-pubertal males. *Med Sci Sports Exerc* 18:629–638, 1986.
38. Wilkins, K.E. The uniqueness of the young athlete: Musculoskeletal injuries. *Am J Sports Med* 8:377–381, 1980.
39. Wilmore, J.H., et al. Physiological deterations consequent to circuit weight training. *Med Sci Sports* 10:79, 1978.
40. Yates, C.K., and Grana, W.A. Adaptation of prepubertal children to exercise. *JAMA* 74:173–177, 1981.

INDEX

Note: Page numbers in *italics* refer to illustrations; numbers followed by (t) indicate tables.

527